MEDICAL ABBREVIATIONS:

30,000 Conveniences at the Expense of Communication and Safety

14th Edition

Neil M Davis, MS, PharmD, FASHP

Professor Emeritus, Temple University
School of Pharmacy, Philadelphia, PA,
Editor Emeritus, Hospital Pharmacy
President, Safe Medication Practices
Consulting, Inc.

published by

Neil M Davis Associates
2049 Stout Drive, B-3
Warminster, PA 18974-3861

Phone (215) 442-7430 or (888) 333-1862
(9 AM-4 PM EST, Mon-Fri)
FAX (215) 442-7432 or (888) 333-4915
E-mail med@neilmdavis.com
Secure Website www.medabbrev.com

First edition, 1983, titled, "1700 Medical Abbreviations:
Conveniences at the Expense of Communications and Safety"
Second edition, 1985, titled, "Medical Abbreviations: 2300
Conveniences at the Expense of Communication and Safety"
Third edition, 1987, titled, "Medical Abbreviations: 4200 ..."
Fourth edition, 1988, titled, "Medical Abbreviations: 5500 ..."
Fifth edition, 1990, titled, "Medical Abbreviations: 7000 ..."
Sixth edition, 1993, titled, "Medical Abbreviations 8600 ..."
Seventh edition, 1995, titled, "Medical Abbreviations 10,000 ..."
Eighth edition, 1997, titled, "Medical Abbreviations: 12,000 ..."
Ninth edition, 1999, titled, "Medical Abbreviations: 14,000 ..."
Tenth edition, 2001, titled, "Medical Abbreviations: 15,000 ..."
Eleventh edition, 2003, titled, "Medical Abbreviations: 24,000 ..."
Twelfth edition, 2005, titled, "Medical Abbreviations: 26,000 ..."
Thirteenth edition, 2007, titled, "Medical Abbreviations 28,000 ..."

Library of Congress Control Number 2008904918

ISBN 978-0-931431-14-2

Warning: The user must exercise care in that the meaning shown in this book may not be the one intended by the writer of the medical abbreviation. When there is doubt, the writer must be contacted for clarification.

Printed in Canada.

Contents

Dedication

This book is dedicated to Julie, my wife, for her support, patience, assistance, and love.

Acknowledgments

The assistance of Evelyn Canizares, Vicki Bell, Gemma Jakeman, Ann Sandt Kishbaugh, Matthew Davis, Robin Miller, and Melissa Miller is gratefully acknowledged.

I would like to express my deep appreciation for the many contributions received from readers for their suggested additions and corrections. Please continue to send these to—

Dr. Neil M Davis
2049 Stout Drive, B-3
Warminster, PA 18974

FAX (215) 442-7432 or (888) 333-4915
E-mail med@neilmdavis.com
Secure Website www.medabbrev.com

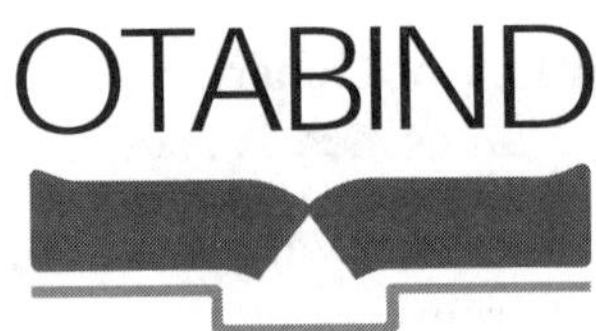

Bound to stay open

The pages in this book open easily and lie flat, a result of the Otabind bookbinding process. Otabind combines advanced adhesive technology and a **free-floating cover** to achieve books that last longer and are bound to stay open.

Preface

Internet-Version Access Information

Along with the purchase of each book, the book owner, at no extra cost, is entitled to a single-user license for access to the Internet version of this 14th edition. This license is valid for 12 months from the date of the initial log-in. Internet Explorer 4.0, Netscape 4.0, or AOL 5.0 as well as the current versions of these 3 browsers, can meet the minimum browser requirement.

Features of the Internet Version

- Updated monthly (suggestions from users are welcomed and will be incorporated).
- Can instantaneously search for the meanings of abbreviations and acronyms.
- Has a reverse-search feature, for example, looking for all the abbreviations that contain the word "laparoscopic."
- Can search for cross-referenced generic and brand names of drugs.
- Can search through the listings of symbols, lists, and normal adult laboratory values.
- Quick access to a "Do Not Use" list of dangerous abbreviations, an explanation as to why they are dangerous, and suggested alternatives to be used. For those facilities that obtain multi-user licenses, they may substitute their own "Do Not Use" list, which they can control and update.
- Can read the full-text of the introductory chapters of the book.

Instructions for the Initial One-time Log-in

- Access the Website at *www.medabbrev.com*
- Click the **Register** button (on the top-left of the screen)
- You must agree to the Single-User License Agreement which is presented.
- You will be asked for the 8-letter access code that appears on the front inside cover of the book. This will be the only time you are asked for this code.
- At this point just follow the directions.
- Note your sign-in name and your self-assigned password. This name/password will only permit one access at a time, so keep this information confidential to ensure your ready access to the site.

Searching for the Meaning of an Abbreviation on the Internet Version

- Use upper OR lower case letters as the search engine is NOT case sensitive.
- Use normal upper OR lower case letters as the search engine is NOT sensitive to whether the letters are **bold-face** or *italicized.*
- Superscripts and subscripts are to be entered as regular text.
- DO NOT enter periods, commas, hyphens, or spaces (enter afib, not a fib).
- For other details, just follow the simple instructions shown on the Website. The Internet version of the book is essentially the same as the print version except for the fact that it is searchable and is updated monthly with about 80 new entries.

Multi-user Site Licenses are Available

A copy of the Multi-User Site License agreement and its price list is available by clicking the "Submit Suggestions" button on *www.medabbrev.com* where you can type a request to receive it or by calling 1 888 333 1862 or 1 215 442 7430. A no-cost, 3-week trial is available.

Extending or Purchasing Internet Access

A 12-month purchase or extension of the Internet version is available. See pricing information on page 377.

Additions, Corrections, and Suggestions are Welcomed

Please send them via any means shown below:

Neil M Davis
2049 Stout Drive, B-3
Warminster PA 18974-3861

FAX 1 888 333 4915 or 1 215 442 7432
Email med@neilmdavis.com
Web site www.medabbrev.com

Thank you for your help in the past.

Have You Used the Internet Version of This Book?

- It is instantaneously searchable for the meanings of abbreviations
- It is reverse searchable (search for all the abbreviations containing a particular word)
- Each month, about 80 new entries are added

See the preface (page vii) for access instructions. A one-year, single-user access is included in the purchase price of the book. Also one-year subscriptions are available for purchase (see page 377).

PDA and BlackBerry Versions are Available

See pricing and ordering information in the pricing section on page 379.

Multi-User Site Licenses are Available

Medical facilities can substitute their own "Do Not Use" list of dangerous abbreviations for the one present. The ability also exists to list abbreviations that are unique to your region and/or organization which would normally not appear in any national list. These lists would be controlled by the facility or company. A no-cost, 3-week trial and pricing information are available by calling 1 888 333 1862 or 1 215 442 7430 or via an e-mail request to ev@neilmdavis.com

Chapter 1
Introduction

Listed are current acronyms, symbols, abbreviations, slang and 30,000 of their possible meanings. This list has been compiled to assist individuals in reading and transcribing medical records, medically-related communications, and prescriptions. The list, although current and comprehensive, represents a portion of abbreviations in use and their many possible meanings as new ones are being coined every day.

WARNING

Abbreviations are a convenience, a time saver, a space saver, and a way of avoiding the possibility of misspelling words. However, a price can be paid for their use. Abbreviations are sometimes not understood. They can be misread, or are interpreted incorrectly. Their use lengthens the time needed to train individuals in the health fields, wastes the time of healthcare workers in tracking down their meaning, at times delays the patient's care, and occasionally results in patient harm.

The publication of this list of abbreviations is not an endorsement of their legitimacy. It is not a guarantee that the intended meaning has been correctly captured, nor is it an indication that the abbreviation is commonly used. The person who uses an abbreviation must take responsibility for making sure that it is properly interpreted. When an uncommon or ambiguous abbreviation is used and it may not be understood correctly, it should be defined by the writer. Where uncertainty exists, the one who wrote the abbreviation must be contacted for clarification.

There are many variations in how an abbreviation can be expressed. Anterior-posterior has been written as AP, A.P., ap, a.p., and A/P. Since there are few standards and those who use abbreviations do not necessarily follow these standards, this book only shows anterior-posterior as AP. This is done to make it easier to find the meaning of an abbreviation as all the meanings of AP are listed together. This elimination of unnecessary duplication also keeps the book at a convenient size, thus enabling it to be sold at a reasonable price.

When an abbreviation is made up of a series of abbreviations, it may not be listed as such. In such instances, the meaning may be determined by looking up each set of abbreviations, as in the example of DTP_a-HIB-PNU-MEN, which means, diphtheria, tetanus toxoids, acellular pertussis; *Haemophilus influenzae* type b conjugate; pneumococcal (*Streptococcus pneumoniae*) conjugate; meningococcal (*Neisseria meningitidis*) conjugate (serogroups unspecified) vaccine.

Lower case letters are used when firm custom dictates as in Ag, Na, mCi, etc. The first letter of brand names are capitalized, whereas nonproprietary names appear in lower case.

The abbreviation ACT is listed as meaning doxorubicin, cyclophosphamide, and paclitaxil. The reason for this apparent disparity is that the official generic names (United States Adopted Names) are shown rather than the brand names Adriamycin and Taxol. In the case of LSD, the official name, lysergide, is given, as well as the chemical name, lysergic acid diethylamide. The Latin derivations for older medical and pharmaceutical abbreviations (*t.i.d., ter in die,* three times daily) may be found in *Remington.*[1]

Some abbreviations which have been encountered or that have been suggested for addition to the book have not been added. Some were obscene or completely insensitive. Slang and drug name abbreviations are shown for informational purposes only and should not be used.

Abbreviations for medical facility names create problems as they are usually not recognized by the readers in other geographic areas. A clue to the fact that one is dealing with such an abbreviation is when it ends with MC, for Medical Center; HS, for Health System; MH, for Memorial Hospital; CH, for Community Hospital; UH, for University Hospital; and H, for Hospital.

If a meaning for an abbreviation with an ending of an S can not be found, look for that abbreviation without the S. SAEs (serious adverse events) would not be found, but SAE (serious adverse event) is listed.

When an abbreviation cannot be found in this book or when the listed meaning(s) do not make sense, there is a possibility that the abbreviation has been misread. As an example, a reader could not find the meaning of HHTS. On closer examination it really was +HTS, not HHTS. Also EWT could not be identified because it was really ENT.

Some common French and Spanish abbreviations are listed in the book. Because of language structure differences, these abbreviations are often reversed, as in the case of HIV, which in Spanish and French is abbreviated as VIH.

Chapter 5 presents a list of 275 of the most commonly used abbreviations. The purpose of this list is to serve as a primer for whose entering a health-related field.

Chapter 9 contains a cross-referenced list of 3,400 generic and brand drug names. The list contains names of commonly prescribed, new drugs, and recently discontinued drugs. Brand names have their first letter capitalized whereas generic names are in lower case. This list will enable readers to obtain the generic name for brand name products or brand names for generic names. It will also serve as a spelling check.

Coded drug names and abbreviations for drug names are found in the chapter on abbreviations (Chapter 6). Abbreviated drug names should not be used as they pose a safety risk.

Chapter 10 is a table of normal laboratory values. Both the conventional and international values are listed. Each laboratory publishes a list of its normal values. These local lists should be reviewed to see if there are significant differences.

The Council of Biology Editors (CBE), in their 1983 edition of the *CBE Style Manual* listed about 600 abbreviations gathered from 15 internationally recognized authorities and organizations.[2] The majority of these symbols and abbreviations tend to be more scientifically oriented than those which would appear in medical records. In the few situations where the CBE abbreviations differ from what is presented in this book, the CBE abbreviation has been placed in parentheses after the meaning. As is the practice in the United States, mL has been used rather than ml and the spelling of liter, meter, etc. is used rather than litre and metre, even though ml, litre, and metre are listed in the *CBE Style Manual*. A new edition of the *CBE Style Manual* was published in 1995.[3] Again, in this edition, emphasis is placed on scientific abbreviations.

Only a few of the acronyms and abbreviations for the major cardiologic trials, such as, TIMI-Thrombosis In Myocardial Infarction (trial), have been included in this book. For a list of 4,200 of these acronyms and abbreviations, consult reference number 4.

An examination of the abbreviations, acronyms, symbols, and their 30,000 meanings is a testimonial to the problems and dangers associated with most undefined abbreviations.

References

1. Hendrickson R, ed. Remington's The Science and Practice of Pharmacy, 21st ed. Phila., PA: Lippincott Williams and Wilkins, 2006.

2. CBE Style Manual, 5th ed. Bethesda, MD: Council of Biology Editors; 1983.

3. Scientific Style and Format: The CBE Manual for Authors, Editors, and Publishers, 6th Ed. Council of Biological Editors-Cambridge University Press. Cambridge UK, New York, Victoria Australia: 1995.

4. Cheng TO, Julian D. Acronyms of cardiologic trials-2002. Int J Cardiol 2003;91:261–351.

Chapter 2

Dangerous, Contradictory, and/or Ambiguous Abbreviations

Healthcare organizations are directed by the Joint Commission on Accreditation of Healthcare Organizations to formulate a "Do Not Use" list of dangerous abbreviations which should NOT be used. An example of such a list, which has been adopted from the Institute of Safe Medication Practice Inc. (ISMP) list, is shown as Table 2.

Many inherent problems associated with abbreviations contribute to or cause errors. Reports of such errors have been published routinely.[1–5]

Table 1. Examples of Abbreviations and Symbols That Have Been Misread or Misinterpreted

(1) "HCT250 mg" was intended to mean hydrocortisone 250 mg but was interpreted as hydrochlorothiazide 50 mg (HCTZ50 mg).

(2) Flucytosine was improperly abbreviated as 5 FU, causing it to be read as fluorouracil. Flucytosine is abbreviated 5 FC and fluorouracil is 5 FU.

(3) Floxuridine was improperly abbreviated as 5 FU, causing it to be read as fluorouracil. Floxuridine is abbreviated FUDR and fluorouracil is 5 FU.

(4) MTX was thought to be mechlorethamine. MTX is methotrexate and mechlorethamine is abbreviated HN2.

(5) **The abbreviation "U" for unit is the most dangerous one in the book, having caused numerous ten-fold insulin and heparin overdoses. The word unit should never be abbreviated.** The handwritten U for unit has been mistaken for a zero, causing tenfold errors. The handwritten U has also been read as the number four, six, and as "cc."

(6) OD, meant to signify once daily, has caused Lugol's solution to be given in the right eye.

(7) OJ meant to signify orange juice, looked like OS and caused saturated solution of potassium iodide to be given in the left eye.

(8) IVP, meant to signify intravenous push (Lasix 20 mg IVP), caused a patient to be given an intravenous pyelogram which is the usual meaning of this abbreviation.

(9) Na Warfarin (sodium warfarin) was read as "No Warfarin."

(10) The abbreviation "s̄" for "without" has been thought to mean "with" (c̄).

(11) The order for PT, intended to signify a laboratory test order for prothrombin time, resulted in the ordering of a physical therapy consultation.

(12) The abbreviation "TAB," meant to signify Triple Antibiotic (a coined name for a hospital sterile topical antibiotic mixture), caused patients to have their wounds irrigated with a diet soda. At another facility, with the same set of circumstances, they did not have TAB®, so they used Diet Shasta.®

(13) A slash mark (/) has been mistaken for a one, causing a patient to receive a 100 unit overdose of NPH insulin when the slash was used to separate an order for two insulin doses:
6 units regular insulin/20 units NPH insulin

(14) Vidarabine, an antiviral agent, was ordered as ara-A; however, ara-C, which is cytarabine, an antineoplastic agent, was given.

(15) On several occasions, pediatric strength diphtheria-tetanus toxoids (DT) have been confused with adult strength tetanus-diphtheria toxoids (Td).

(16) DTP is commonly understood to refer to diphtheria-tetanus-pertussis vaccine, but in some hospitals it is also used as shorthand for a sedative cocktail of Demerol, Thorazine, and Phenergan. Several cases have occurred where a child was vaccinated rather than given the sedative mixture.

(17) What does the abbreviation MR mean? Some will guess measles-rubella vaccine (M-R-Vax II, Merck), while others will assume mumps-rubella vaccine (Biavax II, Merck).

(18) The abbreviation TIW (three times a week) was thought to mean Tuesday and Wednesday when the I was read as a slash mark. Due to confirmation bias (you see what you know), this uncommon abbreviation is seen as the more commonly used TID (three times a day).

(19) PCA, meant to be procainamide, was interpreted as patient-controlled analgesia.

(20) PGE_1 (alprostadil, Caverject) was read as P6 E1 (Alcon's ophthalmic 6% pilocarpine and 1% epinephrine solution).

(21) A nurse transcribed an oral order for the antibiotic aztreonam as AZT, which was subsequently thought to be the antiviral drug zidovudine.

(22) An order for TAC 0.1%, intended to mean triamcinolone cream, was interpreted as tetracaine, Adrenalin, and cocaine solution.

(23) An order for SPA (salt poor albumin) was overlooked because it was not recognized as a drug order.

(24) Therapy was delayed and considerable professional time was wasted when an order for "Bactrim SS q 12 h on S/S" had to be clarified (Bactrim Single Strength every 12 hours on Saturday and Sunday).

(25) A physician wrote an order stating "may take own supply of EPO". The physician meant evening primrose oil, not Epogen (epoetin alfa).

(26) 4-MP was recommended to treat ethylene glycol poisoning. The medical resident mistakenly interpreted this as 6-MP (6-mercaptopurine). 4-MP is fomepizole (4 methylpyrazole) and 6-MP is mercaptopurine (6-mercaptopurine).

(27) An order for lomustine stated it was to be given at "hs". This was misinterpreted as to mean every night. After continuous administration, toxicity resulted in the patient's death. The drug is normally given once every 6 weeks. State complete orders such as "HS × 1 dose today," "HS nightly," or "HS nightly PRN for sleep."

(28) The directions for an order for Cortisporin Otic Solution indicated "Three drops in ® ear TID." The patient was given the drops in the rear rather than the right ear.

(29) There have been mix-ups between IL-2 and IL-11 when IL-2 is expressed as IL-II (Roman numeral 2). The II has been read as "IL eleven," and vice versa. IL-2 (interleukin 2) is aldesleukin (Proleukin) and IL-11 is oprelvekin (Neumega).

(30) A drug was ordered "Q 10 h." It was read as QID (four times daily). Drugs should not be ordered at unusual hourly intervals such as every 10, 18, or 36 hours, as this has resulted in a host of errors. Standard times are every 2, 3, 4, 6, 8, or 12 hours; once, twice, three, or four times daily; every other day, or Monday, Wednesday, and Friday and once weekly.

(31) 6 IU was read 61 units instead of the intended 6 international units.

(32) A dose of phenytoin was modified and expressed as mg/Kg/d. The d was read as "dose" rather than the intended "day" resulting in 3 extra doses being given.

(33) An order appeared as "If no BM in PM, give MOM in AM p.r.n."

(34) Sometimes ambiguous abbreviations cause financial losses to health providers. For example, an insurance provider may pay less for an office visit for mental retardation than it does for mitral regurgitation. This can happen if the coder is faced with the abbreviation MR.

(35) The abbreviation for "q PM" has been read as 9 PM (a one time dose at 9 PM) rather than every night.

(36) An order was written in a hospital, "Cortisporin 3 drops, AS bid." There was a question about the meaning of AS, but since the patient was scheduled for a colonoscopy it was decided that the meaning was "anal sphincter", so the drug was administered rectally rather than in the left ear as intended. When the patient was asked to roll over for their medicine, I suppose they could have protested that there was nothing wrong with their rectum, but then again, maybe this was part of a complex preparation for their colonoscopy!

(37) A liver transplant patient on readmission had an order handwritten, "MMF 1000 mg PO BID (mycophenolate mofetil)." Mycophenolate mofetil is the immunosuppressive agent CellCept which has been abbreviated MMF. The order was misread as 1000 mg twice daily MWF (Monday, Wednesday, and Friday). Several doses of this critical drug were omitted before the error was discovered.

(38) A prescription was written for PTU. PTU normally means propylthiouracil, however Purinethol was dispensed in error causing a fatality. Purinethol is never abbreviated PTU. The error probably occurred because both propylthiouracil and Purinethol are available in 50 mg

tablets and sit side-by-side on the pharmacy shelf. The prescriber contributed to the error by using nonstandard terminology, an abbreviation.

(39) A nurse mistaken administered Chloral Hydrate Syrup intravenously. This syrup is intended for oral administration only. This was done because the label contained the legend C IV. This was interpreted as intravenous when in fact, C IV stands for a class 4 controlled substance. All controlled substances are indicated as Roman numerals, I, II, III, IV, V. Even though 99.99% of nurses know that drugs in screw-capped bottles, labeled "syrup" are not intended for intravenous administration, it would pay to change C IV to C4 on drug company labels.

(40) After performing spinal surgery a surgeon kept his ICU patients NPO (nothing by mouth), until they had flatus and good **b**owel **s**ounds. His order was: "Strict NPO. Check BS Q2H." The patient had "blood sugar" laboratory tests drawn Q2H!

The author would appreciate receiving other examples of abbreviations that have been misinterpreted causing error or delays so that this section can be expanded.

A prescription could be written with directions as follows: "OD OD OD," to mean one drop in the right eye once daily!

Abbreviations should not be used for drug names as they are particularly dangerous. As previously illustrated, there is the possibility that the writer may, through mental error, confuse two abbreviations and use the wrong one. Similarly, the reader may attribute the wrong meaning to an abbreviation. To further confound the problem, some drug name abbreviations have multiple meanings (see ATR, CPM, CPZ, FLU, GEM, NITRO, and PBZ in Table 3). The abbreviation AC has been used for three different cancer chemotherapy combinations to mean Adriamycin and either cyclophosphamide, carmustine, or cisplatin.

See chapter 4 which discusses how medical writers, editors, and health professionals can prevent the coining and use of these ambiguous abbreviations. To avoid the introduction of contradictory or ambiguous abbreviations, before coining a new abbreviation, one must do some research. Check this book and Medline to see other possible meanings that already exist for the planned abbreviation. Secondly, rethink if there is really a need to develop an abbreviation for the term.

Beside causing medication errors and incorrect interpretation of medical records, abbreviations can create problems because treatment is delayed while a health professional seeks clarification for the meaning of the abbreviation used. Abbreviations should not be used to designate drugs. The establishment of abbreviations for drug combinations is an ongoing problem and should require facility/organizational approvals.

Certain meanings of abbreviations in the book are followed by a warning, "this is a dangerous abbreviation." This warning could be placed after many abbreviations, but was reserved for situations where errors have been published because these abbreviations were used or where the meaning is critical and not likely to be known. If no alternative abbreviation is suggested, then the term should be spelled out rather than abbreviated. Such warning statements should also appear after every abbreviation for a drug or drug combination.

References

1. Davis NM, Cohen MR. Medication errors: causes and prevention. Warminster, PA: Neil M Davis Associates; 1983.
2. Cohen MR. Medication error reports. Hosp Pharm (appears monthly from 1975 to the present).
3. Cohen MR. Medication errors. Nursing 2008 (appears monthly, starting in Nursing 77, to the present).
4. Davis NM. Med Errors. Am J Nursing (appears monthly from 1994 to 1995).
5. Cohen MR. Medication Errors. American Pharmacists Assoc. Wash. DC, 2006.

Table 2. Dangerous Abbreviations and Dosage Designations

Problem term	Reason	Suggested term
O.D. for once daily	Interpreted as right eye	Write "once daily"
q.o.d. for every other day	Interpreted as meaning "every once a day" or read as q.i.d.	Write "every other day"
q.d. for once daily	Read or interpreted as q.i.d.	Write "once daily"
q.n. for every night nightly	Read as every hour	Write "every night," "HS" or
q hs for once daily at bedtime, each day	Read as every hour	Use "HS" or "at bedtime"
TIW for three times a week	Interpeted as T/W (Tuesday & Wednesday); as twice a week; as TID (three times daily)	Write "three times a week"
U for Unit	Read as 0, 4, 6, or cc	Write "unit"
O.J. for orange juice	Read as OD or OS	Write "orange juice"
µg (microgram)	When handwritten, misread as mg	Write "mcg"
sq or sub q for subcutaneous	The q is read as every	Use "subcut"
IU for international unit	Misread as IV (intravenous) also the I is is read as a one (6 IU is read as 61 units)	Use "units" or spell out "international units," using a lowercase u.
AU for each ear	Read as OU (each eye)	Spell out "each ear"
ss for sliding scale or half in the Apothecary system	Read as the number 55	Spell out "sliding scale" or "1/2"
Chemical symbols	Not understood or misunderstood	Write full name
cc for expressing liquid measurements	Read as u (unit) or 00	Write "mL" when expressing liquid measurements (drugs, urine, blood, etc.)

Lettered abbreviations for drug names such as MS and MS04 for morphine sulfate or DPH, ASA, APAP, AZT, CPZ, and others and for protocols	Not understood or misunderstood	Use generic or brand name(s). For protocols, follow the facility's procedures.
Apothecary symbols or terms	Not understood or misunderstood	Use metric system
per os for by mouth	OS read as left eye	Use "by mouth," "orally," or "PO"
D/C for discharge	Interpreted as discontinue (orders for discharge medications result in premature discontinuance of current medication)	Write "discharge"
Ṫ/d for one per day	Read as t.i.d.	Use "once daily"
T1D for type 1 diabetes mellitus	Read as TID (three times daily)	Use DM-1
/ (a slash mark) for with, and, or per	Read as a one	Use, "and," "with," or "per"
Roman numerals	Not understood or misinterpreted (iv read as intravenous rather than 4; iii, X, L, and C, are not understood)	Use Arabic numerals (4, 3, 10, 50, 100, etc.)
> and <	Not understood or the meaning is reversed	Use "greater than" or "less than"
Drug name and dosage not separated by space	Inderal40 mg misread as Inderal 140 mg	Always leave a space between a drug name, dose, and unit of measure
Trailing zeros; 1.0 mg	When handwritten decimal point not seen causing tenfold overdose	Omit zero; 1 mg when expressing drug strengths or doses. This does NOT apply to laboratory or other precise values.
Naked decimal point; .5 mL	Decimal point not seen causing tenfold overdose	Add zero; 0.5 mL
Slang	Can be offensive and/or insensitive	Do not use slang in oral or written communication

Table 3. Examples of Abbreviations That Have Contradictory or Ambiguous Meanings

Abbreviation	Meanings
ABP	= ambulatory blood pressure arterial blood pressure
AC	= anticoagulant anticonvulsant
ACU	= acute receiving unit ambulatory care unit
AMI	= amifostine amitriptyline
APC	= advanced pancreatic cancer advanced prostate cancer
ATR	= atropine atracurium
AZT	= zidovudine azathioprine
BD	= behavior disorder Behçet disease bipolar disorder Bowen disease
BM	= bone metastases brain metastases
BNO	= bladder neck obstruction bowels not open
BO	= bowel open bowel obstruction
BT	= bladder tumor brain tumor breast tumor
CARBO	= Carbocaine carboplatin (Paraplatin)
CAS	= carotid artery stenosis cerebral arteriosclerosis coronary artery stenosis
CIA	= chemotherapy-induced amenorrhea chemotherapy-induced anemia
CLD	= chronic liver disease chronic lung disease
CPM	= cyclophosphamide chlorpheniramine maleate
CPZ	= chlorpromazine Compazine
CRU	= cardiac rehabilitation unit catheterization recovery unit clinical research unit
DW	= dextrose in water distilled water deionized water
DXM	= dexamethasone dextromethorphan
ED	= eating disorder(s) elbow disarticulation emotional disorder erectile dysfunction
ESLD	= end-stage liver disease end-stage lung disease
FA	= folic acid folinic acid (leucovorin calcium)
FEC	= fluorouracil, epirubicin, and cyclophosphamide fluorouracil, etoposide, and cisplatin
FGAs	= first generation antihistamines first generation antipsychotics
FLU	= fluconazole (Diflucan) fludarabine (Fludara) flunisolide (Aero Bid) fluoxetine (Prozac) fluticasone propionate (Flonase) influenza
GD	= Graves disease Gaucher disease
GEM	= gemfibrozil gemicitabine
HCC	= hepatocellular carcinoma Hürthle cell carcinoma
HD	= Hansen disease Hirschsprung disease Hodgkin disease Huntington disease
HRF	= hypertensive renal failure hypoxic respiratory failure
HSS	= half-strength saline solution (0.45% sodium chloride injection) hypertonic saline solution (injection), (3, 5, and 7.5% sodium chloride injection

Table 3. Examples of Abbreviations That Have Contradictory or Ambiguous Meanings (*continued*)

Abbreviation	Meaning
ICA	= internal carotid artery intracranial abscess intracranial aneurysm
IAI	= intra-abdominal infection intra-abdominal injury intra-amniotic infection
I & D	= incision and drainage irrigation and debridement
IRDM	= insulin-required diabetes mellitus Insulin resistant diabetes mellitus
IT	= intrathecal intratracheal intratumoral intratympanic
KET	= ketamine ketoconazole
LAPC	= locally-advanced pancreatic cancer locally-advanced prostatic cancer
LF	= left foot Little finger Long finger
LFD	= lactose-free diet low-fat diet low-fiber diet
LL	= left leg left lung lower lid lower limb lower lip
LNE	= lymph node enlargement lymph node excision
LNU	= learned nonuse (splint) lower and upper (heard as L & U)
Ltx	= liver transplant Lung transplant
LVO	= left ventricular opacification left ventricular output left ventricular overactivity
MBC	= male breast cancer metastatic breast cancer
Mon	= Monday Month
MP	= melphalan; prednisone mitoxantrone; prednisone
MPM	= malignant peritoneal mesothelioma malignant pleural mesothelioma
MS	= mental status milk shake mitral sound morning stiffness morphine sulfate multiple sclerosis mitral stenosis musculoskeletal medical student minimal support muscle strength
MTD	= maximum tolerated dose minimum toxic dose
MTZ	= mirtazapine mitoxantrone
MV	= mechanical ventilation manual ventilation
NAF	= Native-American female Negro-American female normal adult female
NBM	= no bowel movement normal bowel movement nothing by mouth
NE	= no effect no enlargement not evaluated
NITRO	= nitroglycerin sodium nitroprusside
OLB	= open-liver biopsy open-lung biopsy
PBL	= primary breast lymphoma primary brain lymphoma
PBZ	= phenylbutazone pyribenzamine phenoxybenzamine
PCU	= palliative care unit primary care unit progressive care unit protective care unit

Table 3. Examples of Abbreviations That Have Contradictory or Ambiguous Meanings (*continued*)

Abbreviation	Meanings
PD	= Paget disease panic disorder Parkinson disease personality disorder
Pit	= Pitocin Pitressin
PORT	= postoperative radiotherapy postoperative respiratory therapy
PVO	= peripheral vascular occlusion portal vein occlusion pulmonary venous occlusion
RS	= Reiter syndrome Rett syndrome Reye syndrome Raynaud disease (syndrome) rumination syndrome
RTI	= reproductive tract infection respiratory tract infection
S & S	= swish and spit swish and swallow
SA	= suicide alert suicide attempt
SAD	= schizoaffective disorder social anxiety disorder seasonal affective disorder
SDBP	= seated, standing, or supine diastolic blood pressure
SGAs	= second generation antihistamines second generation antipsychotics
SJS	= Schwartz-Jampel syndrome Stevens-Johnson syndrome Swyer-James syndrome
SSE	= saline solution enema soapsuds enema
STF	= special tube feeding standard tube feeding
TAC	= tetracaine, Adrenalin, and cocaine solution triamcinolone cream
3TC	= lamivudine (Epivir)
T&C #3	= Tylenol with 30 mg of Codeine
T/E	= testosterone to epitestosterone (ratio) testosterone to estrogen (ratio) trunk-to-extremity skinfold thickness (index)
TICU	= thoracic intensive care unit transplant intensive care unit trauma intensive care unit
TMZ	= temazepam temozolomide
TS	= Tay-Sachs (disease) Tourette syndrome Turner syndrome
tubal	= tubal ligation tubal pregnancy
VAC	= etoposide (VePesid), cytarabine (ara-C, and carboplatin vincristine, dactinomycin (actinomycin D), and cyclophosphamide vincristine, doxorubicin (Adriamycin), and cyclophosphamide
VAD	= vincristine, doxorubicin, (Adriamycin) and dexamethasone vincristine, doxorubicin (Adriamycin) and dactinomycin
VAP	= vincristine, Adriamycin, and prednisone vincristine, Adriamycin, and procarbazine vincristine, actinomycin D, and Platinol AQ vincristine, asparaginase, and prednisone
WS	= Waardenburg syndrome Werner syndrome West Syndrome Williams syndrome

Chapter 3

A Healthcare Controlled Vocabulary

Presently there are no standards for abbreviations used in prescribers' orders, consultations, written prescriptions, standing orders, computer order sets, nurse's medication administration records, pharmacy profiles, hospital formularies, etc. Because in the healthcare field everyone does their own thing, there are many variations. These variations in the way abbreviations are expressed are not always understood and at times are misinterpreted. They cause delays in initiating therapy, cause accidents, waste time for everyone in clarifying these documents, lengthen the time it takes to train those working in the healthcare field, lengthen hospital stays, and waste money.

A controlled vocabulary similar to what is used in the aviation industry is needed. Everyone in the aviation industry "follows the book," and uses a controlled vocabulary. All pilots and air traffic controllers say, "alfa", "bravo", "charlie." See Table 1, the phonetic alphabet. They do not go off on their own and say "adam", "beef", "candy!" They say "one three," not thirteen, because thirteen sounds like thirty. Radio transmission in the aviation industry is not easy to decipher, yet because precision is critical, everything possible is done to eliminate error. To prevent errors all radio transmissions are given only in English, every transmission is given in the same order and must be immediately repeated by the receiver to make sure it was heard correctly. Written and oral communication in the medical professions are just as critical and are also not easy to decipher, so establishing a controlled vocabulary is also necessary in this industry.

Listed below are some of the organizations that have ongoing projects related to standardizing medical terminology:

The United States Pharmacopeial Convention, Inc.
12601 Twinbrook Parkway
Rockville, MD, 20852

National Library of Medicine
Unified Medical Language Systems
8600 Rockville Pike
Bethesda, MD, 20894

Council of Biological Editors, through their Scientific Style and Format: The *CBE Manual for Authors, Editors, and Publishers,* 6th Ed. Council of Biological Editors; Cambridge University Press, Cambridge UK, New York, Victoria Australia: 1995

American Medical Association, through their *AMA Manual of Style, 10th Edition.* AMA, Chicago, 2008

Computer-Based Patient Record Institute, Inc.
1000 East Woodfield Rd. Suite 102
Schuamburg, IL 60173-5921
http://www.CPRI.org

Association for Healthcare Documentation Integrity through their *The Book of Style for Medical Transcription,* 3rd ed., 2008, Association for Healthcare Documentation Integrity, Modesta CA

Listed below (Table 2) is the start of a Healthcare Controlled Vocabulary. The basis for this controlled vocabulary is established standard terminology and the result of 41 years of studying medical errors by this author.

It is anticipated that a Healthcare Controlled Vocabulary, with professional organizations' input and backing, will grow and someday evolve into an "official standard." Your suggestions and comments are vital to this growth and eventual recognition. It is always safest to avoid the use of abbreviations unless they are well known in your work environment.

Table 1. Phonetic Alphabet

The International Civil Aviation Organization phonetic alphabet is used by the aviation industry when communications conditions are such that the information cannot be readily received without their use. Health professionals also should use it when it is necessary to orally spell critical information.

Character	Telephony	Phonic
A	Alfa	(AL-FAH)
B	Bravo	(BRAH-VOH)
C	Charlie	(CHAR-LEE) or (SHAR-LEE)
D	Delta	(DELL-TA)
E	Echo	(ECK-OH)
F	Foxtrot	(FOKS-TROT)
G	Golf	(GOLF)
H	Hotel	(HOH-TEL)
I	India	(IN-DEE-AH)
J	Juliett	(JEW-LEE-ETT)
K	Kilo	(KEY-LOH)
L	Lima	(LEE-MAH)
M	Mike	(MIKE)
N	November	(NO-VEM-BER)
O	Oscar	(OSS-CAH)
P	Papa	(PAH-PAH)
Q	Quebec	(KEH-BECK)
R	Romeo	(ROW-ME-OH)
S	Sierra	(SEE-AIR-RAH)
T	Tango	(TANG-GO)
U	Uniform	(YOU-NEE-FORM) or (OO-NEE-FORM)
V	Victor	(VIK-TAH)
W	Whiskey	(WIS-KEY)
X	X-ray	(ECKS-RAY)
Y	Yankee	(YANG-KEY)
Z	Zulu	(ZOO-LOO)
1	One	(WUN)
2	Two	(TOO)
3	Three	(TREE)
4	Four	(FOW-ER)
5	Five	(FIFE)
6	Six	(SIX)
7	Seven	(SEV-EN)
8	Eight	(AIT)
9	Nine	(NIN-ER)
0	Zero	(ZEE-RO)

Table 2. Examples of a Controlled Vocabulary

Standard	What **not** to use or do	Comments
100 mg (100 space mg)	100mg (100 no space mg)	The USP* standard way of expressing a strength is to leave a space between the number and its units. Leaving this space makes it easier to read the number as can be seen below. 1mg 1 mg 10mg 10 mg 100mg 100 mg
1 mg	1.0 mg	This is a USP standard. When a trailing zero is used, the decimal point is sometimes not seen when working from handwritten copies or when the decimal point falls on a line thus causing a tenfold overdose. These overdoses have caused injury and death. A "trailing zero" may be used only where required to demonstrate the level of precision of the value being reported, such as for laboratory results, imaging studies that report size of lesions, or catheter/tube sizes. It may **NOT** be used in medication orders or other medication-related documentation.
0.1 mL	.1 mL	When the decimal point is not seen, this is read as 1 mL, causing a ten fold overdose.
once daily (Do not abbreviate.)	The abbreviation OD	The classic meaning for OD is right eye. Liquids intended to be given once daily are mistakenly given in the right eye.
	The abbreviation QD	When the Q in QD is dotted too aggressively it looks like Q.I.D. and the medication is given four times daily. When a lower case q is used, the tail of the q has come up between the q and the d to make it look like qid. In the United Kingdom, Q.D. means four times daily
unit (Do not abbreviate. Write "unit" using a lower-case u)	The abbreviation U	The handwritten U is mistaken for a zero when poorly written causing a 10 fold overdose (i.e. 6 U regular insulin is read as 60). The poorly written U has also been read as a 4, 6, and cc. Write "unit," leaving a space between the number and the word unit.
mg (lower case mg with no period)	mg., Mg., Mg, MG, mgm, mgs	The USP standard expression is the mg
mL (lower case m with a capital L, no period)	mL., ml, ml., mls, mLs, cc	The USP standard expression is the mL for the measurement of liquids

Table 2. (cont.)

Standard	What **not** to use or do	Comments
Use generic names or brand names	Do not abbreviate drug names or combinations of drugs, such as CPZ, PBZ, NTG, MS, $MS0_4$, 5FC, MTX, 6MP, MOPP, ASA, HCTZ, etc.	Abbreviated drug names and acronyms are not always known to the reader; at times they have more than one possible meaning, or are thought to be another drug.
		When the chemical name “6 mercaptopurine” has been used, six doses of mercaptopurine have been mistakenly administered. The generic name, mercaptopurine, should be used. $MgS0_4$ (magnesium sulfate) has been read as morphine sulfate.
	Do not use shortened names or chemical names in patient-related documents	When an unofficial shortened version of the name norfloxacin, norflox was used, Norflex was mistakenly given. An order for Aredia was read as Adriamycin, as some professionals abbreviated the name Adriamycin as “Adria” which looks like Aredia.
The metric system	The apothecary system (grains, drams, minims, ounces, etc.)	The Apothecary system is so rarely used it is not recognized or understood. The symbol for minim (♏) is read as mL; the symbol for one dram (ʒ T) is read as 3 tablespoons, and gr (grain) is read as gram.
Use properly placed commas for numbers above 9999, as in 10,000, or 5,000,000	5000000	Some healthcare workers have difficulty in reading large numbers such as 5000000. The use of commas helps the reader to read these numbers correctly.
600 mg When possible, do not use decimal expressions.	0.6 g	A USP standard. The elimination of decimals lessens the chance for error.
25 mcg	0.025 mg	Mistakes are made when reading numbers less than 1 with decimals.
Use specific concentrations and the time in which intravenous potassium chloride should be administered.	Do not use the term “bolus” in conjunction with the administration of potassium chloride injection.	Some physicians will erroneously indicate that potassium chloride injection should be “bolused” or be given “IV push,” vaguely meaning that it should not be dripped in slowly. Many deaths have been reported when prescribers have been taken literally and the potassium chloride was given by bolus or IV push for fluid-restricted patients. Orders should be specific such as, “20 mEq of potassium chloride in 50 mL of 5% dextrose to run over 30 minutes.”

(*continued*)

Table 2. (cont.)

Standard	What **not** to use or do	Comments
use "and"	Do not use a slash (/) mark or the symbol "&"	A slash mark looks like a one. An order written "6 units regular insulin/20 units NPH insulin," was read as 120 units of NPH insulin. The symbol "&" has been read as a 4.
Orally transmitted medical orders should be read back as heard for verification.	Do not assume that one has spoken or heard correctly.	During oral communications, speakers misspeak and/or transcribers mishear. To minimize these errors, the transmitter must speak clearly and slowly, the transcriber must repeat what was transcribed, and the transmitter must listen attentively when this is being done. Errors are less likely to occur when the prescription is complete. When spelling out words, use the phonetic alphabet shown in Table 1. Oral orders should be avoided whenever possible.
When prescriptions are written or orally transmitted they must be complete. • dosage form must be specified • strength must be specified • directions must be specified • included in the directions must be the purpose or indication.	Incomplete orders	Prescribers on occasion think of one drug and mistakenly order another. Nurses and pharmacists on occasion misread prescriptions because of error, poor handwriting or poor oral communications, or look-alike or sound-alike drugs.[1] When the prescription is complete and the purpose or indication is included, these errors are less likely to occur. Listing the purpose or indication on the prescription label will assist in increasing patient adherence.
Written communications must be legible.	Illegible handwriting	Those who cannot or will not write legibly must print (if this would be legible), type, use a computer, or have an employee write for them and then immediately verify and sign the document.
Prescribe specific doses.	Do not prescribe 2 ampuls or 2 vials	There is often more than one size or concentration of drug available. Failing to be specific will lead to unintended doses being administered.
As required by the Joint Commission on Accreditation of Healthcare Organizations, establish a list of dangerous abbreviations which should not be used	Use dangerous abbreviations.	See Chapter 2 of this book "Dangerous, Contradictory, and/or Ambiguous Abbreviations."

Table 2. (cont.)

Standard	What **not** to use or do	Comments
Use h or hr for hour	°	An order written as q 4° has been read as q 40 or the symbol ° has not been understood.
Specify amount of drug to be given in a single dose.[2]	Specify total amount of drug to be administered over a period of time.	Orders such as . . . . 1,600 mg over 4 days have caused death when mistakenly given as a single dose. Order should state . . . . 400 mg once daily for four days (2-1-08 to 2-4-08)

*USP = United States Pharmacopeia

1. Davis NM. Look-alike and sound alike drug names. Hosp Pharm 2006, Supplement Wall-chart (Call 1-800-223-0554)
2. Kohler D. Standardizing the expression & nomenclature of cancer treatment regimens. Am J Health-System Pharm. 1998;55;137–44

Additions, Corrections, and Suggestions are Welcomed

Please send them via any means shown below:

Neil M Davis
2049 Stout Drive, B-3
Warminster PA 18974-3861

FAX 1 888 333 4915 or 1 215 442 7432
Email med@neilmdavis.com
Web site www.medabbrev.com

Thank you for your help in the past.

Have You Used the Internet Version of This Book?

- It is instantaneously searchable for the meanings of abbreviations
- It is reverse searchable (search for all the abbreviations containing a particular word)
- Each month, about 80 new entries are added

See the preface (page vii) for access instructions. A one-year, single-user access is included in the purchase price of the book. Also one-year subscriptions are available for purchase (see page 377).

PDA and BlackBerry Versions are Available

See pricing and ordering information in the pricing section on page 379.

Multi-User Site Licenses are Available

Medical facilities can substitute their own "Do Not Use" list of dangerous abbreviations for the one present. The ability also exists to list abbreviations that are unique to your region and/or organization which would normally not appear in any national list. These lists would be controlled by the facility or company. A no-cost, 3-week trial and pricing information are available by calling 1 888 333 1862 or 1 215 442 7430 or via an e-mail request to ev@neilmdavis.com

Chapter 4

How Medical Writers, Editors, and Health Professionals Can Help Control the Proliferation of Health-Related Abbreviations

I have been collecting medical abbreviations for over 30 years, during which time I cofounded the Institute for safe Medication Practices and authored 14 editions of the book you are currently reading. The current edition contains 30,000 possible meanings for these health-related abbreviations. If there is such a thing as the world's foremost authority on medical abbreviations, then I am it. What I have learned is that abbreviations are a mixed blessing. They are a convenience, a time saver, a space saver, and a way of avoiding the possibility of misspelling words. However, a price is paid for their use. They can be misread or interpreted incorrectly. Their use lengthens the time needed to train individuals in the health fields, wastes the time of healthcare workers in tracking down their meanings, at times delays patient care, and, more often than people suspect, results in patient harm.

This chapter will discuss:

- How and why new abbreviations come into use
- The problems created by the use of abbreviations
- What medical writers, editors, and health professionals can do to prevent or lessen the problems created by medical abbreviations

The Evolution of Abbreviations

Speaking for myself and, I imagine, the great majority of others, we are used to taking shortcuts in our daily work. When we continually make a written record of a long word or phrase for our personal use, it is only natural to abbreviate it; no one else will see our shortcut and we know what it means. Eventually, we start to use these abbreviations to make it quicker and easier to communicate with the people with whom we work. As time goes on, these abbreviations are used in wider and wider circles.

Abbreviations can also be developed for commercial purposes because it is perceived that abbreviating a word or phrase has appeal to readers and customers. Medical writers and editors may also be the developers of a new abbreviation in order to save space or because they believe this will make for easier reading.

It is instructive to look at an example of how an abbreviation works its way into public use. The abbreviation MRI, for *magnetic resonance imaging,* did not appear in the National Library of Medicine's PubMed until 1983. In 1983 it appeared 13 times. In 2007, it appeared 22,292 times. This 1983 date is not quite accurate, as MRI did appear, once in 1977, to mean, *microroughness index*. You would call this a successful abbreviation that has served a useful purpose. New abbreviations appear because of new technology, new equipment, new therapies, new tests, new drug classes, new diseases, new government programs, new insurance programs, new services, etc.

The Problem with Abbreviations

There is a learning curve involved with abbreviations. First, learning occurs within a small group of insiders, those within the company that pioneer the development of a product or medical specialists that work on defining a new disease or syndrome. Whether the masses discern that MRI means *microroughness index* or *magnetic resonance imaging* was not a problem; however if your intention is to communicate, HD does not do it; as it could mean *Hansen disease, Hodgkin disease,* or *Huntington disease*. Yes, CHF means *congestive heart failure* 99% of the time, but other times it means *Crimean hemorrhagic fever, chronic heart failure,* and *congenital hepatic fibrosis*. For examples of other ambiguous abbreviations, see page 8. Some abbreviations are contradictory in their various possible meanings, such as BO for bowel *open* or *bowel obstructed* and S & S for *swish and spit* and also for *swish and swallow*.

Some medical abbreviations have proven to be dangerous, and the Joint Commission on Accreditation of Healthcare Organizations (it is obvious why this is abbreviated, JCAHO) has required healthcare facilities to start campaigns to eliminate their use[1,2]. A list of dangerous abbreviations and alternatives is shown on pages 6 and 7. Some of these abbreviations do not appear dangerous in print, but when they are handwritten, as is routinely done in practice, their danger becomes more apparent. Health professionals learn from what they see in print and they will use what they have seen in print when writing by hand in a medical record or a prescription.

What To Do

Avoid using abbreviations

Before using an abbreviation, ask yourself the question: Is it necessary? I have seen long articles where a term is followed by an abbreviation identifying it, and this abbreviation is never used again in the article. Was it really necessary to develop or show this abbreviation?

Before using an abbreviation, authors and editors should determine what is being gained by its use. How much easier will it be to read the article? Will it save a significant amount of space? How cumbersome is the word or phrase being abbreviated? Is it an abbreviation which most of the readers will already be familiar with?

Medical facilities, when formulating their preprinted order sets, protocols, guidelines, etc. should avoid all but the most widely-known abbreviations.

Always avoid using the abbreviations known to be dangerous (see table which appears on pages 6 and 7).

Test a New Abbreviation Before It Is Introduced

Before a new or unfamiliar abbreviation is coined or used, do some research to see if the abbreviation is also in use with another meaning. If you know that the abbreviation is already commonly in use to mean something else, you should come up with a different abbreviation or not abbreviate the term. I believe the authors and editors of the articles that abbreviated *Crimean hemorrhagic fever and congenital hepatic fibrosis as* CHF, should have known better. One of these problems was resolved when the condition was later referred to in the literature as *Crimean-Congo hemorrhagic fever* (CCHF). The *chronic heart failure* meaning for CHF is more often used outside the Untied States. The possible meanings of abbreviations can be researched on www.medabbrev.com, www.ncbi.nlm.nih.gov/entrez, and www.google.com. www.medabbrev.com (see page vii) is unique in that it also contains abbreviations which are unique to healthcare facilities that would not be found on other search engines

Conclusions

There are abbreviations that are dangerous and should not be used (see Chapter 2, Dangerous, Contradictory, and/or Ambiguous Abbreviations, page 3)

There are abbreviations that have ambiguous or contradictory meanings and therefore are not helpful and may be harmful and should not be used. For examples of such abbreviations, see page 8. There are certain abbreviations, which are so rarely used or used only by a select group of specialists that they will not be understood by the average health professional.

It takes experience and the judgment to predict which new abbreviations will make it into the vocabulary of most healthcare professionals. It is best to err on the side of not assigning an abbreviation to a word or group of words, than to assign one.

A price is paid when health professionals use uncommon or multi-definition abbreviations when communicating and sometimes that price is a human life. Medical writers, editors, researchers, hospital administrators, government agencies, health-related industries, etc., can help by following the recommendations presented above. Healthcare professionals must follow this lead.

Table 1. The rate of appearance of the abbreviation MRI in the National Library of Medicine's PubMed

Year	Number of times MRI appeared
1980–82	0
1983	13
1984	132
1985	471
1986	913
1987	2,002
1989	4,591
2004	15,447
2005	17,404
2006	19,061
2007	22,292

1. Anon. "National Patient Safety Goals" chapter in Comprehensive Accreditation Manual for Hospitals: The Official Handbook, Refreshed Core, January 2005. Joint Commission on Accreditation of Healthcare Organizations, Oakbrook Terrace, IL. 2005. page NPSG-3
2. www.jcaho.org (click Prohibited Abbreviations- See goal 2)

Additions, Corrections, and Suggestions are Welcomed

Please send them via any means shown below:

Neil M Davis
2049 Stout Drive, B-3
Warminster PA 18974-3861

FAX 1 888 333 4915 or 1 215 442 7432
Email med@neilmdavis.com
Web site www.medabbrev.com

Thank you for your help in the past.

Have You Used the Internet Version of This Book?

- It is instantaneously searchable for the meanings of abbreviations
- It is reverse searchable (search for all the abbreviations containing a particular word)
- Each month, about 80 new entries are added

See the preface (page vii) for access instructions. A one-year, single-user access is included in the purchase price of the book. Also one-year subscriptions are available for purchase (see page 377).

PDA and BlackBerry Versions are Available

See pricing and ordering information in the pricing section on page 379.

Multi-User Site Licenses are Available

Medical facilities can substitute their own "Do Not Use" list of dangerous abbreviations for the one present. The ability also exists to list abbreviations that are unique to your region and/or organization which would normally not appear in any national list. These lists would be controlled by the facility or company. A no-cost, 3-week trial and pricing information are available by calling 1 888 333 1862 or 1 215 442 7430 or via an e-mail request to ev@neilmdavis.com

Chapter 5
Medical Abbreviation Primer

When first entering a medically related field, one must learn the language in order to function. Part of learning this language is to learn the meaning of the abbreviations, acronyms, and symbols in use. This chapter is intended to introduce newcomers to this commonly used medically related shorthand.

The determination of which abbreviations (refers also to acronyms and symbols) are most commonly used is based on the selection by the author with the consultation of experts in various health-related fields. The categorizing of the abbreviations is arbitrary, but is intended to represent the most common use, as the abbreviations could have been placed in many different categories.

This list could have been expanded to include many hundreds-more commonly used abbreviations, but then the list would have been too long to serve as a primer. The absence of an abbreviation from this listing does not mean it is not in common use. Each area of practice and specialty could have added their own commonly used abbreviations.

A few of the abbreviations below have more than one meaning listed. This was done when several meanings are in common use. Many abbreviations have more than one meaning and they must be viewed in their clinical context to arrive at their intended meaning. See Chapter 6 of this book for additional meanings for the abbreviations listed below.

In practice, there are inconsistencies as to how abbreviations are written. They may appear in all capital letters, lower case, or in capital letters and lower case. They may or may not have periods after each letter.

The readers are urged to read Chapter 2, Dangerous, Contradictory, and/or Ambiguous Abbreviations.

Two Hundred and Seventy-Five Commonly Used Medical Abbreviations Arranged by Category—a Primer

Physical Examination, History Portion of the Medical Record, and Discharge Summary

Abbreviation	Meaning
C/O	complains of
CC	chief complaint(s)
CTA	clear to auscultation
Dx	diagnosis
F/U	follow-up
FH	family history
H/O	history of
HPI	history of present illness
Hx	history
PE	physical examination pelvic examination pulmonary embolism
PH/SH	personal and social history
PI	present illness
PMH	past medical history
ROS	review of systems
SH	social history
Tx	treatment
CV	cardiovascular
GI	gastrointestinal
GU	genitourinary
EENT	ears, eyes, nose, and throat
HEENT	head, ears, eyes, nose, and throat
Ob/Gyn	obstetrics and gynecology
Peds	pediatrics
UCD	usual childhood diseases
A & P	auscultation and percussion
ADL	activities of daily living
CN III	third cranial nerve (there are CN I to XII)
RCM	right costal margin (there is also a LCM)
RUQ	right upper quadrant (also there is RLQ, LUQ, and LLQ)
TM	tympanic membrane
AAO X 3	alert, awake, and oriented to time, place, and person
BM	bowel movement
BP	blood pressure
CVAT	costovertebral angle tenderness
DTR	deep tendon reflex
EOMI	extraocular muscles intact
HJR	hepatojugular reflux
JVD	jugular venous distention
IBW	ideal body weight
LBW	lean body weight
BSA	body surface area
LMP	last menstrual period
NAD	no apparent distress no apparent disease
NC/AT	normocephalic, atraumatic
NKA	no known allergies
NKDA	no known drug allergies
OD	right eye
OS	left eye
OU	both eyes
PERRLA	pupils equal, round, reactive to light and accommodation
IOP	intraocular pressure
ROM	range of motion
VS	vital signs
P	pulse
T	temperature
RR	respiratory rate; recovery room
HR	heart rate
RRR	regular rate and rhythm (heart)
WDWNWM	well developed, well nourished, white male (also there are abbreviations for females and other races [WF = white female; AAF = African-American female]
YO	year old
DOB	date of birth
+	positive; present; plus
−	negative; absent; minus
$\bar{c}$	with
õ	negative; without
W/O	without

Diseases and Symptoms

AD	Alzheimer disease
AIDS	acquired immunodeficiency syndrome
HIV	human immuno-deficiency virus
AMI	acute myocardial infarction
MI	myocardial infarction
CHF	congestive heart failure
ACS	acute coronary syndrome
HT	hypertension (also HTN) height
DM	diabetes mellitus
AODM	adult onset diabetes mellitus
IDDM	insulin dependent diabetes mellitus
NIDDM	noninsulin-dependent diabetes mellitus
PD	Parkinson disease
AOM	acute otitis media
Ca	cancer
COAD	chronic obstructive airway disease
COPD	chronic obstructive pulmonary disease
DOE	dyspnea on exertion
SOB	shortness of breath
URI	upper respiratory infection
TB	tuberculosis
CVA	cerebrovascular accident; costovertebral angle
DVT	deep vein thrombosis
NV	nausea and vomiting
NVD	nausea, vomiting, and diarrhea neck vein distention
PONV	postoperative nausea and vomiting
PUD	peptic ulcer disease
GERD	gastroesophageal reflux disease
RA	rheumatoid arthritis
OA	osteoarthritis
SLE	systemic lupus erythematosus
TIA	transient ischemic attack
HA	headache
BPH	benign prostatic hypertrophy (hyperplasia)
UTI	urinary tract infection
STD	sexually transmitted disease
MVA	motor vehicle accident

Clinical Laboratory

ANA	antinuclear antibody
Alb	albumin
ALT	alanine aminotransferase
LFT	liver function test
aPTT	activated partial thromboplastin time
AST	aspartate aminotransferase
BG	blood glucose; blood gases
BS	blood sugar bowel sounds breath sounds
BUN	blood urea nitrogen
CK-MB	creatine kinase, MB fraction
CO_2	carbon dioxide
CPK	creatinine phosphokinase
CrCl	creatinine clearance
SCr	serum creatinine
C & S	culture and sensitivity
ESR	erythrocyte sedimentation rate
Gluc	glucose
FBS	fasting blood sugar
HbA_{1c}	glycosylated hemoglobin
CHOL	cholesterol
HDL	high-density lipoprotein
LDL	low-density lipoprotein
LDH	lactic dehydrogenase
Trig	trigylcerides
INR	international normalized ratio
DB	direct bilirubin
TB	total bilirubin
TP	total protein
Ca	Calcium (also Ca^{++})
Cl	Chloride (also Cl^{-})
K	Potassium (also K^{+})
Mg	Magnesium (also Mg^{++})
Na	Sodium (also Na^{+})
OGTT	oral glucose tolerance test
PSA	prostate-specific antigen
UA	urinalysis
VDRL	Venereal Disease Research Laboratory (test for syphilis)
CBC	complete blood count
Diff	differential (blood count)
Eos	eosinophil
Fe	iron
Hct	hematocrit
Hgb	hemoglobin
H&H	hemoglobin and hematocrit
Plt	platelets
MCV	mean corpuscular volume
RBC	red blood cell (count)
Segs	segmented neutrophils
WBC	white blood cell (count)
ABG	arterial blood gases
WNL	within normal limits

Other Diagnostic Tests, Procedures, and Treatments

ECG	electrocardiogram
EEG	electroencephalogram
FEV_1	forced expiratory volume in one second
IPPB	intermittent positive-pressure breathing
PFT	pulmonary function tests
PEEP	positive end-expiratory pressure
MUGA	multigated (radionuclide) angiogram
CT	computer tomography
IVP	intravenous pyelogram
MRI	magnetic resonance imaging
PET	positron emission tomography
US	ultrasound
CABG	coronary artery bypass graft
PCTA	percutaneous transluminal coronary angioplasty
PT	physical therapy
D & C	dilatation and curettage

Physicians' Orders and Prescriptions

ASAP	as soon as possible
OOB	out of bed
BRP	bathroom privileges
CPR	cardiopulmonary resuscitation
DNR	do not resuscitate
DAW	dispense as written
DC or D/C	discharge discontinue
I/O	intake and output
LD	loading dose
NAS	no salt added
NPO	nothing by mouth
PO	by mouth; postoperative
IM	intramuscular
IV	intravenous
SC	subcutaneous
SQ	subcutaneous (SC preferred)
PICC	percutaneous indwelling central catheter
IVPB	intravenous piggyback
NGT	nasogastric tube
cap	capsule
tab	tablet
inj	injection
i	one
ii	two
q	*every (as in q 6 hours)*
h	hour(s)
b.i.d.	*twice daily*
t.i.d.	*three times daily*
q.i.d.	*four times daily*
QAM	every morning
QPM	every evening
AC	*before meals*
PC	*after meals*
HS	*bedtime*
NR	no refills (prescriptions)
PRN	*as required; whenever necessary*
MRx1	may repeat one time
Rx	*prescription* *pharmacy*
OTC	over-the-counter (no prescription required)
Stat	*immediately*
TKO	to keep (vein) open
TO	telephone order
VO	verbal order

Drug Names
(Presented for informational purposes only; they should *not* be used)

APAP	acetaminophen
ASA	aspirin
5D/W	dextrose 5% injection (in water)
Dig	digoxin
ETOH	alcohol (ethyl alcohol)
$FeSO_4$	ferrous sulfate
H_2O	water
H_2O_2	hydrogen peroxide
HCl	hydrochloride (when following a drug name, as in thiamine HCl [thiamine hydrochloride]) hydrochloric acid (when it appears separately [not as part of a drug name])
KCl	potassium chloride
$MgSO_4$	magnesium sulfate
MOM	milk of magnesia
NaCl	sodium chloride
NS	normal saline (0.9% sodium chloride; same as NSS)
NSS	normal saline solution (0.9% sodium chloride)
O_2	oxygen
PCN	penicillin
tPA	tissue plasminogen activator
IVF	intravenous fluids
TPN	total parenteral nutrition
lytes	electrolytes (sodium, potassium, chloride, etc.)

Drug Classes

ABX	antibiotic(s)	PPI	proton pump inhibitor
COX-2 I	cyclooxygenase-2 inhibitor	SSRI	selective serotonin reuptake inhibitor
MAOI	monoamine oxidase inhibitor	TCA	tricyclic antidepressant
NSAID	nonsteroidal anti-inflammatory drug		
OC	oral contraceptive		

Units of Measure

cm	centimeter (2.54 cm = 1 inch)	mEq	milliequivalent
g	gram (28.35 g = 1 ounce)	mg	milligram (1,000 mg = 1 gram [g])
kg	kilogram (1 kg = 2.2 pounds)	mL	milliliter (1,000 mL = 1 liter [L])
L	liter (1 L = 1,000 mL = 1 quart plus about 2 ounces)	mmHg	millimeters of mercury
lb	pound (1 lb = 0.454 Kg)	°C	degrees Centigrade (Celsius)
mcg	microgram (1,000 mcg = 1 milligram [mg])	°F	degrees Fahrenheit

Hospital Locations

CCU	cardiac care unit	OB	obstetrics
DR	delivery room	OR	operating room
ED	emergency department	PACU	postanesthesia care unit
ER	emergency room (same as ED)	PICU	pediatric intensive care unit pulmonary intensive care unit
ICU	intensive care unit	RD	radiology department
L & D	labor and delivery	SICU	surgical intensive care unit
LDR	labor, delivery, and recovery		
MICU	medical intensive care unit		
NICU	neonatal intensive care unit		

Miscellaneous

ARNP	Advanced Registered Nurse Practitioner	MD	Doctor of Medicine
DO	Doctor of Osteopathy	PA	Physician Assistant
LPN	Licensed Practical Nurse	RPh	Registered Pharmacist
MA	Medical Assistant	RN	Registered Nurse
MAR	medication administration record		

Additions, Corrections, and Suggestions are Welcomed

Please send them via any means shown below:

Neil M Davis
2049 Stout Drive, B-3
Warminster PA 18974-3861

FAX 1 888 333 4915 or 1 215 442 7432
Email med@neilmdavis.com
Web site www.medabbrev.com

Thank you for your help in the past.

Have You Used the Internet Version of This Book?

- It is instantaneously searchable for the meanings of abbreviations
- It is reverse searchable (search for all the abbreviations containing a particular word)
- Each month, about 80 new entries are added

See the preface (page vii) for access instructions. A one-year, single-user access is included in the purchase price of the book. Also one-year subscriptions are available for purchase (see page 377).

PDA and BlackBerry Versions are Available

See pricing and ordering information in the pricing section on page 379.

Multi-User Site Licenses are Available

Medical facilities can substitute their own "Do Not Use" list of dangerous abbreviations for the one present. The ability also exists to list abbreviations that are unique to your region and/or organization which would normally not appear in any national list. These lists would be controlled by the facility or company. A no-cost, 3-week trial and pricing information are available by calling 1 888 333 1862 or 1 215 442 7430 or via an e-mail request to ev@neilmdavis.com

Chapter 6

Lettered Abbreviations, Acronyms, and Slang

When an abbreviation contains numbers, symbols, punctuation, spaces, etc., they are *not* considered during alphabetizing. When looking for 6MP, it will be found after the MP listings and H_2O will be found after HO. Abbreviations that only contain numbers (no letters) are found in chapter 7, Symbols and Numbers. Entries beginning with a *Greek letter* are alphabetized where the name of the letter would be found alphabetically.

The letter-by-letter (dictionary) system of alphabetizing is used ("*ad lib*" is listed under ADL).

When an abbreviation ending with an S can not be found, check for the abbreviation without the S as it may be the plural form of one that is listed.

Brand names (proprietary names) have their first letter capitalized, whereas nonproprietary (generic) names are in lower-case letters.

Although shown for informational purposes, drug names should not be abbreviated as the meaning may not be known to the reader or interpreted as intended.

Slang is presented for informational purposes only and should not be used.

The listing of symbols, numbers, and Greek letters can be found in Chapter 7.

Some of the meanings shown are very specialized or new and will not be understood by the majority of health professionals. These very specialized abbreviations are presented for informational purposes and their use in healthcare documentation should be done with assurance that they will be understood. See WARNING in chapter 1.

A

A	accommodation
	Acinetobacter
	adenosine
	age
	alive
	ambulatory
	angioplasty
	anterior
	anxiety
	apical
	arterial
	artery
	Asian
	assessment
	assistance
	auscultation
A+	blood type A positive (A positive is preferred)
A−	blood type A negative (A negative is preferred)
A′	ankle
@	at
(a)	axillary temperature
$\bar{a}$	before
A_1	aortic first heart sound
A_2	aortic second sound
A250	5% albumin 250 mL
A1000	5% albumin 1000 mL

A II	angiotensin II
AA	accelerated approval (FDA)
	acetic acid
	achievement age
	active assistive
	acute asthma
	affected area
	affirmative action
	African American
	Alcoholics Anonymous
	alcohol abuse
	alopecia areata
	alveolar-arterial gradient
	amino acid
	anaplastic astrocytoma
	androgenetic alopecia
	anesthesiologist assistant
	anti-aerobic
	antiarrhythmic agent
	aortic aneurysm
	aplastic anemia
	arachidonic acid
	arm ankle (pulse ratio)
	ascending aorta
	ascorbic acid (vitamin C)
	audiologic assessment
	Australia antigen
	authorized absence
	automobile accident
	cytarabine (ara-C) and doxorubicin (Adriamycin)
aa	of each
A&A	aid and attendance
	albuterol and ipratropium bromide (Atrovent) (this combination is available as Combivent Aerosol and DuoNab inhalation solution)
	arthroscopy and arthrotomy
	awake and aware
A-a	alveolar arterial (gradient)
a/A	arterial-alveolar (gradient)
AIIA	Angiotensin II antagonist
AAA	abdominal aortic aneurysmectomy (aneurysm)
	acute anxiety attack
	apply to affected area
	Area Agencies on Aging
	aromatic amino acids
	arterio-arterial anastomosis
A&AA	active and active assistive
AAAASF	American Association for Accreditation of Ambulatory Surgery Facilities
AAAE	amino acid activating enzyme
AAAHC	Accreditation Association of Ambulatory Health Care
AABB	American Association of Blood Banks
AABR	automated auditory brainstem response
AAC	Adrenalin, atropine, and cocaine
	advanced adrenocortical cancer
	antimicrobial agent-associated colitis
	augmentative and alternative communication
AACD	aging-associated cognitive decline
AACG	acute-angle closure glaucoma
AACLR	arthroscopic anterior cruciate ligament reconstruction
AAD	acid-ash diet
	antibiotic-associated diarrhea
A_1AD	alpha$_1$-antitrypsin deficiency
AADA	Abbreviated Antibiotic Drug Application
[A-a]Do_2	alveolar-arterial oxygen tension gradient
AAE	active assistance exercise
	acute allergic encephalitis
AAECS	amino acid enriched cardioplegic solution
A/AEX	active assistive exercise
AAF	African-American female
	altered auditory feedback
AAFB	alcohol acid-fast bacilli
AAFO	active ankle-foot orthoses
AAG	alpha-1-acid glycoprotein
AAH	acute alcoholic hepatitis
	atypical adenomatous hyperplasia
AAI	acute alcohol intoxication
	arm-ankle index
	atlantoaxial instability
	atrial demand-inhibited (pacemaker)
AAK	atlantoaxial kyphosis
AAL	anterior axillary line
AALNC	Legal Nurse Consultant (American Association of Legal Nurse Consultants)
AAM	African-American male
	amino acid mixture
AAMI	age-associated memory impairment
AAMS	acute aseptic meningitis syndrome
AAN	AIDS-associated neutropenia
	analgesic abuse nephropathy
	analgesic-associated nephropathy
	attending's admission notes
AANA	American Association of Nurse Anesthetists
AAO	alert, awake, & oriented
AAO × 3	alert, awake and oriented to time, place, and person
AAOC	antacid of choice
AAP	acute anterior poliomyelitis
	American Academy of Pediatrics (guidelines)
	assessment adjustment pass

AAPC — antibiotic-associated pseudomembranous colitis
AAPMC — antibiotic-associated pseudomembranous colitis
a/ApO_2 — arterial-alveolar oxygen tension ratio
AAPSA — age-adjusted prostate-specific antigen
AAR — antigen-antiglobulin reaction
automated anesthesia record
AARF — atlantoaxial rotatory fixation (subluxation; dislocation)
AAROM — active-assistive range of motion
AAS — acute abdominal series
alkylating agent score
allergic Aspergillus sinusitis
androgenic-anabolic steroid
Ann Arbor stage (Hodgkin disease staging system)
aortic arch syndrome
Associate's Degree, Applied Science
atlantoaxis subluxation
atomic absorption spectroscopy
atypical absence seizure
AASCRN — amino acid screen
AASH — adrenal androgen-stimulating hormone
AAST — American Association for the Surgery of Trauma (trauma grading)
AAST-OIS — American Association for the Surgery of Trauma—Organ Injury Scale
AASV — antibody-associated systemic vasculitis
AAT — activity as tolerated
alpha-antitrypsin
androgen ablation therapy
at all times
atrial demand-triggered (pacemaker)
atypical antibody titer
automatic atrial tachycardia
A_1AT — $alpha_1$-antitrypsin
A_1AT-P_i — $alpha_1$-antitrypsin (phenotyping)
AAU — acute anterior uveitis
AAV — adeno-associated vector
adeno-associated virus
AAV-GAD — glutamic acid decarboxylase (gene viral transfer with the) adeno-associated virus
AAVV — accumulated alveolar ventilatory volume
AAWD — antiandrogen withdrawal
AB — abortion
Ace® bandage
antibiotic
antibody
Aphasia Battery
apical beat
armboard
attentional blink
products meeting bioequivalence requirements for generic pharmaceuticals
Aβ — beta-amyloid peptide
A/B — acid-base ratio
apnea/bradycardia
A > B — air greater than bone (conduction)
A & B — apnea and bradycardia
assault and battery
AB+ — AB positive blood type (AB positive preferred)
AB− — AB negative blood type (AB negative preferred)
ABA — applied behavioral analysis
ABBI — Advanced Breast Biopsy Instrumentation
ABC — abacavir (Ziagen)
abbreviated blood count
Aberrant Behavior Checklist
absolute band counts
absolute basophil count
activity-based costing
advanced breast cancer
airway, breathing, and circulation
all but code (resuscitation order)
aneurysmal bone cyst
antigen-binding capacity
apnea, bradycardia, and cyanosis
applesauce, bananas, and cereal (diet)
argon-beam coagulator
Aristotle Basic Complexity (Score)
aspiration, biopsy and cytology
artificial beta cells
automated blood count (no differential)
avidin-biotin complex
ABCD — **a**ge, **b**lood pressure, **c**linical features, and **d**uration of symptoms (prognostic score for short term risk of stroke after transient ischemic attack)
amphotericin B cholesteryl sulfate complex (Amphotec; amphotericin B colloid dispersion)
asymmetry, **b**order irregularity, **c**olor variation, and **d**iameter more than 6 mm (melanoma warning signs in a mole)
automated blood count (differential done manually)
ABCDE — botulism toxoid pentavalent
ABCS — Active Bacterial Core Surveillance (CDC)
automated blood count, STKR (differential done by machine)

A

ABCs	**A**$_{1c}$ level (glycosylate hemoglobin A$_{1c}$), **B**lood pressure, and **C**holesterol level (ABCs of diabetes care)
	abstinence, fidelity ("being faithful"), or condom use (ABCs of HIV prevention)
	airway, breathing, and circulation stabilization (ABCs of resuscitation)
	aneurysmal bone cysts
ABD	after bronchodilator
	automated border detection detection
	type of plain gauze dressing
Abd	abdomen
	abdominal
	abductor
ABDCT	atrial bolus dynamic computer tomography
AC followed by D	doxorubicin (Adriamycin) and cyclophosphamide followed by docetaxel
ABD GR	abdominal girth
ABD PB	abductor pollicis brevis
Abd/pel	abdomen/pelvis
ABD PL	abductor pollicis longus
ABE	acute bacteria endocarditis
	adult basic education
	average bioequivalence
	botulism equine trivalent antitoxin
ABECB	acute bacterial exacerbations of chronic bronchitis
ABEP	auditory brain stem-evoked potentials
	aortic blood flow
A-beta42	beta-amyloid 42
ABF	aortobifemoral (bypass)
ABG	air/bone gap
	aortoiliac bypass graft
	arterial blood gases
	axiobuccogingival
ABH	Ativan, Benadryl, and Haldol
ABI	ankle brachial index (ankle-to-arm systolic blood pressure ratio)
	atherothrombotic brain infarction
	auditory brainstem implant
ABID	antibody identification
A Big	atrial bigeminy
ABK	aphakic bullous keratopathy
ABL	abetalipoproteinemia
	allograft bound lymphocytes
	axiobuccolingual
ABLB	alternate binaural loudness balance
ABLC	amphotericin B lipid complex (Abelcet)
ABLV	Australian bat lyssavirus
A/B Mods	apnea/bradycardia moderate stimulation
ABMS	acute bacterial maxillary sinusitis
	autologous bone marrow support
A/B MS	apnea/bradycardia mild stimulation
ABMT	autologous bone marrow transplantation
ABN	abnormality(ies)
	Advance Beneficiary Notice
abnl bld	abnormal bleeding
ABNM	American Board of Nuclear Medicine
abnor.	abnormal
ABO	absent bed occupant
	blood group system (A, AB, B, and O)
ABP	ambulatory blood pressure
	androgen-binding protein
	arterial blood pressure
ABPA	allergic bronchopulmonary aspergillosis
ABPB	axillary brachial plexus block
ABPI	Association of the British Pharmaceutical Industry
ABPM	axillary brachial plexus block
ABPM	allergic bronchopulmonary mycosis
	ambulatory blood pressure monitoring
ABQAURP	American Board of Quality Assurance and Utilization Review Physicians
ABR	absolute bed rest
	auditory brain-stem response
ABRS	acute bacterial rhinosinusitis
ABS	absent
	absorbed
	absorption
	Accuchek® blood sugar
	acute brain syndrome
	admitting blood sugar
	Alterman-Bishop stent
	antibody screen
	at bedside
ABSS	Anderson Behavioral State Scale
A/B SS	apnea/bradycardia self-stimulation
ABT	aminopyrine breath test
	antibiotic therapy
	autologous blood therapy
ABVD	doxorubicin (Adriamycin)®, bleomycin, vinblastine, and dacarbazine (DTIC)
ABW	actual body weight
ABx	antibiotics
AC	abdominal circumference
	acceleration capacity (heart)
	acetate
	acromioclavicular
	activated charcoal
	acute

	African Caribbean
	air conditioned
	air conduction
	anchored catheter
	antecubital
	anticoagulant
	anticonvulsant
	arm circumference
	assist control
	autologous cell
	before meals (*a.c.* preferred)
	doxorubicin (Adriamycin) and cyclophosphamide
a.c.	before meals
A-C	Astler-Coller (stages of colorectal cancer
A/C	anterior chamber of the eye
	assist/control
A & C	alert and cooperative
A_{1C}	glycosylated hemoglobin A_{1C}
5-AC	azacitidine (Vidaza)
9AC	rubitecan (9-aminocamptothecin; Orathecin)
ACA	acrodermatitis chronica atrophicans
	acyclovir
	adenocarcinoma
	against clinical advice
	aminocaproic acid (Amicar)
	anterior cerebral artery
	anterior communicating artery
	anticanalicular antibodies
AC/A	accommodation convergence–accommodation (ratio)
ACABS	acute community-acquired bacterial sinusitis
ACAD	anterior circulation arterial dissection
ACAS	acute community-acquired sinusitis
	asymptomatic carotid artery study
ACAT	acyl coenzyme A: cholesterol acyltransferase
ACB	alveolar-capillary block
	antibody-coated bacteria
	aortocoronary bypass
	before breakfast
AcB	assist with bath
AC & BC	air and bone conduction
ACBE	air contrast barium enema
ACBG	aortocoronary bypass graft
ACBT	active cycle of breathing techniques
ACC	acalculous cholecystitis
	accident
	accommodation
	acinar cell carcinoma
	adenoid cystic carcinomas
	administrative control center
	advanced colorectal cancer
	ambulatory care center
	American College of Cardiology (guidelines)
	amylase creatinine clearance
	anterior cingulate cortex
	automated cell count
ACCE	Academic Clinical Coordinator Educator
ACC-NCDR	American College of Cardiology-National Cardiovascular Data Registry
AcCoA	acetyl-coenzyme A
ACCP	American College of Chest Physicians
ACCR	amylase creatinine clearance ratio
ACCU	acute coronary care unit
ACCU✔	Accucheck® (blood glucose monitoring)
ACD	absolute cardiac dullness
	absorbent cover dressing
	acid-citrate-dextrose
	advanced cervical dilation
	allergic contact dermatitis
	alveolar capillary dysplasia
	anemia of chronic disease
	anterior cervical diskectomy
	anterior chamber depth
	anterior chamber diameter
	anterior chest diameter
	average cost per day
	before dinner
	dactinomycin (actinomycin D; Cosmegen)
ACDC	antibody complement-dependent cytolysis
AC-DC	bisexual (homo- and heterosexual)
ACDDS	Alcoholism/Chemical Dependency Detoxification Service
ACDF	anterior cervical diskectomy and fusion
ACDFs	adult children from dysfunctional families
ACDK	acquired cystic disease of the kidney
ACDs	anticonvulsant drugs
ACE	adrenocortical extract
	adverse clinical event
	aerosol-cloud enhancer
	angiotensin-converting enzyme
	antegrade colonic enema
	antegrade continence enema
	doxorubicin (Adriamycin), cyclophosphamide, and etoposide
ACEI	angiotensin-converting enzyme inhibitor
ACF	aberrant crypt focus
	accessory clinical findings
	acute care facility
	anterior cervical fusion
ACG	accelerography

	adjusted clinical groups
	angiocardiography
ACGME	Accreditation Council for Graduate Medical Education
ACH	adrenal cortical hormone
	aftercoming head
	arm girth, chest depth, and hip width
ACh	acetylcholine
ACHA	air-conduction hearing aid
AChE	acetylcholinesterase
AChEIs	acetylcholinesterase inhibitors
ACHES	abdominal pain, chest pain, headache, eye problems, and severe leg pains (early danger signs of oral contraceptive adverse effects)
AC & HS	before meals and at bedtime
ACI	acceleration index
	adrenal cortical insufficiency
	aftercare instructions
	anabolic-catabolic index
	anemia of chronic illness
	autologous chondrocyte implantation
ACIOL	anterior chamber intraocular lens
ACIP	Advisory Committee on Immunization Practices (of the Centers for Disease Control and Prevention)
ACIS	automated cellular imaging system
ACJ	acromioclavicular joint
A/CK	Accuchek®
ACL	accessory collateral ligament (hand)
	American cutaneous leishmaniasis
	anterior cruciate ligament (knee)
aCL	anticardiolipin (antibody)
ACLA	aclarubicin
ACLF	adult congregate living facility
ACLR	anterior cruciate ligament repair
ACLS	advanced cardiac (cardiopulmonary) life support
	Allen Cognitive Level Screen
ACM	alternative/complementary medicine
	Arnold-Chiari malformation
ACME	arginine catabolic mobile element
	aphakic cystoid macular edema
	Automated Classification of Medical Entities
ACMT	advanced combined modality therapy
ACMV	assist-controlled mechanical ventilation
ACN	acetonitrile
	acute conditioned neurosis
ACNP	Acute Care Nurse Practitioner
ACNU	nimustine HCl (Nidran; Acnu)
ACO	anterior capsular opacification
ACOA	Adult Children of Alcoholics
ACOG	American College of Obstetricians and Gynecologists
A COMM A	anterior communicating artery
ACOS-OG	American College of Surgeons Oncology Group
ACP	accessory conduction pathway
	acid phosphatase
	adamantinomatous craniopharyngioma
	adenocarcinoma of the prostate
	advance care planning
	ambulatory care program
	anesthesia-care provider
	anterior cervical plate
	antrochoanal polyp
ACPA	anticytoplasmic antibodies
AC-PC line	anterior commissure-posterior commissure line
AC-PH	acid phosphatase
ACPO	acute colonic pseudo-obstruction
ACPP	adrenocorticopolypeptide
ACPPD	average cost per patient day
ACPP PF	acid phosphatase prostatic fluid
ACPS	anterior cervical plate stabilization
ACQ	acquired
	Areas of Change Questionnaire
ACQ-5	asthma control questionnaire (5-item symptom and activity version)
ACR	adenomatosis of the colon and rectum
	albumin to creatinine ratio
	American College of Rheumatology
	anterior chamber reformation
	anticonstipation regimen
ACR20	American College of Rheumatology rating scale (20% or more improvement)
ACRC	advanced colorectal cancer
ACRD	acquired cystic renal disease
ACRES	amplification created restriction enzyme site
ACRN	AIDS-Certified Registered Nurse
ACS	anterior compartment syndrome
	acute confusional state
	acute coronary syndromes
	American Cancer Society
	anodal-closing sound
	automated corneal shaper
	before supper
ACSF	anterior cervical spine fixation
	artificial cerebrospinal fluid
ACSL	automatic computerized solvent litholysis
ACSM	American College for Sports Medicine
ACSVBG	aortocoronary saphenous vein bypass graft
ACSW	Academy of Certified Social Workers

ACT	activated clotting time
	aggressive comfort treatment
	allergen challenge test
	anticoagulant therapy
	artemisinin-based combination therapy
	assertive community treatment (program)
	doxorubicin (adriamycin), cyclophosphamide, and paclitaxel (Taxol)
ACT-D	dactinomycin (Cosmegen)
Act Ex	active exercise
ACTG	AIDS Clinical Trial Group
ACTH	corticotropin (adrenocorticotropic hormone)
ACT-Post	activated clotting time post-filter
ACT-Pre	activated clotting time pre-filter
ACTSEB	anterior chamber tube shunt encircling band
ACU	ambulatory care unit
ACUP	adenocarcinoma of unknown primary (origin)
ACUV	air-contrast ultrasound venography
ACV	acyclovir (Zovirax)
	amifostine, cisplatin, and vinblastine
	assist control ventilation
	atrial/carotid/ventricular
A-C-V	A wave, C wave, and V wave
ACVBP	doxorubicin (Adriamycin), cyclophosphamide, vindesine, bleomycin, and prednisone
ACVD	acute cardiovascular disease
ACVP	doxorubicin (Adriamycin), cyclophosphamide, vincristine, and prednisone
ACW	anterior chest wall
	apply to chest wall
acyl-CoA	acyl coenzyme A
AD	accident dispensary
	admitting diagnosis
	advance directive (living will)
	air dyne
	alternating days (this is a dangerous abbreviation)
	Alzheimer disease
	androgen deprivation
	antidepressant
	assistive device
	atopic dermatitis
	autistic disorder
	axillary dissection
	axis deviation
	right ear
A&D	admission and discharge
	alcohol and drug
	ascending and descending
	vitamins A and D
ADA	adenosine deaminase
	American Dental Association
	American Diabetes Association
	Americans with Disabilities Act
	anterior descending artery
	awareness during anesthesia
ADAM	adjustment disorder with anxious mood
ADAS	Alzheimer Disease Assessment Scale
ADAS-COG	Alzheimer Disease Assessment Scale-Cognitive Subscale
ADAT	advance diet as tolerated
ADAU	adolescent drug abuse unit
ADB	amorous disinhibited behavior
ADC	Aid to Dependent Children
	AIDS (acquired immune deficiency syndrome) dementia complex
	anxiety disorder clinic
	apparent diffusion coefficient (radiology)
	average daily census
	average daily consumption
ADCA	autosomal dominant cerebellar ataxia
ADCC	antibody-dependent cellular cytotoxicity
A.D.C. VAAN DIML	mnemonic for formatting physician orders: **A**dmit, **D**iagnosis, **C**ondition, **V**itals, **A**ctivity, **A**llergies, **N**ursing procedures, **D**iet, **I**ns and outs, **M**edication, **L**abs
ADD	adduction
	annual disability density
	arrest in dilation/descent
	attention-deficit disorder
	average daily dose
ADDH	attention-deficit disorder with hyperactivity
ADDL	additional
ADDLs	amyloid-derived diffusible ligands
ADDM	adjustment disorder with depressed mood
ADDP	adductor pollicis
ADDs	AIDS (acquired immune deficiency syndrome)-defining diseases
ADDU	alcohol and drug dependence unit
ADE	acute disseminated encephalitis
	adverse drug event
ADEM	acute disseminating encephalomyelitis
ADE-NOCA	adenocarcinoma
ADEPT	antibody-directed enzyme prodrug therapy
ADFT	atrial defibrillation threshold
ADFU	agar diffusion for fungus
ADG	atrial diastolic gallop

A

Abbreviation	Meaning
	axiodistogingival
ADH	antidiuretic hormone
	atypical ductal hyperplasia
ADHD	attention-deficit hyperactivity disorder
ADHF	acute decompensated heart failure
ADI	acceptable daily intake
	acute diaphragmatic injury
	AIDS (acquired immunodeficiency symdrome) defining illness
	allowable (acceptable) daily intake
	axiodistoincisal
A-DIC	doxorubicin (Adriamycin) and dacarbazine
ADJ	adjusted
Adj Dis	adjustment disorder
Adj D/O	adjustment disorder
ADL	activities of daily living
ADLG	average duration of life gained
ad lib	as desired
	at liberty
ADM	abductor digiti minimi (muscle)
	acceptance of disability modified
	acellular dermal matrix
	administered (dose)
	admission
	adrenomedullin
	doxorubicin (Adriamycin)
ADMA	asymmetrical dimethyl arginine
ADME	absorption, distribution, metabolism, and excretion
ADO	axiodisto-occlusal
ADOA	autosomal-dominant optic atrophy
Ad-OAP	doxorubicin (Adriamycin), vincristine, (Oncovin) cytarabine, (Ara C) and prednisone
ADOL	adolescent
ADON	Assistant Director of Nursing
ADP	arterial demand pacing
	adenosine diphosphate
ADPC	active distance to palmar crease
ADPKD	autosomal dominant polycystic kidney disease
ADPV	anomaly of drainage of pulmonary vein
ADQ	abductor digiti quinti
	adequate
ADR	acute dystonic reaction
	adverse drug reaction
	alternative dispute resolution
	doxorubicin (Adriamycin)
ADRB2	beta-2 adrenergic receptor
ADRD	Alzheimer disease and related disorders
ADRIA	doxorubicin (Adriamycin)
ADRV	adult diarrhea rotavirus
ADS	admission day surgery
	anatomical dead space
	anonymous donor's sperm
	antibody deficiency syndrome
ADs	advance directives (living wills)
AdSD	adductor spasmodic dysphonia
ADSU	ambulatory diagnostic surgery unit
ADT	admission, discharge, and transfer
	alternate-day therapy
	androgen deprivation treatment (therapy)
	anticipate discharge tomorrow
	any damn thing (a placebo)
	Auditory Discrimination Test
ADTP	Adolescent Day Treatment Program
	Alcohol-Dependence Treatment Program
ADTR	Academy of Dance Therapists, Registered
ADU	automated dispensing unit
ADV	adenovirus vaccine, not otherwise specified
adv	adventitious sounds (wheezes and rhonchi)
ADV$_4$	adenovirus vaccine, type 4, live, oral
ADV$_7$	adenovirus vaccine, type 7, live, oral
A5D5W	alcohol 5%, dextrose 5% in water for injection
ADX	audiological diagnostic
AE	above elbow (amputation)
	accident and emergency (department)
	acute exacerbation
	adaptive equipment
	adverse event
	air entry
	androgen excess
	anoxic encephalopathy
	antiembolitic
	arm ergometer
	aryepiglottic (fold)
A&E	accident and emergency (department)
AEA	above-elbow amputation
	anti-endomysium antibody
AEB	as evidenced by
	atrial ectopic beat
AEC	absolute (blood) eosinophil count
	at earliest convenience
AECB	acute exacerbations of chronic bronchitis
AECG	ambulatory electrocardiogram
AECOPD	acute exacerbation of chronic obstructive pulmonary disease
AED	antiepileptic drug
	automated (automatic) external defibrillator
AEDD	anterior extradural defects

AEDF	absent end-diastolic flow (umbilical-artery Doppler ultrasonography)
AEDP	assisted end-diastolic pressure
	automated external defibrillator pacemaker
AEE	asthma-exacerbation episodes
AEEU	admission entrance and evaluation unit
AEFI	adverse events following immunization
AEG	air encephalogram
	Alcohol Education Group
AEIOU TIPS	mnemonic for the diagnosis of coma: **A**lcohol, **E**ncephalopathy, **I**nsulin, **O**piates, **U**remia, **T**rauma, **I**nfection, **P**sychiatric, and **S**yncope
AELBM	after each loose bowel movement
AEM	active electrode monitor
	ambulatory electrogram monitor
	antiepileptic medication
AEP	auditory evoked potential
AEq	age equivalent
AER	acoustic evoked response
	albumin excretion rate
	auditory evoked response
AERD	aspirin-exacerbated respiratory disease
Aer. M.	aerosol mask
AERS	adverse event reporting system
AERs	adverse event reports
Aer. T.	aerosol tent
AES	adult emergency service
	anti-embolic stockings
AEs	adverse events
AET	alternating esotropia
	atrial ectopic tachycardia
AF	acid-fast
	afebrile
	amniotic fluid
	anterior fontanel
	antifibrinogen
	aortofemoral
	ascitic fluid
	atrial fibrillation
AF-AFl	atrial fibrillation and atrial flutter
AFB	acid-fast bacilli
	aorto-femoral bypass
	aspirated foreign body
AFB_1	aflatoxin B_1
AFBG	aortofemoral bypass graft
AFBY	aortofemoral bypass (graft)
AFC	adult foster care
	air filled cushions
	alveolar fluid clearance
AFDC	Aid to Families with Dependent Children
AFE	amniotic fluid embolization
AFEB	afebrile
AFEU	ante partum fetal evaluation unit
AF/FL	atrial fibrillation/atrial flutter
aFGF	acidic fibroblast growth factor
AFH	adult family home
	angiomatoid fibrous histiocytoma
	anterior facial height
AFI	acute febrile illness
	amniotic fluid index
A fib	atrial fibrillation
AFIP	Armed Forces Institute of Pathology
AFKO	ankle-foot-knee orthosis
AFL	air/fluid level
	atrial flutter
AFLP	acute fatty liver of pregnancy
	amplified fragment length polymorphism
A Flu	atrial flutter
AFM	active fetal movement
	acute *Plasmodium falciparum* malaria
	aerosol face mask
	atomic force microscopy
	doxorubicin (Adriamycin), fluorouracil, and methotrexate
AFM×2	double-aerosol face mask
AFO	ankle-fixation orthotic
	ankle-foot orthosis
AFOF	anterior fontanel and open and flat
AFP	acute flaccid paralysis
	alpha-fetoprotein
	anterior faucial pillar
	ascending frontal parietal
AFQT	Armed Forces Qualification Test
AFRD	acute febrile respiratory disease
AFRIMS	Armed Forces Research Institute of Medical Sciences
AFRRI	Armed Forces Radiological Research Institute
AFRS	allergic fungal rhinosinusitis
AFS	allergic fungal sinusitis
	atomic fluorescence spectrometry
Aft/Dis	aftercare/discharge
AFTN	autonomously functioning thyroid nodule
AFV	amniotic fluid volume
AFVSS	afebrile, vital signs stable
AFX	air-fluid exchange
AFx	atypical fibroxanthoma
AG	abdominal girth
	adrenogenital
	aminoglycoside
	Amsler grid
	anaplastic glioma
	anion gap
	antigen
	antigravity
	atrial gallop

A

Ag	silver
A/G	albumin to globulin ratio
AGA	accelerated growth area acute gonococcal arthritis androgenetic alopecia antigliadin antibody appropriate for gestational age average gestational age
AGAS	accelerated graft atherosclerosis
AG/BL	aminoglycoside/beta-lactam
AGC	absolute granulocyte count advanced gastric cancer atypical glandular cells
AGCUS	atypical glandular cells of undetermined significance
AGD	agar gel diffusion
AGE	acute gastroenteritis advanced glycation end product(s) angle of greatest extension anterior gastroenterostomy arterial gas embolism
AGECAT	automatic geriatric examination for computer-assisted taxonomy
AGF	angle of greatest flexion
AGG	agammaglobulinemia
aggl.	agglutination
AGHD	adult growth hormone deficiency
AGI	alpha-glucosidase inhibitor
AGIB	acute gastrointestinal bleeding
AGL	acute granulocytic leukemia
A GLAC-TO-LK	alpha galactoside leukocytes
AGN	acute glomerulonephritis
AGNB	aerobic gram-negative bacilli
$AgNO_3$	silver nitrate
AgNORs	argyrophilic nucleolar organizer regions (staining)
α_1-AGP	alpha$_1$-acid glycoprotein
AGPT	agar-gel precipitation test
AGS	adrenogenital syndrome Alagille syndrome American Geriatric Society (guidelines)
AG SYND	adrenogenital syndrome
AGT	alanine-glyoxylate aminotransferase angiotensinogen
AGTT	abnormal glucose tolerance test
AGU	aspartylglycosaminuria
AGUS	atypical glandular cells of uncertain significance
AGV	Ahmed glaucoma valve
AGVHD	acute graft-versus-host disease
AGVI	Ahmed glaucoma valve implantation
AH	abdominal hysterectomy amenorrhea and hirsutism amenorrhea-hyperprolactinemia antihyaluronidase auditory hallucinations
A&H	accident and health (insurance)
AHA	acetohydroxamic acid (Lithostat®) acquired hemolytic anemia American Health Association (guidelines) autoimmune hemolytic anemia
AHAs	alpha hydroxy acids
AHase	antihyaluronidase
AHB_c	hepatitis B core antibody
AHC	acute hemorrhagic conjunctivitis acute hemorrhagic cystitis Adolescent Health Center alternating hemiplegia of childhood avoidable hospitalization conditions
AHCA	Agency for Healthcare Administration American Healthcare Association
AHCPR	Agency for Health Care Policy and Research
AHCs	academic health centers
AHD	alien-hand syndrome antecedent hematological disorder arteriosclerotic heart disease autoimmune hemolytic disease
AHE	acute hemorrhagic encephalomyelitis amygdalo-hippocampectomy
AHEC	Area Health Education Center
AHF	antihemophilic factor Argentine hemorrhagic fever (Junin virus) vaccine
AHF-M	antihemophilic factor (human), method M, (monoclonal purified)
AHFS	American Hospital Formulary Service
AHG	antihemophilic globulin
AHGS	acute herpetic gingival stomatitis
AHHD	arteriosclerotic hypertensive heart disease
AHI	apnea-hypopnea index
AHJ	artificial hip joint
AHL	apparent half-life
AHM	ambulatory Holter monitoring
AHMO	anterior horizontal mandibular osteotomy
AHN	adenomatous hyperplastic nodule Assistant Head Nurse
AHO	Albright hereditary osteodystrophy
AHP	acute hemorrhagic pancreatitis acute hepatic panel (see page 318) American Herbal Pharmacopeia and Therapeutic Compendium
AHPB	adjusted historic payment base
AhpF	alkyl hydroperoxide reductase, F isomer
AHR	adjusted hazard ratios airway hyperresponsiveness
AHRE	atrial high-rate event
AHRF	acute hypoxemic respiratory failure

AHS	adaptive hand skills allopurinol hypersensitivity syndrome Alpers-Huttenlocher syndrome anticonvulsant hypersensitivity syndrome
AHSA	Assistant Health Services Administrator
AHSCT	autologous hemopoietic stem-cell transplantation
AHSG	fetuin-A (alpha2-Heremans Schmid glycoprotein
AHSP	alpha hemoglobin stabilizing protein
AHST	autologous hematopoietic stem cell transplantation
AHT	alternating hypertropia autoantibodies to human thyroglobulin
AHTG	antihuman thymocyte globulin
AI	accidentally incurred accommodative insufficiency allelic imbalance American Indian allergy index aortic insufficiency apical impulse apnea index artificial insemination artificial intelligence
A & I	Allergy and Immunology (department) auscultation and inspection
AIA	Accommodation Independence Assessment allergen-induced asthma allyl isopropyl acetamide anti-insulin antibody aspirin-induced asthma
AI-Ab	anti-insulin antibody
AIBF	anterior interbody fusion
AIC	amount in controversy
AICA	anterior inferior cerebellar artery anterior inferior communicating artery
AICBG	anterior interbody cervical bone graft
AICD	activation-induced cell death automatic implantable cardioverter/defibrillator
AICM	anti-inflammatory controller medication
AICS	acute ischemic coronary syndromes
AID	absolute iron deficiency acute infectious disease aortoiliac disease artificial insemination donor automatic implantable defibrillator
AIDH	artificial insemination donor husband
AIDKS	acquired immune deficiency syndrome with Kaposi sarcoma
AIDP	acute inflammatory demyelinating polyradiculoneuropathy
AIDS	acquired immunodeficiency syndrome
AIE	acute inclusion body encephalitis
AIED	autoimmune inner-ear Disease
AIEOP	Italian Association of Pediatric Hematology and Oncology (cancer study group)
AIF	aortic-iliac-femoral
AIGHL	anterior band of the inferior glenohumeral ligament
AIH	artificial insemination with husband's sperm autoimmune hepatitis
AIHA	autoimmune hemolytic anemia
AIHD	acquired immune hemolytic disease
AIIRs	airborne infection isolation rooms
AIIS	anterior inferior iliac spine
AILD	angioimmunoblastic lymphadenopathy with dysproteinemia
AILT	angioimmunoblastic T-cell lymphoma
AIM	anti-inflammatory medication
AIMS	Abnormal Involuntary Movement Scale Arthritis Impact Measurement Scales
AIN	acute interstitial nephritis anal intraepithelial neoplasia anterior interosseous nerve
AINS	anti-inflammatory non-steroidal
AIO	all-in-one (lipid emulsion, protein, carbohydrate, and electrolytes combined total parenteral nutrition)
AIOD	aortoiliac occlusive disease
AION	anterior ischemic optic neuropathy
AIP	acute infectious polyneuritis acute intermittent porphyria acute interstitial pneumonia asymptomatic inflammatory prostatitis autoimmune pancreatitis
AIPC	androgen-independent prostate cancer
AIR	accelerated idioventricular rhythm acetylcholine-induced relaxation acute insulin response
AIRE	autoimmune regulator (gene)
AIRR	acute infusion-related reaction
AIS	Abbreviated Injury Score acute ischemic stroke adolescent idiopathic scoliosis

	anti-insulin serum
AISA	acquired idiopathic sideroblastic anemia
AIS/ISS	Abbreviated Injury Scale/ Injury Severity Score
AIT	adoptive immunotherapy
	Advanced Individual Training (Army)
	amiodarone-induced thyrotoxicosis
	auditory integration therapy
AITD	autoimmune thyroid disease
	autoimmune thyroiditis
AITN	acute interstitial tubular nephritis
AITP	autoimmune thrombocytopenia purpura
AIU	absolute iodine uptake
	adolescent inpatient unit
AIVC	absence of the inferior vena cava
AIVR	accelerated idioventricular rhythm
AJ	ankle jerk
AJCC	American Joint Committee on Cancer
AJO	apple juice only
AJR	abnormal jugular reflex
AK	above-knee (amputation)
	actinic keratosis
	artificial kidney
AKA	above-knee amputation
	alcoholic ketoacidosis
	all known allergies
	also known as
a.k.a.	also known as
AKC	acute kidney injury
	atopic keratoconjunctivitis
AKP	anterior knee pain
AKS	alcoholic Korsakoff syndrome
	arthroscopic knee surgery
AKU	artificial kidney unit
AL	acute leukemia
	argon laser
	artemether-lumefantrine (antimalarial drug combination [Riamet; Coarten])
	arterial line
	assisted living
	attachment level (dental)
	axial length
	left ear
Al	aluminum
ALA	adrenalin (epinephrine), lidocaine, and amethocaine (tetracaine)
	alpha-linolenic acid (α-linolenic acid)
	alpha-lipoic acid
	amebic liver abscess
	aminolevulinic acid (Levulan)
	antileukotriene agent
	antilymphocyte antibody
	as long as
ALAC	antibiotic-loaded acrylic cement
ALAD	abnormal left axis deviation
ALA-GLN	alanyl-glutamine
ALARA	as low as reasonably achievable
ALAT	alanine aminotransferase (also ALT; SGPT)
ALAX	apical long axis
ALB	albumin
	albuterol
	anterior lenticular bevel
ALBUMS	aldehyde linker-based ultrasensitive mismatch scanning
ALC	acute lethal catatonia
	alcohol
	alcoholic liver cirrhosis
	allogeneic lymphocyte cytotoxicity
	alternate level of care
	Alternate Lifestyle Checklist
	axiolinguocervical
ALCA	anomalous left coronary artery
ALCL	anaplastic large-cell lymphoma
ALC R	alcohol rub
ALD	adrenoleukodystrophy
	alcoholic liver disease
	aldolase
ALDH	aldehyde dehydrogenase
ALDO	aldosterone
ALDOST	aldosterone
ALF	acute liver failure
	arterial line filter
	assisted living facility
ALFT	abnormal liver function tests
ALG	antilymphoblast globulin
	antilymphocyte globulin
ALGB	adjustable laparoscopic gastric banding
ALH	atypical lobular hyperplasia
ALI	Abbott Laboratories, Inc.
	acute lung injury
	argon laser iridotomy
ALIF	anterior lumbar interbody fusion
A-line	arterial catheter
ALJ	administrative law judge
ALK	alkaline
	anaplastic lymphoma kinase
	anterior lamellar keratoplasty
	automated lamellar keratoplasy
ALK Ø	alkaline phosphatase
ALK ISO	alkaline phosphatase isoenzymes
ALK-P	alkaline phosphatase
ALK PHOS ISO	alkaline phosphatase isoenzyme
ALL	acute lymphoblastic leukemia
	acute lymphocytic leukemia
	allergy
ALLD	arthroscopic lumbar laser diskectomy
ALLO	allogeneic

Allo-BMT allogeneic bone marrow transplantation
Allo-HCT allogenic hematopoietic cell transplant
allo-SCT allogeneic stem cell transplantation
ALM acral lentiginous melanoma
alveolar lining material
autoclave-killed *Leishmania major*
ALMI anterolateral myocardial infarction
ALN anterior lower neck
anterior lymph node
axillary lymph nodes
ALND axillary lymph node dissection
ALNM axillary lymph node metastasis
ALO apraxia of eyelid opening
axiolinguo-occlusal
ALOC altered level of consciousness
$Al(OH)_3$ aluminum hydroxide
ALOS average length of stay
ALP alkaline phosphatase
argon laser photocoagulation
Alupent
Alpha1 (M) Alpha 1 microglobulin
ALPS autoimmune lymphoproliferative syndrome
ALPSA anterior labroligamentous periosteal sleeve avulsion
ALPZ alprazolam (Xanax)
ALR adductor leg raise
ALRI acute lower-respiratory-tract infection
anterolateral rotary instability
ALS acid-labile subunit
acute lateral sclerosis
advanced life support
amyotrophic lateral sclerosis
antilymphocyte serum
ALSG Australian Leukemia Study Group
ALSOB alcohol-like substance on breath
ALT alanine aminotransferase(SGPT)
antibiotic lock technique (catheter infection prevention)
argon laser trabeculoplasty
autolymphocyte therapy
2 *alt* every other day (this is a dangerous abbreviation)
ALTB acute laryngotracheobronchitis
ALTE acute (aberrant, apparent) life threatening event
ALTF anterolateral thigh flap
alt hor every other hour (this is a dangerous abbreviation)
ALTP argon laser trabeculoplasty
ALUP Alupent
ALv attachment level (dental)
ALVAD abdominal left ventricular assist device
ALWMI anterolateral wall myocardial infarct
ALZ Alzheimer disease
AM adult male
aerosol mask
amalgam
anovulatory menstruation
anterior midpapillary
morning (a.m.)
myopic astigmatism
AMA advanced maternal age
against medical advice
American Medical Association
antimitochondrial antibody
AMAC adults molested as children
AMAD activity median aerodynamic diameter
AMBI acute multiple brain infarcts
AM Care brushing teeth, washing face and hands
AMAD morning admission
AM/ADM morning admission
AMAG adrenal medullary autograft
AMAL amalgam
AMAN acute motor axonal neuropathy
AMAP American Medical Accreditation Program
as much as possible
Amask aerosol mask
AMAT anti-malignant antibody test
Arm Motor Ability Test
A-MAT amorphous material
AMAT S/E Arm Motor Ability Test for shoulder/elbow
AMAT W/H Arm Motor Ability Test for wrist/hand
AMB ambulate
ambulatory
amphotericin B (Fungizone)
as manifested by
AMBDs autoimmune mucocutaneous blistering diseases
AMBER advanced multiple beam equalization radiography
Ambu artificial-respiration device consisting of a bag that is squeezed by hand
AMC arm muscle circumference
arthrogryposis multiplex congenita
AM/CR amylase to creatinine ratio
AMD age-related macular degeneration
arthroscopic microdiskectomy
axiomesiodistal
dactinomycin (actinomycin D; Cosmegen)
methyldopa (alpha methyldopa)
AMDR acceptable macronutrient distribution range

AME	agreed medical examination
	anthrax meningoencephalitis
	apparent mineralocorticoid excess (syndrome)
	Aviation Medical Examiner
AMegL	acute megokaryoblastic leukemia
AMES-LAN	American sign language
AMF	aerobic metabolism facilitator
	amifostine (Ethyol)
	amonafide
	autocrine motility factor
AMG	acoustic myography
	aminoglycoside
	axiomesiogingival
	Federal Republic of Germany's equivalent to United States Food, Drug, and Cosmetic Act
AMGA	American Medical Group Association
AMI	acute myocardial infarction
	amifostine (Ethyol)
	amitriptyline
	axiomesioincisal
AMKL	acute megakaryocytic leukemia
AML	acute myelogenous leukemia
	angiomyolipoma
	anterior mitral leaflet
AMLOS	arithmetic mean length of stay
AMLR	auditory midlatency response
	Marketing Authorization Application (French)
AMM	agnogenic myeloid metaplasia
AMML	acute myelomonocytic leukemia
AMMOL	acute myelomonoblastic leukemia
AMN	adrenomyeloneuropathy
amnio	amniocentesis
AMN SC	amniotic fluid scan
AMOL	acute monoblastic leukemia
AMOVA	analysis of molecular variance
AMP	adenosine monophosphate
	ampere
	ampicillin
	ampul
	amputation
	antipressure mattress
AMPLE	allergies, medications, past medical history, last meal, events leading to admission (used for history and physical examination)
AMPPE	acute multifocal placoid pigment epitheliopathy
A-M pr	Austin-Moore prosthesis
AMPS	Assessment of Motor and Process Skills
AMPT	metyrosine (alphamethylpara tyrosine)
AMR	acoustic muscle reflex
	alternating motion rates
	amrubicin
AMRI	anterior medial rotary instability
AMS	accelerator mass spectrometry
	acute maxillary sinusitis
	acute mountain sickness
	aggravated in military service
	altered mental status
	amylase
	aseptic meningitis syndrome
	atypical mole syndrome
	auditory memory span
m-AMSA	amsacrine (acridinyl anisidide)
AMSAN	acute motor sensory axonal neuropathy
AMSIT	portion of the mental status examination: A—appearance, M—mood, S—sensorium, I—intelligence, T—thought process
AMT	abbreviated mental test
	Adolph's Meat Tenderizer
	allogeneic (bone) marrow transplant
	alpha-methyltryptamine
	aminopterin
	amniotic membrane transplantation
	amount
AMTS	Abbreviated Mental Test Score
AMU	accessory-muscle use
AMV	alveolar minute ventilation
	assisted mechanical ventilation
AMY	amylase
AMY/CR	amylase/creatinine ratio
AN	acoustic neuromas
	Alaska Native
	amyl nitrate
	anorexia nervosa
	anticipatory nausea
	Associate Nurse
	avascular necrosis
ANA	American Nurses Association
	antinuclear antibody
ANAD	anorexia nervosa and associated disorders
ANADA	Abbreviated New Animal Drug Application
ANAG	acute narrow angle glaucoma
ANA SWAB	anaerobic swab
ANC	absolute neutrophil count
	antenatal care
ANCA	antineutrophil cytoplasmic antibody
anch	anchored
ANCN	absolute neutrophil count nadir
ANCOVA	analysis of covariance
AND	allow natural death

	anterior nasal discharge
	Associate's Degree in Nursing
	axillary node dissection
ANDA	Abbreviated New Drug Application
anes	anesthesia
ANF	antinuclear factor
	atrial natriuretic factor
ANG	angiogram
	angiotensin
ANG II	angiotensin II
ANGIO	angiogram
ANH	acute normovolemic hemodilution
	artificial nutrition and hydration
	assisted nutrition and hydration
ANISO	anisocytosis
ANK	ankle
	appointment not kept
ANL	acceptable noise level
ANLL	acute nonlymphoblastic leukemia
ANM	Assistant Nurse Manager
ANMAT	Argentina Regulatory Agency
ANN	artificial neural network(s)
	axillary node-negative
ANNA	artificial neural network analysis
ANOVA	analysis of variance
ANP	Adult Nurse Practitioner
	atrial natriuretic peptide (anaritide acetate)
	axillary node–positive
ANPR	advanced notice of proposed rule making
ANS	answer
	autonomic nervous system
ANSER	Aggregate Neurobehavioral Student Health and Education Review
ANSI	American National Standards Institute
ANT	anterior
	anthrax vaccine, not otherwise specified
	enpheptin (2-amino-5-nitrothiazol)
ANT_a	anthrax vaccine, absorbed
ante	before
ANTI A:AGT	anti–blood group A antiglobulin test
Anti bx	antibiotic
anti-D	anti-D immune globulin
anti-GAD	antibodies to glutamic acid decarboxylase
anti-HBc	antibody to hepatitis B core antigen (HBcAg)
anti-HBe	antibody to hepatitis B e antigen (HBeAg)
anti-HBs	antibody to hepatitis B surface antigen (HBsAg)
anti-Sm	anti-*Schistosoma mansoni* (antibody)
ant sag D	anterior sagittal diameter
ANTU	alpha naphthylthiourea
ANUG	acute necrotizing ulcerative gingivitis
ANV	acute nausea and vomiting
ANVISA	National Health Surveillance Agency (Brazil)
ANX	anxiety
	anxious
ANZDATA	Australia and New Zealand Dialysis and Transplant Registry
AO	abdominal obesity
	acridine orange (stain)
	Agent Orange
	Alveolar osteitis (also known as dry socket)
	anaplastic oligodendrogliomas
	anterior oblique
	aorta
	aortic opening
	aortography
	axio-occlusal
	plate, screw (orthopedics)
	right ear
A-O	atlanto-occipital (joint)
A/O	alert and oriented
A & O	alert and oriented
A&O × 3	awake and oriented to person, place, and time
A&O × 4	awake and oriented to person, place, time, and object
AOA	anaplastic oligoastrocytoma
AOAA	aminooxoacetic acid
AOAP	as often as possible
AOAs	adult offspring of alcoholics
AOB	alcohol on breath
AOBC	aortic occlusion balloon catheter
AOBS	acute organic brain syndrome
AOC	abridged ocular chart
	advanced ovarian cancer
	amoxicillin, omeprazole, and clarithromycin
	anode opening contraction
	antacid of choice
	area of concern
AOCD	anemia of chronic disease
AOCL	anodal opening clonus
AOCN	Advanced Oncology Certified Nurse
AOD	adult-onset diabetes
	alcohol and (and/or) other drugs
	alleged onset date
	anaplastic oligodendroglioma
	arterial occlusive disease
	Assistant-Officer-of-the-Day
AODA	alcohol and other drug abuse
AODM	adult-onset diabetes mellitus
AOE	acute otitis externa
A of 1	assistance of one
A of 2	assistance of two

AOFAS American Orthopaedic Foot and Ankle Society (clinical rating scale)
AOI apnea of infancy
area of induration
ao-il aorta-iliac
AOIVM angiographically occult intracranial vascular malformation
AOL augmentation of labor
AOLC acridine-orange leukocyte cytospin
AOLD automated open lumbar diskectomy
AOM acute otitis media
alternatives of management
AONAD alert, oriented, and no acute distress
AOO anodal opening odor
continuous arterial asynchronous pacing
AOP anemia of prematurity
anodal opening picture
aortic pressure
apnea of prematurity
AOR adjusted odds ratio
Alvarado Orthopedic Research
at own risk
auditory oculogyric reflex
AORC arthritis and other rheumatic conditions
AORT REGURG aortic regurgitation
AORT STEN aortic stenosis
AOS ambulatory outpatient surgery
anode opening sound
antibiotic order sheet
aortic ostial stenoses
arrived on scene
AOSC acute obstructive suppurative cholangiotomy
AOSD adult-onset Still disease
AOTB alcohol on the breath
AOTe anodal opening tetanus
AP abdominal pain
abdominoperineal
acute pancreatitis
aerosol pentamidine
alkaline phosphatase
angina pectoris
antepartum
anterior-posterior (x-ray)
aortopulmonary
apical periodontitis
apical pulse
appendectomy
appendicitis
arterial pressure
arthritis panel (see page 318)
atrial pacing
attending physician
doxorubicin (Adriamycin); cisplatin (Platinol)
A&P active and present
anterior and posterior
assessment and plans
auscultation and percussion
A/P accounts payable
ascites/plasma ratio
$A_2 > P_2$ second aortic sound greater than second pulmonic sound
APA aldosterone-producing adenoma
American Psychiatric Association
anticipatory postural adjustment
antiphospholipid antibody
APAA anterior parietal artery aneurysm
APAC acute primary angle closure
APACHE Acute Physiology and Chronic Health Evaluation
APAD anterior-posterior abdominal diameter
APAG antipseudomonal aminoglycosidic
APAP acetaminophen (N acetylpara-aminophenol; Tylenol; paracetamol)
APB abductor pollicis brevis
atrial premature beat
APBI accelerated partial breast irradiation
APBSCT autologous peripheral blood stem cell transplantation
APC absolute phagocyte count
activated protein C
acute pharyngoconjunctiivitis (fever)
adenoidal-pharyngeal-conjunctival
adenomatous polyposis of the colon and rectum
advanced pancreatic cancer
Advance Practice Clinician
advanced prostate cancer
Ambulatory Payment Classification
annual percentage change
antigen-presenting cell
argon plasma coagulator
aspirin, phenacetin, and caffeine (no longer marketed in the US)
asymptomatic prostate cancer
atrial premature contraction
autologous packed cells
APCD adult polycystic disease
APCE affinity probe capillary electrophoresis
APCIs atrial peptide clearance inhibitors
APCKD adult polycystic kidney disease
AP-CT abdominal and pelvic computer tomography
APD acid peptic disease
action potential duration
afferent pupillary defect
anterior-posterior diameter

atrial premature depolarization
automated peritoneal dialysis
pamidronate disodium (aminohydroxypropylidene diphosphate)

APDC Anxiety and Panic Disorder Clinic

AP-DRGs all-patient diagnosis-related groups

APDT acellular pertussis vaccine with diphtheria and tetanus toxoids

APE absolute prediction error
acute psychotic episode
acute pulmonary edema
anterior pituitary extract
doxorubicin (Adriamycin), cisplatin (Platinol-AQ), and etoposide

APECED autoimmune polyendocrinopathy-candidiasis ectodermal dystrophy

APER abdominoperineal excision of the rectum

APG ambulatory patient group
Apgar (score)

Apgar appearance (color), pulse (heart rate), grimace (reflex irritability), activity (muscle tone), and respiration (score reflecting condition of newborn)

APH adult psychiatric hospital
alcohol-positive history
antepartum hemorrhage

APhA American Pharmacists Association

APHIS Animal and Plant Health Inspection Service

API active pharmaceutical ingredients
Asian-Pacific Islander

APIS Acute Pain Intensity Scale

APIVR artificial pacemaker-induced ventricular rhythm

APKD adult polycystic kidney disease
adult-onset polycystic kidney disease

APL abductor pollicis longus
accelerated painless labor
acute promyelocytic leukemia
anterior pituitary-like (hormone) chorionic gonadotropin

AP & L anteroposterior and lateral

APLA antiphospholipid antibody

APLD automated percutaneous lumbar diskectomy

APLS antiphospholipid syndrome

APME acute postinfectious measles encephalitis

APMPPE acute posterior multifocal placoid pigment epitheliopathy

APMS acute pain management service

APN acquired pendular nystagmus
acute panautonomic neuropathy
acute pyelonephritis
Advanced Practice Nurse

APO adverse patient occurrence
apolipoprotein A-1
doxorubicin (Adriamycin), prednisone, and vincristine (Oncovin)

APO(a) apolipoprotein (A)

APOE apolipoprotein E

APOE-4 apolipoprotein-E (gene)

APOLT auxiliary partial orthotopic liver transplantation

APOPPS adjustable postoperative protective prosthetic socket

APP alternating pressure pad
amyloid precursor protein
appetite

APPG aqueous procaine penicillin G (dangerous terminology; since it is for intramuscular use only; write as penicillin G procaine)

APPLA another planned permanent living arrangement

appr. approximate

appt. appointment

APPY appendectomy

APR abdominoperineal resection
acute radiation proctitis
average payment rate

AP & R apical and radial (pulses)

APR-DRGs all-patient refined diagnosis-related groups

APRT abdominopelvic radiotherapy

APRV airway pressure release ventilation

APS acute pain service
Acute Physiology Scoring (system)
adult protective services
Adult Psychiatric Service
antiphospholipid syndrome

APSAC anistreplase (anisoylated plasminogen streptokinase activator complex)

APSD Alzheimer presenile dementia

APSP assisted peak systolic pressure

APSS Associated Professional Sleep Societies

aPTT activated partial thromboplastin time

APU ambulatory procedure unit
antepartum unit

APUD amine precursor uptake and decarboxylation

APV amprenavir (Agenerase)

APVC partial anomalous pulmonary venous connection

APVR aortic pulmonary valve replacement

APVT advanced portal vein thrombosis

APW aortopulmonary window

AQ amodiaquine

aq water

AQ accomplishment quotient

A

aq dest distilled water
AQLQ-J Asthma Quality of Life Questionnaire—Juniper
AQLQ-M Asthma Quality of Life Questionnaire—Marks
AQOL acne quality of life
AQR ain't quite right (slang)
A quad atrial quadrageminy
AR Achilles reflex
acoustic reflex
active resistance
airway resistance
alcohol related
allergic rhinitis
androgen receptor
ankle reflex
aortic regurgitation
apoptotic rate
Argyll Robertson (pupil)
assisted respiration
at risk
aural rehabilitation
autorefractor
Ar argon
A&R adenoidectomy with radium
advised and released
A-R apical-radial (pulses)
A/R accounts receivable
ARA Action Research Arm (test)
adenosine regulating agent
Ara arabinose
ara-A vidarabine (Vira-A)
ara-AC fazarabine
ara-C cytarabine (Cytosar-U)
ARAD abnormal right axis deviation
ARAS ascending reticular activating system
atherosclerotic renal-artery stenosis
ARB angiotensin II receptor blocker
antibiotic-resistant bacteria
any reliable brand
ARBOR arthropod-borne virus
ARBOW artificial rupture of bag of water
ARC abnormal retinal correspondence
adult residential care
AIDS-related complex
Alcohol Rehabilitation Center
anomalous retinal correspondence
American Red Cross
autologous red cells
ARCBS American Red Cross Blood Services
ARD acute respiratory disease
adult respiratory distress
antibiotic removal device
antibiotic retrieval device
aphakic retinal detachment
ARDMS American Registry of Diagnostic Medical Sonographers
ARDS adult respiratory distress syndrome
ARE active-resistive exercises
ARF acute renal failure
acute respiratory failure
acute rheumatic fever
amylase-rich food (flour)
ARFF at risk for falling
ARG alkaline reflux gastritis
arginine
ARGNB antibiotic-resistant gram-negative bacilli
ARH autosomal recessive hypercholesterolemia
ARHL age-related hearing loss
ARHNC advanced resected head and neck cancer
ARI acute renal insufficiency
acute respiratory infection
acute respiratory illness
aldose reductase inhibitor
arousal index
ARIF arthroscopic reduction and internal fixation
ARIMA autoregressive integrated moving average (model)
ARJP autosomal recessive juvenile parkinsonism
ARL acquired immunodeficiency syndrome (AIDS)-related lymphoma
average remaining lifetime
ARLD alcohol-related liver disease
ARM anxiety reaction, mild
artificial rupture of membranes
ARMD age-related macular degeneration
ARMS alveolar rhabdomyosarcoma
amplification refractory mutation system
ARN acute retinal necrosis
ARND alcohol-related neurodevelopmental disorder
ARNP Advanced Registered Nurse Practitioner
AROM active range of motion
artifical rupture of membranes
ARP absolute refractory period
acute radiation proctitis
alcohol rehabilitation program
asparagine-rich protein
ARPE amylase-rich pleural effusion
ARPF anterior release posterior fusion
ARPKS autosomal recessive polycystic kidney disease
ARPN Advanced Practice Registered Nurse
ARPT acid reflux provocation test
ARR absolute risk reduction
anterior rectal resection
arrive

aRR	adjusted rate ratio
ARROM	active resistive range of motion
ARRT	American Registry of Radiologic Technologists
ARS	acute radiation sickness
	antirabies serum
ART	Accredited Record Technician (for newer title, see RHIT)
	Achilles (tendon) reflex test
	acoustic reflex threshold(s)
	anesthesia release time (patient-on-table until release for surgical preparation)
	antiretroviral therapy
	arterial
	assessment, review, and treatment
	assisted reproductive technology
	automated reagin test (for syphilis)
ARTIC	articulation
Art T	art therapy
ARU	acute receiving unit
	alcohol rehabilitation unit
ARV	AIDS-related virus
	antiretroviral
ARVC	arrhythmogenic right ventricular cardiomyopathy
ARVD	arrhythmogenic right ventricular dysplasia
	atherosclerotic renovascular disease
ARVMB	anomalous right ventricular muscle bundles
ARVs	antiretroviral drugs
ARW	Accredited Rehabilitation Worker
ARWY	airway
AS	activated sleep
	alpha-synuclein
	American Samoa
	anabolic steroid
	anal sphincter
	androgen suppression
	Angelman syndromes
	ankylosing spondylitis
	anterior synechia
	anxiety sensitivity
	aortic stenosis
	artesunate (an antimalarial agent)
	Asperger syndrome
	atherosclerosis
	atropine sulfate
	AutoSuture®
	doctor called through answering service
	left ear
ASA	American Society of Anesthesiologists
	American Statistical Association
	angiosarcoma
	argininosuccinate
	aspirin (acetylsalicylic acid)
	as soon as
	atrial septal aneurysm
ASA I	**American Society of anesthesiologists' classification** Healthy patient with localized pathological process
ASA II	A patient with mild to moderate systemic disease
ASA III	A patient with severe systemic disease limiting activity but not incapacitating
ASA IV	A patient with incapacitating systemic disease
ASA V	Moribund patient not expected to live.
	(These are American Society of Anesthesiologists' patient classifications. Emergency operations are designated by "E" after the classification.)
5-ASA	mesalamine (5-aminosalicylic acid; Asacol; Rowasa) (this is a dangerous abbreviation as it is mistaken for five aspirin tablets)
ASAA	acquired severe aplastic anemia
ASACL	American Society of Anesthesiologists Classification (see ASA I)
ASAD	arthroscopic subacromial decompression
aSAH	aneurysmal subarachnoid hemorrhage
AS/AI	aortic stenosis/aortic insufficiency
ASAM PPC-2	Patient Placement Criteria published by the American Society of Addiction Medicine, Second Edition
ASAP	Alcohol and Substance Abuse Program
	as soon as possible
ASAT	aspartate aminotransferase (also AST; SGOT)
ASB	anesthesia standby
	anterior skull base
	asymptomatic bacteriuria
ASBO	adhesive small-bowel obstruction
ASBS	American Society of Bariatric Surgery
ASBs	artificially sweetened beverages
A's & B's	apnea and bradycardia
ASC	active symptom control
	altered state of consciousness
	ambulatory surgery (surgical) center
	anterior subcapsular cataract
	antimony sulfur colloid
	apocrine skin carcinoma
	ascorbic acid (vitamin C)
ASCA	antisaccharomyces cerevisiae

A

ASCAD atherosclerotic coronary artery disease
ASCCC advanced squamous cell cervical carcinoma
ASCCHN advanced squamous cell carcinoma of the head and neck
ASCI acute spinal cord injury
ASCO American Society of Clinical Oncology
ASCR autologous stem cell rescue
ASCS autologous stem cell support
ASCT allogeneic stem cell transplantation
autologous stem cell transplantation
ASCUS atypical squamous cell of undetermined significance
ASCVD arteriosclerotic cardiovascular disease
ASCVR arteriosclerotic cardiovascular renal disease
ASD acute stress disorder
adjacent segment disease
air-space disease
aldosterone secretion defect
androstenedione
annual summary dose (ionizing radiation)
atrial septal defect
autism spectrum disorder(s)
ASD I atrial septal defect, primum
ASD II atrial septal defect, secundum
ASDA American Sleep Disorders Association (criteria)
ASDH acute subdural hematoma
ASDPs antisocial personality disorders
ASE abstinence symptom evaluation
acute stress erosion
ASEX Arizona Sexual Experiences (sexual dysfunction scale)
ASF anterior spinal fusion
asymmetric screen film (radiology)
auditory spatial facilitation
ASFA Adoption and Safe Families Act
ASFR age-specific fertility rate
ASG atrial septal graft
ASH American Society of Hematology (guidelines)
asymmetric septal hypertrophy
AsH hypermetropic astigmatism
ASHD arteriosclerotic heart disease
ASI active specific immunotherapy
Addiction Severity Index
Anxiety Status Inventory
Arterial Stiffness Index
aSi amorphous silicon
ASIA **American Spinal Injury Association (Score)**
A-Complete—No preservation of any motor and/or sensory function below the zone of injury
B-Incomplete—Preserved sensation
C-Incomplete—Preserved motor (nonfunctional)
D-Incomplete—Preserved motor (functional)
E-Complete Recovery
ASIH absent, sick in hospital
ASIMC absent, sick in medical center
ASIS anterior superior iliac spine
ASK antistreptokinase
ASKase antistreptokinase
ASL American Sign Language
antistreptolysin (titer)
ASLO antistreptolysin-O
ASLV avian sarcoma and leukosis virus (Rous virus)
AsM myopic astigmatism
ASMA antismooth-muscle antibody
ASMI anteroseptal myocardial infarction
ASN Associate's of Science in Nursing
ASO accessory sinus ostia
administrative services only (contract)
AIDS (acquired immunodeficiency syndrome) service organization(s)
aldicarb sulfoxide
allele-specific oligodeoxy-nucleotide (probes)
Amplatzer Septal Occluder
antisense oligonucleotides
antistreptolysin-O titer
arterial switch operation
arteriosclerosis obliterans
automatic stop order
As_2O_3 arsenic trioxide (Trisenox)
ASOT antistreptolysin-O titer
ASOTP Affiliate Sex Offender Treatment Provider
ASP acute suppurative parotitis
acute symmetric polyarthritis
antisocial personality
application service provider
asparaginase
aspartic acid
ASPDV anterior superior pancreaticoduodenal vein
ASPVD arteriosclerotic peripheral vascular disease
ASR aldosterone secretion rate
articular surface replacement
automatic speech recognition
ASRA Alcohol Severity Rating Scale
ASRM American Society for Reproductive Medicine (Infertility with endometriosis score/staging)

A

ASS anterior superior supine
aspirin (some European countries)
assessment

ASST autologous serum skin test

asst assistant

AST allergy skin test
androgen suppression therapy
Aphasia Screening Test
aspartate aminotransferase (same as SGOT)
astemizole (Hismanal)
astigmatism

AstdVe assisted ventilation

ASTH asthenopia

ASTI acute soft tissue injury

AS TOL as tolerated

ASTIG astigmatism

ASTM American Society for Testing and Materials

ASTRO American Society for Therapeutic Radiation and Oncology
astrocytoma

ASTZ antistreptozyme test

ASU acute stroke unit
ambulatory surgical unit

ASV antisnake venom

ASVD arteriosclerotic vessel disease

ASYM asymmetric(al)

ASX asymptomatic

AT abdominothoracic
activity therapy (therapist)
Addiction Therapist
anaerobic threshold
antithrombin
applanation tonometry
ataxia-telangiectasia
atraumatic
atrial tachycardia

AT1 angiotensin II type 1

AT 10 dihydrotachysterol (Hytakerol; DHT®)

ATA atmosphere absolute
authority to administer

ATB antibiotic
aquatic therapy bar
atypical tuberculosis

ATBF African tick-bite fever

ATC acute toxic class
aerosol treatment chamber
alcoholism therapy classes
all-terrain cycle
antituberculous chemoprophylaxis
around-the-clock
Arthritis Treatment Center
Athletic Trainer, Certified

ATCC American Type Culture Collection

ATCCS acute traumatic central cord syndrome

ATD antithyroid drug(s)
anticipated time of discharge
aqueous tear deficiency
asphyxiating thoracic dystrophy
autoimmune thyroid disease

ATE adipose tissue extraction

AT-EI assistive technology and environmental interventions

ATEM analytical transmission electron microscopy

ATEs arterial thromboembolic events

ATF Alcohol, Tobacco, and Firearms (Bureau)

At Fib atrial fibrillation

ATFL anterior talofibular ligament

AT III FUN antithrombin III functional

ATG antithymocyte globulin

ATHR angina threshold heart rate

ATI Abdominal Trauma Index
acute traumatic ischemia

ATL Achilles tendon lengthening
adult T-cell leukemia
anterior temporal lobectomy
anterior tricuspid leaflet
antitension line
atypical lymphocytes

ATLL adult T-cell leukemia/lymphoma

ATLP anterior thoracolumbar locking (implant) plate

ATLS acute tumor lysis syndrome
advanced trauma life support

ATM acute transverse myelitis
ataxia telangiectasia mutated (gene)
atmosphere

At ma atrial milliamp

ATN acute tubular necrosis

ATNC atraumatic normocephalic

aTNM autopsy staging of cancer

ATNR asymmetrical tonic neck reflex

ATO arsenic trioxide (Trisenox)

ATOD-C Alcohol, Tobacco and Drugs, Certified

ATP according-to-protocol
addiction treatment program
adenosine triphosphate
anterior tonsillar pillar
antitachycardia pacing
autoimmune thrombocytopenia purpura

ATP III Adult Treatment Panel III

ATPase adenosine triphosphatase

ATPS ambient temperature & pressure, saturated with water vapor

ATR Achilles tendon reflex
atracurium (Tracrium)
atrial
atropine

A

ATRA	all-*trans* retinoic acid (tretinoin-Vesanoid)
atr fib	atrial fibrillation
ATRO	atropine
ATRX	acute transfusion reaction
ATSDR	Agency for Toxic Substances and Disease Registry
ATU	alcohol treatment unit
ATUE	abbreviated therapeutic use exemption
ATV	all-terrain vehicle
ATS	American Thoracic Society (guidelines) antimony trisulfide antitetanic serum (tetanus antitoxin) anxiety tension state
ATSO	admit to (the) service of
ATSO4	atropine sulfate
ATSP	asked to see patient
ATT	alternating triple therapy antitetanus toxoid arginine tolerance test
ATTN	attention
ATTR	amyloid transtyretin
at. wt	atomic weight
ATX	atelectasis
ATZ	anal transitional zone
AU	allergenic (allergy) units arbitrary units both ears (this is a dangerous abbreviation, as it may be seen as OU [both eyes])
Au	gold
A/U	at umbilicus
^{198}Au	radioactive gold
AUA score	American Urological Association—pertains to benign prostatic hypertrophy symptoms
AUB	abnormal uterine bleeding
AuBMT	autologous bone marrow transplant
AUC	analytical ultracentrifugation area under the curve
AUC_t	area under the curve to last time point
AUD	amplifiable units of DNA (deoxyribonucleic acid) arthritis of unknown diagnosis auditory
AUD COMP	auditory comprehension
AUDIT	Alcohol Use Disorders Identification Test
AUG	acute ulcerative gingivitis
AUGIB	acute upper gastrointestinal bleeding
AUIC	area under the inhibitory curve
AUL	acute undifferentiated leukemia
AUR	acute urinary retention
AUS	acute urethral syndrome artificial urinary sphincter auscultation
AuSCT	autologous stem cell transplantation
AutD	autistic disorder
AUTO	autologous
AUTO SP	automatic speech
AV	anteverted anticipatory vomiting arteriovenous atrioventricular auditory visual auriculoventricular
A:V	arterial-venous (ratio in fundi)
AVA	anthrax vaccine, adsorbed aortic valve area aortic valve atresia arteriovenous anastomosis
AVB	atrioventricular block Aventis Behring
AVC	acrylic veneer crown aortic valve classification atrioventricular conduction
AVD	aortic valve disease apparent volume of distribution arteriosclerotic vascular disease atrioventricular delay cerebrovascular accident (French, Spanish)
AVDP	asparaginase, vincristine, daunorubicin, and prednisone avoirdupois
$AVDO_2$	arteriovenous oxygen difference
AVE	aortic valve echocardiogram atrioventricular extrasystole
AVED	ataxia with isolated vitamin E deficiency
AVF	arteriovenous fistula augmented unipolar foot (left leg)
avg	average
AVGS	autologous vein graft stent
AVGs	ambulatory visit groups
AVH	acute viral hepatitis
AVHB	atrioventricular heart block
AVHs	auditory verbal hallucinations
AVJA	atrioventricular junction ablation
AVJR	atrioventricular junctional rhythm
AVL	American visceral leishmaniasis augmented unipolar left (left arm)
AVLT	auditory verbal learning test
AVM	arteriovenous malformation
AVN	arteriovenous nicking atrioventricular node avascular necrosis
AVNB	atrioventricular nodal block
AVNR	atrioventricular nodal re-entry
AVNRT	atrioventricular node recovery time

	atrioventricular nodal re-entry tachycardia
A-VO_2	arteriovenous oxygen difference
AVOC	avocation
AVP	arginine vasopressin
	Aventis Pasteur
AVPU	alert, (responds to) verbal (stimuli), (responds to) painful (stimuli), unresponsive (mnemonic used by EMTs to judge patients' level of consciousness)
AVR	aortic valve replacement
	augmented unipolar right (right arm)
AVRP	atrioventricular refractory period
AVRT	atrioventricular reciprocating tachycardia
AVS	aortic valve sclerosis
	atriovenous shunt
AVSD	atrioventricular septal defect
AVSS	afebrile, vital signs stable
AVT	atrioventricular tachycardia
	atypical ventricular tachycardia
AvWS	acquired von Willebrand syndrome
AW	abdominal wall
	abnormal wave
	airway
A/W	able to work
A&W	alive and well
AWA	alcohol withdrawal assessment
	as well as
A waves	atrial contraction wave
AWB	autologous whole blood
AWD	alcohol withdrawal delirium
	alive with disease
AWDW	assault with a deadly weapon
AWE	acetowhite epithelium
AWI	anterior wall infarct
AWMI	anterior wall myocardial infarction
AWO	airway obstruction
AWOL	absent without leave
AWP	airway pressure
	average wholesale price
AWRU	active wrist rotation unit
AWS	alcohol withdrawal seizures (syndrome)
AWSA	Alcohol Withdrawal Severity Assessment (scale)
AWU	alcohol withdrawal unit
ax	axillary
AXB	axillary block
AXC	aortic cross clamp
ax-fem.fem.	axilla-femoral-femoral (graft)
AXFR	axillofemoral reconstruction
AXND	axillary node dissection
AXR	abdomen x-ray
AxSYM®	immunodiagnostic testing equipment
AXT	alternating exotropia
AY	acrocyanotic (infant color)
AZA	azathioprine (Imuran)
5 AZA-CdR	5-Aza-2′-deoxycitidine (decitabine; Dacogen)
5-AZC	azacitidine (Vidaza)
AzdU	azidouridine
AZE	azelastine hydrochloride (Astelin)
AZM	acquisition zoom magnification
	azithromycin (Zithromaz; Z-Pak)
AZOOR	acute zonal occult outer retinopathy
AZQ	diaziquone
AZT	zidovudine (azidothymidine; Retrovir)
A-Z test	Aschheim-Zondek test (diagnostic test for pregnancy)

B

B	bacillus
	bands
	bilateral
	black
	bloody
	bolus
	both
	botulism (Vaccine B is botulism toxoid)
	brother
	buccal
	See "Plan B"
Ⓑ	both
B+	blood type B positive (B positive is preferred)
B−	blood type B negative (B negative is preferred)
B_1	thiamine HCl
B I	Billroth I (gastric surgery)
B II	Billroth II (gastric surgery)
B_2	riboflavin
B_3	nicotinic acid
b/4	before
B_5	pantothenic acid
B_6	pyridoxine HCl
B_7	biotin
B_8	adenosine phosphate
B_9	benign
B_{12}	cyanocobalamin
B19	parvovirus B19
B52	combined 5 mg of lorazepam (Haldol) IV and 2 mg of haloperidol (Ativan) IV (slang)
BA	backache
	Baker Act (Florida mental health act enabling involuntary commitment)
	Baptist
	benzyl alcohol
	bile acid
	biliary atresia
	bioavailability
	blood agar
	blood alcohol
	Boehler angel
	bone age
	Bourns assist
	branchial artery
	broken appointment
	bronchial asthma
	buccoaxial
	butyric acid
Ba	barium
B > A	bone greater than air
B < A	bone less than air
B & A	brisk and active
BAA	beta-adrenergic agonist
BAAM	Beck airway airflow monitor
Bab	Babinski
BAC	Bacterial Artficial Chromosome
	benzalkonium chloride
	blood-alcohol concentration
	bronchioloalveolar carcinoma
	buccoaxiocervical
BACCA	basal cell cancer
BACE	beta-site APP (amyloid precursor protein)-cleaving enzyme
BACI	bovine anti-cryptosporidium immunoglobulin
BACM	blocking agent corticosteroid myopathy
BACON	bleomycin, doxorubicin, lomustine, vincristine, and mechlorethamine
BACOP	bleomycin, doxorubicin (Adriamycin), cyclophosphamide, vincristine, and prednisone
BACPAC	Bulk Activities Post Approval Change
BACs	bacterial artificial chromosomes
BACT	bacteria
	base-activated clotting time
BAD	Benadryl, Ativan, and Decadron
	bipolar affective disorder
	blunt aortic disruption
BADL	basic activities of daily living
BADLS	Bristol Activities of Daily Living Scale
BaE	barium enema
BAE	bronchial artery embolization
BAEDP	balloon aortic end diastolic pressure
BAEP	brain stem auditory evoked potential
BAERs	brain stem auditory evoked responses
BaEV	baboon endogenous virus
BAG	buccoaxiogingival
BAHA	bone-anchored hearing aids
BAI	blunt abdominal injury
	breath-actuated inhalers
	Brief Assessment Interview
BAIQ	below average intelligence quotient
BAK cage	an interbody fusion system used to stabilize the spine
BAL	balance
	blood-alcohol level
	British antilewisite (dimercaprol)
	bronchoalveolar lavage
BALB	binaural alternate loudness balance
BALF	bronchoalveolar lavage fluid
B-ALL	B cell acute lymphoblastic leukemia
BALP	baseline bone alkaline phosphatase

BALT	bronchus-associated lymphoid tissue
BAM	bony acetabular morphology
	Brain Acoustic Monitor
BaM	barium meal
BAMS	bioaerosol mass spectrometry
BAN	British Approved Name
Banana Bag	a yellow colored intravenous infusion containing a multivitamin product, folic acid, thiamine hydrochloride, and possibly magnesium sulfate in 5% dextrose or 0.9% sodium chloride. Contents can vary. Used for alcoholic patients. (slang)
BAND	band neutrophil (stab)
BANS	back, arm, neck and scalp
BAO	basal acid output
BAoV	bicuspid aortic valve
BAP	blood agar plate
BAPS	balance activation proprioceptive system
	biomechanical ankle platform system
BAPT	Baptist
baPWV	brachial-ankle pulse wave velocity
BAR	biofragmentable anastomotic ring
Barb	barbiturate
BARN	bilateral acute retinal necrosis
BAR Troche	Benadryl, Ativan, and Reglan troche
BAS	balloon atrial septostomy
	Barnes Akathisia Scale
	behavioral activation system
	bile acid sequestrants
	boric acid solution
	bronchial asthma (in) status
BaS	barium swallow
BASA	baby aspirin (81 mg chewable tablets of aspirin)
BASC	Behavior Assessment System for Children
BASIS	Basic Achievement Skills Individual Screener
BASK	basket cells
BASMI	Bath Ankylosing Spondylitis Metrology Index
baso.	basophil
BASO STIP	basophilic stippling
BAT	Behavioral Avoidance Test
	best available therapy
	blunt abdominal trauma
	borreliacidal-antibody test
	brightness acuity tester
BATF	Bureau of Alcohol, Tobacco and Firearms
BATO	boronic acid adduct of technetium oxime
batt	battery
BAVP	balloon aortic valvuloplasty
BAU	bioequivalent allergy units
BAV	bicuspid aortic valve
BAW	bronchoalveolar washing
BB	baby boy
	backboard
	back to back
	bad breath
	bed bath
	bed board
	beta-blocker
	blanket bath
	blood bank
	blow bottle
	blue bloaters
	body belts
	both bones
	breakthrough bleeding
	breast biopsy
	bronchial brushing
	brush biopsy
	buffer base
B&B	bismuth and bourbon
	bowel and bladder
B/B	backward bending
BBA	born before arrival
BBAS	blade and balloon atrial septostomy
BBB	baseball bat beating
	blood-brain barrier
	bundle branch block
BBBB	bilateral bundle branch block
BBC	bilateral breast cancer
	Brown-Buerger cystoscope
BBCS	bumps, bruises, cuts and scrapes (that is no serious injuries) (slang)
BBD	baby born dead
	before bronchodilator
	benign breast disease
BBE	biofield breast examination
BBFA	both bones forearm
BBFF	both bone foreman fracture
BBFP	blood and body fluid precautions
BBI	Bowman Birk inhibitor
BBIC	Bowman Birk inhibitor concentrate
BBL	bottle blood loss
BBM	banked breast milk
BBOW	bulging bag of water
BBP	blood-borne pathogen
	butyl benzyl phthalate
BBR	bibasilar rales
BBS	Bardet-Biedl syndrome
	Berg Balance Scale
	bilateral breath sounds
BBSE	bilateral breath sounds equal
BBSI	Brigance Basic Skills Inventory
BBT	basal body temperature
	Buteyko breathing technique

BB to MM	belly button to medial malleolus
B Bx	breast biopsy
BC	back care
	basket catheter
	battered child
	bed and chair
	beta carotene
	bicycle
	birth control
	bladder cancer
	blood culture
	Blue Cross
	bone conduction
	Bourn control
	breast cancer
	buccocervical
	buffalo cap (cap for intravenous line)
B/C	because
	blood urea nitrogen/creatinine ratio
B&C	bed and chair
	biopsy and curettage
	board and care
	breathed and cried
BCA	balloon catheter angioplasty
	basal cell atypia
	bichloracetic acid
	bicinchoninic acid
	brachiocephalic artery
BCa	breast cancer
BCAA	branched-chain amino acids
BC < AC	bone conduction less than air conduction
BC > AC	bone conduction greater than air conduction
B. cat	*Branhamella catarrhalis*
B-CAVe	bleomycin, lomustine (CCNU), doxorubicin (Adriamycin), and vinblastine (Velban)
BCB	Brilliant cresyl blue (stain)
BCBR	bilateral carotid body resection
BC/BS	Blue Cross/Blue Shield
BCC	basal cell carcinoma
	birth control clinic
BCCa	basal cell carcinoma
BCD	basal cell dysplasia
	bleomycin, cyclophosphamide, and dactinomycin
	borderline of cardial dullness
BCDCSW	Board Certified Diplomate in Clinical Social Work
BCDH	bilateral congenital dislocated hip
BCE	basal cell epithelioma
	beneficial clinical event
BCEDP	breast cancer early detection program
B cell	B lymphocyte
BCETS	Board Certified Expert in Traumatic Stress
BCF	basic conditioning factor
	Baylor core formula
BCG	bacille Calmette-Guérin vaccine
	bicolor guaiac
BCH	benign cephalic histiocytosis
	benign coital headache
BCHA	bone-conduction hearing aid
BChE	butyrylcholinesterase
BCI	blunt carotid injury
BCIE	bullous congenital ichthyosiform erythroderma
BCIR	Barnett continent intestinal reservoir
BCL	basic cycle length
	bio-chemoluminescence
B/C/L	BUN,(blood urea nitrogen), creatinine, lytes (electrolytes)
B-CLL	B-cell chronic lymphocytic leukemia
BCLP	bilateral cleft lip and palate
BCLS	basic cardiac life support
BCM	below costal margin
	birth control medication
	birth control method
	body cell mass
BCMA	bar-code medication administration
BCME	bis (chloromethyl) ether
BCNP	Board Certified Nuclear Pharmacist
BCNU	bacteria-controlled nursing unit
	carmustine (BiCNU; Gliadel)
BCOC	bowel care of choice
	bowel cathartic of choice
BCP	biochemical profile
	birth control pills
	blood cell profile
	carmustine, cyclophosphamide, and prednisone
BCPAP	Broun continuous positive airway pressure
BCPNN	Bayesian Confidence Propagation Neural Network
BCQ	breast central quadrantectomy
BCR	bicaudate ratio
	breakpoint cluster region (gene)
	bulbocavernosus reflex
BCRE	black cohosh root extract
BCRS	Brief Cognitive Rate Scale
BCRT	breast-conservation followed by radiation therapy
BCS	battered child syndrome
	breast-conserving surgery
	Budd-Chiari syndrome
BCSF	bone cell stimulating factor
BCSS	bone cell stimulating substance
BCT	Bag Carrying Test
	breast-conserving therapy
	broad complex tachycardias
BCTP	bi-component triton tri-n-butyl phosphate
BCU	burn care unit
BCUG	bilateral cystourethrogram

BCVA	best corrected visual acuity
BCVI	blunt cerebrovascular injury
BD	band neutrophil
	base deficit
	base down
	behavior disorder
	Behçet disease
	bile duct
	biotinidase deficiency
	bipolar disorder(s)
	birth date
	birth defect
	blood donor
	Bowen disease
	brain dead
	bronchial drainage
	bronchodilator
	buccodistal
	Buerger disease
	1,4-butanediol
	twice daily (in the United Kingdom, Australia, and elsewhere)
bd	twice daily (in the United Kingdom, Australia, and elsewhere)
B-D	Becton Dickinson and Company
BDAE	Boston Diagnostic Aphasia Examination
BDAS	balloon dilation atrial septostomy
BDBS	Bonnet-Dechaume-Blanc syndrome
BDC	burn-dressing change
BDCM	bromodichloromethane
BDD	body dysmorphic disorder
	bronchodilator drugs
BDE	bile duct exploration
	boron dose enhancer
BDF	bilateral distal femoral
	black divorced female
BDI	Beck Depression Inventory
	bile duct incision
	bile duct injury
BDI SF	Beck Depression Inventory-Short Form
BDL	below detectable limits
	bile duct ligation
B-DLCL	diffuse large B-cell lymphoma
BDM	black divorced male
BDNF	brain-derived neurotrophic factor
BDOD	brain-dead organ donor
B-DOPA	bleomycin, dacarbazine, vincristine (Oncovin), prednisone, and doxorubicin (Adriamycin)
BDP	beclomethasone dipropionate (Beconase AQ; QVAR)
	best demonstrated practice
BDR	background diabetic retinopathy
	black dot ringworm
	bronchodilator response
	bulk dose regimen
BDS	bile duct stone(s)
BDUs	battle dress uniforms
BDV	Borna disease virus
BE	bacterial endocarditis
	barium enema
	Barrett esophagus
	base excess
	below elbow
	bioequivalence
	bread equivalent
	breast examination
B ↑ E	both upper extremities
B ↓ E	both lower extremities
B & E	brisk and equal
BEA	below-elbow amputation
BEAC	carmustine (BiCNU), etoposide, cytarabine (ara-C), and cyclophosphamide
BEACOPP	bleomycin, etoposide, doxorubicin (Adriamycin), cyclophosphamide, vincristine (Oncovin), procarbazine, and prednisone
BEAM	brain electrical activity mapping
	carmustine (BCNU), etoposide, cytarabine (ara-C), and methotrexate
BEAR	Bourn electronic adult respirator
BEB	benign essential blepharospasm
BEC	bacterial endocarditis
BECs	bronchial epithelial cells
BECT	barium enema computed tomography
BED	binge-eating disorder
	biochemical evidence of disease
	biological effective dose
	biological equivalent dose
BEE	basal energy expenditure
BEF	bronchoesophageal fistula
BEGA	best estimate of gestational age
BEH	behavior
	benign essential hypertension
Beh Sp	behavior specialist
BEI	bioelectric impedance
	butanol-extractable iodine
BEL	blood ethanol level
BEP	bleomycin, etoposide, and cisplatin (Platinol)
	brain stem evoked potentials
BE-PEG	balanced electrolyte with polyethylene glycol
BEST	bio-electrical stimulation therapy
BET	bacterial endotoxins test
BEV	billion electron volts
	bleeding esophageal varices
BF	biofeedback
	black female
	bone fragment
	boyfriend
	breakfast fed

	breast-fed
B/F	bound-to-free ratio
B & F	back and forth
%BF	percentage of body fat
BFA	baby for adoption
	basilic forearm
	bifemoral arteriogram
BFC	benign febrile convulsion
BFD	blackfoot disease
BFEC	benign focal epilepsy of childhood
bFGF	basic fibroblast growth factor
BFI	Brief Fatigue Inventory
BFL	breast firm and lactating
B-FLY	butterfly
BFM	Berlin-Frankfurt-Munster(cancer study group)
	black married female
	body fat mass
	bright field microscope
BFNC	benign familial neonatal convulsions
BFP	biologic false positive
	blue fluorescent protein
BFR	Backward Functional Reach (test)
	blood filtration rate
	blood flow rate
B. frag	*Bacillus fragilis*
BFs	breast-feeds
BFT	bentonite flocculation test
	biofeedback training
BFU_e	erythroid burst-forming unit
BG	baby girl
	basal ganglia
	blood glucose
	bone graft
B-G	Bender-Gestalt (test)
BGA	Bundesgesundheitsamt (German drug regulatory agency)
B-GA-LACTO	beta galactosidase
BGC	basal-ganglion calcification
BGCT	benign glandular cell tumor
BGDC	Bartholin gland duct cyst
BGDR	background diabetic retinopathy
BGL	blood glucose level
BGM	blood glucose monitoring
bGS	biopsy Gleason score
BGT	Bender-Gestalt test
	blood glucose testing
BGTT	borderline glucose tolerance test
BH	bowel habits
	breath holding
BHA	butylated hydroxyanisole
BHC	benzene hexachloride
	Braxton Hicks contractions
bHCG	beta human chorionic gonadotropin
BHD	carmustine, hydroxyurea, and dacarbazine
BHDS	Birt-Hogg-Dube syndrome
B-HEXOS-A-LK	beta hexosaminidase A leukocytes
BHGI	The Breast Health Global Initiative
BHI	biosynthetic human insulin
	brain-heart infusion
BHL	bilateral hilar lymphadenopathy
BHMCO	behavioral health managed care organization
BHN	bridging hepatic necrosis
BHR	Birmingham hip resurfacing
	bronchial hyperresponsiveness (hyperactivity)
BHP	boarding home placement
	British Herbal Pharmacopeia
BHS	Beck Hopelessness Scale
	beta-hemolytic streptococci
	breath-holding spell
BHT	borderline hypertensive
	breath hydrogen test
	butylated hydroxytoluene
BHWU	Bair Hugger warming unit
BI	Barthel Index
	base in
	bleeding index (dental)
	Boehringer Ingelheim Pharmaceuticals, Inc.
	bowel impaction
	brain injury
Bi	bismuth
BIA	bioelectrical impedance analysis
	biospecific interaction analysis
BIB	brought in by
BIBA	brought in by ambulance
BIC	brain injury center
BICAP	bipolar electrocoagulation therapy
bicarb	bicarbonate
BiCNU®	carmustine
BICROS	bilateral contralateral routing of signals
BICU	burn intensive care unit
BID	brought in dead
BID	twice daily (b.i.d. preferred)
b.i.d.	twice daily
BIDA	amonafide
BiDil®	hydralazine and isosorbide dinitrate
BIDS	bedtime insulin, daytime sulfonylurea
BIF	bifocal
BIG	botulism immune globulin
	Breast International Group
BIGEM	bigeminal
BIG-IV	botulism immune globulin intravenous (human)
BIH	benign intracranial hypertension
	bilateral inguinal hernia
BIL	bilateral
	brother-in-law
BILAT SLC	bilateral short leg case

BILAT SXO	bilateral salpingo-oophorectomy
Bili	bilirubin
BILI-C	conjugated bilirubin
BIL MRY	bilateral myringotomy
BIMA	bilateral internal mammary arteries
BIN	twice a night (this is a dangerous abbreviation)
BIND	Biological Investigational New Drug
BIO	binocular indirect ophthalmoscopy
BIOF	biofeedback
BIP	bipolar affective disorder bleomycin, ifosfamide, and cisplatin (Platinol) bleomycin-induced pneumonitis brain injury program
BIPA	Benefits Improvement and Protection Act
BiPAP	bilevel (biphasic) positive airway pressure
BiPD	biparietal diameter
BIPP	bismuth iodoform paraffin paste
BIR	back internal rotation
BI-RADS	Breast Imaging Reporting and Data System (American College of Radiology)
BIRB	Biomedical Institutional Review Board
BIS	behavioral inhibition system Bispectral Index
Bi-SLT	bilateral, sequential single lung transplantation
bisp	bispinous diameter
BIT	behavioral inattention test burp in transit (gas seen in the stomach on an abdominal film) (slang)
BITA	bilateral internal thoracic artery
BiV	biventricular pacing
BIVAD	bilateral ventricular (biventricular) assist device
BIW	twice a week (this is a dangerous abbreviation)
BIZ-PLT	bizarre platelets
BJ	Bence Jones (protein) biceps jerk body jacket bone and joint
BJE	bone and joint examination bones, joints, and extremities
BJI	bone and joint infection
BJLO	Benton Judgment Line Orientation (test)
BJM	bones, joints, and muscles
BJOA	basal joint osteoarthritis
BJP	Bence Jones protein
BJR	Bezold-Jarisch reflex
BK	below knee (amputation) bradykinin bullous keratopathy
BKA	below-knee-amputation
BKC	blepharokeratoconjunctivitis
bkft	breakfast
Bkg	background
BKTT	below-knee to toe (cast)
BKV	BK polyomavirus
BKWC	below-knee walking cast
BKWP	below-knee walking plaster (cast)
BL	balloon laryngoplasty baseline (fetal heart rate) bioluminescence bland blast cells blood level blood loss blue bronchial lavage Burkitt lymphoma
B/L	brother-in-law
BLA	Biological License Application blood-loss anemia
BLB	Boothby-Lovelace-Bulbulian (oxygen mask) bronchoscopic lung biopsy
BLBK	blood bank
BLBS	bilateral breath sounds
BL = BS	bilateral equal breath sounds
bl cult	blood culture
B-L-D	breakfast, lunch, and dinner
bldg	bleeding
bld tm	bleeding time
BLE	both lower extremities
BLEED	ongoing *b*leeding, *l*ow blood pressure, *e*levated prothrombin time, *e*rratic mental status, and unstable comorbid *d*isease (risk factors for continued gastrointestinal bleeding)
BLEO	bleomycin sulfate
BLESS	bath, laxative, enema, shampoo, and shower
BLG	bovine beta-lactoglobulin
BLI	blast lung injury
BLIC	beta-lactamase inhibitor combination
BLIP	beta-lactamase inhibiting protein
BLL	bilateral lower lobe blood lead level brows, lids, and lashes
BLLS	bilateral leg strength
BLM	bleomycin sulfate
BLN	bronchial lymph nodes
BLOBS	bladder obstruction
BLOC	brief loss of consciousness
BLOKS	Boston Leeds Osteoarthritis Knee Score

Abbreviation	Meaning
BLPB	beta-lactamase-producing bacteria
BLPO	beta-lactamase-producing organism
BLQ	below the limit of quantification
	both lower quadrants
BLR	blood flow rate
BLS	basic life support
	Bureau of Labor Statistics
BLT	bilateral lung transplantation
	blood-clot lysis time
	brow left transverse
B.L. unit	Bessey-Lowry units
BLV	bovine leukemia virus
BM	bacterial meningitis
	black male
	bone marrow
	bone metastases
	bowel movement
	brain metastases
	breast milk
	bullous myringitis
BMA	biomedical application
	bismuth subsalicylate, metronidazole, and amoxicillin
	bone marrow aspirate
	British Medical Association
BMAT	basic motor ability test(s)
BMB	bone marrow biopsy
BMBF	German Ministry of Education and Research
BMC	bone marrow cells
	bone marrow culture
	bone mineral content
BMCS	balloon-mounted coronary stents
BMD	Becker muscular dystrophy
	benchmark dose
	bipolar manic depressive
	bipolar mood disorder
	bone marrow depression
	bone mineral density
BMDC	bone marrow-derived (stem) cells
BME	basal medium Eagle (diploid cell culture)
	biomedical engineering
	brief maximal effort
BMET	basic metabolic panel (see page 318)
BMF	between meal feedings
	black married female
BMFDS	Burke-Marsden-Fahn dystonia rating scale
BMG	benign monoclonal gammopathy
BMH	bone marrow harvest
BMI	body mass index
BMJ	bones, muscles, joints
BMK	birthmark
BML	bone marrow lesion
BMM	black married male
	bone marrow metastases
	bone marrow micrometastases
BMMC	bone marrow mononuclear T cells
BMMM	bone marrow micrometastases
B-MODE	brightness modulation
BMP	basic metabolic profile (panel) (see page 318)
	behavior management plan
	bone morphogenetic protein
BMPC	bone marrow plasmacytosis
BMPs	bone-morphogenic proteins
BMQ	Beliefs about Medicines Questionnaire
BMR	basal metabolic rate
	best motor response
BMRM	bilateral modified radical mastectomy
BMS	bare-metal stents
	Bristol-Myers Squibb Company
	burning mouth syndrome
BMSC	bone marrow-derived stem cells
BMT	bilateral myringotomy and tubes
	bismuth subsalicylate, metronidazole, and tetracycline
	bone marrow transplant
BMTH	bismuth, metronidazole, tetracycline, and a histamine H_2-receptor antagonist
BMTN	bone marrow transplant neutropenia
BMTT	bilateral myringotomy with tympanic tubes
BMTU	bone marrow transplant unit
BMU	basic multicellular unit
BMY	Bristol-Myers Squibb
BN	battalions
	bladder neck
	bulimia nervosa
BNBAS	Brazelton Neonatal Behavioral Assessment
BNC	binasal cannula
	bladder neck contracture
BNCT	boron neutron capture therapy
BND	bloody, near dead (slang)
BNE	but not exceeding
BNF	British National Formulary
BNI	blind nasal intubation
BNL	below normal limits
	breast needle localization
Bn M	bone marrow
B-NHL	B-cell non-Hodgkin lymphoma
BNO	bladder neck obstruction
	bowels not open
BNP	brain natriuretic peptide
	B-type natriuretic peptide (nesiritide [Natrecor])
BNPA	binasal pharyngeal airway
BNR	bladder neck retraction
BNS	benign nephrosclerosis
BNT	back to normal
	Boston Naming Test
BO	base out

	because of
	behavior objective
	body odor
	bowel obstruction
	bowel open
	bucco-occlusal
B & O	belladonna & opium (suppositories)
BOA	behavioral observation audiometry
	born on arrival
	born out of asepsis
BOB	ball-on-back
BOC	beats of clonus
BOCF	baseline observation carried forward
BOD	bilateral orbital decompression
	burden of disease
BODE	body mass index, airflow obstruction, dyspnea, and exercise capacity (index)
Bod Units	Bodansky units
BOE	bilateral otitis externa
BOH	Board of Health
	bundle of His
BOLD	bleomycin, vincristine (Oncovin), lomustine, and dacarbazine
	blood oxygenation level-dependent
BOM	benign ovarian mass
	bilateral otitis media
BOMA	bilateral otitis media, acute
BOME	bilateral otitis media with effusion
BOMP	bleomycin, vincristine (Oncovin), mitomycin, and cisplatin (Platinol)
BoNTA	botulinum toxin type A
BOO	bladder outlet obstruction
BOOP	bronchitis obliterans-organized pneumonia
BOP	bleeding on probing
BOR	bortezomib (Velcade)
	bowels open regularly
	bronchia-oto-renal (syndrome)
BORN	State Board of Registration in Nursing
BORospA	borreliosis (Lyme disease, *Borrelia* sp.) vaccine, outer surface protein A
BOS	base of support
	bronchiolitis obliterans syndrome
BOSS	Becker orthopedic spinal system
BOT	base of tongue
	borderline ovarian tumors
BOU	burning on urination
BOUGIE	bougienage
BOVR	Bureau of Vocational Rehabilitation
BOW	bag of water
BOW-I	bag of water–intact
BOW-R	bag of water–ruptured
BP	bathroom privileges
	bed pan
	bench press
	benzoyl peroxide
	biological parent(s)
	bipolar
	birthplace
	blood pressure
	bodily pain
	body powder
	British Pharmacopeia
	bullous pemphigoid
	bypass
bp	base pair(s) (genetics)
BP-200	Bourn Infant Pressure Ventilator
BPA	birch pollen allergy
	bisphenol A
BPAD	bipolar affective disorder
BPAR	biopsy-proven actue rejection
BPb	whole blood lead concentration
BPC	British Pharmaceutical Codex
BPCF	bronchopleural cutaneous fistula
BPI	bipolar disorder, Type I
BPII	bipolar type II disorder
BPD	benzoporphyrin derivative
	biparietal diameter
	borderline personality disorder
	bronchopulmonary dysplasia
BPd	diastolic blood pressure
BPD/DS	biliopancreatic diversion with a duodenal switch (surgery for obesity)
BPE	benign enlargement of the prostate
BPF	Brazilian purpuric fever
	bronchopleural fistula
BPH	benign prostatic hypertrophy
BPG	bypass graft
	penicillin G benzathine (Bicillin L-A; Permapen) for IM use only
BPI	bactericidal/permeability increasing (protein)
	Brief Pain Inventory
BPIG	bacterial polysaccharide immune globulin
BPL	benzylpenicilloylpolylysine
	bone probing length (dental)
BPLA	blood pressure, left arm
BPLND	bilateral pelvic lymph node dissection
BPM	beats per minute
	breaths per minute
BPN	bacitracin, polymyxin B, and neomycin sulfate
BPO	benign prostatic obstruction
	benzoyl peroxide
	bilateral partial oophorectomy
BPOC	barcode point-of-care
BPOP	bizarre parosteal osteochondromatous proliferation (Nora's Lesion)

BPP biophysical profile
BPPP bilateral pedal pulses present
BP,P,R,T, blood pressure, pulse, respiration, and temperature
BPPV benign paroxysmal positional vertigo
BPR beeper
blood per rectum
blood pressure recorder
BPRS Brief Psychiatric Rating Scale
BPS bilateral partial salpingectomy
blood pump speed
BPs systolic blood pressure
BPSD behavioral and psychological symptoms of dementia
bronchopulmonary segmental drainage
BPSO bilateral prophylactic salpingo-oophorectomy
BPT BioPort Corporation
BPV benign paroxysmal vertigo
benign positional vertigo
bovine papilloma virus
BPW bilateral pick-up walker
Bq becquerel
BQL below quantifiable levels
BQR brequinar sodium
BR bathroom
bedrest
Benzing retrograde
birthing room
blink rate
blink reflex
bowel rest
brachioradialis
breast
breast reconstruction
breech
bridge
bright red
brown
Br bromide
bromine
BRA bananas, rice (rice cereal), and applesauce
brain
BrAC breath alcohol content
BRCA1 breast cancer gene 1
BRCA2 breast cancer gene 2
BRADY bradycardia
BRANCH branch chain amino acids
BRAO branch retinal artery occlusion
BRAS bilateral renal artery stenosis
BRAT bananas, rice (rice cereal), applesauce, and toast
Baylor rapid autologous transfuser
blunt thoracic abdominal trauma
BRATT bananas, rice (rice cereal), applesauce, tea, and toast
BRB blood-retinal barrier
bright red blood
BRBR bright red blood per rectum
BRBPR bright red blood per rectum
BRC bladder reconstruction
BrCa breast cancer
BRCM below right costal margin
BrdU bromodeoxyuridine
BRex breathing exercise
Br Fdg breast-feeding
BRFS biochemical relapse-free survival
BRFSS Behavioral Risk Factor Surveillance System (CDC)
BRJ brachial radialis jerk
BRM biological response modifiers
BRN brown
BRO brother
BROM back range of motion
BRONK bronchoscopy
BRP bathroom privileges
BRR Bannayan-Riley-Ruvalcaba (syndrome)
BR RAO branch retinal artery occlusion
BR RVO branch retinal vein occlusion
BRS baroreceptor reflex sensitivity
BrS breath sounds
BRSV bovine respiratory syncytial virus
BRU basic remodeling unit (osteon)
brucellosis (*Brucella melitensis*) vaccine
BRVO branch retinal vein occlusion
BS barium swallow
bedside
before sleep
Behçet syndrome
Bennett seal
blind spot
blood sugar
Blue Shield
bone scan
bowel sounds
breath sounds
B & S Bartholin and Skene (glands)
bending and stooping
Brown and Sharp (suture sizes)
BS×4 bowel sounds in all four quadrants
BSA body surface area
bowel sounds active
Brief Scale of Anxiety
BSAB Balthazar Scales of Adaptive Behavior
BSAb broad-spectrum antibiotics
BSAP bone-specific alkaline phosphatase
BSB bedside bag
body surface burned
BSC basosquamous (cell) carcinoma
bedside care
bedside commode

	best supportive care
	biological safety cabinet
	Biomedical Science Corps
	burn scar contracture
BSCC	bedside commode chair
	Bjork-Shiley convexo-concave (valves)
BSCVA	best spectacle-corrected visual acuity
BSD	baby soft diet
	bedside drainage
BSE	bovine spongiform encephalopathy
	breast self-examination
BSEC	bedside easy chair
BSepF	black separated female
BSepM	black separated male
BSER	brain stem evoked responses
BSF	black single female
	busulfan (Myleran)
BSG	Bagolini striated glasses
	brain stem gliomas
BSGA	beta streptococcus group A
BSGI	breast-specific gamma imaging
BSI	bloodstream infection
	body substance isolation
	brain stem injury
	Brief Symptom Inventory
BSL	baseline
	Biological Safety Level
	blood sugar level
BSL-1	Biosafety Level 1
BS L base	breath sounds diminished, left base
BSM	black single male
	blood safety module
	body surface mapping
BSN	Bachelor of Science in Nursing
	bowel sounds normal
BSNA	bowel sounds normal and active
BSNMT	Bachelor of Science in Nuclear Medicine Technology
BSNT	breast soft and nontender
BSNUTD	baby shots not up to date
BSO	bilateral salpingo-oophorectomy
	l-buthionine sulfoximine
bSOD	bovine superoxide dismutase
BSOM	bilateral serous otitis media
BSP	body substance precautions
	bone sialoprotein
	Bromsulphalein®
BSPA	bowel sounds present and active
BSPM	body surface potential mapping
BSR	body stereotactic radiosurgery
	bowels sounds regular
BSRI	Bem Sex Role Inventory
BSRT (R)	Bachelor of Science in Radiologic Technology (Registered)
BSS	Baltimore Sepsis Scale
	bedside scale
	bismuth subsalicylate
	black silk sutures
BSS®	balanced salt solution
BSSG	sitogluside
BSSO	bilateral sagittal split osteotomy
BSSRO	bilateral sagittal split-ramus osteotomy
BSSS	benign sporadic sleep spikes
BSST	breast self-stimulation test
BST	bedside testing
	bovine somatotropin
	brain-stem tumors
	brief stimulus therapy
BSU	Bartholin, Skene, urethra (glands)
	behavioral science unit
BSu	blood sugar
BSUTD	baby shots up to date
	Base Service Unit
BSW	Bachelor of Social Work
	bedscale weight
BT	bedtime
	behavioral therapy
	bituberous
	bladder tumor
	Blalock-Taussig (shunt)
	bleeding time
	blood transfusion
	blood type
	blue tongue
	blunt trauma
	bowel tones
	brain tumor
	breast tumor
	bronchial thermoplasty
Bt	*Bacillus thuringiensis*
B-T	Blalock-Taussig (shunt)
B/T	between
Bt#	bottle number
BTA	below the ankle
	bladder tumor antigen
	bladder tumor-associated analytes
	botulinum toxic type A (Botox)
BTA-A	botulinum toxin type A (Botox)
BTB	back to bed
	beat-to-beat (variability)
	breakthrough bleeding
BTBV	beat-to-beat variability
BTC	behind-the-counter (drugs)
	bilateral tubal cautery
	biliary tract cancer
	bladder tumor check
	by the clock
BTE	Baltimore Therapeutic Equipment
	behind-the-ear (hearing aid)
	bisected, totally embedded
BTF	blenderized tube feeding
BTFS	breast tumor frozen section
BTG	beta thromboglobulin
B-Thal	beta thalassemia

B

BTHOOM	beats the hell out of me (better stated as "differed diagnosis")
BTI	biliary tract infection
	bitubal interruption
BTKA	bilateral total knee arthroplasty
BTL	bilateral tubal ligation
BTM	bilateral tympanic membranes
	bismuth subcitrate, tetracycline, and metronidazole
BTMEAL	between meals
BTO	bilateral tubal occlusion
BTP	bismuth tribromophenate
	breakthrough pain
BTPABA	bentiromide
BTPS	body temperature pressure saturated
BTR	bladder tumor recheck
BTS	Blalock-Taussig shunt
BTSH	bovine thyrotropin
BTT	bridge to transplant
BTU	behavior therapy unit
BTW	back to work
	between
	by-the-way
BTW M	between meals
BTX	Botulinum toxin type A (Botox)
BtxA	botulinum toxin type A (Botox)
BU	base up (prism)
	below umbilicus
	Bodansky units
	burn unit
	busulfan (Myleran)
BUA	broadband ultrasound attenuation
BUCAT	busulfan, carboplatin, and thiotepa
BuCy	busulfan and cyclophosphamide
BUD	budesonide (Rhinocort)
BUdR	bromodeoxyuridine
BUE	both upper extremities
BUFA	baby up for adoption
BULB	bilateral upper lid blepharoplasty
BUN	blood urea nitrogen
	bunion
BUO	bleeding of undetermined origin
BUPE	buprenorphine and naloxone (Suboxone) (slang)
Bupi	bupivacaine (Marcaine, Sensorcaine)
BUR	back-up rate (ventilator)
Burd	Burdick suction
BUS	Bartholin, urethral, and Skene glands
	bladder ultrasound
	bulbourethral sling
BUSV	Bartholin urethral Skeins vagina
BUT	biopsy urease test
	break up time
Butt Paste	16% Zinc Oxide ointment. Contents and strength can vary. (slang and a commercial product)
BV	bacterial vaginitis
	bevacizumab (Avastin)
	biological value
	blood volume
BVAD	biventricular assist device
BVAS	Birmingham Vasculitis Activity Score
BVD	bovine viral diarrhea
BVDU	bromovinlydeoxyuridine (brivudin)
BVE	blood volume expander
BVF	bulboventricular foramen
BVH	biventricular hypertrophy
BVL	bilateral vas ligation
BVM	bag valve mask
BVMG	Bender Visual-Motor Gestalt (test)
BVO	branch vein occlusion
BVR	Bureau of Vocational Rehabilitation
BVRO	bilateral vertical ramus osteotomy
BVRT	Benton Visual Retention Test
BVT	basilica vein transposition
	bilateral ventilation tubes
BVZ	bevacizumab (Avastin)
BW	bandwidth (radiology)
	birth weight
	bite-wing (radiograph)
	body water
	body weight
B & W	Black and White (milk of magnesia & aromatic cascara fluidextract)
BWA	bed-wetter admission
BWC	bladder-wash cytology
BWCO	baby won't come out (needs Caesarian) (slang)
BWCS	bagged white cell study
BWF	Blackwater fever
BWFI	bacteriostatic water for injection
BWidF	black widowed female
BWidM	black widowed male
BWS	battered woman syndrome
	Beckwith-Wiedemann syndrome
BWs	bite-wing (x-rays)
BWSE	black widow spider envenomation
BWSTT	body weight-supported treadmill training
BWT	bowel wall thickness
BWX	bite-wing x-ray
Bx	behavior
	biopsy
B × B	back-to-back
BX BS	Blue Cross and Blue Shield
BXM	B-cell crossmatch
BXO	balanitis xerotica obliterans
ΦBZ	phenylbutazone
BZD	benzodiazepine
BZDZ	benzodiazepine
BZP	benzyl piperazine (known as 1-benzylpiperazine, A2, Frenzy, Nemesis, Lovely and Lovelies)

C

C	ascorbic acid (Vitamin C)
	carbohydrate
	Catholic
	Caucasian
	Celsius
	centigrade
	Chlamydia
	clubbing
	conjunctiva
	constricted
	cyanosis
	cytidine
	hundred
$\bar{c}$	with
C'	cervical spine
C+	with contrast
C−	without contrast
C 1	cyclopentolate 1% ophthalmic solution (Cyclogyl)
C_1–C_7	cervical vertebra 1 through 7
C_1–C_8	cervical nerves 1 through 8
C_1–C_9	precursor molecules of the complement system
C_1–C_{12}	cranial nerves 1 to 12
C3	complement C3
C4	complement C4
CI-CV	Drug Enforcement Agency scheduled substances class one through five
C_{II}	second cranial nerve
CA	cancelled appointment
	cancer
	cancer antigen
	Candida albicans
	carcinoma
	cardiac arrest
	carotid artery
	celiac artery
	cellulose acetate (filter)
	Certified Acupuncturist
	chronologic age
	competent authority
	Cocaine Anonymous
	community-acquired
	compressed air
	continuous aerosol
	coronary angioplasty
	coronary artery
Ca	calcium
	cancer
C/A	conscious, alert
Ca++	calcification
	calcium
CA 125	cancer antigen 125
C&A	Clinitest® and Acetest®
CAA	cerebral amyloid angiopathy
	coloanal anastamosis
	crystalline amino acids
CAAP-1	Certified Associate Addiction Professional Level 1
CAB	catheter-associated bacteriuria
	cellulose acetate butyrate
	combined androgen blockade
	complete abortion
	complete atrioventricular block
	Consumer Affairs Branch (FDA)
	coronary artery bypass
CAB-BAGE	coronary artery bypass graft (CABG)
CABG	coronary artery bypass graft
CaBI	calcium bone index
CaBP	calcium-binding protein
CABS	coronary artery bypass surgery
CAC	cardioacceleratory center
	carotid artery calcification
	Certified Alcohol Counselor
	Community Action Center
	computer-assisted coding
	computerized autocoding
	coronary artery calcification
CACB	chronic angle closure glaucoma
CA-ChEIs	centrally acting cholinesterase inhibitors
CACI	computer-assisted continuous infusion
$CaCl_2$	calcium chloride
$CaCO_3$	calcium carbonate
CACP	cisplatin
CACS	cancer-related anorexia/cachexia
CAD	cadaver (kidney donor)
	calcium alginate dressing
	cervical artery dissection
	computer-aided diagnosis
	computer-aided dispatch
	coronary atherosclerotic disease
	coronary artery disease
CaD	calcium and vitamin D (fortified milk)
CADAC	Certified Alcohol and Drug Abuse Counselor
CADASIL	cerebral autosomal dominant arteriopathy with subcortical infarcts and leukoencephalopathy
CADD®	Computerized Ambulatory Drug Delivery (pump)
CADL	communication activities of daily living (speech/ cognitive test)
CADP	computer-assisted design of prosthesis
CADRF	coronary artery disease risk factors
CADXPL	cadaver transplant
CAE	cellulose acetate electrophoresis

coronary artery endarterectomy
cyclophosphamide, doxorubicin (Adriamycin), and etoposide

CAEC cardiac arrhythmia evaluation center
Cook airway exchange catheter

CaEDTA calcium disodium edetate

CAERS CFSAN (Center for Food Safety and Applied Nutrition) Adverse Events Reporting System (FDA)

CAEV caprine arthritis encephalitis virus

CAF chronic atrial fibrillation
controlled atrial flutter/fibrillation
coronary artery fistula
cyclophosphamide, doxorubicin (Adriamycin), and fluorouracil

CAFF controlled atrial fibrillation/flutter

CAFT Clinitron® air fluidized therapy

CAG chronic atrophic gastritis
closed angle glaucoma
continuous ambulatory gamma globin (infusion)
coronary arteriography
critical angle of Gissane

CaG calcium gluconate

CAGE a questionnaire for alcoholism evaluation C Have you ever felt the need to cut down on your drinking? A Have you ever felt annoyed by criticism of your drinking? G Have you ever felt guilty abut your drinking? E Have you ever taken a drink (eye opener) first thing in the morning?

CAH chronic active hepatitis
chronic aggressive hepatitis
congenital adrenal hyperplasia

CAHB chronic active hepatitis B

CAI carbonic anhydrase inhibitors
carboxyamide aminoimidazoles
carotid artery injury
computer-assisted instructions

'caid Medicaid

CAIRO CApecitabine, IRinotecan, and Oxaliplatin

CAIV cold-adapted influenza virus vaccine

CAL callus
calories (cal)
chronic airflow limitation
clinical attachment level (dental)

C_{alb} albumin clearance

cal ct calorie count

CALD chronic active liver disease

CALGB Cancer and Leukemia Group B

CALI chromophore-assisted laser inactivation

CALLA common acute lymphoblastic leukemia antigen

CAM campylobacter vaccine
Caucasian adult male
cell adhesion molecules
child abuse management
complementary and alternative medicine
confusion assessment method
controlled ankle motion
cystic adenomatoid malformation

CAMA Chronic and Acute Medical Assistance
corrected-arm-muscle area

CAMCOG Cambridge Cognitive Examination

CAMD computer-aided molecular design

CAMF cyclophosphamide, Adriamycin, methotrexate, and fluorouracil

CAMP cyclophosphamide, doxorubicin (Adriamycin), methotrexate, and procarbazine

cAMP cyclic adenosine monophosphate

CA-MRSA community-associated methicillin-resistant *Staphylococcus aureus*

CAMs cell adhesion molecules

CA-MSSA community-acquired methicillin-susceptible *Staphylococcus aureus*

CAMT congenital amegakaryocytic thrombocytopenia

CAN cardiovascular autonomic neuropathy
Certified Nurse Assistant
chronic allograft nephropathy
contrast-associated nephropathy
cord around neck

CA/N child abuse and neglect

CAN-A Certified Nursing Assistant-Advanced

CANC cancelled

c-ANCA antineutrophil cytoplasmic antibody

CANDA computer-assisted new drug application

CAN-KLB *Candida albicans, Klebsiella pneumoniae* vaccine

CANP Certified Adult Nurse Practitioner

CAO chronic airway (airflow) obstruction

CaO_2 arterial oxygen concentration

$Ca(OH)_2$ calcium hydroxide

CAOS computer-assisted orthopedic surgery

CaOx calcium oxalate

CAP cancer of the prostate
capsule
cellulose acetate phthalate
Certified Addiction Professional
cervical acid phosphatase
chaotic atrial tachycardia
chemistry admission profile
chloramphenicol
College of American Pathologists (cancer checklist)
community-acquired pneumonia
compound action potentials

	cyclophosphamide, doxorubicin (Adriamycin), and cisplatin
CaP	cancer of the prostate
Ca/P	calcium to phosphorus ratio
CA4P	combretastatin A4 prodrug
CAPA	Certified Ambulatory Perianesthesia Nurse
	Corrective and Preventive Action (related to FDA)
CAPB	central auditory processing battery
CAPD	central auditory processing disorder
	continuous ambulatory peritoneal dialysis
CAPLA	computer-assisted product license application
CaPPS	calcium pentosan polysulfate
CAPS	aspects of **c**ognition, **a**ffective state, **p**hysical condition, and **s**ocial factors (patient assessment; parameters)
	caffeine, alcohol, pepper, and spicy food (dietary restrictions)
CAPS-SX	Clinical Administered PTSD (Post-traumatic Stress Disorder) Scale–One Week Symptom Version
CAPWA	computerized arterial pulse waveform analysis
CAR	cancer-associated retinopathy
	cardiac ambulation routine
	carotid artery repair
	carotid artery rupture
	coronary artery revascularization
	Coxsackie adenovirus receptor
CA-RA	common adductor-rectus abdominis
CARB	carbohydrate
CARBO	Carbocaine
	carboplatin (Paraplatin)
CARD	Cardiac Automatic Resuscitative Device
CARES	Cancer Rehabilitation Evaluation System
CARF	Commission on Accreditation of Rehabilitation Facilities
CARM	Centre for Adverse Reactions Monitoring (New Zealand)
C-arm	fluoroscopy image intensifier
CARN	Certified Addiction Registered Nurse
CARN-AP	Certified Addictions Registered Nurse - Advanced Practice
CARS	Childhood Autism Rating Scale
	coherent anti-Stokes Raman scattering
CART	classification and regression tree
CARTI	community-acquired respiratory tract infection(s)
CAS	carotid angioplasty and stenting
	carotid artery stenosis (stenting)
	cerebral arteriosclerosis
	Chemical Abstracts Service
	Clinical Asthma Score
	collision avoidance system
	combined androgen suppression
	computer-assisted surgery
	coronary artery stenosis
CASA	cancer-associated serum antigen
	Center on Addiction and Substance Abuse
	computer-assisted semen analysis
	court appointed special advocate
CaSC	carcinoma of the sigmoid colon
CASH	chemotherapy-associated steatohepatitis
CASHD	coronary arteriosclerotic heart disease
CA-SAI	community-acquired *Staphylococcus aureus* infections
CASL	continuous arterial spin labeled
CASP	Child Analytic Study Program
CASS	computer-aided sleep system
CAST®	color allergy screening test
CASWCM	Certified Advanced Social Work Case Manager
CAT	Cardiac Arrest Team
	carnitine acetyl transferase
	cataract
	Children's Apperception Test
	coital alignment technique
	computed axial tomography
	methcatinone
CATH	catheter
	catheterization
	Catholic
CATS	catecholamines
CATSHL	camptodactyly, tall stature, and hearing loss (syndrome)
CATT	card agglutination test with stained trypanosomes
CAU	Caucasian
CAUTI	catheter-associated urinary tract infection
CAV	cardiac allograft vasculopathy
	computer-aided ventilation
	congenital absence of vagina
	cyclophosphamide, doxorubicin (Adriamycin), and vincristine
CAV-1	canine adenovirus type 1
CAVB	complete atrioventricular block
CAVC	common artrioventricular canal
	complete atrioventricular canal
CAVE	Content Analysis of Verbatim Explanation
	cyclophosphamide, doxorubicin, (Adriamycin) vincristine, and etoposide
CAVH	continuous arteriovenous hemofiltration

CAVHD continuous arteriovenous hemodialysis
CAVM cerebral arteriovenous malformation
CAV-P-VP cyclophosphamide, doxorubicin (Adriamycin), vincristine, cisplatin, and etoposide
CAVR continuous arteriovenous rewarming
CAVS calcific valve stenosis
CAVSD complete atrioventricular septal defect
CAVU continuous arteriovenous ultrafiltration
CAW carbonaceous-activated water (Willard Water)
CAX central axis
Ca x P calcium times phosphorus product
CB cerebellopontine
cesarean birth
chronic bronchitis
code blue
conjugated bilirubin (direct)
(umbilical) cord blood
c/b complicated by
C & B chair and bed
crown and bridge
CB1 cannabinoid receptor, type 1
CBA chronic bronchitis and asthma
cost-benefit analysis
County Board of Assistance
CBAPF Certified Board ofAddiction Professionals
CBASP Cognitive Behavioral Analysis System of Psychotherapy
CBAVD congenital bilateral absence of the vas deferens
CBC carbenicillin
complete blood count
contralateral breast cancer
CBCDA carboplatin
CBCL Child Behavior Checklist
CBCT community based clinical trials
cone-beam computed tomography
CBD closed bladder drainage
common bile duct
corticobasal degeneration
CBDE common bile duct exploration
CBDS common bile duct stone(s)
CBE Changes Being Effected (FDA regulatory term)
charting by exception
child birth education
clinical breast examination
CBEFM Clear-blue Easy Fertility Monitor
CBER Center for Biologics Evaluation and Research (FDA)
CBF cerebral blood flow
CBFS cerebral blood flow studies
CBFV cerebral blood flow velocity
CBG capillary blood glucose
CBGM capillary blood glucose monitor
CBH collimated beam handpiece (for laser)
CBI Caregiver Burden Index
continuous bladder irrigation
CBLI cumulative blood lead index
CBM cryopreserved bone marrow
CBN chronic benign neutropenia
collected by nurse
CBP chronic benign pain
copper-binding protein
CBPP contagious bovine pleuropneumonia
CBPS Community Based Prevention Services
congential bilateral perisylvian syndrome
coronary bypass surgery
CBR carotid bodies resected
chronic bedrest
clinical benefit rate
clinical benefit responders
complete bedrest
CB1R cannabinoid-1 receptor
CBRAM controlled partial rebreathing-anesthesia method
CBRN chemical, biological, radiological, or nuclear (agents)
CB RRR s M/R/G cardiac beat, regular rhythm and rate without murmurs, rubs, or gallops
CBrS clear breath sounds
CBS Caregiver Burden Screen
Charles Bonnet syndrome
chronic brain syndrome
coarse breath sounds
corticobasal syndrome
Cruveilhier-Baumgarten syndrome
CBT cognitive behavioral therapy
CBU cumulative breath units
CBV central blood volume
cyclophosphamide, carmustine (BiCNu), and etoposide (VePesid)
CBZ carbamazepine (Tegretol)
CBZE carbamazepine epoxide
CC cardiac catheterization
Catholic
cerebral concussion
cervical cancer
chart check (as in 24 hour CC)
chief complaint
choriocarcinoma
chronic complainer
chronic constitpation
circulatory collapse
clean catch (urine)
comfort care
complications and comorbidity

	coracoclavicular
	cord compression
	corpus callosum
	creatinine clearance
	critical condition
	cubic centimeter (cc); Note, mL is the standard designation for expressing liquid measurements. It is preferred as a poorly written cc looks like the dangerous abbreviation for unit "u" or 00
	with correction (with glasses)
C_c	concentration of drug in the central compartment
C/C	cholecystectomy and operative cholangiogram
	complete upper and lower dentures
CCII	Clinical Clerk–2nd year
C & C	cold and clammy
CCA	calcium-channel antagonist
	Certified Coding Associate
	cholangiocarcinoma
	circumflex coronary artery
	common carotid artery
	concentrated care area
	countercurrent chromatography
	critical care area
CCAM	congenital cystic adenomatoid malformation (of the lung)
CCAP	capsule cartilage articular preservation
CCAT	common carotid artery thrombosis
C-CATODSW	Certified Clinical Alcohol, Tobacco and Other Drugs Social Worker
CCAVC	complete common atrioventricular canal
CCB	calcium channel blocker(s)
	Community Care Board
	corn, callus, and bunion
CCBT	Certified Cognitive Behavioral Therapist
CCC	Cancer Care Center
	central corneal clouding (Grade 0+ to 4+)
	Certificate of Clinical Competency
	child care clinic
	cholangiocellular carcinoma
	circulating cancer cells
	closed chest compressions
	Comprehensive Cancer Center
	continuous curvilinear capsulorrhexis
	Coricidin Cough and Cold (slang)
C/cc	colonies per cubic centimeter
CC & C	colony count and culture
CCC-A	Certificate of Clinical Competence in Audiology
CCCE	Clinical Center Coordinator Educator
CCCN	Certified Continence Care Nurse
CCC-SP	Certificate of Clinical Competence in Speech-Language Pathology
CCD	charged-coupled device
	childhood celiac disease
	chin-chest distance
	clinical cardiovascular disease
	colpocystodefecography
CCDC	Certified Chemical Dependency Counselor
CCDC-1	Certified Chemical Dependency Counselor, Level One
CCDS	color-coded duplex sonography
CCE	clubbing, cyanosis, and edema
	colon capsule endoscopy
	countercurrent electrophoresis
CC-EMG	corpus cavernosum electromyography
CCF	cephalin cholesterol flocculation
	Cleveland Clinic Foundation
	compound comminuted fracture
	congestive cardiac failure
	crystal-induced chemotactic factor
CCFA	cycloserine cefoxitin fructose agar
CCFE	cyclophosphamide, cisplatin, fluorouracil, and estramustine
CCFs	chronic-care facilities
CCG	Children's Cancer Group
CCH	chronic community care home
	Cook County Hospital
	cluster headache
CCHB	congenital complete heart block
CCHD	complex congenital heart disease
	cyanotic congenital heart disease
CCHF	Congo-Crimean hemorrhagic fever
CCHO	consistent carbohydrate
CCHS	congenital central hypoventilation syndrome
CCI	chronic coronary insufficiency
	Correct Coding Initiative
	corrected count increment
CCJAP	Certified Criminal Justice Addiction Professional
CCJAS	Certified Criminal Justice Addiction Specialist
CCK	cholecystokinin
CCK-OP	cholecystokinin octapeptide
CCK-PZ	cholecystokinin pancreozymin
CCL	cardiac catheterization laboratory
	critical condition list
CCl_4	carbon tetrachloride
CCLE	chronic cutaneous lupus erythematosus
CCM	calcium citrate malate
	cerebral cavernous malformation
	Certified Case Manager

	children's case management
	country coordinating mechanism
	cyclophosphamide, lomustine (CCNU; CeeNU), and methotrexate
CCMHC	Certified Clinical Mental Health Counselor
CCMSU	clean catch midstream urine
CCMU	critical care medicine unit
CCN	continuing care nursery
	cyr61, ctfg, nov (family of proteins)
CCNS	cell cycle-nonspecific
	Certified Clinical Nurse Specialist
CCNU	lomustine (CeeNu)
CCO	continuous cardiac output
	Corporate Compliance Officer
CCOHTA	Canadian Coordinating Office for Health Technology Assessment
C-collar	cervical collar
CCP	crystalloid cardioplegia
	cyclic citrullinated peptide
CCPD	continuous cycling (cyclical) peritoneal dialysis
CCPs	Corporate Compliance Programs
CCR	California Cancer Registry
	cardiac catheterization recovery
	complete cytogenetic remission
	Continuity of Care Record
	continuous complete remission
	counterclockwise rotation
C_{cr}	creatinine clearance
cCR	complete clinical remission
CCRC	Certified Clinical Research Coordinator
	continuing care residential community
CC-RCC	clear-cell renal-cell carcinoma
CCRN	Certified Critical Care Registered Nurse
CCRT	combined chemoradiotherapy
CCRU	critical care recovery unit
CCS	California Children's Services
	cell cycle-specific
	certified coding specialist
	color contrast sensitivity
CC & S	cornea, conjunctiva, and sclera
CCSA	Canadian Cardiovascular Society Angina (score)
CCSK	clear cell sarcoma of the kidney
CCSP	Certified Chiropractic Sports Physician
	Clara cell secretory protein
CCS-P	Certified Coding Specialist, Physician-Based
CCSS	Childhood Cancer Survivor Study
CCSV	cell-cultured smallpox vaccine
CCT	calcitriol
	carotid compression tomography
	central corneal thickness
	Certified Cardiographic Technician
	closed cerebral trauma
	closed cranial trauma
	collision cell technology
	congenitally corrected transposition (of the great vessels)
	Critical Care Technician
	crude coal tar
CCTGA	congenitally corrected transposition of the great arteries
CCT in PET	crude coal tar in petroleum
CCTV	closed circuit television
CCU	coronary care unit
	critical care unit
CCUA	clean catch urinalysis
CCUP	colpocystourethropexy
CCV	Critical Care Ventilator (Ohio)
	critical closing volume
CCW	childcare worker
	counterclockwise
CCWR	counterclockwise rotation
CCX	complications
CCY	cholecystectomy
CD	cadaver donor
	candela
	Castleman disease
	celiac disease
	cervical dystonia
	cesarean delivery
	character disorder
	chemical dependency
	childhood disease
	chlorproguanil-dapsone (Lapdap)
	chronic dialysis
	circular dichroism
	closed drainage
	Clostridium difficile
	clusters of differentiation
	common duct
	communication disorders
	complementarity-determining
	complicated delivery
	conduct disorder
	conjugate diameter
	contact dermatitis
	continuous drainage
	conventional denture
	convulsive disorder
	cortical dysplasia
	Crohn disease
	cumulative doses
	cycle day, referring to cycle day number of the menstrual cycle; e.g.: CD#1, first day of menstrual cycle
	cyclodextran
	cytarabine and daunorubicin

Cd cadmium
concentration of drug
C/D cigarettes per day
cup-to-disc ratio
CD4 antigenic marker on helper/inducer T cells (also called OKT 4, T4, and Leu3)
CD8 antigenic marker on suppressor/cytotoxic T cells (also called OKT 8, T8, and Leu 8)
C&D curettage and desiccation
cystectomy and diversion
cytoscopy and dilatation
CDA Certified Dental Assistant
chenodeoxycholic acid (chenodiol)
congenital dyserythropoietic anemia
2-CDA cladribine (Leustatin; chlorodeoxyadenosine)
CDAD *Clostridium difficile*-associated diarrhea
CDAI Crohn Disease Activity Index
CDAK Cordis Dow Artificial Kidney
CDAP continuous distended airway pressure
CDB cough and deep breath
CDC calculated day of confinement
cancer detection center
carboplatin, doxorubicin, and cyclophosphamide
Centers for Disease Control and Prevention
Certified Drug Counselor
chenodeoxycholic acid (chenodiol)
Clostridium difficile colitis
CDCA chenodeoxycholic acid (chenodiol)
CDCC complement-dependent cellular cytotoxicity
CDCP Centers for Disease Control and Prevention (CDC is official abbreviation)
CDCR conjunctivodacryocystorhinostomy
CdCS Cri du Chat syndrome
CDD Certificate of Disability for Discharge
Clostridium difficile disease
cytidine deaminase
CDDN Certified Developmental Disabilities Nurse
CDDP cisplatin (Platinol)
CDE canine distemper encephalitis
Certified Diabetes Educator
common data element
common duct exploration
CDER Center for Drug Evaluation and Research (FDA)
CDFI color Doppler flow imaging
CDG carbohydrate-deficient glycoprotein
congenital disorders of glycosylation
CDGE constant denaturant gel electrophoresis
CDGP constitutional delay of growth and puberty
CDGS carbohydrate-deficient glycoprotein syndrome
CDH chronic daily headache
congenital diaphragmatic hernia
congenital dislocation of hip
congenital dysplasia of the hip
CDHP 5-chloro-2 4-dihydroxypyridine
CDI Children's Depression Inventory
clean, dry, and intact
Clostridium difficile infection
color Doppler imaging
conformation-dependent immunoassay
Cotrel Duobosset Instrumentation
CDIC *Clostridium difficile*-induced colitis
C Dif *Clostridium difficile*
C Diff *Clostridium difficile*
CDJ choledochojejunostomy
CDK climatic droplet keratopathy
cyclin-dependent kinase
CDKI cyclin-dependent kinase inhibitor
CDK2 cyclin-depenent kinases 2
CDLC continuous double-loop closure
CDLE chronic discoid lupus erythematosus
CdLS Cornelia de Lange syndrome
CDM charge description master
clinical development monitor
CDMS Certified Disability Management Specialist
clinically definite multiple sclerosis
CDO cartilage disorder
CDONA/LTC Certified Director of Nursing Administration in Long-Term Care
CDP cancer detection program
chemical dependence profile
Chemical Dependency Professional
Child Development Program
clinical development plan
complete decongestive physiotherapy
crystalline degradation product
cytidine diphosphate
CDQ corrected development quotient
CDR cancer detection rate
Cause of Death Registry
clinical data repository
Clinical Dementia Rating
cognitive dietary restraint
commonly deleted region
continuing disability review
CDRH Center for Devices and Radiological Health
CDR(H) cup-to-disc ratio horizontal
CDRs complementary determining regions
CDRS Children's Depression Rating Scale

CDR(V)	cup-to-disc ratio vertical
CDS	Chemical Dependency Specialist
	Chronic Disease Score
	closed-door seclusion
	color Doppler sonography
	continuous dopamine stimulation
CDSC	Communicable Disease Surveillance Centre (United Kingdom)
CDSPIES	congestive heart failure, drugs, spasm, pneumothorax, infection, embolism, and secretions (differential diagnosis mnemonic)
CDSR	Cochrane Database of Systematic Reviews
CDSS	Cervical Dystonia Severity Scale
CDSSs	clinical decision support systems
CDT	carbohydrate-deficient transferrin
	catheter-directed thrombolysis
	Chemical Dependency Technician
	clinical development team
	Clock-Drawing Test
	complete decongestive therapy (for lymphedema)
	connecting discourse tracking (measure of speech perception)
	cystic dysplasia of the testis
	current dental terminology
	cytolethal distending toxin
CDTA	cyclohexane-1,2-diaminetetraacetic acid
CDTM	collaborative drug therapy management
CDU	chemical dependency unit
	color-coded duplex ultrasonography
CDV	canine distemper virus
	cardiovascular
	cyclophosphamide, doxorubicin, and vincristine
CDX	chlordiazepoxide (Librim)
cDXA	central dual-energy X-ray absorptiometry
cdyn	dynamic compliance
CE	California encephalitis
	capillary electrophoresis
	capsule endoscopy
	carboplatin and etoposide
	cardiac enlargement
	cardiac enzymes
	cardioesophageal
	Carpentier-Edwards (heart-valve prosthesis)
	cataract extraction
	central episiotomy
	chemoembolization
	chest expansion
	cholesterol ester
	community education
	Conformité Europène (an indication of compliance to all EU directives)
	conjugated estrogens
	consultative examination
	continuing education
	contrast echocardiology
	cystic echinococcosis
C&E	consultation and examination
	cough and exercise
	curettage and electrodesiccation
CEA	carcinoembryonic antigen
	carotid endarterectomy
	continuous epidural anesthesia
	cost-effectiveness analysis
CEB	calcium entry blocker
	carboplatin, etoposide, and bleomycin
CEBV	chronic Epstein-Barr virus
CEC	capillary electrochromatography
	Council for Exceptional Children
CECA	Childhood Experience of Care and Abuse (interview)
CECD	congenital endothelial corneal dystrophy
CE$\bar{c}$/IOL	cataract extraction with intraocular lens
CECT	contrast-enhanced computed tomography
CED	Camurati-Engelmann disease
	clinically effective dose
	convection-enhanced delivery
	cystoscopy-endoscopy dilation
CEDS	Certified Eating Disorders Specialist
CEE	Central European encephalitis
	conjugated equine estrogen (Premarin; conjugated estrogen)
CEF	chick embryo fibroblast
	cyclophosphamide, epirubicin, and fluorouracil
CEFM	continuous external fetal monitoring
CEFOT	cefotaxime (Claforan)
CEFOX	cefoxitin (Mefoxtin)
CEFTAZ	ceftazidime
CEFUR	cefuroxime
CEI	continuous extravascular infusion
	converting enzyme inhibitor
CEJ	cementoenamel junction (dental)
	cervical-enamel junction (dental)
CEL	cardiac exercise laboratory
CELIP	Claims Expansion Line-item Processing
CELP	chronic erosive lichen planus
CEM	Clinical Event Manager
CEMD	consultative examination by physician
CE-MRA	contrast-enhanced magnetic resonance angiography
ceMRI	contrast-enhanced magnetic resonance imaging
CEN	Certified Emergency Nurse

Abbreviation	Meaning
	European Committee for Standardization
CENOG	computerized electroneuro-ophthalmogram
CEO	chief executive officer
CEOT	calcifying epithelial odontogenic tumor
CEP	cardiac enzyme panel
	chronic eosinophilic pneumonia
	cognitive evoked potential
	congenital erythropoietic porphyria
	countercurrent electrophoresis
	cyclophosphamide, etoposide, and cisplatin (Platinol AQ)
CEPE	cataract extraction by phacoemulsification
CEPH	cephalic
	cephalosporin
CEPH FLOC	cephalin flocculation
CEPP (B)	cyclophosphamide, etopside, procarbazine, prednisone, and bleomycin
CER	conditioned emotional response
CE&R	central episiotomy and repair
CERA	continuous erythropoiesis receptor activator (methoxy polyethylene glycol-epoetin beta [MICERA])
	cortical evoked response audiometry
CERAD	Consortium to Establish a Registry for Alzheimer Disease
CERD	chronic end-stage renal disease
CERT	Comprehensive Error Rate Testing
CERULO	ceruloplasmin
CERV	cervical
CES	Cauda equina syndrome
	central excitatory state
	cognitive environmental stimulation
	estrogen, conjugated (conjugated estrogen substance)
CESB	chronic electrical stimulation of the brain
CES-D	Center for Epidemiologic Studies – Depression
CESI	cervical epidural steroid injection
CET	common extensor tendon
CETC	circulating epithelial tumor cells
CETN	Certified Enterostomal Therapy Nurse
CETP	cholesteryl ester transfer protein
CEU	Utah residents with ancestry from northern and western European ancestry (populations included in HapMap - see HapMap)
CEUS	contrast-enhanced ultrasonography
CEV	cyclophosphamide, etoposide, and vincristine
CE w/IOL	cataract extraction with intraocular lens
CF	calcium leucovorin (citrovorum factor)
	cancer-free
	cardiac failure
	Caucasian female
	Christmas factor
	cisplatin and fluorouracil
	complement fixation
	contractile force
	count fingers
	cystic fibrosis
C3F8	perfluoropropane
C&F	cell and flare
	chills and fever
CFA	common femoral artery
	complete Freund adjuvant
	cryptogenic fibrosing alveolitis
	cystic fibrosis anthropathy
CFAC	complement-fixing antibody consumption
C-factor	cleverness factor
CFCF	carbon fiber composite frame cage
CFCs	chlorofluorocarbons
CFD	color-flow Doppler
	computational fluid dynamics
CFDS	color flow Doppler sonography
CFEOM	congenital fibrosis of the extraocular muscles
CFF	critical fusion (flicker) frequency
CFFT	critical flicker fusion threshold
CFG	comfort function goal (guideline for pain tolerance)
	convergent functional genomics
CFH	chemical fume hood
	complement factor H
CFI	chemotherapy-free intervals
	confrontation fields intact
CFIDS	chronic fatigue immune dysfunction syndrome
CFL	cadaveric fascia lata
	calcaneofibular ligament
	cisplatin, fluorouracil, and leucovorin calcium
CFLX	ciprofloxacin (Cipro)
	circumflex
CFM	cerebral function monitor
	close fitting mask
	craniofacial microsomia
	cyclophosphamide, fluorouracil, and mitoxantrone
CFNS	chills, fever, and night sweats
CFOI	Census of Fatal Occupational Injuries (US Bureau of Labor Statistics report)
CFP	cystic fibrosis protein
CFPT	cyclophosphamide, fluorouracil, prednisone, and tamoxifen
CFR	case-fatality rates

	Code of Federal Regulations
	coronary flow reserve
CFRB	critical findings read back
CFRN	Certified Flight Registered Nurse
CFRP	carbon-fiber reinforced polymer
CFS	cancer family syndrome
	Child and Family Service
	childhood febrile seizures
	chronic fatigue syndrome
	congenital fibrosarcoma
	craniofacial surgery
CFSAN	Center for Food Safety and Applied Nutrition (FDA)
CFT	capillary filling time
	chronic follicular tonsillitis
	chronic food toxicity (obesity) (slang)
	complement fixation test
CFTR	cystic fibrosis transmembrane (conductance) regulator
	cystic fibrosis transmembrane receptor
CFU	colony-forming units
CFU-E	colony-forming unit–erythroid
CFU-G	colony-forming unit–granulocyte
CFU-G/M	colony-forming unit–granulocyte/macrophage
CFU-M	colony-forming unit–macrophage
CFU-Mk	colony-forming unit–megakaryocyte
CFU-S	colony-forming unit–spleen
CFV	common femoral vein
CFVR	coronary flow velocity reserve
CFX	circumflex artery
CG	cardiogreen (dye)
	caregiver
	cholecystogram
	contact guarding
	contralateral groin
CGA	clonal group A
	comprehensive geriatric assessment
	contact guard assist
	corrected gestation age
CGB	chronic gastrointestinal (tract) bleeding
CGCG	central giant-cell granuloma
CGCR	Clinical Global Consensus Rating
CGD	chronic glycogen deficit
	chronic granulomatous disease
	cobalt gray equivalent
CGF	continuous gavage feeding (infant feeding)
CGI	Clinical Global Impressions (scale)
CGIC	Clinical Global Impression of Change
CGI-S	Clinical Global Impressions, Severity of Illness
CGL	chronic granulocytic leukemia

	with correction/with glasses
CGM	continuous glucose monitoring
	cortical gray matter
CGMP	Current Good Manufacturing Practices
cGMP	cyclic guanosine monophosphate
CGN	Certified Gastroenterology Nurse
	chronic glomerulonephritis
cGN	crescentic glomerulonephritis
C-GRD	coffee-ground
CGRN	Certified Gastroenterology Registered Nurse
CGRP	calcitonin gene-related peptide
CGS	cardiogenic shock
	catgut suture
	centimeter-gram-second system
CGTT	cortisol glucose tolerance test
cGVHD	chronic graft-versus-host disease
cGy	centigray
CH	Caribbean Hispanic
	chest
	chief
	child (children)
	chronic
	cluster headache
	concentric hypertrophy
	congenital hypothyroidism
	convalescent hospital
	crown-heal
C_h	hepatic clearance
ch^1	Christ Church chromosone
CH_{50}	total hemolytic complement
C&H	cocaine and heroin
CHA	compound hypermetropic astigmatism
	congenital hypoplastic anemia
CHAD	cyclophosphamide, altretamine, (hexamethylmelamine), doxorubicin (Adriamycin), and cisplatin (DDP)
CHADS	an index that quantifies baseline risk of stroke for individuals with atrial fibrillation (congestive heart failure, hypertension, age greater than 75, diabetic, and history of stroke)
CHAI	Commission for Healthcare Audit and Inspection (United Kingdom)
	continuous hepatic artery infusion
CHAID	Chi Square Automatic Interaction Detection
CHAM-OCA	cyclophosphamide, hydroxyurea, dactinomycin, methotrexate, vincristine, leucovorin, and doxorubicin
CHAM-PUS	Civilian Health and Medical Program of the Uniformed Services

CHAMPVA	Civilian Health and Medical Program-Veterans Administration
Chandelier sign	used to describe a patient who experiences extreme pain during a physical examination (slang)
CHAP	child health associate practitioner
	cyclophosphamide, altretamine, (hexamethylmelamine), doxorubicin (Adriamycin), and cisplatin (Platinol)
CHAQ	childhood health assessment questionnaire
CHARGE	coloboma (of eyes), hearing deficit, choanal atresia, retardation of growth, genital defects (males only), and endocardial cushion defect
CHART	complaint, history, assessment, Rx (treatment), transport
	continuous hyperfractionated accelerated radiotherapy
	Craig Handicap Assessment and Reporting Technique
CHB	chronic hepatitis B
	complete heart block
	congenital heart block
	Han Chinese from Beijing (populations included in HapMap - see HapMap)
CHBHA	congenital Heinz body hemolytic anemia
CHC	community health center
	concentric hypertrophic cardiomyopathy
CH_3–CCNU	semustine
CHCT	caffeine-halothane contracture test
cHct	central hematocrit
CHD	center hemodialysis
	changed diaper
	childhood diseases
	chronic hemodialysis
	common hepatic duct
	congenital heart disease
	coordinate home care
CHE	chronic hepatic encephalopathy
	comprehensive health examination
CHEDDAR	Chief Compliant; History: social and physical as well as contributing factors; Examination; Details of problems and complaints; Drugs and dosage—list current meds; Assessment, diagnostic process, total impression; Return visit information or referral (format of documentation)
CHEF	clamped homogeneous electric field
ChEI	cholinesterase inhibitor
CHEM 7	see page 318
CHEMO	chemotherapy
ChemoRx	chemotherapy
chemo/XRT	chemotherapy with radiation therapy
CHEOPS	Children's Hospital of Eastern Ontario Pain Scale
CHEP	cricohyoidoepiglottopexy
CHESS	chemical shift suppression
CHF	chronic heart failure
	congestive heart failure
	Crimean hemorrhagic fever
CHFV	combined high-frequency of ventilation
CHG	change
	chlorhexidine gluconate
CHI	chikungunya virus vaccine
	closed head injury
	Consolidated Health Informatics
	contrast harmonic imaging
	creatinine-height index
	crushing head injury (injuries)
CHIBLOC	closed head injury, brief loss of consciousness
CHID	Combined Health Information Database
CHIK	Chikungunya (virus)
CHIKV	Chikungunya virus
CHILD	congenital hemidysplasia with ichthyosiform nevus and limb defects (syndrome)
CHIN	community health information network
CHIP	Children's Health Insurance Program
	comprehensive health insurance plan
	iproplatin
ChIP	chromatin immunoprecipitation
CHIR	Chiron Corporation
Chix	chickenpox
CHL	conductive hearing loss
CHLC	Cooperative Human Linkage Center
ChloMP	chlorambucil, mitoxantrone, and prednisolone
ChlVPP	chlorambucil, vinblastine, procarbazine, and prednisone
CHM	complete hydatidiform mole
CHMP	Committee for Medicinal Products for Human Use (EMEA)
CHN	central hemorrhagic necrosis
	Certified Hemodialysis Nurse
	Chinese herb nephropathy
	Community Health Nurse
	community nursing home
CHO	carbohydrate
	Chemical Hygiene Officer
	Chinese hamster ovary
–CHO	aldehyde

C_{H_2O}	free-water clearance
CHO_a	cholera vaccine, attenuated live (oral)
CHOC	chocolate
CHO_{cn}-LPS	cholera vaccine, lipopolysaccharide-toxin conjugate
C_2H_5OH	alcohol (ethyl alcohol)
$CHO_{i\text{-}w}$	cholera vaccine, inactivated whole cell
$CHO_{i\text{-}w\text{-}BS}$	cholera vaccine, inactivated whole cell, B subunit
chol	cholesterol
$\bar{c}$ hold	withhold
Chole	cholecystectomy
CHO_o	cholera, oral vaccine
CHOP	cyclophosphamide, doxorubicin (hydroxy-daunorubicin), vincristine (Oncovin), prednisone
CHOP-Bleo	cyclophosphamide, doxorubicin (hydroxydaunorubicin), vincristine (Oncovin), prednisone, and bleomycin
CHO_{tox}	cholera toxin/toxoid vaccine
CHP	Certification in Healthcare Privacy
CHPB	Canadian Health Protection Branch (the equivalent of the U.S. Food and Drug Administration)
CHPN	Certified Hospice and Palliative Nurse
CHPV	Codman Hakim programmable valve
CHPX	chickenpox
CHR	Cercaria-Hullen reaction
	chronic
	complete hematological response
ChronoHAI	circadian-based hepatic artery infusion
CHRN	Certified Hyperbaric Registered Nurse
CHRPE	congenital hypertrophy of the retinal pigment epithelium
CHRS	congenital hereditary retinoschisis
CHS	Chediak-Higashi syndrome
	contact hypersensitivity
CHT	Certified Hand Therapist
	Certified Hyperbaric Technician
	Certified Hypnotherapist
	chemotherapy
	closed head trauma
ChT	chemotherapy
CHTN	chronic hypertension
CHU	closed head unit
CHUC	Certified Health Unit Coordinator
CHVP	cyclophosphamide, doxorubicin (hydroxydaunorubicin), teniposide (VM26), and prednisone
CHW	community health workers
CHWG	chewing gum
CHX	chlorhexidine (Peridex; Periogard)
CI	cardiac index
	cerebral infarction
	cesium implant
	Clinical Instructor
	cochlear implant
	cognitively impaired
	colon inertia
	commercial insurance
	complete iridectomy
	confidence interval
	continuous infusion
	contraindications
	convergence insufficiency
	core imprint (cytology)
	coronary insufficiency
Ci	curie(s)
CI30	cumulative incidence at 30 years
CIA	calcaneal insufficiency avulsion
	chemotherapy-induced amenorrhea
	chemotherapy-induced anemia
	chronic idiopathic anhidrosis
	collagen-induced arthritis
CIAA	competitive insulin autoantibodies
CIACS	cocaine-induced acute coronary syndrome
CIAED	collagen-induced autoimmune ear disease
cIAI	complicated intraabdominal infections
CIB	Carnation Instant Breakfast®
	crying-induced bronchospasm
	cytomegalic inclusion bodies
CIBD	chronic inflammatory bowel disease
CIBI	Clinician Interview-Based Impression (of change)
CIBIC	Clinician Interview-Based Impression of Change
CIBIC-plus	Clinician Interview-Based Impression of Change with Caregiver Input
CIBP	chronic intractable benign pain
C-IBS	constipated predominant irritable bowel syndrome
CIC	cardioinhibitory center
	Certified in Infection Control
	circulating immune complexes
	clean intermittent catheterization
	completely in-the-canal (hearing aid)
	coronary intensive care
CICE	combined intracapsular cataract extraction
CICU	cardiac intensive care unit
CICVC	centrally inserted central venous catheter
CID	Center for Infectious Diseases (CDC)
	Central Institute for the Deaf

	cervical immobilization device
	chemotherapy-induced diarrhea
	collision-induced dissociation
	combined immunodeficiency
	cytomegalic inclusion disease
CIDP	chronic inflammatory demyelinating polyradiculoneuropathy (polyneuropathy)
CIDS	cellular immunodeficiency syndrome
	continuous insulin delivery system
CIE	capillary immunoelectrophoresis
	chemotherapy-induced emesis
	congenital ichthyosiform erythroderma
	counterimmunoelectrophoresis
	crossed immunoelectrophoresis
CIEA	continuous infusion epidural analgesia
CIEF	capillary isoelectric focusing
CIEP	counterimmunoelectrophoresis
	crossed immunoelectrophoresis
CIFN	chemotherapy-induced fever and neutropenia
CI 5-FU	continuous infusion of fluorouracil
CIG	cigarettes
CIH	Certified in Industrial Health
	continuous infusion haloperidol
CIHD	chronic ischemic heart disease
CIHI	Canadian Institute for Health Information
CIHR	Canadian Institutes of Health Research
CII	continuous insulin infusion
CIIA	common internal iliac artery
CIL	carbamazepine-induced lupus
CIM	change in menses
	chemotherapy-induced mucositis
	constraint-inducedmovement
	convective interaction media
	corticosteroid-induced myopathy
	critical illness myopathy
CIMCU	cardiac intermediate care unit
CIMT	carotid (artery) intimamedia thickness
	constraint-induced movement therapy
CIN	cervical intraepithelial neoplasia
	chemotherapy-induced neutropenia
	chronic interstitial nephritis
C_{IN}	insulin clearance
CIN3+	cervical intraepithelial neoplasia grade 3 or worse
CINAHL	Cumulative Index to Nursing and Allied Health
CIND	cognitive impairment, no dementia
CINE	chemotherapy-induced nausea and emesis
	cineangiogram
CINV	chemotherapy-induced nausea and vomiting
CIO	corticosteroid-induced osteoporosis
CIOMS	The Council for International Organization of Medical Sciences
CIP	Cardiac Injury Panel
	critical illness polyneuropathy
CIPD	chronic intermittent peritoneal dialysis
CIPN	chemotherapy-induced peripheral neuropathy
CipRGC	ciprofloxacin-resistant *Neisseria gonorrhoeae*
CIR	continent intestinal reservoir
CIRB	central institutional review board
Circ	circulation
	circumcision
	circumference
	circumflex
circ. & sen.	circulation and sensation
CIRF	cocaine-induced respiratory failure
CIRM	California Institute of Regenerative Medicine
CIRS-G	Cumulative Illness Rating Scale-Geriatric
CIRT	carbon ion radiotherapy
CIS	Cancer Information Service (National Cancer Institute)
	carcinoma in situ
	clinically isolated syndrome
	Commonwealth of Independent States
	continuous interleaved sampling
CI&S	conjunctival irritation and swelling
CISC	clean intermittent self-catheterization
CISCA	cisplatin, cyclophosphamide, and doxorubicin (Adriamycin)
CISCOM	The Centralized Information Service for Complementary Medicine
CISD	critical incident stress debriefing (used by EMTs)
Cis-DDP	cisplatin (Platinol)
CISH	chromogen in situ hybridization
CISM	critical incident stress management (debriefing used by EMTs)
CIS-R	Clinical Interview Schedule, Revised
CISS	constructive interface in steady state (imaging)
CI-Stim	cochlear implant stimulation
CIT	chemotherapy-induced toxicities
	cold ischemia time
	constraint-induced therapy (protocol)
	conventional immunosuppressive therapy
	conventional insulin therapy
CIT IDS	citation identifiers (National Library of Medicine)
CITP	capillary isotachophoresis

C

CIU	chronic idiopathic urticaria crisis intervention unit
CIV	common iliac vein continuous intravenous (infusion)
CIVD	cold-induced vasodilatation
CIVI	continuous intravenous infusion
CIXU	constant infusion excretory urogram
CIWA-Ar	Clinical Institute Withdrawal Assessment for Alcohol–revised
CJD	Creutzfeldt-Jakob disease
cJET	congenital junctional ectopic tachycardia
CJR	centric jaw relation
CJS	chronic joint symptoms
CK	check conductive keratoplasty creatine kinase
CK-BB	creatine kinase BB band (primarily in brain)
CKC	cold-knife conization
CKD	chronic kidney disease
CK-ISO	creatine kinase isoenzyme
CK-MB	creatine kinase MB fraction (primarily in cardiac muscle)
CK MM	creatine kinase MM fraction (primarily in skeletal muscle)
CKW	clockwise
Cl	chloride (Cl^-)
CL	central line chemoluminescence clear liquid cleft lip cloudy confidence limits contact lens critical list cutaneous leishmaniasis cycle length lung compliance
C_L	compliance of the lungs
C-L	consultation-liaison
CLA	community living arrangements congenital lactic acidosis congenital laryngeal atresia conjugated linoleic acid
CLABSI	central line-associated bloodstream infection
C lam	cervical laminectomy
CLAMSS	cleavage- and ligation-associated mutation-specific sequencing
CLAP	contact laser ablation of prostate
CLARE	contact lens-associated acute red eye
CLAS	Cancer Linear Analogue Scale congenital localized absence of skin
CLASS	computer laser-assisted surgical system
CLASS I	congestive heart failure with no limitation with ordinary activity (New York Heart Association Classification)
CLASS II	congestive heart failure with slight limitation of physical activity
CLASS III	congestive heart failure with marked limitation of physical activity
CLASS IV	congestive heart failure with inability to engage in any physical activity without symptoms
Clav	clavicle
CLB	chlorambucil (Leukeran) coccidian-like body
CLB_{atx}	*Clostridium botulinum* antitoxin
CLBBB	complete left bundle branch block
CLBD	cortical Lewy body disease
CLBP	chronic low back pain
CLB_{tox}	*Clostridium botulinum* toxoid vaccine
CLC	cork leather and celastic (orthotic)
CL/CP	cleft lip and cleft palate
CLD	central lung distance chronic liver disease chronic lung disease *Clostridium difficile* vaccine
Cl_d	dialysis clearance
CLE	centrilobular emphysema congenital lobar emphysema constant-load exercise continuous lumbar epidural (anesthetic)
CLED	cysteine lactose electrolyte-deficient (agar)
CLEIA	chemiluminescent enzyme immunoassay
CLEP	college level examination program
CLF	cholesterol-lecithin flocculation
CLG	clorgyline
CLH	chronic lobular hepatitis
C_h	hepatic clearance
CLI	central lymphatic irradiation clomipramine (Anafranil) critical leg (limb) ischemia
CLIA	chemiluminescent immunoassay Clinical Laboratory Improvement Act
CLINDA	clindamycin (Cleocin)
Cl_{int}	intrinsic clearance
CLL	chronic lymphocytic leukemia
CLLE	columnar-lined lower esophagus
cl liq	clear liquid
CLM	colorectal liver metastases cutaneous larva migrans
CLN	centrolobular necrosis
CLNC	Certified Legal Nurse Consultant
Cl_{nr}	nonrenal clearance
CLO	Campylobacter-like organism

close
cod liver oil
CLOX clock-drawing task (cognitive impairment test)
CL & P cleft lip and palate
CL PSY closed psychiatry
CLPU contact lens-induced peripheral ulceration
Cl_r renal clearance
CLRB clinical laboratory (results) read back
Cl Red closed reduction
CLRO community leave for reorientation
CLS capillary leak syndrome
community living skills
CLSE calf-lung surfactant extract (Infasurf)
CLSI Clinical and Laboratory Standards Institute
CLSM confocal laser scanning microscopy
CLT chronic lymphocytic thyroiditis
complex lymphedema therapy
cool lace tent
Cl_T total body clearance
CLV cuff-leak volume
cutaneous leukocytoclastic vasculitis
CL VOID clean voided specimen
CLW_c *Clostridium welchii* type C (Pigbel) toxoid vaccine
clysis hypodermoclysis
CLZ clozapine (Clozaril)
cm centimeter (2.54 cm = 1 inch)
CM capreomycin (Capastat)
CarboMedics (heart valve prosthesis)
cardiac monitor
cardiomegaly
cardiomyopathy
case management
case manager
Caucasian male
centimeter (cm)
cerebral malaria
Chiari malformation
chondromalacia
chronic migraine (headache)
cochlear microphonics
common migraine
continuous microwave
continuous murmur
contrast media
costal margin
cow's milk
culture media
cutaneous melanoma
cystic mesothelioma
tomorrow morning (this is a dangerous abbreviation)
cM centimorgan (one one-hundredth of a morgan; the unit of distance on a linkage map)
CM-I Chiari malformation Type I
cm1 circumflex marginal 1
cm2 circumflex marginal 2
cm^2 square centimeters
cm^3 cubic centimeter
CMA Certified Medical Assistant
Certified MovementAnalyst
compound myopic astigmatism
cost-minimization analysis
cow's milk allergy
CMAF centrifuged microaggregate filter
CMAI Cohen-Mansfield Agitation inventory
CMAP compound muscle action potential
CMAPs compound muscle action potentials
C_{max} maximum concentration of drug
CMB carbolic methylene blue
CMBBT cervical mucous basal body temperature
CMC carboxymethylcellulose
carpal metacarpal (joint)
chloramphenicol
chronic mucocutaneous candidiasis
clinically meaningful change
closed mitral commissurotomy
CMCD carboxymethylcellulose dressing
CMCN Certified Managed Care Nurse
CMD congenital muscular dystrophy
corrected mass defect
cytomegalic disease
CMDRH Center for Medical Devices and Radiological Health (of the Food and Drug Administration)
CME cervicomediastinal exploration (examination)
continuing medical education
cystoid macular edema
CMER current medical evidence of record
CMF chondromyxoid fibroma
cyclophosphamide, methotrexate and fluorouracil
CMFP cyclophosphamide, methotrexate, fluorouracil, and prednisone
CMFT cyclophosphamide, methotrexate, fluorouracil, and tamoxifen
CMFVP cyclophosphamide, methotrexate, fluorouracil, vincristine, and prednisone
CMG cystometrogram
CMGM chronic megakaryocytic granulocytic myelosis
CMGN chronic membranous glomerulonephritis
CMGs case-mix groups
CMH Cochran Mantel Haenszel
current medical history
CMHC Certified Mental Health Counselor
Community Mental Health Center

	Community Migrant Health Center
CMHN	Community Mental Health Nurse
CMI	case mix index
	cell-mediated immunity
	clomipramine (Anafranil)
	collagen meniscus implant
	Consumer Medicine Information (Australia)
	Cornell Medical Index
CMID	cytomegalic inclusion disease
C_{min}	minimum concentration of drug
CMIR	cell-mediated immune response
CMJ	carpometacarpal joint
	cervicomedullary junction
CMK	congenital multicystic kidney
CML	cell-mediated lympholysis
	chronic myelogenous leukemia
	chronic myeloid leukemia
CML5	lower second premolar
CML-BP	blastic phase chronic myeloid leukemia
CMM	Comprehensive Major Medical (insurance)
	continuous metabolic monitor
	cutaneous malignant melanoma
CMME	chloromethyl methyl ether
CMML	chronic myelomacrocytic leukemia
CMMS	Columbia Mental Maturity Scale
CMN	Certificate of Medical Necessity
	congenital melanocytic nevi
	congenital mesoblastic nephroma
CMO	cardiac minute output
	cetyl myristoleate
	Chief Medical Officer
	comfort measures only (resuscitation order)
	consult made out
CMO 1	corticosterone methyl oxidase type 1
CMOP	cardiomyopathy
C-MOPP	cyclophosphamide, mechlorethamine, vincristine (Oncovin), procarbazine, and prednisone
CMP	cardiomyopathy
	chondromalacia patellae
	comprehensive (complete) metabolic profile (see page 318)
	cushion mouthpiece
CMPA	cow's milk protein allergy
CMPF	cow's milk, protein-free
CMPS	chronic myofascial pain syndrome
CMPT	cervical mucous penetration test
CMR	cardiometabolic risk
	cardiovascular magnetic resonance
	cerebral metabolic rate
	chief medical resident
	child (1-4 years) mortality rates
	chloroform-methanol residue
	crude mortality rate
CMRI	cardiac magnetic resonance imaging
CMRIT	combined modality radioimmunotherapy
CMRNG	chromosomally mediated resistant *Neisseria gonorrhoeae*
CMRO	chronic multifocal recurrent osteomyelitis
$CMRO_2$	cerebral metabolic rate for oxygen
CMS	cardiometabolic syndrome
	Centers for Medicare and Medicaid Services (replaces Health Care Financing Administration [HCFA])
	children's medical services
	circulation motion sensation
	chocolate milkshake
	constant moderate suction
	continuous motion syndrome
CMSC	Certified Medical Staff Coordinator
CMSUA	clean midstream urinalysis
CMT	carpometatarsal (joint)
	Certified Massage Therapist
	Certified Medication Technician
	Certified Medical Transcriptionist
	Certified Music Therapist
	cervical motion tenderness
	Charot-Marie-Tooth (phenotype) (disease)
	Chiropractic manipulative treatment
	choline magnesium trisalicylate (Trilisate)
	combined modality therapy
	continuing medication and treatment
	cutis marmorata telangiectasia
CMTX	chemotherapy treatment
CMUA	continuous motor unit activity
CMV	cisplatin, methotrexate, and vinblastine
	controlled mechanical ventilation
	conventional mechanical ventilation
	cool mist vaporizer
	cytomegalovirus
	cytomegalovirus vaccine
CMVIG	cytomegalovirus immune globulin
CMVS	culture midvoid specimen
CN	charge nurse
	congenital nystagmus
	cranial nerve
	tomorrow night (this is a dangerous abbreviation)
Cn	cyanide
C/N	contrast-to-noise ratio
CN II–XII	cranial nerves 2 through 12
CNA	Certified in Nursing Administration
	Certified Nursing Assistant
	chart not available
C_{Na}	sodium clearance

CNAA	Certified in Nursing Administration, Advanced
CNAG	chronic narrow angle glaucoma
CNAP	continuous negative airway pressure
CNB	core-needle biopsy
CNC	clinical nurse coordinator
	Community Nursing Center
	Consonant-Vowel Nucleus-Consonant (Maryland CNC word list)
CNCbl	cyanocobalamin (vitamin B_{12})
CND	canned
	cannot determine
	chronic nausea and dyspepsia
CNDC	chronic nonspecific diarrhea of childhood
CNE	Chief Nurse Executive
	chronic nervous exhaustion
	continuing nursing education
	could not establish
	culture-negative endocarditis
CNEP	continuous negative extrathoracic pressure
C-NES	conversion nonepileptic seizures
CNF	cyclophosphamide, mitoxantrone (Novatantrone), and fluorouracil
CNG	complete, no growth
CNH	central neurogenic hypernea
	contract nursing home
CNHC	chronodermatitis nodularis helicis chronicus
	community nursing home care
CNI	calcineurin inhibitors
CNL	chemonucleolysis
	chronic neutrophilic leukemia
	Connaught Laboratories
CNLCP	Certified Nurse Life Care Planner
CNLD	chronic neonatal lung disease
CNLSD	condensation nucleation light scattering detection
CNM	certified nurse midwife
CNMP	chronic nonmalignant pain
CNMT	Certified Nuclear Medicine Technologist
CNN	Certified in Nephrology Nursing
	congenital nevocytic nevus
CNNP	Certified Neonatal Nurse Practitioner
CNO	Chief Nursing Officer
	community nursing organization
CNOP	cyclophosphamide, mitoxantrone (Novantrone), vincristine (Oncovin), and prednisone
CNOR	Certified Nurse, Operating Room
CNP	capillary nonprofusion
CNPB	continuous negative pressure breathing
CNPS	cardiac nuclear probe scan
CNR	contrast-to-noise ratio (radiology)
CNRN	Certified Neurosurgical Registered Nurse
CNS	central nervous system
	Certified Nutrition Specialist
	Clinical Nurse Specialist
	coagulase-negative staphylococci
	Crigler-Najjar syndrome
CNSC	Certified Nutrition Support Clinician
CNSD	Certified Nutrition Support Dietitian
CNSHA	congenital nonspherocytic hemolytic anemia
CNSN	Certified Nutrition Support Nurse
CNT	could not tell
	could not test
CNTA	combined neurosurgical and transfacial approach
CNTF	ciliary neurotrophic factor
CNV	choroidal neovascularization
	copy number variations
CNVM	choroidal neovascular membrane
CO	carbon monoxide
	cardiac output
	castor oil
	centric occlusion
	Certified Orthoptist
	cervical orthosis
	corneal opacity
	corn oil
	court order
Co	cobalt
C/O	check out
	complained of
	complaints
	under care of
^{60}Co	radioactive isotope of cobalt
CO_2	carbon dioxide
CO_3	carbonate
COA	children of alcoholic
	coenzyme A
	condition on admission
CoA	coarctation of the aorta
COAD	chronic obstructive airway disease
	chronic obstructive arterial disease
COAG	chronic open angle glaucoma
COAGSC	coagulation screen
COAP	cyclophosphamide, vincristine (Oncovin), cytarabine (ara-C), and prednisone
COAR	coarctation
COARCT	coarctation
COB	cisplatin, vincristine (Oncovin), and bleomycin
	coordination of benefits
COBE	chronic obstructive bullous emphysema

C

C

COBRA Consolidated Omnibus Budget Reconciliation Act of 1985
COBS chronic organic brain syndrome
COBT chronic obstruction of biliary tract
COC calcifying odontogenic cyst
chain of custody
combination oral contraceptive
continuity of care
COCCIO coccidioidomycosis
COCM congestive cardiomyopathy
COCN Certified Ostomy Care Nurse
CoCr cobalt-chromium alloy
COD carotid occlusive disease
cataract, right eye
cause of death
chronic oxygen dependency
codeine
coefficient of oxygen delivery
condition on discharge
CODAS chronotherapeutic oral drug absorption system
CODE 99 patient in cardiac or respiratory arrest
Code Blue patient in cardiac or pulmonary arrest
Code Brown a patient's bed containing feces (slang)
Code Yellow a patient's bed containing urine (slang)
CODES Crash Outcome Data Evaluation System (National Highway Traffic Safety Administration-sponsored)
COD-MD cerebro-oculardysplasia muscular dystrophy
CODO codocytes
COE court-ordered examination
COEPS cortically originating extrapyramidal symptoms
COER-24 24-hour controlled-onset, extended-release (dosage form)
COFS cerebro-oculo-facioskeletal
COG center of gravity
Central Oncology Group
Children's Oncology Group
cognitive function tests
COGN cognition
COGTT cortisone-primed oral glucose tolerance test
COH carbohydrate
controlled ovarian hyperstimulation
COHb carboxyhemoglobin
COHN Certified Occupational Health Nurse
COHN/CM Certified Occupational Health Nurse/Case Manager
COHN-S Certified Occupational Health Nurse - Specialist
COHN-S/CM Certified Occupational Health Nurse - Specialist Case Manager
COI conflict of interest
Coke Coca-Cola®
cocaine
COL colonoscopy
COLD chronic obstructive lung disease
Computer Output to Laser Disk
COLD A cold agglutin titer
Collyr eye wash
col/mL colonies per milliliter
colp colporrhaphy
COLTRU *colletotrichum truncatum*
COM calcium oxalate monohydrate
center of mass
chronic otitis media
COMBO combination ultrasound with electrical stimulation
COME chronic otitis media with effusion
COMF comfortable
COMLA cyclophosphamide, vincristine (Oncovin), methotrexate, calcium leucovorin, and cytarabine (ara-C)
COMM E Committee E, a German Federal Health Agency committee for the evaluation of herbal remedies
COMP Committee on Orphan Medicinal Products (EMEA)
compensation
complications
composite
compound
compress
cyclophosphamide, vincristine (Oncovin), methotrexate, and prednisone
CO-MRSA community-onset methicillin-resistant *Staphylococcus aureus*
COMS clinical outcomes management system
COMT catechol-*O*-methyl-transferase
Certified Ophthalmic Medical Technologist
COMTA Commission on Message Therapy Accreditation
CON catheter over a needle
certificate of need
conservatorship
CON A concanavalin A
conc. concentrated
CONEP National Commission for Ethics in Research (Brazil)
CONG congenital
gallon
CONJ conjunctiva
CONPA-DRI I cyclophosphamide, vincristine, doxorubicin, and melphalan
CONPA-DRI II conpadri I plus high-dose methotrexate

CONPA-DRI III	conpadri I plus intensified doxorubicin
CoNS	coagulase-negative staphylococci
CONT	continuous
	contusions
CON-TRAL	contralateral
CONTU	contusion
CONV	conversation
Conv. ex.	convergence excess
ConvRX	conventional therapy
–COOH	carboxylic acid
CO-Ox	Co-oximetry
COP	center of pressure
	change of plaster
	cicatricial ocular pemphigoid
	Colibacilosis porcina vaccine
	colloid osmotic pressure
	complaint of pain
	cryptogenic organizing pneumonia
	cycophosphamide, vincristine (Oncovin), and prednisone
CoP	Communities of Practice
	Conditions of Participation
COP 1	copolymer 1
COPA	cuffed oropharyngeal airway
COPAdM	cyclophosphamide, vincristine (Oncovin), prednisone, doxorubicin (Adriamycin) and methotrexate
COP-BLAM	cyclophosphamide, vincristine (Oncovin), prednisone, bleomycin, doxorubicin (Adriamycin), and procarbazine (Matulane)
COPD	chronic obstructive pulmonary disease
COPE	chronic obstructive pulmonary emphysema
COPP	cyclophosphamide, vincristine, procarbazine, and prednisone
COPS	community outpatient service
COPT	circumoval precipitin test
CoQ10	coenzyme Q_{10}
COR	coefficient of reproducibility
	conditioned orientation response
	coronary
CoR	custodian of records
CORA	conditioned orientation reflex audiometry
CORBA	Common-Object Request Broker Architecture
CORE	cardiac or respiratory emergency
CORF	Comprehensive Outpatient Rehabilitation Facility
CORLN	Certified Otorhinolaryngology and Head/Neck Nurse
COR P	cor pulmonale
CORT	Certified Operating Room Technician
COS	cataract, left eye
	change of shift
	Chief of Staff
	clinically observed seizure
	controlled ovarian stimulation
	Crisis Outpatient Services
C_{osm}	osmolal clearance
COSTART	<u>Co</u>ding <u>s</u>ymbols for a <u>t</u>hesaurus of <u>a</u>dverse <u>r</u>eaction <u>t</u>erms
COT	content of thought
	court-ordered treatment
COTA	Certified Occupational Therapy Assistant
COTE	comprehensive occupational therapy evaluation
COTT CH	cottage cheese
COTX	cast-off, to x-ray
COU	cardiac observation unit
	cataracts, both eyes
COV	coefficient of variation
COW	circle of Willis
COWA	controlled oral word association
COWAT	Controlled Oral Word Association Test
COWS	Clinical Opioid Withdrawal Scale
	cold to the **o**pposite and **w**arm to the **s**ame
COX	Coxsackie virus
	cyclo-oxygenase
	cytochrome C oxidase
COX-2	cyclo-oxygenase-2
CP	centric position
	cerebellopontine (angles)
	cerebral palsy
	Certified Paramedic
	chemical peel
	chemistry profiles
	chest pain
	chloroquine-primaquine
	chondromalacia patella
	chronic pain
	chronic pancreatitis
	cleft palate
	clinical pathway
	closing pressure
	cold pack
	constrictive pericarditis
	convenience package
	cor pulmonale
	creatine phosphokinase
	cyclophosphamide and cisplatin (Platinol)
	cystopanendoscopy
	process capability
C_p	concentration of drug plasma
	phosphate clearance

C

Cp	*Chlamydia pneumoniae*
C/P	carbohydrate-to-protein ratio
C&P	compensation and pension
	complete and pain-free (range of motion)
	complete and pushing
	cystoscopy and pyelography
CPA	cardiopulmonary arrest
	carotid photoangiography
	cerebellar pontile angle
	chest pain alert
	child protection agency
	color power angiography
	conditioned play audiometry
	congenital primary aphakia
	costophrenic angle
	cyclophosphamide (Cytoxan)
	cyproterone acetate (Androcur)
CPAF	chlorpropamide-alcohol flush
C_{PAH}	para-amino hippurate clearance
CPAN	Certified Postanesthesia Nurse
CPAP	continuous positive airway pressure
CPB	cardiopulmonary bypass
	cisplatin, cyclophosphamide, and carmustine (BiCNU)
	competitive protein binding
CPBA	competitive protein-binding assay
CPBP	cardiopulmonary bypass
CPC	cancer prevention clinic
	cerebral palsy clinic
	Certified Professional Coder
	cetylpyridinium chloride
	chronic passive congestion
	clinicopathologic conference
	coil planet centrifuge
	continue plan of care
CPC 1	Cerebral Performance Category 1 (There are also Categories 2 to 5)
CPC-H	Certified Procedural Coder, Hospital-Based
CP-CML	chronic phase chronic myeloid leukemia
CP/CPPS	chronic prostatitis/chronic pelvic pain syndrome
CPCR	cardiopulmonary-cerebral resuscitation
CPCS	clinical pharmacokinetics consulting service
CPCs	calcium phosphate cements
CPD	cephalopelvic disproportion
	chorioretinopathy and pituitary dysfunction
	chronic peritoneal dialysis
	citrate-phosphate-dextrose
CPDA-1	citrate-phosphate-dextrose-adenine-one
CPDA-2	citrate-phosphate-dextrose-adenine-two

CPDD	calcium pyrophosphate deposition disease
CPDG2	carboxypeptidase-G2
CPDN	Certified Peritoneal Dialysis Nurse
CPDR	Center for Prostate Disease Research (Department of Defense)
CPE	cardiogenic pulmonary edema
	chronic pulmonary emphysema
	Clinical Pastoral Education
	Clostridium perfringens enterotoxin
	clubbing, pitting, or edema
	complete physical examination
	continuing professional education
	cytopathic effect
CPEB	cytoplasmic polyadenylation element binding (protein)
CPE-C	cyclopentenylcytosine
CPEFM	Clear-Plan Easy Fertility Monitor
CPEO	chronic progressive external ophthalmoplegia
CPER	chest pain emergency room
CPET	cardiopulmonary exercise testing
CPETU	chest pain evaluation and treatment unit
CPF	cerebral perfusion pressure
	chlorpyrifos (an insecticide)
CPFT	Certified Pulmonary Function Technologist
CPFX	ciprofloxacin (Cipro)
CPG	clinical practice guidelines
CPG2	carboxypeptidase G2
CPGN	chronic progressive glomerulonephritis
CPH	chronic persistent hepatitis
CPHQ	Certified Professional in Healthcare Quality
CPhT	Certified Pharmacy Technician
CPI	chronic public inebriate
	constitutionally psychopathia inferior
CPID	chronic pelvic inflammatory disease
CPIP	chronic pulmonary insufficiency of prematurity
CPK	creatine phosphokinase (BB, MB, MM are isoenzymes)
CPK-1	creatine phosphokinase MM fraction
CPK-2	creatine phosphokinase MB fraction
CPK-BB	creatine phosphokinase BB fraction
CPKD	childhood polycystic kidney disease
CPK-MB	creatine phosphokinase of muscle band
CPL	criminal procedure law
CPM	cancer pain management
	central pontine myelinolysis
	chlorpheniramine maleate
	chronic progressive myelopathy
	Clinical Practice Model
	continue present management
	continuous passive motion

counts per minute
cycles per minute
cyclophosphamide (Cytoxan)

CPmax peak serum concentration

CPMDI computerized pharmacokinetic model-driven drug infusion

CPmin trough serum concentration

CPMM constant passive motion machine

CPMP Committee for Proprietary Medicinal Products (of the European Union)

CPN Certified Pediatric Nurse
chronic pyelonephritis
common peroneal nerve

CPNA Certified Pediatric Nurse Associate

CPNB continuous peripheral nerve block

CPNI common peroneal nerve injury

CPO chief privacy officer
continue present orders

CPOE computerized physician (prescriber) order entry

CPOM continuous pulse oximeter monitoring

CPON Certified Pediatric Oncology Nurse

CPOX chicken pox

CPP central precocious puberty
cerebral perfusion pressure
chronic pelvic pain
coronary perfusion pressure
cryo-poor plasma

CPPB continuous positive pressure breathing

CPPD calcium pyrophosphate dihydrate
cisplatin

CP & PD chest percussion and postural drainage

CPPS chronic pelvice pain syndrome

CPPV continuous positive pressure ventilation

CPQ Conner Parent Questionnaire

CPR cardiopulmonary resuscitation
computer-based patient records
computerized patient record
customary, prevailing and reasonable (charge payment method)
tablet (French)

CPR-1 all measures except cardiopulmonary resuscitation

CPR-2 no extraordinary measures (to resuscitate)

CPR-3 comfort measures only

CPRAM controlled partial rebreathing anesthesia method

CP/ROMI chest pain, rule out myocardial infarction

CPRS Categorical Pain Relief Scale

CPRS-OCS Comprehensive Psychiatric Rating Scale, Obsessive-Compulsive Subscale

CPRU cardiac procedure recovery unit

CPS carbamyl phosphate synthetase
cardiopulmonary support
Center for Prevention Services (CDC)
cervical pedicle screw
chest pain syndrome
child protective services
Chinese paralytic syndrome
chloroquine-pyrimethamine sulfadoxine
chronic paranoid schizophrenia
clinical performance score
clinical pharmacokinetic service
CoaguChek® Plus System
coagulase-positive staphylococci
complex partial seizures
counts per second
cumulative probability of success

CPs clinical pathways

CPS I carbamyl phosphate synthetase I

cPSA complexed prostate-specific antigen

CPSC Consumer Product Safety Commission

CPSI Chronic Prostatitis Symptom Index

CPSN Certified Plastic Surgical Nurse

CPSP central post-stroke pain

CPT camptothecin
carnitine palmitoyl transferase
chest physiotherapy
child protection team
chromo-perturbation
chronic paranoid type
cold pressor test
Continuous Performance Test
corticosteroid pulse treatment
current perception threshold
Current Procedural Terminology (coding system)

CPT-2007 Current Procedural Terminology, 2007 Edition

CPT-11 irinotecan hydrochloride (Camptosar)

CPTA Certified Physical Therapy Assistant

CPT/C current perception threshold, computerized

CPTH chronic post-traumatic headache

CPU children's psychiatric unit
clinical pharmacology unit

CPUE chest pain of unknown etiology

CPUM Certified Professional in Utilization Management

CPV canine parvovirus
cowpox virus

CPX complete physical examination

CPZ chlorpromazine
Compazine® (CPZ is a dangerous abbreviation as it could be either)

CQ chloroquine

C

CQDS	cumulative quality disruption score
CQI	continuous quality improvement
CR	caloric restrictions
	capillary refill
	cardiac rehabilitation
	cardiorespiratory
	case reports
	chief resident
	chorioretinal
	clockwise rotation
	closed reduction
	colon resection
	complete remission
	contact record
	controlled release
	cosmetic rhinoplasty
	creamed
	credentialing
	crutches
	cycloplegia retinoscopy
Cr	caloric restrictions
	chromium
	creatinine
C/R	conscious, rational
C & R	convalescence and rehabilitation
	cystoscopy and retrograde
CR_1	first cranial nerve
CRA	central retinal artery
	chronic rheumatoid arthritis
	cis-retinoic acid (isotretinion, Accutane®)
	Clinical Research Associate
	colorectal anastomosis
	Contract Research Assistant
	corticosteroid-resistant asthma
CRABP	cellular retinoic acid binding protein
CRAbs	chelating recombinant antibodies
CRADA	Cooperative Research and Development Agreement (with NIH)
CRAG	cerebral radionuclide angiography
CrAg	cryptococcal antigen
CRAMS	circulation, respiration, abdomen, motor, and speech
CRAN	craniotomy
CRAO	central retinal artery occlusion
CRAX	crackers
CRB	Clinical Review Board
CRBBB	complete right bundle branch block
CRBIs	catheter-related bloodstream infections
CRBP	cellular retinol-binding protein
CRBSI	catheter-related bloodstream infections
CRC	case review committee
	child-resistant container
	clinical research center
	Clinical Research Coordinator
	colorectal cancer
CR & C	closed reduction and cast
CrCl	creatinine clearance
CRCLM	colorectal cancer liver metastases
CRCS	colorectal cancer screening
CRD	childhood rheumatic disease
	chronic renal disease
	chronic respiratory disease
	colorectal distension
	cone-rod dystrophy
	congenital rubella deafness
	crown-rump distance
CRE	cumulative radiation effect
CREAT	serum creatinine
CREC	ciprofloxacin-resistant *Escherichia coli*
CREF	cycloplegic refraction
CRELM	screening tests for Congo-Crimean, Rift Valley, Ebola, Lassa, and Marburg fevers
CREP	crepitation
CREST	calcinosis, Raynaud disease, esophageal dysmotility, sclerodactyly, and telangiectasia
CRF	cancer-related fatigue
	cardiac risk factors
	case report form
	chronic renal failure
	corticotrophin-releasing factor
CRFs	clinical risk factors
CRG-L2	Cancer related gene-Liver 2
CRH	corticotropic-releasing hormone
CRFZ	closed reduction of fractured zygoma
CRH	corticotropin-releasing hormone
CRHCa	cancer-related hypercalcemia
CRI	Cardiac Risk Index
	catheter-related infection
	chronic renal insufficiency
CRIB	Clinical Risk Index for Babies
CRIE	crossed radioimmunoelectrophoresis
CRIF	closed reduction and internal fixation
CRIM	cross-reacting immunologic material
CRIMF	closed reduction/intermaxillary fixation
CRIS	controlled-release infusion system
crit	hematocrit
CRKL	crackles
CRL	crown rump length
CRM	circumferential resection margins
	continual reassessment method
	cream
	cross-reacting mutant
CRM +	cross-reacting material positive
CRMD	children with retarded mental development
CRMO	chronic recurrent multifocal osteomyelitis

CRN	Certified Radiologic Nurse
	crown
CRNA	Certified Registered Nurse Anesthetist
CRNFA	Certified Registered Nurse, First Assistant
CRNH	Certified Registered Nurse in Hospice
CRNI	Certified Registered Nurse Intravenous
CRNL	Certified Registered Nurse - Long-Term Care
CRNO	Certified Registered Nurse in Ophthalmology
CRNP	Certified Registered Nurse Practitioner
CRO	cathode ray oscilloscope
	contract research organization(s)
CROACC	cannot rule out anything, correlate clinically (slang)
CROM	cervical range of motion
	chronic refractory osteomyelitis
CROMY	chronic refractory osteomyelitis
Crook-U	a prison ward in a hospital (slang)
CROS	contralateral routing of signals
CRP	canalith repositioning procedure
	chronic relapsing pancreatitis
	coronary rehabilitation program
	C-reactive protein
C&RP	curettage and root planning
CRPA	C-reactive protein agglutinins
CRPC	castration-refractory prostate cancer
CRPD	chronic restrictive pulmonary disease
CRPF	chloroquine-resistant *Plasmodium falciparum*
CRPP	closed reduction and percutaneous pinning
CRPS	complex regional pain syndromes
CRPS I	complex regional pain syndrome type I
CRQ	Chronic Respiratory (Disease) Questionnaire
CRR	community rehabilitation residence
CRRN	Certified Rehabilitation Registered Nurse
CRRN-A	Certified Rehabilitation Registered Nurse - Advanced
CRRT	continuous renal replacement therapy
CRS	Carroll Self-Rating Scale
	catheter-related sepsis
	Center for Scientific Review (NIH)
	Chemical Reference Substances
	child restraint system(s)
	Chinese restaurant syndrome
	chronic rhinosinusitis
	cocaine-related seizure(s)
	colon-rectal surgery
	congenital rubella syndrome
	continuous running suture
	cryoreductive surgery
	cytokine-release syndrome
CRSD	circadian rhythm sleep disorder
CRST	calcification, Raynaud phenomenom, scleroderma, and telangiectasia
CRT	cadaver renal transplant
	capillary refill time
	Cardiac Rescue Technician
	cardiac resynchronization therapy
	cartilage roof triangle
	cathode ray tube
	central reaction time
	Certified Rehabilitation Therapist
	chemoradiotherapy
	choice reaction time
	circuit resistance training
	copper reduction test
	cranial radiation therapy
CRT-D	cardiac resynchronization therapy defibrillator
Cr Tr	crutch training
CRTs	case report tabulations
CRTT	Certified Respiratory Therapy Technician
CRTX	cast removed take x-ray
CRTx	chemoradiotherapy
CRU	cardiac rehabilitation unit
	catheterization recovery unit
	clinical research unit
CRV	central retinal vein
CRVF	congestive right ventricular failure
CRVO	central retinal vein occlusion
CRx	chemotherapy
CIIRx	Century II Bicarbonate Dialysis Machine
CRYO	cryoablation
	cryosurgery
CRYST	crystals
CS	cardiogenic shock
	cardioplegia solution
	cat scratch
	cervical spine
	cesarean section
	chest strap
	cholesterol stone
	chlorobenzylidene malononitrile
	cigarette smoker
	clinically significant
	Clinical Specialist
	clinical stage
	close supervision
	conditionally susceptible
	congenital syphilis
	conjunctiva-sclera
	consciousness
	conscious sedation

	consultation
	consultation service
	coronary sinus
	corticosteroid(s)
	cranial setting
	Cushing syndrome
	cycloserine
	o-chlorobenzylidene malononitrile
C&S	conjunctiva and sclera
	cough and sneeze
	culture and sensitivity
C/S	cesarean section
	consultation
	culture and sensitivity
CSA	central sleep apnea
	childhood sexual abuse
	compressed spectral activity
	Controlled Substances Act
	controlled substance analogue
	corticosteroid-sensitive asthma
	cryosurgical ablation
CsA	cyclosporine (cyclosporin A)
CsA-ME	cyclosporine microemulsion (Neoral)
CSAP	cryosurgical ablation of the prostate
CSB	caffeine sodium benzoate
	Cheyne-Stokes breathing
	Children's Services Board
CSBF	coronary sinus blood flow
CSBM	complete spontaneous bowel movements
CSBO	complete small bowel obstruction
CSC	central serous chorioretinopathy
	cornea, sclera, and conjunctiva
	cryogen spray cooling
	cryopreserved stem cells
CSCI	continuous subcutaneous infusion
CSCR	central serous chorioretinopathy
CSD	cat scratch disease
	celiac sprue disease
	cortical spreading depression
C S&D	cleaned, sutured, and dressed
CSDD	Center for the Study of Drug Development
CSDH	chronic subdural hematoma
	combined systolic and diastolic hypertension
CSE	combined spinal/epidurals
	cross-section echocardiography
CSEA	combined spinal-epidural anesthesia
C sect.	cesarean section
CSF	cerebrospinal fluid
	colony-stimulating factors
CSFELP	cerebrospinal fluid electrophoresis
CSFP	cerebrospinal fluid pressure
CSGIT	continuous-suture graft-inclusion technique
C-Sh	chair shower
CSH	carotid sinus hypersensitivity
	chronic subdural hematoma
	combat surgical hospital(s)
CSHQ	Children's Sleep Habits Questionnaire
CSI	chemical shift imaging
	Computerized Severity Index
	continuous subcutaneous infusion
	coronary stent implantation
	corticosteroid injection
	craniospinal irradiation
CsI	cesium iodide
CSICU	cardiac surgery intensive care unit
CSID	congenital sucrase-isomaitase deficiency
CSII	continuous subcutaneous insulin infusion
CSIO	continuous subcutaneous infusion of opiates
CS IV	clinical stage 4
CSL	chemical safety level
CSLO	confocal scanning laser ophthalmoscopy
CSLU	chronic status leg ulcer
CSM	carotid sinus massage
	cerebrospinal meningitis
	cervical spondylotic myelopathy
	circulation, sensation, and movement
	Committee on Safety of Medicines (United Kingdom)
CSMC	Cedars-Sinai Medical Center (Los Angeles, CA)
CSME	cotton-spot macular edema
CSMN	chronic sensorimotor neuropathy
CSN	Certified School Nurse
	cystic suppurative necrosis
CSNB	congenital stationary night blindness
CSNRT	corrected sinus node recovery time
CSNS	carotid sinus nerve stimulation
CSO	Chief Security Officer
	Consumer Safety Officer (FDA)
	copied standing orders
CSOM	chronic serous otitis media
	chronic suppurative otitis media
CSP	cellulose sodium phosphate
	cervical spine pain
	chiral stationary phase
C-SPI	Certified Specialist in Poison Information
C-spine	cervical spine
CSR	central supply room
	Cheyne-Stokes respiration
	clinical statistical report
	combat stress reaction
	corrected sedimentation rate
	corrective septorhinoplasty
C-S RT	craniospinal radiotherapy

CSS	Canadian Stroke Scale (score)
	carotid sinus stimulation
	Central Sterile Services
	chemical sensitivity syndrome
	chewing, sucking, and swallowing
	child safety seats
	Churg-Strauss syndrome
C_{ss}	concentration of drug at steady-state
CSSD	closed system sterile drainage
CSSS	coronary subclavian steal syndrome
CSSSIs	complicated skin and skin-structure infections
CSSU	cardiac short-stay unit
CST	cardiac stress test
	castration
	central sensory conducting time
	cerebroside sulfotransferase
	Certified Surgical Technologist
	cesarean section prior to labor at term
	contraction stress test
	convulsive shock therapy
	cosyntropin stimulation test
	static compliance
CSTAT	static lung compliance
CSTD	closed-system (drug) transfer device
CSTE	Council of State and Territorial Epidemiologists
CSTO	cat smarter than owner (Veterinary slang)
CSU	cardiac surgery unit
	cardiac surveillance unit
	cardiovascular surgery unit
	casualty staging unit
	catheter specimen of urine
CSVD	cerebral small-vessel disease
CSVT	cerebral sinovenous thrombosis
CSW	cerebral salt-wasting (syndrome)
	Clinical Social Worker
	commercial sex worker
CSWCM	Certified Social Work Case Manager
CSWD	conservative sharp wound debridement
	corticosteroid withdrawal
CSWs	commercial sex workers
CSWSS	continuous spike-waves during slow sleep
CSX	cardiac syndrome X
CT	calcitonin
	calf tenderness
	cardiothoracic
	carpal tunnel
	cellulose triacetate (filter)
	cervical traction
	chemotherapy
	chest tube
	Chlamydia trachomatis
	circulation time
	client
	clinical trial
	clotting time
	coagulation time
	coated tablet
	compressed tablet
	computed tomography
	Coomb test
	corneal thickness
	corneal transplant
	corrective therapy
	cytarabine and thioguanine
	cytoxic drug
C_t	concentration of drug in tissue
C/T	compared to
CTA	catamenia (menses)
	clear to auscultation
	composite tissue allograft
	computed tomographic angiography
CTAB	clear to auscultation, bilaterally
C-TAB	cyanide tablet
CTAP	clear to auscultation and percussion
	computed tomography during arterial portography
CTB	ceased to breathe
	cholera toxin B
CTC	Cancer Treatment Center
	circular tear capsulotomy
	circulating tumor cells
	Clinical Trial Certificate (United Kingdom's equivalent to the Investigational New Drug Application)
	Common Toxicity Criteria
	computed tomographic colonography
	cyclophosphamide, thiotepa, and carboplatin
CTCAE v3.0	Common Terminology Criteria for Adverse Events, version 3.0 (National Cancer Institute grading system for treatment-related toxicities; grade 1 = mild, grade 2 = moderate, grade 3 = severe, grade 4 = life-threatening or disabling, grade 5 = death related to adverse event)
CTCL	cutaneous T-cell lymphoma (mycosis fungoides)
CTCOFR	Composite Time to Complete Organ Failure Resolution
CT & DB	cough, turn & deep breath
CTD	carboxy-terminal domain
	carpal tunnel decompression
	chest tube drainage
	Common Technical Document
	connective tissue disease
	corneal thickness depth
	cumulative trauma disorder

CTDI	computed tomography dose index
CTDW	continues to do well
CTE	chronic traumatic encephalopathy
CTEP	Cancer Therapy Evaluation Program Center for Therapy Evaluation Programs (National Cancer Institute)
CTF	clanging tuning fork (test) Colorado tick fever continuous tube feeding
CTG	cardiotocography
C/TG	cholesterol to triglyceride ratio
CTGA	complete transposition of the great arteries corrected transposition of the great arteries
CTGF	connective tissue growth factor
CTH	clot to hold
CTHA	computed tomography hepatic arteriography
CTI	cavotricuspid isthmus certification of terminal illness
cTI	cardiac troponin I
CTIBL	cancer treatment-induced bone loss
CTICU	cardiothoracic intensive care unit
CTID	chemotherapy-induced diarrhea
CTL	cervical, thoracic, and lumbar chronic tonsillitis control (subjects) cytotoxic T-lymphocytes
CTLM	computed tomography-laser mammography
CTLSO	cervicothoracic-lumbosacral orthosis
CTM	Chlor-Trimeton clinical trials materials computed tomographic myelography
CT/MPR	computed tomography with multiplanar reconstructions
CTMS	clinical trial management systems
CTN	calcitonin Certified Transcultural Nurse
C & T N, BLE	color and temperature normal, both lower extremities
cTnC	cardiac troponin C
cTnI	cardiac troponin I
cTNM	clinical-diagnostic staging of cancer
CTnT	cardiac troponin T
CTO	chronic total (coronary) occlusion
CTP	comprehensive treatment plan
CTPA	clear to percussion and auscultation
CTPN	central total parenteral nutrition
CTR	capsular tension ring carpal tunnel release carpal tunnel repair Certified Tumor Registrar cosmetic transdermal reconstruction
CTRB	Clinical Trial Review Board critical tests read back
CTRS	Certified Therapeutic Recreation Specialist Conners Teachers Rating Scale
CT-RT	chemo-radiotherapy
CTS	cardiothoracic surgeon carpal tunnel syndrome closed-tube sampling
CTSP	called to see patient
CTT	congenital trigger thumb cotton-thread test
CTTH	chronic tension-type headache
CTU	computed tomographic urography
CTW	central terminal of Wilson
CTX	cerebrotendinous xanthomatosis cervical traction chemotherapy cyclophosphamide (Cytoxan)
CTXN	contraction
CTZ	chemoreceptor trigger zone co-trimoxazole (sulfamethoxazole and trimethoprin)
CU	cause undetermined cause unknown chronic undifferentiated clinical units color unit convalescent unit Cuprophan (filter)
Cu	copper
C_u	urea clear clearance
C/U	checkup creatinine/urea ratio
CUA	Certified Urologic Associate clean urinalysis cost-utility analysis
CUC	chronic ulcerative colitis Clinical Unit Clerk
CUCNS	Certified Urologic Clinical Nurse Specialist
CUD	cause undetermined controlled unsterile delivery
CUFCM	Century Ultrafiltration Control Machine
CUG	cystourethrogram
Cu-IUD	copper intrauterine device
CUNP	Certified Urologic Nurse Practitioner
CUOG	Canadian Urologic Oncology Group
CUP	carcinoma of unknown primary (site)
CUPS	carcinoma of unknown primary site
CUR	curettage cystourethrorectocele
CURN	Certified Urologic Registered Nurse
CUS	carotid ultrasound chronic undifferentiated schizophrenia compression ultrasonography contact urticaria syndrome

CUSA	Cavitron ultrasonic suction aspirator
CUT	chronic undifferentiated type (schizophrenia)
CUTA	congenital urinary tract anomaly
CV	cardiovascular
	cell volume
	cisplatin and etoposide (VePesid)
	coefficient of variation
	color vision
	common ventricle
	consonant vowel
	contrast venography
	curriculum vitae
C/V	cervical/vaginal
CVA	cerebrovascular accident
	costovertebral angle
	cough-variant asthma
CVAAS	cold vapor atomic absorption spectrometry
CVAD	central venous access device
CVAH	congenital virilizing adrenal hyperplasia
CVAT	costovertebral angle tenderness
CVB	chronic villi biopsy
	group B coxsackievirus
CVC	central venous catheter
	chief visual complaint
	consonant-vowel-consonant
CVD	cardiovascular disease
	collagen vascular disease
CVDU	chronic ventilator-dependent unit
CVEB	cisplatin, vinblastine, etoposide, and bleomycin
CVENT	controlled ventilation
CVEs	cerebrovascular events
CVF	cardiovascular failure
	cardiovascular fitness
	central visual field
	cervicovaginal fluid
	cobra venom factor
	colovesical fistula
CVG	cochleovestibular ganglion
	coronary vein graft
	cutis verticis gyrata
CVHD	chronic valvular heart disease
CVI	carboplatin, etoposide, ifosfamide, and mesna uroprotection
	cerebrovascular insufficiency
	chronic venous insufficiency
	common variable immunodeficiency (disease)
	continuous venous infusion
CVICU	cardiovascular intensive care unit
CVID	common variable immune deficiency
CVINT	cardiovascular intermediate
CVL	central venous line
	cervicovaginal lavage
	clinical vascular laboratory
CVLP	chimeric virus-like particles
CVLT	California Verbal Learning Test
CVM	Center for Veterinary Medicine (NIH)
CVMP	Committee for Medicinal Products for Veterinary Use (EMEA)
CVMT	cervical-vaginal, motion tenderness
CVN	central venous nutrient
	Certified Vascular Nurse
CVNSR	cardiovascular normal sinus rhythm
CVO	central vein occlusion
	conjugate diameter of pelvic inlet
CvO_2	mixed venous oxygen content
CVOD	cerebrovascular obstructive disease
CVOR	cardiovascular operating room
CVP	central venous pressure
	cyclophosphamide, vincristine, and prednisone
CVPP	lomustine, vinblastine, procarbazine, and prednisone
CVR	cerebral vascular resistance
	cerebrovascular resuscitation
	coronary vascular reserve
CVRI	coronary vascular resistance index
CVRS	Cardiovascular-Respiratory Score
CVS	cardiovascular surgery
	cardiovascular system
	challenge virus standard
	chorionic villi sampling
	clean voided specimen
	continuing vegetative state
CVSCU	cardiovascular special care unit
CVSD	congenital ventricular septal defect
CVST	cardiovascular stress test
	cerebral venous sinus thrombosis
CVSU	cardiovascular specialty unit
CVT	calf vein thrombosis
	cephalic vein transposition
	cerebral venous thrombosis
CVTC	central venous tunneled catheter
CVU	clean voided urine
CVUG	cysto-void urethrogram
CVVH	continuous venovenous hemofiltration
CVVHDF	continuous venovenous hemodiafiltration
CW	careful watch
	case worker
	chest wall
	clockwise
	compare with
C/W	consistent with
	crutch walking
CWA	chemical warfare agents
CWAF	Chemical Withdrawal Assessment Flowsheet

C

CWAP continuous wave arthroscopy pump
CWCN Certified Wound Care Nurse
CWD canal-wall down
cell-wall defective
change wet dressing
chronic wasting disease
CWE cotton-wool exudates
CWL Caldwell-Luc
CWM comprehensive weight management
CWMS color, warmth, movement, and sensation
CWOCN Certified Wound, Ostomy and Continence Nurse
CWP centimeters of water pressure
childbirth without pain
coal worker's pneumoconiosis
cold wet packs
cWPW concealed Wolff-Parkinson-White syndrome
CWR clockwise rotation
CWS Certified Wound Care Specialist
comfortable walking speed
cotton-wool spots
CWT compensated work training
CWV closed wound vacuum
CX cancel
cervix
chronic
circumflex
circumflex artery
culture
cylinder axis
cystectomy
Cx consultation
CXA circumflex artery
CxBx cervical biopsy
CxMT cervical motion tenderness
CXR chest x-ray
CXTX cervical traction
CY calendar year
cyclophosphamide (Cytoxan)
C&Y Children with Youth (program)
CYA cover your ass
CyA cyclosporine
CyADIC cyclophosphamide, doxorubicin (Adriamycin), and dacarbazine
CYC cyclophosphamide
Cyclo C cyclocytidine HCl
CYL cylinder
CYP cytochrome P-450 system
CYP450 cytochrome P450 system
CYRO cryoprecipitate
CYSTA cystathionine
CYSTO cystogram
cystoscopy
CYT cyclophosphamide (Cytoxan)
CYTA cytotoxic agent
CYVA DIC cyclophosphamide, vincristine, Adriamycin, and dacarbazine (DTIC)
CZ central zone (prostate needle biopsy location)
CZE capillary zone electrophoresis
CZI crystalline zinc insulin (regular insulin)
CZP clonazepam (Klonopin)

D

D	daughter
	day
	dead
	decay
	dependent
	depression
	dextrose
	dextro
	diarrhea
	diastole
	dictated
	dilated
	diminished
	Dinamap (blood pressure monitor)
	diopter
	distal
	distance
	divorced
	dream
D+	note has been dictated/look for report
D−	note not dictated, save chart for doctor
$D_{0(2/7/07)}$	Day zero (the day treatment begins, February 7th, 2007)
D_1	day one (first day of treatment)
	first diagonal branch (coronary artery)
D-1 . . . . D-12	dorsal vertebrae 1 to 12
	dorsal nerves 1-12
D_2	second diagonal branch (coronary artery)
	ergocalciferol
2/d	twice a day (this is a dangerous abbreviation)
2-D	two-dimensional
3-D	three-dimensional
D_3	cholecalciferol
D-3+7	cytarabine and daunorubicin
4D	4 prism diopters
4-D	four-dimensional
D5	dextrose 5% injection
5xD	five times a day (this is a dangerous abbreviation)
D-15	Farnsworth panel D-15 color vision test
D50	50% dextrose injection
$D_{5/.45}$	dextrose 5% in 0.45% sodium chloride injection
DA	darbepoetin alfa (Aranesp)
	dark adaptation (test)
	Debtors Anonymous
	degenerative arthritis
	delivery awareness
	Dental Assistant
	diagnostic arthroscopy
	diastolic augmentation
	direct admission
	direct agglutination
	disk areas
	diversional activity
	dopamine
	drug addict
	drug aerosol
Da	daltons
D/A	discharge and advise
DAA	dead after arrival
	dissection aortic aneurysm
DA/A	drug/alcohol addiction
DAB	days after birth
	diamino benzidine
DABA	Diplomate of the American Board of Anesthesiology
DAC	day activity center
	decitabine
	disabled adult child
	Division of Ambulatory Care
DACL	Depression Adjective Checklists
DACS	density-adjusted cell sorting
DACT	dactinomycin (Cosmegen)
DAD	diffuse alveolar damage
	diode array detector
	Disability Assessment of Dementia
	dispense as directed
	drug administration device
	father
DADS	distal acquired demyelinating symmetrical (neuropathy)
DAE	diving air embolism
DAEC	diffuse-adherence *Entamoeba coli*
DAF	decay-accelerating factor
	delayed auditory feedback
DAFE	Dial-A-Flow Extension®
DAFM	double-aerosol face mask
DAFNE	dose adjustment for normal eating
DAG	diacylglyerol
	dianhydrogalactitol
DAH	diffuse alveolar hemorrhage
	disordered action of the heart
DAI	diffuse axonal injury
DAIDS	Division of AIDS (of the National Institute of Allergy and Infectious Diseases, NIH)
DAL	diffuse aggressive lymphomas
	drug analysis laboratory
DALE	disability-adjusted life expectancy
DALK	deep anterior lamellar keratoplasty
DALM	dysplasia-associated lesion or mass
DALY	disability-adjusted life year(s)
DAM	diacetylmonoxine

DAMA	discharged against medical advice
DAMP	deficits in attention, motor control, and perception
DAN	diabetic autonomic neuropathy
DANA	drug-induced antinuclear antibodies
DAo	descending aorta
DAOM	depressor anguli oris muscle
DAP	dapsone
	diabetes-associated peptide
	diastolic augmentation pressure
	distending airway pressure
	Draw-A-Person
DAPT	Draw-A-Person Test
DAR	daily affective rhythm
	data, action, response
DARB	darbepoetin alfa (Aranesp)
DARE	data, action, response, and evaluation
DARP	drug abuse rehabilitation program
	drug abuse reporting program
DARPA	Defense Advanced Research Projects Agency (US Department of Defense)
DARQ	diarylquinoline
D/ART	depression/awareness, recognition and treatment
DAS	day of admission surgery
	developmental apraxia of speech
	died at scene
	disease activity score
	distractive auditory stimuli
	dynamometer anchoring station
DAs	daily activities
DASE	dobutamine-atropine stress echocardiography
DASH	Dietary Approaches to Stop Hypertension (diet)
	Disabilities of the Arm, Shoulder and Hand (questionnaire/rating)
DASI	Duke Activity Status Index
DAST	Drug Abuse Screening Test
DAT	daunorubicin, cytarabine, (ara-C), and thioguanine
	definitely abnormal tracing (electrocardiogram)
	dementia of the Alzheimer type
	diet as tolerated
	diphtheria antitoxin
	direct agglutination test
	direct amplification test
	direct antiglobulin test
DAU	daughter
	drug abuse urine
DAUNO	daunorubicin
DAVA	vindesine sulfate (Eldisine; desacetyl vinblastine amide sulfate)
DAVE	The Data Assessment and Verification program
DAVM	dural arteriovenous malformation
DAV SEP	deviated septum
DAW	dispense as written
DAWN	Drug Abuse Warning Network
dB	decibel
DB	database
	date of birth
	Decision Board
	deep breathe
	demonstration bath
	dermabrasion
	diaphragmatic breathing
	difficulty breathing
	direct bilirubin
	double blind
DBA	Diamond-Blackfan anemia
dBA	decibel, weighted according to the A scale
DB & C	deep breathing and coughing
DBD	mitolactol (dibromodulicitol)
DBDS	Dementia Behavior Disturbance Scale
DBE	deep breathing exercise
	double-balloon endoscopy
DBED	penicillin G benzathine (for IM use only; Bicillin L-A)
dBEMCL	decibel effective masking contralateral
D_5BES	dextrose in balanced electrolyte solution
DBI	documented by initials
DBI®	phenformin HCl
DBIL	direct bilirubin
DBKT	Diabetes: Basic Knowledge Test
DBL	double beta-lactam
DBM	dibenzoylmethane
DBMT	displacement bone marrow transplantation
DBP	D-binding protein
	diastolic blood pressure
	dibutyl phthalate
DBPCFC	double-blind, placebo-controlled food challenge
DBPT	dacarbazine (DTIC), carmustine (BCNU), cisplatin (Platinol), and tamoxifen
DBQ	debrisoquin
DBS	deep brain stimulation
	desirable body weight
	diminished breath sounds
	dorsal blocking splint
	dried blood stain
DBSs	dietary botanical supplements
DBT	dialectical behavior therapy
DBW	dry body weight
DBZ	dibenzamine
DC	daunorubicin and cytarabine
	daycare
	deceleration capacity (heart)

decrease
dendritic cells
dextrocardia
diagonal conjugate
direct Coombs (test)
direct current
discharge (This is a dangerous abbreviation as it is read as discontinue)
discomfort
displacement chromatography
Doctor of Chiropractic
dorsal compartment

D&C dilatation and curettage
direct and consensual

D/C disconnect
discontinue

DCA dichloroacetate
directional coronary atherectomy
disk/condyle adhesion
double-cup arthroplasty
sodium dichloroacetate

DCAG double-coronary artery graft

DCAP-BTLS deformities, contusions, abrasions, and punctures/penetrations, burns, tenderness, lacerations, and swelling (an assessment mnemonic used by EMTs)

DC-ART disease controlling anti-rheumatic therapy

DC&B dilation, currettage, and biopsy

DCBE double-contrast barium enema

DCC day care center(s)
diabetes care clinic
direct current cardioversion

DCCF dural carotid-cavernous fistula

DCCs day care centers

DCCT Diabetes Control and Complications Trial (questionnaire)

DCD developmental coordination disorder
donation after cardiac death

DC'd discontinued

DCE delayed contrast-enhancement
designated compensable event
detection-controlled estimation
distal clavicle excision

D&C&E dilation, curettage, and evacuation

DCE-MRI dynamic contrast enhanced magnetic resonance imaging

DCF data collection form
Denomination Commune Francaise (French-approved nonproprietary name)
docetaxel, cisplatin, and fluorouracil
pentostatin (Nipent; 2′ deoxycoformycin)

DCFS Department of Children and Family Services

DCG diagnostic cardiogram

DCH delayed cutaneous hypersensitivity

DCI decompression illness

DCIA deep circumflex iliac artery (flap)

DCIS ductal carcinoma *in situ*

DCL diffuse cutaneous leishmaniasis

DC-LAMP dendritic cell-lysosomal-associated membrane protein

DCLHb diaspirin cross-linked hemoglobin

DCM dementia care mapping
dilated cardiomyopathy

DCMP dilated cardiomyopathy

DCMXT dichloromethotrexate

DCN Darvocet N

DCNU chlorozotocin

DCO damage control orthopedics
death certificates only (cases known only from death certificates)
diffusing capacity of carbon monoxide

DCP dynamic compression plate

DCP® calcium phosphate, dibasic

DCPM daunorubicin, cytarabine, prednisolone, and mercaptopurine

DCPN direction-changing positional nystagmus

DCR dacryocystorhinostomy
delayed cutaneous reaction
distal clavicle resection

DCRC disseminated colorectal cancer

DCRF data case report forms

3DCRT three-dimensional conformal radiation therapy

DCS damage-control surgery
decompression sickness
dorsal column stimulator

DCSA double-contrast shoulder arthrography

dcSSc diffuse cutaneous systemic sclerosis

DCSW Diplomate in Clinical Social Work

DCT daunorubicin, cytarabine, and thioguanine
decisional conflict theory
deep chest therapy
direct (antiglobulin) Coombs test
dynamic contour tonometry

DCTM delay computer tomographic myelography

DCU day care unit

DCUS duplex-color ultrasonography

DCVC dual-channel virus counter

DCW direct care worker

DCYS Department of Children and Youth Services

DD delayed diarrhea
delivery date
dependent drainage
Descemet detachment

detrusor dyssynergia
developmentally delayed
developmental disabilities
developmental dyslexia
developmentally disabled
dialysis dementia
died of the disease
differential diagnosis
disc diameter
discharge diagnosis
Doctor of Divinity
dose-dense
double dose (used by Radiology)
down drain
dry dressing
dual disorder
Duchenne dystrophy
due date
dysthymic disorder

D/D diarrhea/dehydration
D → D discharge to duty
D & D debridement and dressing
diarrhea and dehydration
divorced and desperate (middle aged female who visits doctor weekly just for male attention) (slang)
drilling and drainage
DDA dideoxyadenosine
DDAH dimethylarginine dimethylaminohydrolase
DDAVP® desmopressin acetate
DDC dose-dense chemotherapy
zalcitabine (dideoxy-cytidine; Hivid)
DDCI dopadecarboxylase inhibitor
DDD defined daily doses
degenerative disk disease
dense deposit disease
fully automatic pacing
DDDR pacemaker code (D = chamber paced-**d**ual, D = chamber sensed-**d**ual, D = response to sensing-**d**ual, R = programmability-**r**ate modulation)
DDDR-70 dual-chamber rate responsive pacing at 70/minute
DDE dichlorodiphenylethylene
DDGB double-dose gallbladder (test)
DDH developmental dysplasia of the hip
DDHT double-dissociated hypertropia
DDI didanosine (dideoxyinosine; Videx)
dressing dry, intact
DDIs drug-drug interactions
DDis developmental disorder
DDiv Doctor of Divinity
DDMAC Division of Drug Marketing, Advertising and Communications (FDA)
DDMC diabetes disease management clinic
DDNS digestive disease and nutrition service
DDP cisplatin (Platinol)
DDRA dead despite resuscitation attempt
DDRE Division of Drug Risk Evaluation (FDA)
DDRUL dorsal distal radioulnar ligament
DDS Denys-Drash Syndrome
dialysis disequilibrium syndrome
Doctor of Dental Surgery
double-decidual sac (sign)
4, 4-diaminodiphenyl-sulfone (dapsone)
D & Ds death and doughnuts (morbidity and mortality conferences) (slang)
DDST Denver Development Screening Test
DDT chlorophenothane
DDTP drug dependence treatment program
DDx differential diagnosis
DE dermal epidermal (junction)
digitalis effect
diminished emotionality
D_5E_{48} 5% Dextrose and Electrolyte 48
D_5E_{75} 5% Dextrose and Electrolyte 75
2-DE two-dimensional echocardiography
two-dimentional gel electrophoresis
3-DE three-dimensional echocardiography
D&E dilation and evacuation
DEA# Drug Enforcement Administration number (physician's federal narcotic number)
DEAE diethylaminoethyl
DEB diepoxybutane (test)
dystrophic epidermolysis bullosa
DEC deciduous (primary teeth)
decrease
diethylcarbamazine (Hetrazan)
Drug Evaluation and Classification (a standardized curriculum to train police officers)
DECA nandrolone decanoate (Deca-Durabolin)
DECAFS Department of Children and Family Services
DECEL deceleration
decub decubitus
DED diabetic eye disease
died in emergency department
DEEDS drugs, exercise, education, diet, and self-monitoring
DEEG depth electroencephalogram
deteriorating electroencephalogram
DEET diethyltoluamide
DEF decayed, extracted, or filled
defecation
deficiency
2-DEF two-dimensional echo-derived ejection fraction

DEFIB	defibrillate
DEFT	defendant
	driven equilibrium Fourier transform (technique)
DEG	diethylene glycol
degen	degenerative
DEHP	diethylhexyl phthalate
DEJ	dentin-enamel junction
DEL	delivered
	delivery
	deltoid
DELM	digital epiluminescence microscopy
DEM	drug evaluation matrix
DEMRI	dynamic enhanced magnetic resonance imaging
Denver II	Denver Developmental Screening Test - second edition
DEPs	diesel exhaust particles
DEP ST SEG	depressed ST segment
DER	disulfiram-ethanol reaction
DERM	dermatology
DES	desflurane (Supreme)
	diethylstilbestrol
	diffuse esophageal spasm
	disequilibrium syndrome
	Dissociative Experience Scale
	drug eluting stent
	dry-eye syndrome
	dysfunctional elimination syndrome (urology)
DESAT	desaturation
DESF	desflurane (Suprane)
DESI	Drug Efficacy Study Implementation
DET	diethyltryptamine
	dipyridamole echocardiography test
DETOX	detoxification
DEV	deviation
	duck embryo vaccine
DEVR	dominant exudative vitreoretinopathy
DEX	dexamethasone
	dexrazoxane (Zinecard)
	dexter (right)
	dexverapamil
DEXA	dual-energy x-ray absorptiometry
DF	day frequency (of voiding)
	decayed and filled
	deferred
	defibrotide
	degree of freedom
	dengue fever
	dexfenfluramine
	diabetic father
	diastolic filling
	dietary fiber
	dorsiflexion
	drug-free
	dye-free
DFA	delayed feedback audiometry
	diet for age
	difficulty falling asleep
	direct fluorescent antibody
	distal forearm
DFCI	Dana-Farber Cancer Institute
DFD	defined formula diets
	degenerative facet disease
DFE	dilated fundus examination
	distal femoral epiphysis
DFG	direct forward gaze
DFI	disease-free interval
DFLE	disability-free life expectancy
DFM	decreased fetal movement
	deep finger massage
	deep friction massage
DFMC	daily fetal movement count
DFMR	daily fetal movement record
DFO	deferoxamine (Desferal)
DFOM	deferoxamine (Desferal)
DFP	diastolic filling period
	isoflurophate (diisopropyl flurophosphate)
DFR	diabetic floor routine
DFRC	deglycerolized frozen red cells
DFS	disease-free survival
	Division of Family Services
	Doppler flow studies
DFSP	dermatofibrosarcoma protuberans
DFT	defibrillation threshold (testing)
DFU	dead fetus in uterus
	diabetic foot ulcer
DFV	D'Aoust Fineman virus
	dengue fever vaccine
	diarrhea, fever, and vomiting
DFW	Dexide face wash
DFWO	dorsiflexory wedge osteotomy
DFYS	Division of Family and Youth Services (government agency)
DG	diagnosis
	dorsal glides
	downward gaze
DGA	DiGeorge anomaly
	disseminated granuloma annulare
DGC	dystrophin-glycoprotein complex
DGE	delayed gastric emptying
DGF	delayed graft function
DGGE	denaturing gradient gel electrophoresis
DGI	disseminated gonococcal infection
DGL	deglycyrrhizinated licorice
DGR	duodenogastric reflux
DGM	ductal glandular mastectomy
DGS	DiGeorge syndrome
DGs	documentation guidelines
DGT	decaffeinated green tea
DH	delayed hypersensitivity
	Dental Hygienist

	dermatitis herpetiformis
	developmental history
	diaphragmatic hernia
D+H	delusions and hallucinations
D-H	Dimon-Hughston (intertrochanteric osteotomy technique)
DHA	dihydroxyacetone
	docosahexaenoic acid
DHAC	dihydro-5-azacytidine
DHAD	mitoxanthrone HCl (Novantrone)
DHANP	Diplomate of the Homeopathic Academy of Naturopathic Physicians
DHAP	dexamethasone, high-dose cytarabine, (ara-A) cisplatin (Platinol)
	docosahexaenoic acid-paclitaxel
DHA-TP	dihydroartemisinin, trimethoprim, and piperaquine
DHBV	duck hepatitis B virus
DHCA	deep hypothermia circulatory arrest
DHCC	dihydroxycholecalciferol
DHD	dissociated horizontal deviation
DHE	dental health education
DHE 45®	dihydroergotamine mesylate
DHEA	dehydroepiandrosterone
DHEAS	dehydroepiandrosterone sulfate
DHF	dengue hemorrhagic fever
	diastolic heart failure
DHFR	dihydrofolate reductase
DHHS	Department of Health and Human Services
DHI	Dizziness Handicap Inventory
	dynamic hyperinflation
DHIC	detrusor hyperactivity with impaired contractility
DHL	diffuse histocytic lymphoma
DHP	dental hygiene program
	dihydropyridine
DHP-1	dehydropeptidase-1
DHPG	ganciclovir
DHPLC	denaturing high-performance liquid chromatography
DHPR	dihydropteridine reductase
DHPS	dihydopteroate synthase
DHR	delayed hypersensitivity reaction
DHS	Department of Human Services
	duration of hospital stay
	dynamic hip screw
DHST	delayed hypersensitivity test
DHT	dihydrotachysterol (Hytakeral; DHT®)
	dihydrotestosterone
	dissociated hypertropia
	Dobhoff tube
DHTF	Dobhoff tube feeding
DI	(Beck) Depression Inventory
	date of injury
	Debrix Index
	detrusor instability
	diabetes insipidus
	diagnostic imaging
	Disability Index
	dorsal interossei
	drug interactions
D&I	debridement and irrigation
	dry and intact
DIA	drug-induced agranulocytosis
	drug-induced amenorrhea
	Drug Information Association
diag.	diagnosis
DIAM	drug-induced aseptic meningitis
DIAP-PERS	(causes of transient incontinence) **d**elirium/confusion, **i**nfection, (urinary), **a**trophic urethritis/ vaginitis, **p**harmaceuticals, **p**sychological, **e**xcessive excretion (e.g., CHF, hyperglycemia) **r**estricted mobility, and **s**tool impaction
DIAS	diastolic
DIAS BP	diastolic blood pressure
Diath SW	diathermy short wave
DIAZ	diazepam (Valium)
DIB	disability insurance benefits
DIBC	drug-induced blood cytopenias
DIBD	drug-induced behavioral disinhibition
DIB-R	Diagnostic Interview for Borderlines (personality disorders)-Revised
DIBS	dead-in-bed syndrome
D-IBS	diarrhea-predominant irritable bowel syndrome
DIC	dacarbazine (DTIC-Dome)
	diagnostic imaging center
	differential interference contrast
	disseminated intravascular coagulation
	drug information center
DICC	dynamic infusion cavernosometry and cavernosography
DICE	dexamethasone, ifosfamide, cisplatin, and etopside, with mesna
DICLOX	dicloxacillin (Dynapen)
DICP	demyelinated inflammatory chronic polyneuropathy
DICT	dose-intensive chemotherapy
DID	death(s) from intercurrent disease
	delayed ischemia deficit
	dissociative identity disorder
	drug-induced disease
di,di	dichorionic, diamniotic
DIE	died in emergency department
	drug-induced esophagitis
DIEA	deep inferior epigastric artery (flap)
DIED	died in emergency department
DIEP	deep inferior epigastric perforator

DIF differentiation-inducing factor
DIFF differential blood count
DIFFC dropped in for friendly chat (no medical problem) (slang)
DIG digoxin (this is a dangerous abbreviation)
DIH died in hospital
DIHS Division of Immigration Health Services
drug-induced hypersensitivity syndrome
DIJOA dominantly inherited juvenile optic atrophy
DIL daughter-in-law
dilute
drug-induced lupus
drug information leaflet
DILC dose-intensity limiting criterium
DILD diffuse infiltrative lung disease
drug-induced liver disease
DILE drug-induced lupus erythematosus
DILI drug-induced liver injury
DILS drug-induced lupus syndrome
DIM diminish
D_5IMB Ionosol MB with 5% dextrose injection
DIMD drug-induced movement disorders
DIMOAD diabetes insipidus, diabetes mellitus, optic atrophy, and deafness
DIMS disorders of initiating and maintaining sleep
DIN disease impact number
ductal intraepithelial neoplasia
DIND delayed ischemic neurologic deficit
DINK a patient who did not keep (appointment)
DIOS distal ileal obstruction syndrome
distal intestinal obstruction syndrome
DIP desquamative interstitial pneumonia
diphtheria toxoid vaccine
diplopia
distal interphalangeal
drip infusion pyelogram
drug-induced parkinsonism
urinalysis dipstick (slang)
DIP_{ant} diphtheria antitoxin
DIPC dynamic infusion pharmacocavemosometry
DIPJ distal interphalangeal joint
DIR directions
DIRD drug-induced renal disease
DIS Diagnostic Interview Schedule (questionnaire)
digital imaging spectrophotometer
dislocation
DISA disseminated autonomy
DISC disabled infectious single cycle (virus)
dynamic integrated stabilization chair
disch. discharge
DISCUS Dyskinesia Indentification System Condensed User Scale
DISH diffuse idiopathic skeletal hyperostosis
DISI dorsal intercalated segmental (segment) instability
DISIDA diisopropyl iminodiacetic acid
D_5ISOM 5% Dextrose and Isolyte M
D_5ISOP 5% Dextrose and Isolyte P
DISR drug-induced skin reactions
DIST distal
distilled
DIT diiodotyrosine
drug-induced thrombocytopenia
DIU death in utero
diuretic(s)
DIV double-inlet ventricle
DIVA digital intravenous angiography
Div ex divergence excess
DIVP dilute intravenous Pitocin
DJD degenerative joint disease
DK dark
diabetic ketoacidosis
diseased kidney
DKA diabetic ketoacidosis
didn't keep appointment
DKB deep knee bends
DKC double knee to chest
dyskeratosis congenita
D-K-S Damus-Kaye-Stansel (operation/procedure)
DL danger list
deciliter (dL; 100 mL)
diagnostic laparoscopy
direct laryngoscopy
drug level
dual lumen
ductal lavage
dL deciliter (100 mL)
D_L maximal diffusing capacity
DLAR direct low-anterior resection
DLB dementia with Lewy bodies
direct laryngoscopy and bronchoscopy
DLBCL diffuse large B-cell lymphoma
DLBD diffuse Lewy body disease
DLBL diffuse large B-cell lymphoma
DLC double-lumen catheter
DLCL diffuse large cell lymphoma
DLCO sb diffusion capacity of carbon monoxide, single breath
DLD date of last drink
DLE decrement-load exercise
discoid lupus erythematosus
disseminated lupus erythematosis

D

DLEK	deep lamellar endothelial keratoplasty
DLF	digitalis-like factor ductal lavage fluid
DLI	donor leukocyte infusions
DLIF	digoxin-like immunoreactive factors
DLIS	digoxin-like immunoreactive substance
DLMP	date of last menstrual period
DLNG	dl-norgestrel
DLNMP	date of last normal menstrual period
DLNs	distant lymph nodes
DLP	dislocation of patella double-limb progression
DLPD	diffuse lymphocytic poorly differentiated
DLPFC	dorsolateral prefrontal cortex
DLQI	Dermatology Life Quality Index
D5LR	dextrose 5% in lactated Ringer injection
DLROW	a test used in mental status examinations (patient is asked to spell WORLD backwards)
DLRT	dogleg radiotherapy
DLS	daily living skills digitalis-like substances dynamic light scattering
DLSC	double-lumen subclavian catheter
DLST	drug-induced lymphocyte stimulation test
DLT	dose-limiting toxicity double-lung transplant
DLTT	dosing least toxic time
DLU	diffused lung uptake
DLV	delavirdine (Rescriptor)
DLW	doubly labeled water
DM	dehydrated and malnourished dermatomyositis dextromethorphan diabetes mellitus diabetic mother diastolic murmur disease management
DM-1	diabetes mellitus type 1
DM-2	diabetes mellitus type 2
DMA	Director of Medical Affairs
Dmab	denosumab
DMAC	disseminated *Mycobacterium avium* complex
DMAD	disease-modifying antirheumatic drug
DMAE	dimethylaminoethanol
DMAIC	disseminated *Mycobacterium avium-intracellulare* complex
DMARD	disease modifying antirheumatic drug
DMAS	Drug Management and Authorization Section
DMAT	disaster medical assistance team
DMB	data monitoring board
DMBA	dimethylbenzanthracene
DMC	dactinomycin, methotrexate, and cyclophosphamide data monitoring committee diabetes management center
DMCS	Dyggve-Melchior-Clausen syndrome
DMD	Descemet membrane detachment disciform macular degeneration Doctor of Dental Medicine drowsiness monitoring device Duchenne muscular dystrophy
DMD w/ SRNM	disciform macular degeneration with subretinal neovascular membrane
DME	diabetic macular edema Director of Medical Education durable medical equipment
DMEC	data-monitoring and ethics committee
DMEM	Dulbecco Modified Eagle Medium
DMEPOS	durable medical equipment, prosthetics, orthotics, and supplies
DMERC	Durable Medical Equipment Regional Carrier
DMEs	drug-metabolizing enzymes
DMETS	Division of Medication Errors and Technical Support (FDA)
DMF	decayed, missing, or filled dimethylformamide distant metastases-free Drug Master File
DMFI	distant metastases free interval
DMFS	decayed, missing, or filled surfaces distant metastases free survival
DMFT	decayed, missing, and filled teeth
DMH	Department of Mental Health
DMI	desipramine (Norpramin) diabetic muscle infarction diaphragmatic myocardial infarction
DM Isch	diaphragmatic myocardial ischemia
DMKA	diabetes mellitus ketoacidosis
DMM	destabilization of the medial meniscus
DMN	dysplastic melanocytic nevus
DMO	dimethadone
DMOADs	disease-modifying osteoarthritis drugs
DMOOC	diabetes mellitus out of control
DMORTs	Disaster Mortuary Operational Response Teams
DMP	data monitoring plan dimethyl phthalate
DMPA	depot-medroxypro-gesterone acetate
DMPC	dimyristoylphosphatidyl choline
DMPG	dimyristoylphosphatidyl glycerol
d-MPH	dexmethylphenidate (Focalin)

DMPK	drug metabolism and pharmacokinetics
DMPM	diffuse malignant peritoneal mesothelioma
DMPS	dimercaptopropane-sulfonic acid
D-MRI	dynamic magnetic resonance imaging
DMS	dimethylsulfide
DMSA	succimer (dimercaptosuccinic acid; Chemet)
DMSO	dimethyl sulfoxide
DMT	dimethyltryptamine
DMTU	dimethylthiourea
DMV	disk, macula, and vessels
	Doctor of Veterinary Medicine
DMVP	disc, macula, vessel, periphery
DMX	diathermy, massage, and exercise
DN	denuded
	diabetic nephropathy
	dicrotic notch
	down
	dysplastic nevus (nevi)
D & N	distance and near (vision)
DNA	deoxyribonucleic acid
	did not answer
	did not attend
	does not apply
DNA ds	deoxyribonucleic acid double-stranded
DNAR	do not attempt resuscitation
DNase	deoxyribonuclease
DNA ss	deoxyribonucleic acid single-stranded
DNCB	dinitrochlorobenzene
DNC	Dermatology Nurse, Certified
	did not come
	dilatation and curettage (usually written as D&C)
DND	died a natural death
DNE	diabetes nurse educator
DNEPTE	did not exist prior to enlistment
DNET	dysembryoplastic neuroepithelial tumor
DNFB	Discharged, No Final Bill (report)
DNFC	does not follow commands
DNI	do not intubate
DNIC	diffuse noxious inhibitory control
DNIF	duties not including flying
DNKA	did not keep appointment
DNMT	DNA (desoxyribonucleic acid) methyltransferase
DNN	did not nurse
DNP	did not pay
	dinitrophenylhydrazine
	do not publish
DNR	daunorubicin
	did not respond
	do not report
	do not resuscitate
	dorsal nerve root
DNS	deviated nasal septum
	Director of Nursing Services
	Doctorate, Nursing Science
	doctor did not see patient
	do not show
	dysplastic nevus syndrome
D_5 1/4 NS	dextrose 5% in 1/4 normal saline (0.225% sodium chloride) injection
D_5 1/2NS	dextrose 5% in 0.45% sodium chloride injection
D_5NS	5% dextrose in normal saline (0.9% sodium chloride) injection
DNT	did not test
	dysembryoplastic neuroepithelial tumor
DNW	did not wait
DO	detrusor overactivity
	diet order
	dissolved oxygen
	distocclusal
	distraction osteogenesis
	Doctor of Osteopathy
	doctor's order
D/O	disorder
✓DO	check doctor's order
DO_2	oxygen delivery
DOA	date of admission
	dead on arrival
	dominant optic atrophy
	driver of automobile
	duration of action
DOA-DRA	dead on arrival despite resuscitative attempts
DOB	dangle out of bed
	date of birth
	Dobrava hantavirus
	dobutamine
	doctor's order book
DOC	date of conception
	diabetes out of control
	died of other causes
	diet of choice
	docetaxel (Taxotere)
	drug of choice
	Drug Optimization Clinic
DOCA	desoxycorticosterone acetate
DOCP	desoxycorticosterone pivalate
DOD	date of death
	dead of disease
	Department of Defense
	drug overdose
DODD	demand oxygen delivery device
DOE	date of examination
	disease-oriented evidence
	dyspnea on exertion
DOES	disorders of excessive somnolence

DOH	Department of Health
DOI	date of implant (pacemaker)
	date of injury
	digital object identifier
DO$_2$I	oxygen delivery index
DOJ	Department of Justice
DOL	days of life
DOL #2	second day of life
DOLV	double-outlet left ventricle
DOM	Doctor of Oriental Medicine
	domiciliary
	domiciliary care
DOMS	delayed-onset muscle soreness
DON	Director of Nursing
	donepezil HCl (Aricept)
DONFL	dissociated optic nerve fiber layer
DOOC	diabetes out of control
DOOR	deafness, onychodystrophy, osteodystrophy, and mental retardation (syndrome)
DOP	degenerate oligonucleotide-primed
	dopamine
DOPS	diffuse obstructive pulmonary syndrome
	dihydroxyphenylserine
	Director of Pharmacy Service(s)
DOR	date of release
DORV	double-outlet right ventricle
DORx	date of treatment
DOS	date of surgery
	dead on scene
	doctor's order sheet
DOSA	day of surgery admission
DOSAK	Central Tumor Registry operated by the German-Austrian-Swiss Association for Head and Neck Tumors
DOSS	docusate sodium (dioctyl sodium sulfosuccinate)
DOT	date of transcription
	date of transfer
	died on table
	directly observed therapy
	Directory of Occupational Titles
	Doppler ophthalmic test
DOTS	directly observed treatment, short course
Doughnut	computed tomography (CT) scanner (slang)
DOV	date of visit
	distribution of ventilation
DOX	doxepin
	doxorubicin (Adriamycin)
DOXY	doxycycline
doz	dozen
DP	dental prosthesis
	depersonalization
	diastolic pressure
	disability pension
	discharge planning
	docetaxel and cisplatin
	dorsalis pedis (pulse)
D/P	dialysate-to-plasma ratio
DPA	Department of Public Assistance
	dipropylacetic acid
	D-penicillamine (penicillamine; Cuprimine)
	dual photon absorptiometry
	durable power of attorney
DPAP	diastolic pulmonary artery pressure
DPB	days postburn
	diffuse panbronchiolitis
DPBS	Dulbecco phosphate-buffered saline
DPC	delayed primary closure
	discharge planning coordinator
	distal palmar crease
DPCP	diphenylcyclopropenone (diphencyprone)
DPD	dihydropyrimidine dehydrogenase
DPDL	diffuse poorly differentiated lymphocytic lymphoma
DPE	Division of Pharmacovigilance and Epidemiology (FDA)
DPEJ	direct percutaneous endoscopic jejunostomy
DPF	docetaxel, cisplatin, (Platinol) and fluorouracil
2,3-DPG	2,3-diphosphoglyceric acid
DPH	Department of Public Health
	diphenhydramine (Benadryl)
	Doctor of Public Health
	phenytoin (diphenylhydantoin; Dilantin)
DPI	days postinfection
	dietary protein intake
	Doppler perfusion index
	dry powder inhaler
	dry powder for inhalation
DPIL	dextrose (percentage), protein (grams per kilogram) Intralipid® (grams per kilogram)
DPJ	dislocation of prosthetic joint
DPL	diagnostic peritoneal lavage
D5PLM	dextrose 5% and Plasmalyte M® injection
DPM	distintegrations per minute (dpm)
	Doctor of Podiatric Medicine
	drops per minute
DPN	^{11}C-diprenorphine
	deep peroneal nerve
	dermatosis papulosa nigra
	diabetic peripheral neuropathy
	diabetic polyneuropathy
DPNP	diabetic peripheral neuropathic pain
DPOA	durable power of attorney
DPOAE	distortion-product otoacoustic emission

DPOAHC durable power of attorney for health care

DPP dentine phosphoproteins
dorsalis pedal pulse
duration of positive pressure

DPP-4 dipeptidyl peptidase IV

DPP-IV dipeptidyl peptidase IV

DPPC colfosceril palmitate (dipalmitoylphosphatidylcholine)

DPPE tesmilifene (diethyl phenylmethyl phenoxy ethanamine)

DPR Department of Professional Regulation
diagnostic procedure room

DPS diaphragm pacing stimulation
disintegration per second

DPSS Department of Public Social Service

DPsy Doctor of Psychology

DPT Demerol, Phenergan, and Thorazine (this is a dangerous abbreviation)
diphtheria, pertussis, and tetanus (immunization)
Driver Performance Test

DPTPM diphtheria, pertussis, tetanus, poliomyelitis, and measles

DPU delayed pressure urticaria

DPUD duodenal peptic ulcer disease

DPVSs dilated perivascular spaces

DPXA dual-photon x-ray absorptiometry

DQ developmental quotients

D/Q deep quiet

D&Q deep and quiet

DQA Data Quality Audit

DQM data quality manager

DQOL diabetes quality of life

DQOLS Dermatology Quality of Life Scales

DQRS Drug Quality Reporting System (FDA)

Dr doctor

DR delivery room
diabetic retinopathy
diagnostic radiology
dining room
diurnal rhythm
drug resistant

DRA Deficit Reduction Act of 2005
distal rectal adenocarcinoma
drug-related admissions

DRAPE drug-related adverse patient event

DRC dose-response curve

DRE digital rectal examination
Drug Recognition Expert (for detection of impaired drivers)

DREAM downstream regulatory element antagonistic modulator (gene)

DRESS depth resolved surface coil spectroscopy
drug rash with eosinophilia and systemic symptoms

DREZ dorsal root entry zone

DRG diagnosis-related groups
dorsal root ganglia

DRGE drainage

DRI defibrillation response interval
Dietary Reference Intakes
Disability Rating Index
Discharge Readiness Index
dopamine reuptake inhibitor

DRIL distal revascularization internal ligation

DRM drug-related morbidity

DRN dorsal raphe nucleus
drug-related neutropenia

DrotAA drotrecogin alfa (activated) (Xigris)

DRP data review plan
drug-related problem

DRPLA dentatorubral-pallidolluysian atrophy

DRPn drug-resistant *Streptococcus pneumoniae*

DRR drug regimen review

DRS Delirium Rating Scale
designated record set
Disability Rating Scale
disease-related symptoms
Duane retraction syndrome

DRSG dressing

DRSI disease-related symptom improvement

DRSP drug-resistant *Streptococcus pneumoniae*

DRT drug-related thrombocytopenia

DrTPar diphtheria toxoid (reduced antigen quantity for adults), tetanus toxoid, and acellular pertussis (reduced antigen quantity for adults) vaccine, for adult use

DRUB drug screen-blood

DRUJ distal or radial ulnar joint

dRVVT diluted Russell viper venom time

DS deep sleep
Dextrostix
dietary supplement
discharge summary
disoriented
distant supervision
double-stapled (suture)
double strength
Down syndrome
drug screen

D/S 5% dextrose and 0.9% sodium chloride (saline) injection

%DS percent diameter stenosis

D&S diagnostic and surgical
dilation and suction

D5S dextrose 5% in 0.9% sodium chloride (saline) injection
D_5-1/2S 5% dextrose in 0.45% sodium chloride (saline) injection
18Ds Special Operations Forces medics
DSA digital subtraction angiography (angiocardiography)
Donor Sperm Archive
DSAEK descemet stripping and automated endothelial keratoplasty
DSAP disseminated superficial actinic porokeratosis
DSB drug-seeking behavior
DSBs double-strand (DNA) breaks
DSC differential scanning calorimeter
Down syndrome child
dynamic susceptibility contrast
DSD degenerative spinal disease
detrusor sphincter dyssynergia
digital selenium drum (radiology)
discharge summary dictated
dry sterile dressing
DSDB direct self-destructive behavior
ds DNA double-stranded desoxyribonucleic acid
DSE dobutamine stress echocardiography
DSF doxorubicin, streptozocin, and fluorouracil
DSG desogestrel
dressing
DSG deoxyspergualin
DSHEA Dietary Supplement Health and Education Act of 1994
DSHR delayed skin hypersensitivity reaction
DSHS Department of Social and Health Services
DSI deep shock insulin
Depression Status Inventory
DSIAR double-stapled ileoanal reservoir
DSM disease state management
drink skim milk
DSM-IV Diagnostic and Statistical Manual of Mental Disorders, 4th edition
DSM-IV-TR Diagnostic and Statistical Manual of Mental Disorders 4th Edition—Text Revision
dSMA distal spinal muscular atrophy
DSMB Data and Safety Management Board
Data and Safety Monitoring Board
DSMC Data Safety and Monitoring Committee
DSMO Designated Standard Maintenance Organization
DSO distal subungual onychomycosis
DSP diabetic sensorimotor polyneuropathy
digital signal processor
distal symmetrical polyneuropathy
DSPC distearoylphosphatidyl choline
DSPD dangerous severe personality disorder
D-SPINE dorsal spine
DSPN distal symmetric polyneuropathy
DSPS delayed sleep phase syndrome
DSRCT desmoplastic small round cell tumor
DSRF drainage subretinal fluid
dsRNA double-stranded deoxyribonucleic acid
DSS dengue shock syndrome
Department of Social Services
Disability Status Scale
discharge summary sheet
disease-specific survival
distal splenorenal shunt
docusate sodium (dioctyl sodium sulfosuccinate)
DSSLR double, seated straight leg raise
DSSN distal symmetric sensory neuropathy
DSSP distal symmetric sensory polyneuropathy
DSST Digit-Symbol Substitution Test
DST daylight saving time
dexamethasone suppression test
digit substitution test
donor-specific (blood) transfusion
DSTO dog smarter than owner (Veterinary slang)
DSU day stay unit
day surgery unit
DSUH direct suggestion under hypnosis
D/Sum discharge summary
DSV digital subtraction ventriculography
DSVP Dietary Supplement Verification Program (United States Pharmacopeia Purity Compliance)
DSW Doctorate in Social Work
DSWI deep sternal wound infection
deep surgical wound infection
DSX dysmetabolic syndrome X
DT deceleration time
delirium tremens
dietary thermogenesis
dietetic technician
diphtheria and tetanus toxoids, adsorbed, pediatric strength
discharge tomorrow
docetaxel (Taxotere)
D/T date/time
due to
d/t due to
d4T stavudine (Zerit)
D & T diagnosis and treatment
dictated and typed
DTaP diphtheria and tetanus toxoids with acellular pertussis vaccine
DTBC tubocurarine (D-tubocurarine)
DTBE Division of Tuberculosis Elimination

DTC day treatment center
differentiated thyroid cancer
direct-to-consumer (advertising)
diticarb (diethyldithio-carbamate)
tubocurarine (D-tubocurarine)
DTCA direct-to-consumer advertising
DTD diastropic dysplasia
DTD #30 dispense 30 such doses
DTF deep transverse friction
DTH delayed-type hypersensitivity
DTI deep tissue injury
Department of Trade and Industry (United Kingdom)
diffusion-tensor imaging
Doppler tissue imaging
DTIC dacarbazine (DTIC-Dome)
D TIME dream time
DTIs direct thrombin inhibitors
DTM deep tissue massage
dermatophyte test medium
DTMS drug therapy management service
DTO danger to others
deodorized tincture of opium (warning: this is *NOT* paregoric)
DTOGV dextral-transposition of great vessels
DTP differential time to positivity
diphtheria, tetanus toxoids, pertussis (antigens unspecified) vaccine
distal tingling on percussion (+Tinel sign)
DTPA pentetic acid (diethylenetriaminepentaacetic acid)
DTP_a diphtheria, tetanus toxoids, acellular pertussis vaccine, for pediatric use
DTPa-HIB diphtheria toxoid, tetanus toxoid, acellular pertussis, and *Haemophilus influenzae* type b conjugate vaccine
DTPa-HIB-IPV diphtheria toxoid, tetanus toxoid, acellular pertussis, *Haemophilus influenzae* type b conjugate, and poliovirus inactivated vaccine
DTP_w diphtheria, tetanus toxoids, whole-cell pertussis vaccine
DTR Dance Therapist, Registered
deep tendon reflexes
Dietetic Technician Registered
dtr daughter
DTs delirium tremens
DTS danger to self
digital tomosynthesis
donor specific transfusion
3D TSE three-dimensional turbo-spin echo (images)
DTT diphtheria tetanus toxoid
dithiothreitol
DTUS diathermy, traction, and ultrasound
DTV due to void
DTVP Developmental Test of Visual Perception
DTwP diphtheria and tetanus toxoids with whole-cell pertussis vaccine
DTX detoxification
DU decubitus ulcer
depleted uranium
developmental unit
diabetic urine
diagnosis undetermined
duodenal ulcer
duroxide uptake
DUB Dubowitz (score)
dysfunctional uterine bleeding
DUBI dysfunctional urinary bladder instability
DUCL dorsal ulnocarpal ligament
DUD dihydrouracil dehydrogenase
DUE drug use evaluation
D&UE dilation and uterine evacuation
DUF Doppler ultrasonic flowmeter
DUI driving under the influence
DUID driving under the influence of drugs
DUII driving under the influence of intoxicants
DUIL driving under the influence of liquor
DUKM dialysate urea kinetic modeling
DUM drug use monitoring
DUN dialysate urea nitrogen
DUNHL diffuse undifferentiated non-Hodgkins lymphoma
DUO Duotube®
DUR drug utilization review
duration
DUS digital ultrasound
distal urethral stenosis
Doppler ultrasound stethoscope
duplex ultrasonography
3DUS three-dimensional ultrasound
DUSN diffuse unilateral subacute neuroretinitis
DV distance vision
domestic violence
double vision
D&V diarrhea and vomiting
disc and vessels
DVA Department of Veterans Affairs
directional vacuum-assisted (biopsy)
distance visual acuity
vindesine (Eldisine; desacetyl vinblastine amide sulfate)
DVAB directional vacuum-assisted biopsy
DVC direct visualization of vocal cords
D V® Cream dienestrol vaginal cream
DVD dissociated vertical deviation
double-vessel disease

D

D

DVG	double vein graft
DVH	dose-volume histogram
DVI	atrioventricular sequential pacing digital vascular imaging direct visual inspection
DVIU	direct vision internal urethrotomy
DVLA	Driver and Vehicle Licensing Agency (United Kingdom)
DVPX	divalproex sodium (Depakote)
DVM	Doctor of Veterinary Medicine
DVMP	disc, vessels, and macula periphery
DVP	digital volume pulse divalproex (Depakote)
dVP	da Vinci (robotic) prostatectomy
DVPA	daunorubicin, vincristine, prednisone, and asparaginase
DVR	Division of Vocational Rehabilitation dose-volume relationship double-valve replacement
DVSA	digital venous subtraction angiography
DVT	deep vein thrombosis digital volume tomography
DVTS	deep venous thromboscintigram
DVVC	direct visualization of vocal cords
DW	daily weight deionized water detention warrant dextrose in water diffusion-weighted (imaging) distilled water doing well double wrap
D/W	dextrose in water discussed with
D-W	Dandy-Walker (deformity/malformation) Danis-Weber (classification for ankle fractures)
D_5W	5% dextrose (in water) injection
D10W	10% dextrose (in water) injection
D20W	20% dextrose (in water) injection
D50W	50% dextrose (in water) injection
D70W	70% dextrose (in water) injection
5 DW	5% dextrose (in water) injection
DWDL	diffuse well-differentiated lymphocytic lymphoma
DWI	diffusion-weighted (magnetic resonance) imaging driving while intoxicated driving while impaired
DWI/PI	diffusion-weighted imaging/ perfusion imaging
DWMRI	diffusion-weighted magnetic resonance imaging
DWR	deep water running
DWRT	delayed work recall test
DWSCL	daily-wear soft contact lens
DWSMB	Dean-Woodcock Sensory Motor Battery (measures of sensory-motor functioning)
DWV	Dandy-Walker variant (a congenital anomaly)
DWW	dynamic wall walk
Dx	diagnosis diagnostic evaluation disease
DXA	dual-energy x-ray absorptiometry
DXG	dioxalane guanine
DxLS	diagnosis responsible for length of stay
DXM	dexamethasone dextromethorphan
DXR	delayed xenograft rejection
DXT	deep x-ray therapy
DXRT	deep x-ray therapy
DXS	Dextrostix®
DY	dusky (infant color) dysprosium
DYF	drag your feet (author's note: see you in court)
DYFS	Division of Youth and Family Services
DysD	dysthymic disorder
DYTRO	dynamic tone-reducing orthosis
DZ	diazepam (valium) disease dizygotic dozen
DZP	diazepam (Valium)
DZT	dizygotic twins
DZX	dexrazoxane (Zinecard)

E

E	East (as in the location e.g., 2E, would be second floor, East wing)
	edema
	effective
	eloper
	enema
	engorged
	eosinophil
	Escherichia
	esophoria for distance
	ethambutol [part of tuberculosis regimen, see RHZ(E/S)/HR]
	evaluation
	evening
	expired
	eye
	methylenedioxy-methamphetamine (MDMA; Ecstasy)
E′	elbow
	esophoria for near
E_1	estrone
E_2	estradiol
E_3	estriol
4E	4 plus edema
E11	Echovirus 11
	embryonic day 11 (11-day-old embryo)
E20	Enfamil 20®
E → A	say E,E,E, comes out as A,A,A upon auscultation of lung showing consolidation
EA	early amniocentesis
	elbow aspiration
	electroacoustic analysis
	electroacupuncture
	enteral alimentation
	epidural anesthesia
	episodic ataxia
	esophageal atresia
E/A	ratio of peak mitral early diastolic and atrial contraction velocity
	European American
E&A	evaluate and advise
EAA	electrothermal atomic absorption
	essential amino acids
	extrinsic allergic alveolitis
EAB	elective abortion
	Ethical Advisory Board
EAC	erythema annulare centrifugum
	esophageal adenocarcinoma
	external auditory canal
EACA	aminocaproic acid (epsilon-aminocaproic acid)
	esophageal adenocarcinoma
EADL	extended activities of daily living
EADs	early after-depolarizations
EAE	experimental allergic encephalomyelitis
	experimental autoimmune encephalomyelitis
EAEC	enteroaggregative *Escherichia coli*
eAG	estimated average glucose
EAggEC	enteroaggregative *Escherichia coli*
EAHF	eczema, allergy, and hay fever
EAL	electronic artificial larynx
EAM	external auditory meatus
EAP	Early Access Program (premarketing use of drug)
	Employment (Employee) Assistance Programs
	erythrocyte acid phosphatase
	etoposide, doxorubicin (Adriamycin), and cisplatin (Platinol)
EAR	estimated average requirement
	excess absolute risk
EARLIES	early decelerations
EART	extended abdominal radiation therapy
EAR OX	ear oximetry
EAS	external anal sphincter
EASC	endoscopic ambulatory surgery center
EASE	Estimation and Assessment of Substance Exposure (model)
EAST	external rotation, abduction stress test
EAT	Eating Attitudes Test
	ectopic atrial tachycardia
EATL	enteropathy-associated T-cell lymphoma
EAU	experimental autoimmune uveitis
EB	eosinophilic bronchitis
	epidermolysis bullosa
	Epstein-Barr (virus)
EBA	epidermolysis bullosa acquisita
EBB	electron beam boosts
	equal breath bilaterally
EBBS	equal bilateral breath sounds
EBC	early (stage) breast cancer
	endoscopic brush cytology
	esophageal balloon catheter
EBCPGs	evidence-based clinical practice guidelines
EBCT	electron-beam computed tomography
EBCTCG	Early Breast Cancer Trialists' Collaborative Group
EBD	endocardial border delineation
	endoscopic balloon dilation
	evidence-based decision (making)
EBE	equal bilateral expansion
EBEA	Epstein-Barr (virus) early antigen

EBF	erythroblastosis fetalis
EBG	evidence-based (practice) guidelines
EBL	endoscopic band ligation estimated blood loss
EBL-1	European bat lyssavirus 1
EBLV	European bat lyssavirus
EBM	evidence-based medicine expressed breast milk
EBMT	European Bone Marrow Transplant (registry group)
EBNA	Epstein-Barr (virus) nuclear antigen
EBO	evidence-based outcomes
EBOS	early-onset benign occipital seizure
EBOV	Ebola virus
EBO-Z	Ebola Zaire virus
EBP	electric breast pump epidural blood patch
EBR	external beam radiotherapy eye-blink rate
EBRs	evidence-based recommendations
EBRT	external beam radiation therapy
EBS	empiric Bayesian screening epidermolysis bullosa simplex
EBSB	equal breath sounds bilaterally
EBT	electron beam tomography erythromycin breath test
EBUS	endobronchial ultrasonography (ultrasound)
EBUS-TBNA	endobronchial ultrasound-guided transbronchial needle aspiration
EBV	Epstein-Barr virus
EBVCA	Epstein-Barr viral capsid antigen
EBVEA	Epstein-Barr virus, early antigen
EBVNA	Epstein-Barr virus, nuclear antigen
EC	ejection click electrical cardioversion electrocautery emergency contraception endocervical enteric coated *Escherichia coli* esophageal candidiasis ethics committee etopside and carboplatin European Community extracellular eye care eyes closed
E_2C	estradiol cypionate
E & C	education and counseling
ECA	enteric coated aspirin (tablets) Epidemiological Catchment Area ethacrynic acid external carotid artery
ECAD	extracorporeal albumin dialysis
e-CAM	electronic Compilation of Analytical Methods
ECASA	enteric coated aspirin (tablets)
ECBD	exploration of common bile duct
ECBO	enterocytopathogenic bovine orphan (virus)
ECC	early childhood caries edema, clubbing, and cyanosis embryonal cell cancer emergency cardiac care Emergency Communications Center endocervical curettage estimated creatinine clearance external cardiac compression extracorporeal circulation
ECCE	extracapsular cataract extraction
ECD	electron capture dissociation endocardial cushion defect equivalent current dipole Erdheim-Chester disease expanded criteria donor
E-CD	E-cadherin
ECDB	encourage to cough and deep breathe
ECDC	European Centre for Disease Prevention and Control
ECDPC	European Centre for Disease Prevention and Control (EDCD is used)
ECE	endothelin-converting enzyme extracapsular extension
ECEMG	evoked compound electromyography
ECF	epirubicin, cisplatin, and fluorouracil extended care facility extracardiac Fontan (procedure) extracellular fluid
ECF-A	eosinophil chemotactic factors of anaphylaxis
ECFV	extracellular fluid volume
ECG	electrocardiogram
ECGE	extracorporeal gas exchange
ECHINO	echinocyte
ECHO	echocardiogram enterocytopathogenic human orphan (virus) etoposide, cyclophosphamide, doxorubicin (hydroxydaunomycin), and vincristine (Oncovin)
ECHO (2D)	echocardiogram (2-dimensional)
EChoG	electrocochleography
ECHO/RV	echocardiography/ radionuclide ventriculography
ECI	extracorporeal irradiation
ECIB	extracorporeal irradiation of blood
ECIC	external carotid and internal carotid extracranial to intracranial (anastamosis)
EC/IC	extracranial/intracranial
ECID	European Centre for Infectious Disease

E

ECK1	*Escherichia coli* K1
ECL	electrochemiluminescence enterochromaffin-like extend of cerebral lesion extracapillary lesions
ECLA	extracorporeal lung assist
ECLP	extracorporeal liver perfusion
ECM	erythema chronicum migrans esophagocardiomyotomy extracellular mass extracellular matrix
ECM/BCM	extracellular mass, body cell mass ratio
ECMO	enterocytopathogenic monkey orphan (virus) extracorporeal circulation membrane oxygenation (oxygenator)
ECN	extended care nursery
ecNOS	endothelial constitutive nitric oxide synthetase
ECochG	electrocochleography
ECOG	Eastern Cooperative Oncology Group
ECoG	electrocochleography electrocorticogram
E coli	*Escherichia coli*
ECO_{tox}	*Escherichia coli* (heat-labile toxin) vaccine
ECP	effective conduction period emergency care provider emergency contraceptive pills eosinophil cationic protein external counterpulsation extracorporeal photochemotherapy extracorporeal photopheresis
ECPL	endocavitary pelvic lymphadenectomy
ECPD	external counterpressure device
ECPP	extracorporeal photophoresis
ECR	emergency chemical restraint extensor carpi radialis
ECRB	extensor carpi radialis brevis
ECRL	extensor carpi radialis longus
ECS	elective cosmetic surgery electrocerebral silence endometrial-cancer-specific
ECT	electroconvulsive therapy emission computed tomography enhanced computed tomography
ECTb	Emory Cardiac Toolbox
ECTR	endoscopic carpal tunnel release
ECU	electrocautery unit emergency care unit emotional care units environmental control unit extensor carpi ulnaris eternal care unit (morgue) (slang)
ECV	emergency center visits external cephalic version (obstetrics)
ECVD	extracellular volume depletion
ECVE	extracellular volume expansion
ECVP	extracellular volume depletion (dehydration)
ECW	extracellular water
ECWHSP	Enhanced Coal Workers' Health Surveillance Program (CDC)
ED	eating disorder(s) education effective dose elbow disarticulation emergency department emotional disorder epidural erectile dysfunction ethynodiol diacetate every day (this is a dangerous abbreviation) extensive disease extensor digitorum
ED_{50}	median effective dose
EDA	elbow disarticulation
EDAC	early definitive abdominal closure Early Detection of Alcohol Consumption (test)
EDAM	edatrexate
EDAP	Emergency Department Approved for Pediatrics etoposide, dexamethasone, cytarabine, (Ara-C and cisplatin (Platinol)
EDAS	encephalodural arterio-synangiosis
EDAT	Emergency Department Alert Team
EDAX	energy-dispersive analysis of x-rays
EDB	ethylene dibromide extensor digitorum brevis
EDC	effective dynamic compliance electrodesiccation and curettage electronic data capture end diastolic counts estimated date of conception estimated date of confinement estramustine, docetaxel, and carboplatin extensor digitorum communis
ED&C	electrodesiccation and curettage
EDCF	endothelium-derived constricting factor
EDCP	eccentric dynamic compression plates
EDCTP	European and Developing Countries Clinical Trials Partnership
EDD	endothelium-dependent dilation esophageal detector device expected date of delivery

E

EdD	Doctor of Education
EDENT	edentulous
EDF	elongation, derotation, and flexion
EDH	epidural hematoma extradural hematoma
EDHF	endothelium-derived hyperpolarizing factor
EDI	Eating Disorders Inventory electrodeionization
EDITAR	extended-duration topical arthropod repellent
EDL	extensor digitorum longus
ED/LD	emotionally disturbed and learning disabled
EDLF	endogenous digitalis-like factors
EDLS	endogenous digitalis-like substance
EDM	early diastolic murmur esophageal Doppler monitor extensor digiti minimi
EDMD-AD	autosomal dominate Emery-Dreifuss muscular dystrophy
EDNO	endothelium-related nitric oxide
ED-OU	emergency department/observation unit
EDP	emergency department physician end-diastolic pressure
EDQ	extensor digiti quinti (tendon)
EDQM	European Directorate for the Quality of Medicines
EDQV	extensor digiti quinti five
EDR	edrophonium (Tensilon) escalating dose regimen extreme drug resistance
EDRF	endothelium derived relaxing factor (nitric oxide)
EDS	Ehlers-Danlos syndrome excessive daytime somnolence
EDSS	Expanded Disability Status Scale (Score)
EDT	exposure duration threshold
EDTA	edetic acid (ethylenediaminetetraacetic acid)
EDTU	emergency diagnostic and treatment unit
EDU	education eating disorder unit
EDUC	education
EDV	end-diastolic velocity end-diastolic volume epidermal dysplastic verruciformis
EDW	estimated dry weight
EDX	edatrexate electrodiagnostic energy-dispersive X-ray (analysis)
EDXRF	energy-dispersive x-ray fluorescence
EE	emetic episodes emotional exhaustion end to end energy expenditure equine encephalitis erosive esophagitis esophageal endoscopy ethinyl estradiol exchange efficiency (units) expressed emotion external ear
E & E	eyes and ears
EEA	electroencephalic audiometry elemental enteral alimentation end-to-end anastomosis energy expended with activity
EEC	ectrodactyly-ectodermal dysplasia (cleft syndrome) endogenous erythroid colony
EECP	enhanced external counter-pulsation
EEE	eastern equine encephalomyelitis edema, erythema, and exudate external eye examination
EEG	electroencephalogram
EELS	electron energy loss spectrometry
EEN	estimated energy needs
EENT	eyes, ears, nose, and throat
EEP	end expiratory pressure
EER	extended endocardial resection extraesophageal reflux
EERD	extraesophageal reflux disease
EES	extraosseous Ewing sarcoma
EES®	erythromycin ethylsuccinate
EET	early exercise testing
EEUS-NA	endoscopic esophageal ultrasound-guided needle aspiration
EEV	encircling endocardial ventriculotomy
EF	eccentric fixation ejection fraction endurance factor erythroblastosis fetalis extended-field (radiotherapy)
EFA	essential fatty acid estimated fetal age
EFAD	essential fatty acid deficiency
E-FAP	Emory Functional Ambulation Profile
EFBW	estimate fetal body weight
EFD	episode free day
EFE	endocardial fibroelastosis epidemic fatal encephalopathy
EFF	effacement
EFI	extended-field irradiation
EFHBM	eosinophilic fibrohistiocytic lesion of bone marrow
EFM	electronic fetal monitor(ing) external fetal monitoring
EFMM	external fetal maternal monitor
EFMT	electric field mediated transfer
EFN	effusion

EFPIA	European Federation of Pharmaceutical Industries and Associations
EFR	effective filtration rate
EFS	event-free survival
EFV	efavirenz (Sustiva)
EFW	estimated fetal weight
EF/WM	ejection fraction/wall motion
e.g.	for example
EGA	esophageal gastric (tube) airway
	estimated gestational age
EGB	endoscopic grasp biopsy
EGb	extract of *Ginkgo biloba*
EGBUS	external genitalia, Bartholin, urethral, and Skene glands
EGC	early gastric carcinoma
EGCG	epigallocatechin gallate
EGFR	epidermal growth factor receptor
EGD	esophagogastroduodenoscopy
EGDT	early goal-directed therapy
	esophagogastric devascularization and transection
EGF	epidermal growth factor
EGF-R	epidermal growth factor receptor
EGG	electrogastrography
EGJ	esophagogastric junction
EGL	eosinophilic granuloma of the lung
EGS	ethylene glycol succinate
EGSs	external guide sequences
EGTA	esophageal gastric tube airway
	ethyleneglycoltetracetic acid
EH	eccentric hypertrophy
	educationally handicapped
	enlarged heart
	essential hypertension
	extramedullary hematopoiesis
Eh	*Entamoeba histolytica*
EHB	elevate head of bed
	extensor hallucis brevis
EHBA	extrahepatic biliary atresia
EHBF	extrahepatic blood flow
EHC	enterohepatic circulation
EHD	electronic home detention
EHDA	etidronate sodium
EHDP	etidronate disodium (Didronel)
EHE	epithelioid hemangioendothelioma
EHEC	enterohemorrhagic *Escherichia coli*
EHF	epidemic hemorrhagic fever
	extremely high frequency
EHH	episodic hypothermia with hyperhidrosis
	esophageal hiatal hernia
EHI	exertional heat illness
EHL	electrohydraulic lithotripsy
	extensor hallucis longus
EHN	ethotoin
EHO	extrahepatic obstruction
EHPH	extrahepatic portal hypertension
EHR	electronic health record(s)
2EHRZ/6HE	daily ethambutol, isoniazid, rifampicin, and pyrazinamide for 2 months, followed by isoniazid and ethambutol for 6 months
2[EHRZ]$_3$/6HE	the same as 2EHRZ/6HE but given three times weekly in the initial intensive phase
2EHRZ/4HR	The same as 2EHRZ/6HE, followed by 4 months of daily isoniazid and rifampicin
EHS	Early Head Start (program)
	electrical hypersensitivity
	employee health service
	Engelbreth-Holm-Swarm (tumor)
	exertional heat stroke
EHT	electrohydrothermosation
	essential hypertension
EI	early intervention
	entry inhibitor
	environmental illness
	enzyme immunoassay
	extensor indicis
E/I	expiratory to inspiratory (ratio)
E & I	endocrine and infertility
EIA	enzyme immunoassay
	exercise-induced asthma
EIAB	extracranial-intracranial arterial bypass
EIAC	enzyme-inducing anticonvulsants
EIACD	enzyme-inducing anticonvulsant drug
EIAD	extended-interval aminoglycoside dosing
EIAV	equine infectious anemia virus
EIB	exercise-induced bronchospasm
EIC	early ischemic change(s)
	electrical impedance cardiography
	endometrial intraepithelial carcinoma
	epidermal inclusion cyst
	extensive intraductal component
EICA	extra-intracranial artery (bypass)
EID	electroimmunodiffusion
	electronic infusion device
EIDC	extreme intervertebral disk collapse
EIEC	enteroinvasive *Escherichia coli*
EIL	elective induction of labor
EIN	Employer Identification Number
eIND	Electronic Investigational New Drug (application)
EIOA	excessive intake of alcohol
EIP	Early Intervention Program
	elective interruption of pregnancy
	end-inspiratory pressure
	extensor indicis proprius
eIPV	enhanced inactivated polio vaccine
EIR	entomological inoculation rate
EIS	electrical impedance scanning

	endoscopic injection scleropathy
EISR	expanded international search report
EIT	electrical impedance tomography
EITB	enzyme-linked immuno-electrotransfer blot
EIV	external iliac vein
EJ	ejection
	elbow jerk
	external jugular
EJB	ectopic junctional beat
EJN	extended jaundice of newborn
EJP	excitatory junction potential
EJV	external jugular vein
EK	Ektachem 400 (see page 318)
	erythrokinase
EKC	epidemic keratoconjunctivitis
EKG	electrocardiogram
EKO	echoencephalogram
EKY	electrokymogram
EL	exercise limit
	exploratory laparotomy
E-L	external lids
ELA	Establishment License Application
ELAD	extracorporeal liver-assist device
ELAFF	extended lateral arm free flap
ELAM	endothelial leukocyte adhesion molecule
ELAMS	Electronic Laboratory Animal Monitoring System
ELB	early light breakfast
	elbow
ELBW	extremely low birth weight (less than 1000 g)
ELC	earlobe creases
ELCA	excimer laser coronary angioplasty
ELD	end-of-life decision(s)
ELDs	end-of-life decisions
ELDU	extralabel drug use
ELEC	elective
ELF	elective low forceps
	endoscopic laser foraminotomy
	epithelial lining fluid
	etoposide, leucovorin, and fluorouracil
	extremely low frequency
ELFA	enzyme-linked fluorescent immunoassay
ELG	endolumenal gastroplication
	endoluminal graft
ELH	endolymphatic hydrops
ELI	endomyocardial lymphocytic infiltrates
ELIG	eligible
ELIOT	electron intraoperative treatment
ELISA	enzyme-linked immunosorbent assay
ELISPOT	enzyme-linked immunospot
ELITT	endometrial laser intrauterine thermal therapy
Elix	elixir
ELLIP	ellipotocytosis
ELM	epiluminescent microscopy
	external laryngeal manipulation
ELM scale-2	Early Language Milestone Scale - second edition
ELND	elective lymph node dissection
ELOP	estimated length of program
ELOS	estimated length of stay
ELP	electrophoresis
	eruptive lingual papillitis
ELPS	excessive lateral pressure syndrome
ELR	elevating leg rests (wheelchair description)
ELS	Eaton-Lambert syndrome
	Editor in the Life Sciences
	endolymphatic sac
ELSD	evaporative light scattering detection
ELSI	ethical, legal, and social implications
ELSS	emergency life support system
ELST	endolymphatic sac tumor
ELT	endoscopic laser therapy
	euglobulin lysis time
ELTR	European Liver Transplant Registry
ELVIS™	Enzyme-Linked Virus Inducible System
EM	early memory
	ejection murmur
	electron microscope
	emergency medicine
	emmetropia
	eosinophilia-myalgia (syndrome)
	erythema migrans
	erythema multiforme
	erythromelalgia
	esophageal manometry
	estramustine (Emcyt)
	extensive metabolizers
	external monitor
E/M	Evaluation and Management (coding system)
EMA	early morning awakening
	endomysial antibody
EMA-CO	etoposide, methotrexate, dactinomycin (actinomycin-D), cyclophosphamide, and vincristine (Oncovin)
eMAR	electronic medication administration record
EMB	endometrial biopsy
	endomyocardial biopsy
	eosin-methylene blue (agar)
	ethambutol (Myambutol)
	Explanation of Medicare Benefits
EMBx	endomyocardial biopsy
EMC	encephalomyocarditis
	endometrial currettage
	essential mixed cryoglobulinemia

	extraskeletal myxoid chondrosarcoma
EMD	electromechanical dissociation
EMDA	electromotive drug administration
EMDR	eye movement desensitization and reprocessing
EME	extreme medical emergency
EMEA	European Medicines Evaluation Agency
EMF	elective midforceps
	electromagnetic field(s)
	electromagnetic flow
	electromotive forces
	endomyocardial fibrosis
	erythrocyte maturation factor
	evaporated milk formula
EMG	electromyograph
	emergency
	essential monoclonal gammopathy
EMI	educably mentally impaired
	elderly and mentally infirm
	electromagnetic interference
EMIC	emergency maternity and infant care
E-MICR	electron microscopy
EMIT	enzyme-multiplied immunoassay technique (test)
EML	essential medicines lists (World Health Organization)
EMLA®	eutectic mixture of local anesthetics (lidocaine and prilocaine in an emulsion base)
EMLB	erythromycin lactobionate
EMMA	eye-movement measuring apparatus
EMMV	extended mandatory minute ventilation
EMo	ear mold
EmOC	emergency obstetric care
EMP	electromolecular propulsion
	estramustine phosphate (Emcyt)
EMPD	extramammary Paget disease
EMPI	enterprise master patient index
EMR	Eastern Mediterranean Region (WHO)
	educable mentally retarded
	electrical muscle stimulation
	electronic medical record
	emergency mechanical restraint
	empty, measure, and record
	endoscopic mucosal resection
	eye-movement recording
EMS	early morning specimen
	early morning stiffness
	electrical muscle stimulation
	emergency medical services
	eosinophilia myalgia syndrome
EMSA	electrophoretic mobility shift assay
EMSU	early morning specimen of urine
EMT	emergency medical technician
	epithelial-mesenchymal transformation (transition)
	estramustine (Emcyt)
EMTA	Emergency Medical Technician, Advanced
EMTALA	Emergency Medical Treatment and Labor Act
EMTC	emergency medical trauma center
EMT-D	emergency medical technician-defibrillation
EMTP	Emergency Medical Technician, Paramedic
EMU	early morning urine
	electromagnetic unit
	epilepsy monitoring unit
EMV	equine morbilli virus
	eye, motor, verbal (grading for Glasgow Coma Scale)
EMVC	early mitral valve closure
EMW	electromagnetic waves
EMZL	extranodal marginal-zone (B-cell) lymphoma
EN	enema
	enteral nutrition
	erythema nodosum
E/N	eggnog
E 50% N	extension 50% of normal
ENA	extractable nuclear antigen
ENB	esthesioneuroblastoma
ENC	encourage
eNDA	Electronic New Drug Application
ENDO	endodontia
	endodontics
	endoscopy
	endotracheal
EndoCAB	plasma antiendotoxin core antibody
ENF	Enfamil
ENF c Fe	Enfamil with iron
ENG	electronystagmogram
	engorged
ENL	enlarged
	erythema nodosum leprosum
ENMG	electroneuromyography
ENMT	ears, nose, mouth, and throat
ENOG	electroneurography
eNOS	endothelial nitric oxide synthase
ENP	extractable nucleoprotein
ENRD	endoscopy-negative reflux disease
ENS	enteric nervous system
	exogenous natural surfactant
ENT	ears, nose, throat
ENTIS	European Network of Teratology Information Services
ENTV	enzootic nasal tumor virus
ENVD	elevated new vessels on the disk
ENVE	elevated new vessels elsewhere

ENVT	environment
ENZ	enzastaurin
EO	elbow orthosis
	embolic occlusion
	eosinophilia
	ethylene oxide
	eyes open
E & O	errors and omissions
EOA	erosive osteoarthritis
	esophageal obturator airway
	examine, opinion, and advice
	external oblique aponeurosis
EOAE	evoked otoacoustic emissions
EOB	edge of bed
	end of bed
	explanation of benefits
EOC	Emergency Operations Center
	enema of choice
	epithelial ovarian cancer
EOD	early-onset disease
	end of day
	end organ damage
	every other day (this is a dangerous abbreviation)
	extent of disease
EOE	Equal Opportunity Employer
EOFAD	early-onset form of familial Alzheimer disease
E of I	evidence of insurability
EOG	electro-oculogram
	electro-olfactogram
	Ethrane, oxygen, and gas (nitrous oxide)
EOGBS	early-onset group B streptococcal (sepsis)
EOIT	end of initial treatment
EOLC	end-of-life-care
EOM	error of measurement
	external otitis media
	extraocular movement
	extraocular muscles
EOMB	explanation of Medicare benefits
EOMG	early-onset myasthenia gravis
EOMI	extraocular movements intact
	extraocular muscles intact
EOO	external oculomotor ophthalmoplegia
EOP1	end-of-phase 1
EOP2	end-of-phase 2
EOR	emergency operating room
	end of range
EORA	elderly onset rheumatoid arthritis
EORTC	European Organization for Research and the Treatment of Cancer
EOS	end of session
	end of study
	eosinophil
EP	ectopic pregnancy
	electronic prescribing
	electrophysiologic
	elopement precaution
	endogenous pyrogen
	Episcopalian
	esophageal pressure
	etoposide and cisplatin (Platinol)
	evoked potentials
E&P	estrogen and progesterone
EPA	eicosapentaenoic acid
	Environmental Protection Agency
EPAB	extracorporeal pneumoperititoneal access bubble
E-Panel	electrolyte panel (See page 318)
EPAP	expiratory positive airway pressure
EPB	extensor pollicis brevis
EPBD	endoscopic papillary balloon dilatation
EPC	erosive prephloric changes
	external pneumatic compression
EPCA	early prostate cancer antigen
Ep-CAM	epithelial cell adhesion molecule
EPCs	endothelial progenitor cells
EPCV	engineering, procurement, construction, and validation
EPD	electrode placement device
	equilibrium peritoneal dialysis
EPDS	Edinburgh Postnatal Depression Scale
EPEC	enteropathogenic *Escherichia coli*
EPEG	etoposide (VePesid)
EPEs	extrapyramidal effects
EPF	endoscopic plantar fasciotomy
	Enfamil Premature Formula®
	extrapyramidal features
EPG	electronic pupillography
	Episodic Payment Group
EPHI	electronic protected health information
EPI	echoplanar imaging
	epinephrine
	epirubicin (Ellence)
	epitheloid cells
	exercise pressure index
	exocrine pancreatic insufficiency
	Expanded Program of Immunizations, (World Health Organization)
	Eysenck Personality Inventory
EPIC	etoposide, prednisolone, ifosfamide, and cisplatin
EPID	epidural
epiDX	epirubicin (4′-epidoxorubicin; Ellence)
EPIG	epigastric
EPIS	epileptic postictal sleep
	episiotomy
epith.	epithelial
EPL	effective patent life

extensor pollicis longus (tendon)
EPM electronic pacemaker
EPMR electronic patient medical record
EPN emphysematous pyelonephritis
ependymoma
estimated protein needs
EPO epoetin alfa (erythropoietin; Epogen)
evening primrose oil
exclusive provider organization
EPOCH etoposide, prednisone, vincristine (Oncovin), cyclophosphamide, doxorubicin (hydroxydaunorubicin)
EPP erythropoietic protoporphyria
extrapleural pneumonectomy
EPPID electronic positive patient and specimen identification
EPPK epidermolytic palmoplantar keratoderma
EPPROM extremely preterm premature rupture of the membranes (less than or equal to 24 weeks)
EPQ Exercise Participation Questionnaire
EPQ-R Eysenck Personality Questionnaire—Revised
EPR electronic prescription record
electron paramagnetic (spin) resonance
electrophrenic respiration
emergency physical restraint
epirubicin (Ellence)
estimated protein requirement
EPS electrolyte-polyethyleneglycol solution
electrophysiologic study
expressed prostatic secretions
extrapulmonary shunt
extrapyramidal syndrome (symptom)
EPSA evoked potential signal averaging
EPSCCA extrapulmonary small cell carcinoma
EPSDT early periodic screening, diagnosis, and treatment
EPSE extrapyramidal side effects
EPSP excitatory postsynaptic potential
EPSS E point septal separation
EPT electroporation therapy
endpoint temperature
EPT® early pregnancy test
EPTE existed prior to enlistment
EPTS existed prior to service
EQC equivalent quality control
EQ-5D European Quality of life scale (EuroQol-5) (includes single item measures of: mobility, self-care, usual activities, pain/discomfort, and anxiety/depression)
ER emergency room
end range
estrogen receptors
extended release
external resistance
external rotation
E & R equal and reactive
examination and report
ER+ estrogen receptor-positive
ER− estrogen receptor-negative
ERA environmental risk assessment
estrogen receptor assay
evoked response audiometry
%ERAD eradication rates
ERAS Electronic Residency Application Service
erbB1 estrogen receptor (tyrosine kinase family) type B1
ERBD endoscopic retrograde biliary drainage
ER by ICA estrogen receptor immunocytochemistry assay
ERC endoscopic retrograde cholangiography
ERCP endoscopic retrograde cholangiopancreatography
ERCT emergency room computerized tomography
ERD early retirement with disability
erectile dysfunction
ERE external rotation in extension
EREM extended-release epidural morphine
ERF external rotation in flexion
ERFC erythrocyte rosette forming cells
ERG electroretinogram
ERI elective replacement indicator
ERIG equine-rabies immune globulin
ERL effective refractory length
ERLND elective regional lymph node dissection
ERM epiretinal membrane
ERMBT erythromycin breath testing
ERMS embryonal rhabdomyosarcoma
exacerbating-remitting multiple sclerosis
ERN error-related negativity (signal)
ERNA equilibrium radionuclide angiocardiography
ERO effective regurgitant orifice (cardiology)
EROS event-related optical signal
ERP effective refractory period
emergency room physician
endocardial resection procedure
endoscopic retrograde pancreatography
event-related potentials
estrogen receptor protein
exposure and ritual prevention
ERPF effective renal plasma flow

ER/PR	estrogen receptor/progesterone receptor
ERS	endoscopic retrograde sphincterotomy
	evacuation of retained secundines (afterbirth)
	extended, rotated, side bent (position of the spine)
ERSR	Electronic Regulatory Submission and Review
ERS-TM	Event Reporting System - Transfusion Medicine
ERT	estrogen replacement therapy
	external radiotherapy
ERTD	emergency room triage documentation
ERUS	endorectal ultrasound
ERV	early revascularization
	expiratory reserve volume
e-Rx	electronic prescription
Er:YAG	Erbium: yttrium aluminum garnet (laser)
ERYTH	erythromycin
ES	electrical stimulation
	Eleutherococcus senticosus (Siberian Ginseng)
	embryonic stem (cells)
	emergency service
	endoscopic sclerotherapy
	endoscopic sphincterotomy
	end-to-side
	ever-smokers
	Ewing sarcoma
	excessive sleepiness
	ex-smoker
	extra strength
ESA	early systolic acceleration
	end-to-side anastomosis
	ethmoid sinus adenocarcinoma
ESADDI	estimated safe and adequate daily dietary intake
ESAP	evoked sensory (nerve) action potential
ESAS	Edmonton Symptom Assessment System
ESAs	erythropoietin-stimulating agents
ESAT	extrasystolic atrial tachycardia
ESBL	extended-spectrum beta-lactamases
ESBLKP	extended-spectrum beta-lactamase-producing *Klebsiella pneumoniae*
ESC	embryonic stem cells
	end systolic counts
ESCC	esophageal squamous cell carcinoma
ESCOP	European Scientific Cooperative on Phytotherapy
ESCS	electrical spinal cord stimulation
ESD	early supported discharge
	Emergency Services Department
	esophagus, stomach, and duodenum
ESE	exon splice enhancer
ES EOC	early-stage epithelial ovarian cancer
eSET	elective single embryo transfer
ESF	external skeletal fixation
ESFT	Ewing sarcoma family of tumors
ESHAP	etopside, methylprednisolone (Solu-Medrol), high-dose cytarabine (ara-C), and cisplatin (Platinol)
ESI	electric source imaging
	electrospray ionization
	epidural steroid injection
ESI-MS	electrospray ionization-mass spectrometry
ESIN	elastic stable intramedullary nailing
ESKD	end-stage kidney disease
ESL	English as a second language
ESLD	end-stage liver disease
	end-stage lung disease
ESM	ejection systolic murmur
	endolymphatic stromal myosis
	ethosuximide (Zarontin)
ESMO	European Society of Medical Oncology
ESN	educationally subnormal
ESN(M)	educationally subnormal-moderate
ESN(S)	educationally subnormal-severe
ESO	esophagus
	esotropia
ESO/D	esotropia at distance
ESO/N	esotropia at near
ESP	endometritis, salpingitis, and peritonitis
	end-systolic pressure
	especially
	extrasensory perception
ESPAC	European Study Group for Pancreatic Cancers
ES/PNET	Ewing sarcomas and peripheral neuroectodermal tumor
ESR	early sheath removal
	electron spin resonance
	erythrocyte sedimentation rate
ESRD	end-stage renal disease
ESRF	end-stage renal failure
ESRS	Extrapyramidal Symptom Rating Scale
ESS	emotional, spiritual, and social
	endometrial stromal sarcoma
	endoscopic sinus surgery
	Epworth Sleepiness Scale
	essential
	euthyroid sick syndrome
EST	Eastern Standard Time
	endodermal sinus tumor
	endoscopic spincterotomy
	electroshock therapy
	electrostimulation therapy

E

established patient
estimated
exercise stress test
expressed sequence tag

E-stim electrical stimulation

ESTs expressed sequence tags

ESU electrosurgical unit

ESWL extracorporeal shock wave lithotripsy

ESWT extracorporeal shockwave therapy

ET ejection time
embryo transfer
endocrine therapy
endometrial thickness
endothelin
endotoxin
endotracheal
endotracheal tube
enterostomal therapy (therapist)
epirubicin and paclitaxel (Taxol)
esotropia
essential thrombocythemia
essential tremor
eustachian tube
Ewing tumor
exchange transfusion
exercise treadmill
exposure time

et and

ET′ esotropia at near

E(T) intermittent esotropia at infinity

E(T′) intermittent esotropia at near

ET-1 endothelin-1

2ET two embryo transfer

ET @ 20′ esotropia at 6 meters (infinity)

ETA endotracheal airway
ethionamide (Trecator-SC)

ETAAS electrothermal atomic absorption spectrometry

ETAC early treatment of the allergic child

et al and others

ETBD etiology to be determined

EtBr ethidium bromide

ETC and so forth
electrothermal capsulorrhaphy
Emergency and Trauma Center
endoscopic tissue culture
epirubicin, paclitaxel (Taxol), and cyclophosphamide
estimated time of conception

ETCH-C Evaluation Tool of Children's Handwriting-Cursive

$ETCO_2$ end-tidal carbon dioxide

ETD electron transfer dissociation
endoscopic transformational diskectomy
eustachian tube dysfunction
eye-tracking dysfunction

ETDLA esophageal-tracheal double lumen airway

ETE end-to-end

ETEC enterotoxigenic *Escherichia coli*

ETF early treatment failure
eustachian tubal function

ETFN empiric therapy in a febrile neutropenic (patient)

ETG Episodic Treatment Group

ETGT equal to or greater than

ETH elixir terpin hydrate
ethanol
Ethrane

ETHc̄C elixir terpin hydrate with codeine

ETI ejective time index
endotracheal intubation

ETKTM every test known to man

ETL echo train length (radiology)

ETLE extratemporal lobe epilepsy

ETLT equal to or less than

ETO estimated time of ovulation
ethylene oxide
etoposide (VePesid)
eustachian tube obstruction

EtOH alcohol (ethyl alcohol)
alcoholic

ETOP elective termination of pregnancy

ETP elective termination of pregnancy
electronic transmission of prescriptions

ETS elevated toilet seat
endoscopic transthoracic sympathectomy
endotracheal suction
end-to-side
environmental tobacco smoke
erythromycin topical solution

ETT endotracheal tube
endurance treadmill test
esophageal transit time
exercise tolerance test
exercise treadmill test (time)
extrathyroidal thyroxine

ETT-Tl exercise treadmill test with thallium

ETU emergency and trauma unit
emergency treatment unit

ETV endoscopic third ventriculostomy

ETX edatrexate

ETYA eicosatetraynoic acid

EU Ehrlich units
endotoxin units
equivalent units
esophageal ulcer
etiology unknown
European Union
excretory urography

EUA examine under anesthesia

E

EUCD — emotionally unstable character disorder
EUD — external urinary device
EUG — extrauterine gestation
EUL — extra uterine life
EUM — external urethral meatus
EUP — Experimental Use Permit
extrauterine pregnancy
EuroSIDA — a prospective observational cohort study to assess the impact of antiretroviral drugs on the outcome of the general population of 14,200 patients HIV-infected patients living in Europe
EUS — endoscopic ultrasonography
esophageal ultrasound
external urethral sphincter
EUS-FNA — endoscopic ultrasonography with fine-needle aspiration
EUTH — euthanasia
EV — epidermodysplasia verruciformis
esophageal varices
etoposide and vincristine
eversion
eV — electron volt (unit of radiation energy)
EV71 — enterovirus-71
EVA — Entry and Validation Application
ethylene vinyl acetate
etoposide, vinblastine, and doxorubicin (Adriamycin)
EVAC — evacuation
EVAc — ethylene-vinyl acetate copolymer
eval — evaluate (evaluation)
EVAR — endovascular aneurysm repair
EVC — Ellis-van Creveld (syndrome)
EVD — external ventricular (ventriculostomy) drain
extraventricular drain
EVE — endoscopic vascular examination
evening
EVER — eversion
EVG — endovascular grafting
EVH — endoscopic (saphenous) vein harvesting
EVI — Exposure to Violence Interview
EVL — endoscopic variceal ligation
EVLT — endovenous laser therapy
EVS — endoscopic variceal sclerosis
EVUS — endovaginal ultrasound
EW — expiratory wheeze
elsewhere
EWB — emotional well-being
estrogen withdrawal bleeding
EWBH — extracorporeal whole body hyperthermia
EWCL — extended-wear contact lens
EWE — Eastern and Western encephalomyelitis vaccine
EWHO — elbow-wrist-hand orthosis
EWL — estimated weight loss
EWS — Early Warning Score
Ewing sarcoma
EWSCLs — extended-wear soft contact lenses
EWT — erupted wisdom teeth
ex — examined
example
excision
exercise
exam. — examination
ExB — excisional biopsy
EXC — excision
EXE — exemestane (Aromasin)
EXEC 22 — Executive 22 chemistry profile (see page 318)
EXECHO — exercise echocardiography
EXEF — exercise ejection fraction
EXGBUS — external genitalia, Bartholin (glands), urethral (glands), and Skene (glands)
EXH VT — exhaled tidal volume
EXIT — Ex-Utero Intrapartum Treatment
EXIT 25 — Executive Interview (cognitive impairment test)
EXL — elixir
EXOPH — exophthalmos
EXP — experienced
expired
exploration
expose
expect — expectorant
exp. lap. — exploratory laparotomy
EXT — extension
extensor (tendon)
external
extract
extraction
extremities
extremity
Ext mon — external monitor
extrav — extravasation
ext. rot. — external rotation
EXTUB — extubation
EX U — excretory urogram
EZ — Edmonston-Zagreb (vaccine)
EZ-HT — Edmonston-Zagreb high-titer (vaccine)

F

F — facial; Fahrenheit; fair; false; fasting; father; feces; female; finger; firm; flow; fluoride; French; Friday; fundi; fundus

F/ — full upper denture

/F — full lower denture

(F) — final

°F — degrees Fahrenheit

F= — firm and equal

F_1 — offspring from the first generation

F_2 — offspring from the second generation

F_3 — Fluothane

14 F — 14-hour fast required

F II-F XIII — factor 2 through 13

FA — Fanconi anemia; fatty acid; femoral acetabular; femoral artery; fetus active; fibroadenoma; first aid; fludarabine (Fludara); fluorescein angiogram; fluorescent antibody; folic acid; folinic acid (leucovorin calcium) (this is a dangerous abbreviation); forearm; Friedreich ataxia; functional activities

FAA — febrile antigen agglutination; folic acid antagonist

FAAAAI — Fellow of the American Academy of Allergy, Asthma & Immunology

FAAD — Fellow American Academy of Dermatology

FAAH — fatty acid amide hydrolase

FAAN — Food Allergy and Anaphylaxis Network

FAAP — family assessment adjustment pass

FAAPM — Fellow, American Academy of Pain Management

FAA SOL — formalin, acetic, and alcohol solution

FAAN — Fellow of the American Academy of Nursing

FAAP — Fellow of the American Academy of Pediatrics

FAB — digoxin immune Fab (Digibind); French-American-British Cooperative group; functional arm brace

FABACs — fatty acid bile acid conjugates

FABER — flexion, abduction, and external rotation

FABF — femoral artery blood flow

FABIANS — Felt awful but I'm alright now syndrome (slang)

FAC — ferrite ammonium citrate; fluorouracil, doxorubicin (Adriamycin), and cyclophosphamide; fractional area change; fractional area concentration; functional aerobic capacity

FACA — Fellow of the American College of Anaesthetists

FACAG — Fellow of the American College of Angiology

FACAL — Fellow of the American College of Allergists

FACAN — Fellow of the American College of Anesthesiologists

FACAS — Fellow of the American College of Abdominal Surgeons

FACC — Fellow of the American College of Cardiology

FACCP — Fellow of the American College of Chest Physicians

FACCPC — Fellow of the American College of Clinical Pharmacology & Chemotherapy

FACD — Fellow of the American College of Dentists

FACE — Fatality Assessment and Control Evaluation (National Institute for Occupational Safety and Health report)

FACEM — Fellow of the American College of Emergency Medicine

FACEP — Fellow of the American College of Emergency Physicians

FACES — pain scale for assessing pain intensity

FACG — Fellow of the American College of Gastroenterology

FACH — forceps to after-coming head

FACIT-F — Functional Assessment of Chronic Illness Therapy Fatigue Subscale

FACLM Fellow of the American College of Legal Medicine

FACN Fellow of the American College of Nutrition

FACNP Fellow of the American College of Neuropsychopharmacology

FACO Fellow of the American College of Otolaryngology

FACOG Fellow of the American College of Obstetricians & Gynecologists

FACOS Fellow of the American College of Orthopedic Surgeons

FACP Fellow of the American College of Physicians

FACPRM Fellow of the American College of Preventive Medicine

FACR Fellow of the American College of Radiology

FACS Fellow of the American College of Surgeons
fluorescent-activated cell sorter

FACSM Fellow of the American College of Sports Medicine

FACT focused appendix computed tomography

FACT-An Functional Assessment of Cancer Therapy-Anemia

FACT-B ....-Breast

FACT-F ....-Fatigue

FACT-G ....-General

FACT-L ....-Lung

FACT-O ....-Ovarian

FACT-P ....-Prostate

FAD familial Alzheimer disease
Family Assessment Device
fetal abdominal diameter
fetal activity determination
flavin adenine dinucleotide

FAE fetal alcohol effect

FAEE fatty acid ethyl ester

FAF frequency-altered feedback

FAFSA Free Application for Federal Student Aid

FAGA full-term appropriate for gestational age

FAH fumarylacetoacetase hydrolase

FAI Functional Assessment Inventory

FAK focal adhesion kinase

FAL femoral arterial line

FALL fallopian

FALS familial amyotrophic lateral sclerosis

FAM family
fluorouracil, doxorubicin (Adriamycin), and mitomycin
full allosteric modulators

FAMA fluorescent antibody to membrane antigen

FAME fluorouracil, doxorubicin (Adriamycin), and semustin (methyl CCNU)

FAMMM familial atypical multiple mole melanoma

FAM-S fluorouracil, doxorubicin (Adriamycin), mitomycin, and streptozotocin

FAMTX fluorouracil, doxorubicin (Adriamycin), and methotrexate

FANA fluorescent antinuclear antibody

FANG fluorescent angiography

FANSS&M fundus anterior, normal size and shape and mobile

FAO fatty acid oxidation
Food and Agriculture Organization

FAP Facility Admission Profile
familial adenomatous polyposis
familial amyloid polyneuropathy
femoral artery pressure
fibrillating action potential
functional ambulation profile

FAQ frequently asked question(s)

FAR frontal arousal rhythm

F-ara-A fludarabine phosphate (Fludara)

f-ARPV fosamprenavir (Lexiva)

FARS Fatality Analysis Reporting System

FAS fetal alcohol syndrome

FASAY functional analysis of separated alleles in yeast

FASC fluorescent-activated substrate conversion (assay)
fasciculations

FASD fetal alcohol spectrum disorder

FASHP Fellow of the American Society of Health-System Pharmacists

FASPS familial advanced sleep-phase syndrome

FAST fetal acoustic stimulation testing
flow-assisted short-term
fluorescent allergosorbent technique
focused assessment with sonography for trauma

FAT Fetal Activity Test
fluorescent antibody test
food awareness training

FAV facio-auricular vertebral

FAZ foveal avascular zone

FB fasting blood (sugar)
finger breadth
flexible bronchoscope
foreign body

F/B followed by
forward/backward
forward bending

FBC full (complete) blood count

FBCOD foreign body, cornea, right eye

FBCOS foreign body, cornea, left eye

FBD familial British dementia
fibrocystic breast disease
functional bowel disease
FBF forearm blood flow
FBG fasting blood glucose
foreign-body-type granulomata
FBH hydroxybutyric dehydrogenase
FBHH familial benign hypocalciuric hypercalcemia
FBI flossing, brushing, and irrigation
full bony impaction
FBL fecal blood loss
FBM felbamate (Felbatol)
fetal breathing motion
foreign body, metallic
FBO for the benefit of
FBP frontal bite plane (dental)
FBRCM fingerbreadth below right costal margin
FBS failed back syndrome
fasting blood sugar
fetal bovine serum
foreign body sensation (eye)
FBSS failed back surgery syndrome
FBU fingers below umbilicus
FBW fasting blood work
FC family conference
febrile convulsion
female child
fever, chills
film coated (tablets)
financial class
finger clubbing
finger counting
flexion contractor
flow compensation (radiology)
flucytosine (Ancobon)
foam cuffed (tracheal or endotrachael tube)
Foley catheter
follows commands
foster care
French Canadian
functional capacity
functional class
F/C film coated (tablet)
F + C flare and cells
F & C foam and condom
5FC flucytosine (this is a dangerous abbreviation as it can be seen as 5FU)
FCA Federal False Claims Act
femoral cortical allograft
FCAS familial cold autoinflammatory syndrome
F. cath. Foley catheter
FCBD fibrocystic breast disease
FCC familial cerebral cavernoma
familial colonic cancer
family centered care
femoral cerebral catheter
follicular center cells
fracture compound comminuted
FCCA Final Comprehensive Consensus Assessment
FCCC fracture complete, compound, and comminuted
FCCL follicular center cell lymphoma
FCCM Fellow, American College of Critical Care Medicine
FCCU family centered care unit
FCD feces collection device
fibrocystic disease
FCDB fibrocystic disease of the breast
FCE fluorouracil, cisplatin, and etoposide
functional capacity evaluation
FCFD fluorescence capillary-fill device
FCH familial combined hyperlipidemia
fibrosing cholestatic hepatitis
FCHL familial combined hyperlipemia
FCI flow cytometric immunophenotyping
FCL fibular collateral ligament
F-CL fluorouracil and calcium leucovorin
FCM facial choreic movements
flow cytometry
FCMC family centered maternity care
FCMD Fukiyama congenital muscular dystrophy
FCMN family centered maternity nursing
FCNV fever, cough, nausea, and vomiting
FCOU finger count, both eyes
FCP formocresol pulpotomu
FCR flexor carpi radialis
fractional catabolic rate
FCRB flexor carpi radialis brevis
FCRT fetal cardiac reactivity test
focal cranial radiation therapy
FCS fever, chills, and sweating
FCSNVD fever, chills, sweating, nausea, vomiting, and diarrhea
FCSRT Free and Cued Selective Reminding Test
FCT fever-clearance time
FCU flexor carpi ulnaris (tendon)
FCV feline calicivirus
FD familial dysautonomia
fetal demise
fetal distress
focal distance
food diary
forceps delivery
Forestier Disease
free drain
full denture
fully dilated
functional deficits

F & D	fixed and dilated
FDA	Food and Drug Administration
	fronto-dextra anterior
FDB	first-degree burn
	flexor digitorum brevis
FDBL	fecal daily blood loss
FDC	familial dilated cardiomyopathy
	fixed-dose combination (preparations)
FDCA	Food, Drug, and Cosmetic Act
FDCs	follicular dendritic cells
FDE	fixed-drug eruption
FDEIA	food-dependent, exercise-induced anaphylaxis
FDF	flexor digitorum profundus (tendon)
FDG	feeding
	fluorine-18-labeled deoxyglucose (^{18}fluorodeoxyglucose)
FDGB	fall down, go boom
FDG-PET	positron emission tomography with ^{18}fluorodeoxyglucose
FDGS	feedings
FDI	first dorsal interosseous
	food-drug interaction
	Functional Disability Index
FDIP	fourth dorsal interosseus pedis (muscle)
FDIU	fetal death in utero
FDL	flexor digitorum longus
FDLMP	first day of last menstrual period
FDM	feline diabetes mellitus
	fetus of diabetic mother
	flexor digiti minimi
FDP	fibrin-degradation products
	fixed-dose procedure
	flexor digitorum profundus
FDPCA	fixed-dose patient-controlled analgesia
FD-PET	fluorodopa-positron emission tomography
FDQB	flexor digiti quinti brevis
FDR	first-dose reaction
FDS	flexor digitorum superficialis
	for duration of stay
FDT	frequency-doubling technology (perimetry for visual field screening)
	fronto-dextra transversa (right frontotransverse)
	Functional Dexterity Test
FE	field echo (radiology)
	frequency encode (radiology)
Fe	female
	iron
F & E	full and equal
FEB	febrile
FEC	fluorouracil, epirubicin, and cyclophosphamide
	fluorouracil, etoposide, and cisplatin
	forced expiratory capacity
FECG	fetal electrocardiogram
FeCh	ferrochelatase
FECP	free erythrocyte coproporphyrin
FeCrNi	iron-chromium-nickel alloy
FECT	fibroelastic connective tissue
FED	fish eye disease
FEE	Far-Eastern equine encephalitis
FEES	fiberoptic endoscopic evaluation (examination) of swallowing
FEESST	flexible endoscopic evaluation of swallowing with sensory testing
FEF	forced expiratory flow rate
FEF$_{25\%-75\%}$	forced expiratory flow during the middle half of the forced vital capacity
FEF$_{x-y}$	forced expiratory flow between two designated volume points in the forced vital capacity
FEHBP	Federal Employee Health Benefits Plan
FEL	familial erythrophagocytic lymphohistiocytosis
	free electron laser
FeLV	feline leukemia virus
FEM	femoral
FEMA	Federal Emergency Management Agency
FEM-FEM	femoral femoral (bypass)
FEMG	facial electromyography
FEM-POP	femoral popliteal (bypass)
FEM-TIB	femoral tibial (bypass)
femto	prefix for units denoting a factor of 10^{-15} or 0.000,000,000,000,001 (symbol f)
FERGs	focal electroretinograms
FEN	fluid, electrolytes, and nutrition
FENa	fractional extraction of sodium
FENIB	familial encephalopathies with neuroserpin inclusion bodies
FEN-PHEN	fenfluramine and phentermine
FENS	field-electrical neural stimulation
FEOM	full extraocular movements
FEP	first-episode psychosis
	free erythrocyte porphyrins
	free erythrocyte protoporphorin
	functional exercise program
FER	flexion, extension, and rotation
FERPA	Family Educational Rights and Privacy Act
FERR	serum ferritin
FES	fat embolism syndrome
	floppy eyelid syndrome
	forced expiratory spirogram
	functional electrical stimulation
FeSO$_4$	ferrous sulfate

FESS functional endonasal sinus surgery
functional endoscopic sinus surgery
FET familial essential tremor
fixed erythrocyte turnover
frozen embryo transfer
FETI fluorescence (fluorescent) energy transfer immunoassay
FEU fibrinogen equivalent units
FEUO for external use only
FEV familial exudative vitreoretinopathy
FEV_1 forced expiratory volume in one second
FEVC forced expiratory vital capacity
$FEV_{1\%VC}$ forced expiratory volume in one second as percent of forced vital capacity
FEVR familial exudative vitreoretinopathy
FF fat free
fecal frequency
filtration fraction
finger-to-finger
five-minute format
flat feet
force fluids
formula fed
forward flexion
foster father
Fox-Fordyce (disease)
fundus firm
further flexion
F/F face-to-face
F&F filiform and follower
fixes and follows
F→F finger to finger
FF1/U fundus firm 1 cm above umbilicus
FF2/U fundus firm 2 cm above umbilicus
FF@u fundus firm at umbilicus
FFA free fatty acid
fundus fluorescein angiogram
fusiform face area
FFAT Free Floating Anxiety Test
FFB flexible fiberoptic bronchoscopy
FFCD French Foundation for Digestive Cancerology
FFD fat-free diet
focal-film distance
FFDM freedom from distant metastases
full-field digital mammography
FFE free-flow electrophoresis
FFF field-flow fractionation
freedom from (biochemical and/or clinical) failure
FFI fast food intake
fatal familial insomnia
FFL flexible fiberoptic laryngoscopy
FFM fat-free mass
Five-Factor Model (of personality)
five-finger movement
freedom from metastases
FFN fetal fibronectin
FFOV functional field of view
FFP free from progression
fresh frozen plasma
FFPE formalin-fixed, paraffin-embedded
FFQ food frequency questionnaire
FFR freedom from relapse
Forward Functional Reach (test)
FFROM full, free range of motion
FFS failure-free survival
fee-for-service
Fight For Sight
flexible fiberoptic sigmoidoscopy
FFT fast-Fourier transforms
flicker fusion threshold
FFTC fast-Fourier Transform Convolution
FFTDWB flat foot touchdown weight bearing
FFTP first full-term pregnancy
FFU/1 fundus firm 1 cm below umbilicus
FFU/2 fundus firm 2 cm below umbilicus
FG fibrin glue
fusiform gyrus
FGAs first-generation antihistamines
first-generation antipsychotics
FGC familial gigantiform cementoma
female genital cutting
full gold crown
FGF fibroblast growth factor
FGID functional gastrointestinal disorder(s)
FGM female genital mutilation
FGM/C female genital mutilation/cutting
FGP fundic gland polyps
FGR fetal growth restriction
FGS fibrogastroscopy
focal glomerulosclerosis
FH familial hypercholesterolemia
family history
favorable histology
fetal head
fetal heart
fundal height
FH+ family history positive
FH− family history negative
FHA filamentous hemagglutinin
FHB flexor hallucis brevis
FHBL familial hypobetalipoproteinemia
FHC familial hypertrophic cardiomyopathy
family health center
FHCIC Fuchs heterochromic iridocyclitis
FHD family history of diabetes
FHF fulminant hepatic failure
FHH familial hypocalciuric hypercalcemia
fetal heart heard
FHI fibrous hamartoma of infancy
frontal horn index

F

	Fuchs heterochromic iridocyclitis
FHL	flexor hallucis longus
	functional hallux limitus
FHM	familial hemiplegic migraine
FHN	family history negative
FHNH	fetal heart not heard
FHO	family history of obesity
FHP	family history positive
FHR	fetal heart rate
FHRB	fetal heart rate baseline
FHRV	fetal heart rate variability
FHS	fetal heart sounds
	fetal hydantoin syndrome
FHT	fetal heart tone
FHVP	free hepatic vein pressure
FHX	fluorouracil, hydroxyurea, and radiotherapy
FHx	family history
FI	fecal incontinence
	feeding intolerance
	fiscal intermediary
FIA	familial intracranial aneurysms
	Family Independence Agency (formerly Department of Social Services)
FIAC	fiacitabine
FIAU	fialuridine
FIB	fibrillation
	fibula
	focused ion-beam
FICA	Federal Insurance Contributions Act (Social Security)
$FiCO_2$	fraction of inspired carbon dioxide
FICS	Fellow of the International College of Surgeons
FID	father in delivery
	free induction decay
FIESTA	fast imaging employing steady-state acquisition (imaging)
FIF	forced inspiratory flow
FiF	Functional Intact Fibrinogen (test)
FIGE	field inversion gel electrophoresis
FIGLU	formiminoglutamic acid
FIGO	International Federation of Gynecology and Obstetrics
FIH	first-in-human (trial)
FIL	father-in-law
	Filipino
FIM	functional independence measure
FIN	flexible intramedullary nail
FIND	follow-up intervention for normal development
FiO_2	fraction of inspired oxygen
FIP	feline infectious peritonitis
	flatus in progress
FIRI	fasting insulin resistance index
FISH	fluorescent (fluorescence) *in situ* hybridization
FISH-MD	fluorescence *in situ* hybridization microdissection
FISP	fast imaging with steady state precision
FIT	fecal immunochemical test
	functional inferior turbinoplasty
FITC	fluorescein isothiocyanate conjugated
FIV	feline immunodeficiency virus
	in vitro fertilization (French)
FIVC	forced inspiratory vital capacity
FIX	factor IX (nine)
FJB	facet joint block
FJN	familial juvenile nephrophthisis
FJP	familial juvenile polyposis
FJROM	full joint range of motion
FJS	finger joint size
FJV	first jejunal vein
FK506	tacrolimus (Prograf)
FKA	failed to keep appointment
	formally known as
FKBP	FK-506 binding protein (tacrolimus; Prograf)
FKD	Kinetic Family Drawing
FKE	full-knee extension
FKGL	Flesh-Kincaid Grade Level (score)
FL	fatty liver
	femur length
	fetal length
	fluid
	fluorescein
	fluorouracil and leucovorin
	flutamide and leuprolide acetate
	focal laser
	focal length
	follicular lymphoma
	full liquids
	functional limitations
fL	femtoliter (10^{-15} liter)
F/L	father-in-law
FLA	free-living amebic (ameba)
	low-friction arthroplasty
FLACC	Face, Legs, Activity, Cry, and Consolability (pain assessment scale)
FLAG	**fl**udarabine, **a**ra-C (cytarabine), and **G-**CSF (filgrastim)
FLAIR	fluid-attenuated inversion recovery
FLAP	fluorouracil, leucovorin, doxorubicin (Adriamycin), and cisplatin (Platinol)
	5-lipoxygenase activating protein
FLASH	fast low-angle shot
FLAVO	flavopiridol
FLB	funny looking beat
FLBS	funny looking baby syndrome (see note under FLK)
FLC	follicular large cell lymphoma
	fuzzy logic control

FLD	fatty liver disease
	fluid
	flutamide and leuprolide acetate depot
	full lower denture
FL Dtr	full lower denture
FLE	frontal lobe epilepsy
FLe	fluorouracil and levamisole
flexsig	flexible sigmoidoscopy
FLF	funny looking facies (see note under FLK)
FLGA	full-term, large for gestational age
FLIC	Functional Living Index– Cancer
FLIE	Functional Living Index– Emesis
FLIPI	Follicular Lymphoma International Prognostic Index
FLK	funny looking kid (should never be used: unusual facial features, is a better expression)
FLM	fetal lung maturity
fl. oz.	fluid ounce
FLP	fasting lipid profile
	Functional Limitations Profile
FL REST	fluid restriction
FLS	fibroblast-like synoviocytes
	flashing lights and/or scotoma
	flu-like symptoms
FLT	fluorothymidine
FLU	fluconazole (Diflucan)
	fludarabine (Fludara)
	flunisolide (Aero Bid)
	fluoxetine (Prozac)
	fluticasone propionate (Flonase)
	influenza
FLU A	influenza A virus
FLUO	Fluothane
fluoro	fluoroscopy
FLUT	flutamide (Eulexin)
FLV	Friend leukemia virus
FLW	fasting laboratory work
FLZ	flurazepam (Dalmane)
FM	face mask
	fat mass
	fetal movements
	fibromyalgia (syndrome)
	fine motor
	floor manager
	fluorescent microscopy
	foster mother
F & M	firm and midline (uterus)
F-MACHOP	fluorouracil, methotrexate, cytarabine (ara-C), cyclophosphamide, doxorubicin (hydroxydaunorubicin), vincristine (Oncovin), and prednisone
FMC	fetal movement count
	fine motor coordination
FMD	family medical doctor
	fibromuscular dysplasia
	flow-mediated dilatation
	foot-and-mouth disease
FMDV	foot-and-mouth disease virus
FME	Frühsommer-meningoenzephalitis vaccine
	full-mouth extraction
FMEA	failure mode effects analysis
FMEN-1	familial multiple endocrine neoplasia, type 1
FMF	familial Mediterranean fever
	fetal movement felt
	forced midexpiratory flow
FMG	fine mesh gauze
	foreign medical graduate
FMH	family medical history
	fibromuscular hyperplasia
FM 100-hue	Farnsworth-Munsell 100-hue test
FmHx	family history
FML	familial multiple lipomatosis
FML®	fluorometholone
FMLA	Family and Medical Leave Act of 1993
FMN	first malignant neoplasm
	flavin mononucleotide
FMOA	full-mouth odontectomy and alveoloplasty
FMOL	femtomole (10^{-15} mole)
FMP	fasting metabolic panel
	first menstrual period
	functional maintenance program
FMPA	full-mouth periapicals
FMR	fetal movement record
	focused medical review
	functional magnetic resonance (imaging)
	functional mitral regurgitation
FMR1	fragile X mental retardation 1
FMRD	full-mouth restorative dentistry
fMRI	functional magnetic resonance imaging
FMRP	fragile X mental retardation protein(s)
FMS	fibromyalgia syndrome
	fluorouracil, mitomycin, and streptozocin
	full-mouth series
F & MS	frontal and maxillary sinuses
FMT	fluorescein meniscus time (dry-eye test)
	functional muscle test
FMTC	familial medullary thyroid carcinoma
FMU	first morning urine
FMV	flow-mediated vasodilation
	fluorouracil, semustine (methyl-CCNU), and vincristine
FMX	full-mouth x-ray
FMZ	flumazenil (Romazicon)
FN	facial nerve

false negative
febrile neutropenia
femoral neck
finger-to-nose (test)
flight nurse

F/N fluids and nutrition

F to N finger-to-nose

FNA femoral neck anteversion
fine-needle aspiration

FNa filtered sodium

FNAB fine-needle aspiration biopsy

FNAC fine-needle aspiratory cytology

FNB femoral nerve block

FNC Family Nurse Clinician

FNCJ fine-needle catheter jejunostomy

FND fludarabine, mitoxantrone (Novantrone), and dexamethasone
focal neurological deficit

FNF femoral-neck fracture
finger-nose-finger (test)

FNH focal nodular hyperplasia

FNHL follicular non-Hodgkin lymphoma

FNMTC familial nonmedullary thyroid carcinoma

FNP Family Nurse Practitioner

FNR false-negative rate

FNS food and nutrition services
functional neuromuscular stimulation

F/NS fever and night sweats

FNT finger-to-nose (test)

FNTC fine-needle transhepatic cholangiography

FO foot orthosis
foramen ovale
foreign object
fronto-occipital

FOB father of baby
fecal occult blood
feet out of bed
fiberoptic bronchoscope
foot of bed

FOBT fecal occult blood test

FOC father of child
fluid of choice
fronto-occipital circumference

FOCF first observation carried forward

FOD fixing right eye
free of disease

FOEB feet over edge of bed

FOF fell on floor

FOG Fluothane, oxygen and gas (nitrous oxide)
full-on gain

FOH family ocular history

FOI fiberoptic intubation
flight of ideas

FOIA Freedom of Information Act

FOID fear of impending doom

FOK feeling-of-knowing (episodic memory procedure)

FOL fiberoptic laryngoscopy

FOLFIRI leucovorin, (**fol**inic acid) fluorouracil, and **iri**notecan

FOLFOX leucovorin calcium (folinic acid), fluorouracil, and oxaliplatin

FOM floor of mouth

FOMi fluorouracil, Oncovin, (vincristine), and mitomycin

FONSI finding of no significant impact

FOO family of origin

FOOB fell out of bed

FOOSH fell on outstretched hand

FOP fasting office profile
fibrodysplasia ossificans progressiva

FOPS fiberoptic proctosigmoidoscopy

FORMIL foreign military

FOS fiberoptic sigmoidoscopy
fixing left eye
force of stream (urology)
fosphenytoin (Cerebyx)
fructooligosaccharides
future order screen

FOSC freestanding outpatient surgery center

FOT forced oscillation technique
form of thought
frontal outflow tract

FOV field of view

FOVI field of vision intact

FOW fenestration of oval window

FOZ functional optical zone

FP fall precautions
false positive
familial porencephaly
family planning
family practice
family practitioner
family presence
fibrous proliferation
flat plate
fluorescence polarization
fluticasone propionate
food poisoning
frozen plasma

F/P fluid/plasma (ratio)

F-P femoral popliteal

fpA fibrinopeptide A

FPAL full term, premature, abortion, living

FPB femoral-popliteal bypass
flexor pollicis brevis

FPC familial polyposis coli
family practice center

FPD feto-pelvic disproportion
fixed partial denture

FPDL flashlamp-pumped pulsed dye laser

FPE first-pass effect

FPG	fasting plasma glucose
FPHx	family psychiatric history
FPIA	fluorescence-polarization immunoassay
FPIES	food protein-induced enterocolitis syndrome
FPL	federal poverty level
	final printed labeling (FDA document)
	flexor pollicis longus (tendon)
	final printed labeling
FPLD	familial partial lipodystrophy
FPLV	feline panleucopenia virus
FPM	full passive movements
FPN	ferroportin
FPNA	first-pass nuclear angiocardiography
FPNP	Family Planning Nurse Practitioner
FPO	fetal pulse oximetry
FPOR	follicle puncture for oocyte retrieval
FPPI	first postpacing interval
FPU	family participation unit
FPV	fosamprenavir (Lexiva)
FPZ	fluphenazine (Prolixin; Permitil)
FPZ-D	fluphenazine decanoate (Prolixin Decanoate)
FQ	fluoroquinolones
	frequency
FR	fair
	father
	Father (priest)
	Federal Register
	first responder
	flow rate
	fluid restriction
	fluid retention
	fractional reabsorption
	freestyle, no head or lower-extremity fixation (aquatic therapy)
	frequent relapses
	Friends
	frothy
	full range
Fr	French (catheter gauge)
F/R	fire/rescue
F & R	force and rhythm (pulse)
FRA	fall risk assessment
	femoral ring allograft
	fluorescent rabies antibody
FRAC	fracture
FRACTS	fractional urines
FRAG	fragment
FRAG-X	Fragile X Syndrome
FRAP	family risk assessment program
	fluorescence recovery after photobleaching
FRC	frozen red cells
	functional residual capacity
FRCPC	Fellow of the Royal College of Physicians of Canada
FRCPE	Fellow of the Royal College of Physicians of Edinburgh
FRCSC	Fellow of the Royal College of Surgeons of Canada
FRCSE	Fellow of the Royal College of Surgeons of Edinburgh
FRCSI	Fellow of the Royal College of Surgeons of Ireland
FRE	flow-related enhancement
FRET	fluoresence resonance energy transfer
FRF	filtration replacement fluid
FRG	Functional Related Groups
FRH	febrile-range hyperthermia
FRJM	full range of joint movement
FRN	fetal rhabdomyomatous nephroblastoma
FRNT	focus-reduction neutralization test
FROA	full range of affect
FROM	full range of motion
FROMAJE	functioning, reasoning, orientation, memory, arithmetic, judgment, and emotion (mental status evaluation)
FRP	follicle regulatory protein
	functional refractory period
FRS	first-rank symptoms
	flexed, rotated, side-bent (position of the spine)
	Framingham risk scores
	Functional Rating Scale
FRSN	fluoroquinolone-resistant *Streptococcus pneumoniae*
FRSS	forward resuscitative surgery system
FS	fetoscope
	fibromyalgia syndrome
	fingerstick
	flexible sigmoidoscopy
	foreskin
	fractional shortenings
	frozen section
	full strength
	functional status
F & S	full and soft
FSA	Family Services Association
FSAD	female sexual arousal disorder(s)
FSALO	Fletcher suite after loading ovoids
FSALT	Fletcher suite after loading tandem
FSB	fetal scalp blood
	full spine board
FSBG	fingerstick blood glucose
FSBM	full-strength breast milk
FSBS	fingerstick blood sugar
FSC	Fatigue Symptom Checklist
	flexible sigmoidoscopy
	Forensic Science Center

	fracture, simple, and comminuted
	fracture, simple, and complete
FSCC	fracture, simple, complete, and comminuted
FSD	female sexual dysfunction
	focal-skin distance
	fracture, simple, and depressed
FSE	fast spin-echo
	fetal scalp electrode
FSF	fibrin stabilizing factor
FSG	fasting serum glucose
	focal and segmental glomerulosclerosis
FSGA	full-term, small for gestational age
FSGN	focal segmental glomerulonephritis
FSGS	focal segmental glomerulosclerosis
FSH	facioscapulohumeral
	follicle-stimulating hormone
FSHD	facioscapulohumeral (muscular) dystrophy
FSHMD	facioscapulohumeral muscular dystrophy
FSIQ	Full-Scale Intelligence Quotient (part of Wechsler test)
FSL	fasting serum level
FSM	functional status measures
F-SM/C	fungus, smear and culture
FSME	Frühsommer-meningoencephalitis
FSO	for screws only (prosthetic cups)
	frontal sinus obliteration
FSOP	French Society of Pediatric Oncology
FSP	Family Service Plan
	fibrin split products
FSR	fractionated stereotactic radiosurgery
	fusiform skin revision
FSRP	Framingham Stroke Risk Profile
FSRS	fractionated stereotactic radiosurgery
FSRT	fractionated stereotactic radiotherapy
FSS	Fatigue Severity Scale
	federal supply schedule (cost source)
	fetal scalp sampling
	fetal scalp stimulation
	Flinders Symptom Score
	Forensic Science Service (United Kingdom)
	Freeman-Sheldon syndrome
	French steel sound (dilated to #24FSS)
	frequency-selective saturation
	full-scale score
	functional somatic symptoms
FST	forward surgical team(s)
FSW	feet of sea water (pressure)
	field service worker
FT	family therapy
	fast-twitch
	feeding tube
	filling time
	finger tip
	flexor tendon
	fluidotherapy
	follow through
	foot (ft)
	Fourier transform (radiology)
	free testosterone
	full-term
F_3T	trifluridine (Viroptic)
FT_3	free triiodothyronine
FT_4	free thyroxine
FT_4I	free thyroxine index
FTA	femorotibial angle
	fluorescent titer antibody
	fluorescent treponemal antibody
FTA-ABS	fluorescent treponemal antibody absorption
FTAGA	full-term average gestational age
FTB	fingertip blood
FTBD	full-term born dead
FTBI	fractionated total body irradiation
FTC	emtricitabine (Emtriva)
	fallopian tube carcinoma
	Federal Trade Commission
	follicular thyroid carcinoma
	frames to come
	full to confrontation
FTD	failure to descend
	frontotemporal degeneration
	frontotemporal dementia
	full-term delivery
FTE	failure to engraft
FTEs	full-time equivalents
FTF	failure to fly (for attempted suicide) (slang)
	finger-to-finger
	free thyroxine fraction
FTFTN	finger-to-finger-to-nose
FTG	full-thickness graft
FTI	farnesyltransferase inhibitor
	force-time integral
	free thyroxine index
FTICR-MS	Fourier-transform ion cyclotron resonance-mass spectrometry
F TIP	finger tip
FTIR	Fourier-transform infrared spectroscopy
FTIUP	full-term intrauterine pregnancy
FTKA	failed to keep appointment
FTLB	full-term living birth
FTLD	frontotemporal lobar degeneration
	frontotemporal lobar dementia
FTLFC	full-term living female child
FTLMC	full-term living male child
FTM	female-to-male (transmission)
	fluid thioglycollate medium
FTMH	full-thickness macular hole(s)

Abbreviation	Meaning
FTMS	Fourier-transform mass spectrometer
FTN	finger-to-nose
	full-term nursery
FTNB	full-term newborn
FTND	Fagerstrom Test for Nicotine Dependence
	full-term normal delivery
FTNSD	full-term, normal, spontaneous delivery
FTO	full-time occlusion (eye patch)
FTOZ	frontotemporal orbitozygomatic
FTOZ1	one-piece frontotemporal orbitozygomatic
FTP	failure to progress
	full-term pregnancy
FTR	father
	failed to report
	failed to respond
	for the record
FTRAM	free transverse rectus abdominis myocutaneous (flap)
FTSD	full-term spontaneous delivery
FTSG	full-thickness skin graft
FTT	failure to thrive
	fetal tissue transplant
	Finger-Tapping Test
Ftube	feeding tube
FTUPLD	full-term uncomplicated pregnancy, labor, and delivery
FTV	Fortovase (saquinavir, soft gel cap)
	functional trial visit
FTW	failure to wean
FU	fraction unbound
	fluorouracil
F & U	flanks and upper quadrants
F/U	follow-up
	fundus at umbilicus
F↑U	fingers above umbilicus
F↓U	fingers below umbilicus
5-FU	fluorouracil
FUA	flat and upright (x-ray of the) abdomen
FUB	functional uterine bleeding
FUCO	fractional uptake of carbon monoxide
FUD	fear, uncertainty, and doubt
	frequency, urgency, and dysuria
	full upper denture
FUDR(r)	floxuridine
FU Dtr	full upper denture
FUFA	fluorouracil and leucovorin (folinic acid)
FU/FL	full upper denture, full lower denture
FUFOL	fluorouracil and leucovorin calcium (folinic acid)
Fugl	Fugl-Meyer Assessment of Motor Recovery After Stroke
FUL	federal upper limit (price list)
FULG	fulguration
5FU/LV	fluorouracil and leucovorin
FUN	follow-up note
FUNASA	Fundão Naçional de Sade (Brazil's national health agency)
FUNG-C	fungus culture
FUNG-S	fungus smear
FUO	fever of undetermined origin
FUOV	follow-up office visit
FU/LP	full upper denture, partial lower denture
FUP	follow-up
FUS	fusion
FUT	fibrinogen update test
FUV	follow-up visit
FV	femoral vein
F & V	fruits and vegetables
FVBG	free vascularized bone graft
FVC	false vocal cord(s)
	forced vital capacity
FVCA	four-vessel cerebral angiography
FVD	fever, vomiting, and diarrhea
FVFR	filled voiding flow rate
FVH	focal vascular headache
F VIII	factor VIII (factor eight; antihemophilic factor)
FVL	factor V-Leiden (mutation)
	femoral vein ligation
	flow volume loop
	functional visual loss
FVM	fetal ventriculomegaly
FVP	foot venous pressure
FVR	feline viral rhinotracheitis
	forearm vascular resistance
FW	fetal weight
F/W	followed with
F waves	fibrillatory waves
	flutter waves
FVWs	flow-velocity waveforms (umbilical artery Doppler)
FWB	fetal well-being
	free water bolus
	fresh whole blood
	full-weight bearing
	functional well-being
FWCA	functional work capacity assessment
FWD	fairly well developed
FWHM	full-width at half maximum (radiology)
FWS	fetal warfarin syndrome
FWW	front-wheel walker
Fx	fractional urine
	fracture
FXa	activated factor X
FXaI	activated factor X inhibitor
Fx-BB	fracture both bones
Fx-dis	fracture-dislocation

F XI	Factor XI (eleven)
FXL	functional
FXN	function
FXR	fracture
FXS	fragile X syndrome
FXTAS	fragile X associated tremor/ataxia syndrome
FY	fiscal year
FYC	facultative yeast carrier
FYI	for your information
FZ	flutamide and goserelin acetate (Zoladex)
FZRC	frozen red (blood) cells

F

G

G	gallop
	gastrostomy
	gauge
	gauss (a unit of magnetic flux density in radiology)
	gavage feeding
	gingiva
	good
	grade
	gram (g) (28.35 g = 1 ounce)
	gravida
	guaiac
	guanosine
	riboflavin (vitamin G)
G +	gram-positive
	guaiac positive
G −	gram-negative
	guaiac negative
↑g	increasing
↓g	decreasing
G1-4	grade 1-4
G-11	hexachlorophene
GA	Gamblers Anonymous
	gastric analysis
	general anesthesia
	general appearance
	gestational age
	ginger ale
	glycyrrhetinic acid
	granuloma annulare
	glucose/acetone
Ga	gallium
^{67}Ga	gallium citrate Ga 67
GAA	alpha-glucosidase (gene)
	glacial acetic acid
GABA	gamma-aminobutyric acid
GABHS	group A beta hemolytic streptococci
GABS	group A beta (hemolytic) streptococci
GAD	generalized anxiety disorder
	glutamic acid decarboxylase
GAE	granulomatous amebic encephalitis
GAEB	good air entry bilaterally
GAF	geographic adjustment factors
	Global Assessment of Functioning (scale)
GAG	glycosaminoglycan
GAGS	global acne grading system
GAHM	genioglossus advancement and hyoid myotomy
GAGPS	glycosaminoglycan polysulfate
GAGS	global acne grading system

GAHM genioglossus advancement and hyoid myotomy

GAL galanthamine hydrobromide (Razadyne)
gallon (1 gallon US = 3.8 L; 1 gallon UK = 4.5 L)
Guardian *ad Litem* (court appointed guardian)

G'ale ginger ale

GALI-PUT galactose-1-phosphate uridye transferase enzyme

GALT galactose-1-phosphate uridyltransferase (gene)
gut-associated lymphoid tissue

GAM Gamma Knife
gene-activated matrices

Gamma-GT gamma-glutamyl transpeptidase

GAMT guanidinoacetate methyltransferase

GAN giant axonal neuropathy

GAO General Accounting Office

GAP GTPase activating protein

GAP-43 growth-associated protein-43

GAR gonnococcal antibody reaction

GARFT glycinamide ribonucleotide formyl transferase

GAS general adaption syndrome
ginseng-abuse syndrome
Glasgow Assessment Schedule
Global Assessment Scale
group A streptococcal (*Streptococcus pyogenes*) disease vaccine
group *A* streptococci

Gas Anal F&T gastric analysis, free and total

Ga scan gallium scan

Gastroc gastrocnemius

GAT geriatric assessment team
Goldmann applanation tonometry
group adjustment therapy

GATB General Aptitude Test Battery

GAU geriatric assessment unit

GAVE gastric antral vascular ectasia

Gaw airway conductance

GB gallbladder
gingival bleeding
Ginkgo biloba
Guillain-Barré (syndrome)

G & B good and bad

GBA gingivobuccoaxial
ganglionic-blocking agent

GBBS group B beta hemolytic streptococcus

GBD global burden of disease

GBE *Ginkgo biloba* extract

GBEF gallbladder ejection fraction

GBG gonadal-steroid binding globulin

GBH gamma benzene hexachloride (lindane)

GBIA Guthrie bacterial inhibition assay

GBL gamma butyrolactone

GBM glioblastoma multiforme
glomerular basement membrane

GBMI guilty but mentally ill

GBP gabapentin (Neurontin)
gastric bypass
gated blood pool (imaging)

GBPS gated blood pool scan

GBR gamma band response (audiology)
good blood return
guided bone regeneration

GBS gallbladder series
gastric bypass surgery
group B streptococcal (*Streptococcus agalactiae*) disease vaccine
group B streptococci
Guillain-Barré syndrome

GBV-C GB virus type C (also known as hepatitis G virus)

GBW generalized body weakness

GBX gall bladder extraction (cholecystectomy)

GC gas chromatography
gastric cancer
geriatric chair (Gerichair)
gingival curettage
gliomatosis cerebri
glucocorticoid
gonococci (gonorrhea)
good condition
graham crackers

G−C gram-negative cocci

G+C gram-positive cocci

GCA ghost cell ameloblastoma
giant cell arteritis

GCBP gated cardiac blood pool

GCC glassy cell carcinoma
guanylyl cyclase C

GCE general conditioning exercise

GCDFP gross cystic disease fluid protein

GCF giant cell fibroblastoma
gingival crevicular fluid

GC/FID gas chromatography/flame ionization detection

GCI General Cognitive Index

GCIIS glucose control insulin infusion system

GCL generalized congenital lipodystrophy

GCM giant cell myocarditis
good central maintained

GCMD generalized cardiovascular metabolic disease

GCMN giant congenital melanocytic nevus

GC-MS gas chromatography-mass spectroscopy

GC-O gas chromatography-olfactometry

GCP	gentamicin, clindamycin, and polymyxin topical preparation good clinical practice
GCPS	Greig cephalopolysyndactyly syndrome
GCR	gastrocolonic response glucocerebrosidase
GCS	Glasgow Coma Scale glucocorticosteroid(s) graduated compression stockings
GCSE	generalized convulsive status epilepticus
G-CSF	filgrastim (granulocyte colony-stimulating factor)
GCST	Gibson-Cooke sweat test
GCT	general care and treatment germ-cell tumor giant-cell tumor glucose challenge test granulosa cell tumor
GCU	gonococcal urethritis
GCV	ganciclovir (Cytovene) great cardiac vein
GCVF	great cardiac vein flow
GD	gastric distension Gaucher disease gemcitabine (Gemzar) and docetaxel (Taxotere) generalized delays gestational diabetes good gravely disabled Graves disease
Gd	gadolinium
G & D	growth and development
GDA	gastroduodenal artery
GDB	Guide Dogs for the Blind
Gd-BOPTA	gadolinium benzyloxypropionic tetra acetate
GDC	Guglielmi detachable coil
GDD	glaucoma drainage devices
Gd-DTPA	gadopentetate (Magnevist)
Gd-DTPA-BMA	gadodiamide (Omniscan)
GdE	gadolinium enhancing
GD FA	grandfather
GDH	glutamic dehydrogenase
Gd-HPD03A	gadoteridol
GDJ	gastroduodenal junction
g/dl	grams per deciliter
GDM	gestational diabetes mellitus
GDM A-1	gestational diabetes mellitus, insulin controlled, Type I
GDM A-2	gestational diabetes mellitus, diet controlled, Type II
GD MO	grandmother
Gd-MRI	gadolinium-enhanced magnetic resonance imaging
GDNF	glial (cell line) derived neurotrophic factor
GDP	gamma-detecting probe gel diffusion precipitin
GDPs	general dental practitioners
GDR	glucose disposal rate
GDS	Geriatric Depression Scale Global Deterioration Scale
GDS-15	15-item Geriatric Depression Scale
GDx®	a scanning laser polarimeter
GE	gainfully employed gastric emptying gastroenteritis gastroesophageal group exercise
GEA	gastroepiploic artery
GEC	galactose elimination capacity
GED	General Educational Development (Test) General Equivalency Diploma
GEE	gait energy expenditure generalized estimating equations (statistics) Global Evaluation of Efficacy glycine ethyl ester graft-enteric erosion
GEF	graft-enteric fistula
GEH	generalized eruptive histiocytosis
GEICAM	Grupo Español de Investigacion en Cancer de Mama (the Spanish Group for the Investigation of Breast Cancer)
GEJ	gastroesophageal junction
GEL	giant esophageal leiomyoma
GEM	gemcitabine (Gemzar) gemfibrozil (Lopid) general equivalence mapping generalized erythema multiforme
GEMOX	gemcitabine and oxaliplatin
GEMU	geriatric evaluation and management unit
GEN	general anesthesia genital
GenD	genetic doping
GEN/ENDO	general anesthesia with endotracheal intubation
GENT	gentamicin
GENTA/P	gentamicin-peak
GENTA/T	gentamicin-trough
GEP	gastroenteropancreatic gene expression profiles
GEQ	generic equiavalent
GER	gastroesophageal reflux
GERD	gastroesophageal reflux disease
GES	gastric emptying scintigraphy

GEST	gestational
GET	gastric emptying time
	graded exercise test
GET 1/2	gastric emptying half-time
GETA	general endotracheal anesthesia
GETS	Glasgow and Edinburgh Throat Scale
GETV	gadolinium-enhancing tumor volume
GEU	geriatric evaluation unit
GF	gastric fistula
	gluten free
	grandfather
GFAAS	graphite furnace atomic absorption spectrometry
GFAP	glial fibrillary acidic protein
GF-BAO	gastric fluid, basal acid output
GFCL	Goldmann fundus contact lens
GFD	gluten-free diet
GFFF	gravitational field-flow fractionation
GFJ	grapefruit juice
GFM	good fetal movement
GFP	green fluorscent protein
GFR	glomerular filtration rate
	grunting, flaring, and retractions
GFS	glaucoma filtering surgery
GG	gamma globulin
	Gates-Glidden (dental drills)
	guaifenesin (glyceryl guaiacolate)
G=G	grips equal and good
GGDS	global genome damage score
GGE	Gastrografin enema
	generalized glandular enlargement
GGF	great grandfather
GGM	great grandmother
GGO	ground-glass opacity
GGS	glands, goiter, and stiffness
	group G streptococci
GGT	gamma-glutamyl-transferase
GGTP	gamma-glutamyl-transpeptidase
GH	general health
	genetic hemochromatosis
	gingival hyperplasia
	glenohumeral
	good health
	group home
	growth hormone
GH_3	Gerovital
GHAA	Group Health Association of America
GHB	gamma hydroxybutyrate (sodium oxybate; Xyrem)
GHb	glycosylated hemoglobin
GHD	growth hormone deficiency
GHDA	growth hormone deficiency (syndrome) in adults
GHG	greenhouse gases
GHI	growth hormone insufficiency
GHJ	glenohumeral joint
G-H jt	glenohumeral joint
GHLC	glenohumeral ligament complex
GHP(S)	gated heart pool (scan)
GHQ	General Health Questionnaire
GHQ-30	General Health Questionnaire
GHRF	growth hormone releasing factor
GI	gastrointestinal
	gingival index (dental)
	glycemic index
	granuloma inguinale
GIA	gastrointestinal anastomosis
GIB	gastric ileal bypass
	gastrointestinal bleeding
GIC	general immunocompetence
	Global Impression of Change
GID	gastrointestinal distress
	gender identity disorder
GIDA	Gastrointestinal Diagnostic Area
GIFD #3	colonoscope
GIFT	gamete intrafallopian (tube) transfer
GIH	gastrointestinal hemorrhage
GIK	glucose-insulin-potassium
GIL	gastrointestinal (tract) lymphoma
GING	gingiva
	gingivectomy
G1K	greater than one thousand
GIO	glucocorticoid-induced osteoporosis
GIOP	glucocorticoid-induced osteoporosis
GIP	gastric inhibitory peptide
	giant cell interstitial pneumonia
	glucose-dependent insulinotropic polypeptide
GIPU	gastrointestinal procedure unit
GIR	glucose infusion rate
GIRDCA	Gruppo Italiano Ricerca Dermatiti da Contatto e Ambientali (patch test series)
GIS	gas in stomach
	gastrointestinal series
GISA	glycopeptide intermediate-resistant *Staphylococcus aureus*
GIST	gastrointestinal stromal tumor
GIT	gastrointestinal tract
GITS	gastrointestinal therapeutic system
	gut-derived infectious toxic shock
GITSG	Gastrointestinal Tumor Study Group
GITT	glucose insulin tolerance test
GIWU	gastrointestinal work-up
giv	given
GJ	gastrojejunal
	gastrojejunostomy
	grapefruit juice
GJH	generalized joint hypermobility
GJIC	gap junction intercellular communication
GJT	gastrojejunostomy tube

G1K greater than one thousand
GK Gamma Knife
GKRS gamma-knife radiosurgery
GKS gamma-knife surgery
GKT gamma-knife thalamotomy
GL gastric lavage
glaucoma
greatest length
GLA gamolenic acid
gingivolinguoaxial
glucose-lowering agents
GLB Graham-Leach-Bliley Act of 1999
GLC gas-liquid chromatography
GLD Glanders (*Actinobacillus mallei*) vaccine
GLF ground-level fall
GLIO glioblastoma
GLL green-light laser
GLM general linear model
GLN glomerulonephritis
GLOC gravity-induced loss of consciousness
GLP Gambro Liendia Plate
Good Laboratory Practice (Principles of)
group-living program
GLP-1 glucagon-like peptide-1
GLR gravity lumbar reduction
GLU glucose
GLU 5 five-hour glucose tolerance test
GLUC glucose
GLYCOS Hb glycosylated hemoglobin
GM gastric mucosa
general medicine
genetically modified
geometric mean
gram (g)
grand mal
grandmother
gray matter
G-M Geiger-Müller (counter)
GM + gram-positive
GM − gram-negative
gm % grams per 100 milliliters
GmbH *Gesellschaft mit beschränkter Haftung* (a corporation with restricted liability or a private limited liability company)
GMC general medical clinic
general medical condition
geometric mean concentration
gross-motor coordination
GMCD grand mal convulsive disorder
GM-CSF sargramostim (granulocyte-macrophage colony-stimulating factor; Leukine)
GME gaseous microemboli
graduate medical education
GMF general medical floor
GMFCS Gross Motor Function Classification System
GMFM gross motor function measure
GMH germinal matrix hemorrhage
GML gingival margin levels (dental)
GMLOS geometric mean length of stay
GMOs genetically modified organisms
GMP general medical panel (see page 318)
Good Manufacturing Practices
guanosine monophosphate
GMR gallop, murmur or rub
GMS galvanic muscle stimulation
general medical services
general medicine and surgery
Gomori methenamine silver (stain)
GM&S general medicine and surgery
GMSPS Glasgow Meningococcal Septicemia Prognostic Score
GMTs geometric mean antibody titers
GN glomerulonephritis
graduate nurse
gram-negative
GNA *Galanthus nivalis* agglutinin
GNB ganglioneuroblastoma
gram-negative bacilli
gram-negative bacteremia
GNBM gram-negative bacillary meningitis
GNC gram-negative cocci
GND gram-negative diplococci
GNDS Guy Neurological Disability Scale
GNG gluconeogenesis
go/no-go (frontal executive function test)
GNID gram-negative intracellular diplococci
GNP Gerontological Nurse Practitioner
GNR gram-negative rods
GnRH gonadotropin-releasing hormone
GNS gram-negative sepsis
oblimersen sodium (Genasense)
GnSAF gonadotropin surge attenuating factor
GNT Graduate Nurse Technician
GNYHA Greater New York Hospital Association
GO Graves ophthalmopathy
Greek Orthodox
GOAT Galveston Orientation and Amnesia Test
GOBI growth monitoring, *o*ral rehydration, *b*reast feeding, and *i*mmunization
GOCS Global Obsessive-Compulsive Scale
GOD glucose oxidase
GOG Gynecologic Oncology Group

GOJ	gastro-oesophageal junction (UK and other countries)
GOK	God only knows (slang)
GOLD	Global Initiative for Chronic Obstructive Lung Disease (guidelines)
GOM	granular osmiophilic material
GOMER	get out of my emergency room
GON	gonococcal ophthalmia neonatorum
	greater occipital nerve
	greater occipital neuritis
GONA	glaucomatous optic nerve atrophy
GONIO	gonioscopy
GOO	gastric outlet obstruction
GOR	gastro-oesophageal reflux (United Kingdom)
	general operating room
GORD	gastro-oesophageal reflux disease (United Kingdom)
GORK	God only really knows (slang)
GOS	gadolinium oxyorthosilicate
	galactose oxidase and Schiff reagent (test)
	Glasgow Outcome Scale
GOSE	Glasgow Outcome Scale-Extended
GOT	glucose oxidase test
	glutamic-oxaloacetic transaminase (aspartate aminotransferase)
	goals of treatment
GOX	glucose oxidation
GP	gabapentin (Neurontin)
	general practitioner
	globus pallidus
	glucose polymers
	glycoprotein
	gram-positive
	grandparent
	gutta percha
G/P	gravida/para
G_4P_{3104}	four pregnancies (gravid), 3 went to term, one premature, no abortion (or miscarriage), and 4 living children (p = para)
GPA	gelatin particle agglutination
	global program on AIDS
G#P#A#	gravida (number of pregnancies) para (number of live births) abortion (number of abortions)
G6Pase	glucose-6-phosphatase
GPB	gram-positive bacilli
GPC	gel-permeation chromatography
	giant papillary conjunctivitis
	glycerophosphorylcholine
	G-protein coupled
	gram-positive cocci
GPCL	gas-permeable contact lens
GPCR	G protein-coupled receptors
GPC/TP	glycerylphosphorylcholine to total phosphate
G6PD	glucose-6-phosphate dehydrogenase
GPGL	gamma probe guided lymphoscintigraphy
GPI	general paralysis of the insane
	glucose-6-phosphate isomerase
	glycoprotein IIb/IIIa receptor inhibitor(s)
GPi	globus pallidus interna
G-PLT	giant platelets
GPMAL	gravida, para, multiple births, abortions, and live births
GPN	General Pediatric Nurse
	glossopharyngeal neuralgia
	graduate practical nurse
GPO	group purchasing organization
GPP	Good Programming Practice
GPRD	General Practice Research Database (United Kingdom)
GPS	Goodpasture syndrome
GPS™	Gravitational Platelet Separation (System)
GPT	glutamic pyruvic transaminase
	Grooved Pegboard Test (of hand function)
GPVP	good pharmacovigilance process
GPX	glutathione peroxidase
GPx-1	glutathione peroxidase-1
GR	gastric resection
	growth rate
gr	grain (approximately 65 mg) (this is a dangerous abbreviation)
G−R	gram-negative rods
G+R	gram-positive rods
GRA	granisetron (Kytril)
	glucocorticoid remediable aldosteronism
gravida 6, para 4-0-2-3	6 pregnancies resulting in 4-full term deliveries with 0 premature births and 2 abortions or miscarriages and 3 living children
GRAS	generally recognized as safe
GRASE	Generally Recognized as Safe and Effective
GRASS	gradient recalled acquisition in a steady state
Grav.	gravid (pregnant)
GRC	gastric remnant cancers
GRD	gastroesophageal reflux disease
GRD DTR	granddaughter
GRD SON	grandson
GRE	glycopeptide-resistant enterococci
	graded resistive exercise
	gradient-recalled echo

G

	gradient refocused echo
GR-FR	grandfather
GRKP	gentamicin-resistant *Klebsiella pneumoniae*
GR-MO	grandmother
GRN	granules
	green
GRO	growth-related oncogene
GRP	Good Regulatory Practice
	group
$Gr_1P_0AB_1$	one pregnancy, no births, and one abortion
GRP HM	group home
GRR	gross reproduction rate
GRT	gastric residence time
	glandular replacement therapy
	Graduate Respiratory Therapist
	grasp and release test
	group-randomized trial
GRTT	Graduate Respiratory Therapist Technician
GRV	gastric residual volume
GS	gallstone
	generalized seizure
	general surgery
	Gleason score
	gliosarcoma
	glucosamine sulfate
	gluteal sets
	Gram stain
	grip strength
G/S	5% dextrose (glucose) and 0.9% sodium chloride (saline) injection
G & S	gait and stance
GSAP	greatest single allergen present
G-SAS	Gambling Symptom Assessment Scale
GS-Cbl	glutathionylcobalamin
GSCU	geriatric skilled care unit
GSD	gallstone disease
	globule-size distribution
	glucogen storage disease
GSD-1	glycogen storage disease, type 1
GSE	genital self-examination
	gluten sensitive enteropathy
	grip strong and equal
GSH	glutathione
GSI	genuine stress incontinence
GSIS	glucose-stimulated insulin secretion
GSK	GlaxoSmithKline
GSM	Global System of Mobile Communication
	grey-scale median
GSMD	gestational sack and maternal date
GSP	generalized social phobia
	general survey panel
	Good Statistical Practice
GSPN	greater superficial petrosal neurectomy
GSR	galvanic skin resistance (response)
	gastrosalivary reflex
GSS	genotypic-sensitivity scores
	Gerstmann-Straüssler-Scheinker (syndrome)
GST	glutathione S-transferase
	gold sodium thiomalate (Myochrysine)
GSTM	gold sodium thiomalate (Myochrysine)
GSUI	genuine stress urinary incontinence
GSV	greater saphenous vein
GSW	gunshot wound
GSWA	gunshot wound to abdomen
GT	gait
	gait training
	gastrostomy
	gastrotomy tube
	gene therapy
	glucose tolerance
	great toe
	greater trochanter
	green tea
	group therapy
GTA	glutaraldehyde
GTB	gastrointestinal tract bleeding
GTC	generalized tonic-clonic (seizure)
GTCS	generalized tonic-clonic seizure
GTD	gestational trophoblastic disease
GTE	general therapeutic exercise
	Green tea extract
GTF	gastrostomy tube feedings
	glucose tolerence factor
GTH	gonadotropic hormone
GTN	gestational trophoblastic neoplasms
	glomerulo-tubulo-nephritis
	glyceryl trinitrate (name for nitroglycerin in the United Kingdom)
GTO	Golgi tendon organ(s)
GTP	glutamyl transpeptidase
	green tea polyphenols
	guanosine triphosphate
GTPAL	gestation, term, preterm, abortion and living
GTR	granulocyte turnover rate
	gross total resection
	guided tissue regeneration
GTS	Gilles de la Tourette syndrome
gtt.	drops
GTT	gestational transient thyrotoxicosis
	gestational trophoblastic tumor
	glucose tolerance test
GTT agar	gelatin-tellurite-taurocholate agar
GTT3H	glucose tolerence test, 3 hours (oral)
gtts.	drops

G-tube	gastrostomy tube
GU	gastric upset
	genitourinary
	gonococcal urethritis
GUAR	guarantor
GUD	genital ulcer disease
GUI	genitourinary infection
GUM	Genitourinary Medicine (clinics)
GUS	genitourinary sphincter
	genitourinary system
GUSTO	Global Utilization of Streptokinase and TPA for Occluded Arteries
GV	gentian violet
	growth velocity
GVF	Goldmann visual fields
	good visual fields
GVG	vigabatrin (gamma-vinyl GABA)
GVH	generalized visceral hypersensitivity
GVHD	graft-versus-host disease
GVL	graft-versus leukemia
GVM	Graft-versus malignancy
GVN	gentamicin, vancomycin, and nystatin
GVS	gastric vertical stapling
GVSDS	growth velocity standard deviation score
GVT	graft-versus-tumor
G/W	dextrose (glucose) in water
G&W	glycerin and water (enema)
GWA	genome-wide association
	gunshot wound of the abdomen
GWBI	General Well-Being Index
GWD	Guinea-worm disease
GWMFT	Graded Wolf Motor Function Test
GWS	Gulf-war syndrome
GWT	gunshot wound of the throat
GWTG	Get With The Guidelines (American Heart Association program)
GWX	guide-wire exchange
GXP	graded exercise program
GXT	graded exercise test
Gy	gray (radiation unit)
GYN	gynecology
GZTS	Guilford-Zimmerman Temperament Survey

H

H	*Haemophilis*
	Haldol (haloperidol); as in vitamin H (slang)
	head
	heart
	height
	Helicobacter
	heroin
	Hispanic
	hour
	husband
	hydrogen
	hyperopia
	hypermetropia
	hyperphoria
	hypodermic
	isoniazid [part of tuberculosis regimen, see RHZ(E/S)/HR]
	objective angle
	trastuzumab (Herceptin)
H′	hip
Ⓗ	hypodermic injection
H^2	hiatal hernia
H_2	hydrogen
3H	high, hot, and a helluva lot
H24	24 hour
356h	Application to Market a New Drug, Biologic or an Antibiotic Drug for Human Use (FDA form number)
HA	headache
	hearing aid
	heart attack
	hemadsorption
	hemagglutination
	hemolytic anemia
	Hispanic American
	hospital-acquired
	hospital admission
	hyaluronan
	hyaluronic acid
	hyperalimentation
	hypermetropic astigmatism
	hypothalmic amenorrhea
H/A	head-to-abdomen (ratio)
	holding area
HA-1A®	nebacumab
HAA	haloacetic acid
	hepatitis-associated antigen
HAAB	hepatitis A antibody
HAAF	hypoglycemia-associated autonomic failure
HAART	highly active antiretroviral treatment
HABF	hepatic artery blood flow

HAC	hydroxyapatite cement
HAc	acetic acid
HACA	human antichimeric antibodies
HACCP	Hazard Analysis Critical Control Point(s)
HACE	hepatic artery chemoembolization high-altitude cerebral edema
HACEK group	*Haemophilus parainfluenzae, H. aphrophilus,* and *H. paraphrophilus, Actinobacillus actinomycetemcomitans, Cardiobacterium hominis, Eikenella corrodens,* and *Kingella kingae*
HACS	hyperactive child syndrome
HAD	HIV (human immunodeficiency virus)-associated dementia human adjuvant disease hypertonic acetate dextran
HADH	the reduced form of nicotinamide-adenine dinucleotide (hydride donors in biochemical redox reactions)
HADS	Hospital Anxiety and Depression Scale
HAE	hearing aid evaluation hepatic artery embolization herb-related adverse event hereditary angioedema
HAEC	Hirschprung associated enterocolitis
HAF	hyperalimentation fluid
HAFM	hospital-acquired *Plasmodium falciparum* malaria
HAGG	hyperimmune antivariola gamma globulin
HAGHL	humeral avulsion of the glenohumeral ligament
HAGL	humeral avulsion of the glenohumeral ligament
HAH	high-altitude headache
HAI	hemagglutination inhibition assay hepatic arterial infusion
HAIC	hepatic arterial infusional chemotherapy
HAK	hyperalimentation kit
HAL	hemorrhoidal artery ligation hip axis length hyperalimentation
HALC	hand-assisted laparoscopic colectomy
HALDN	hand-assisted laparoscopic donor nephrectomy
HALE	health-adjusted life expectancy
HALN	hand-assisted laparoscopic (radical) nephrectomy
HALO	halothane (Fluothane) hours after light onset
HALRI	hospital-acquired lower respiratory infections
HALRN	hand-assisted laparoscopic radical nephrectomy
HALS	hand-assisted laparoscopic surgery
HALSR	hand-assisted laparoscopic sigmoid resection
HAM	Haldol, Ativan, and morphine high-dose cytarabine (ara-C) and mitoxantrone HTLV-1-associated myelopathy human albumin microspheres
HAMA	human antimurine antibody
HAM-A	Hamilton Anxiety (scale)
HAM D	Hamilton Depression (scale)
HAMLET	human alpha-lactalbumin made lethal to tumor cells
HAMS	hamstrings
HAN	heroin-associated nephropathy
HANE	hereditary angioneurotic edema
HAO	hearing aid orientation
HAP	hearing aid problem heredopathia atactica polyneuritiformis hospital-acquired pneumonia hydroxyapatite
HAPC	hospital-acquired penetration contact
HAPD	home-automated peritoneal dialysis
HAPE	high-altitude pulmonary edema
HapMap	A catalog of common genetic variants that occur in human beings. It describes what these variants are, where they occur in our DNA, and how they are distributed among people within populations and among populations in different parts of the world. (The International Haplotype Map Project) (www.hapmap.org)
HAPS	hepatic arterial perfusion scintigraphy
HAPTO	haptoglobin
HAQ	Headache Assessment Questionnaire Health Assessment Questionnaire
HAR	high-altitude retinopathy hyperacute rejection
HARDI	high-angular resolution diffusion-weighted imaging
HARH	high-altitude retinal hemorrhage
HARP	hypoprebetalipoproteinemia, acanthocytosis, retinitis pigmentosa, and pallidale degeneration (syndrome)
HARS	Hamilton Anxiety Rating Scale HIV-associated adipose redistribution syndrome
HAS	Hamilton Anxiety (Rating) Scale

	headache associated with sexual activity
	hemangiosarcoma
	Holmes-Adie syndrome
	home assessment service
	hyperalimentation solution
HASCI	head and spinal cord injury
HASCVD	hypertensive arteriosclerotic cardiovascular disease
HASHD	hypertensive arteriosclerotic heart disease
HASTE	half-Fourier acquisition single-shot turbo spin-echo
HAT	head, arms, and trunk
	hepatic artery thrombosis
	heterophile antibody titer
	histone acetyltransferase
	hormone ablative therapy
	hospital arrival time
	human African trypanosomiasis (sleeping sickness)
HAV	hallux abducto valgus
	hepatitis A vaccine
	hepatitis A virus
HAV-HBV	hepatitis A virus, and hepatitis B virus vaccine
HAZWOPER	Hazardous Waste Operations and Emergency Response
HB	heart-beating (donor)
	heart block
	heel-to-buttock
	hemoglobin (Hb)
	hepatitis B
	high calorie
	hold breakfast
	housebound
	hydrocodone bitartrate
1°HB	first degree heart block
HB1°	first degree heart block
HB2°	second degree heart block
HB3°	third degree heart block
HBAB	hepatitis B antibody
Hb A_{1c}	glycosylated hemoglobin
HBAC	hyperdynamic beta-adrenergic circulatory
HbAS	sickle cell trait
HBBW	hold breakfast for blood work
HBC	health and beauty care
	hereditary breast cancer
	hit by car
HBcAb	hepatitis B core antibody (antigen)
HBc AB	hepatitis B core antibody
HBc Ag	hepatitis B core antigen
HbCO	carboxyhemoglobin
HB core	hepatitis B core antigen
HBC	hit by car
HbCV	*Haemophilus* b conjugate vaccine
HBD	has been drinking
	hydroxybutyrate dehydrogenase
HBDH	hydroxybutyrate dehydrogenase
HBE	hepatitis B epsilon
	human bronchial epithelial (cells)
	hypopharyngoscopy, bronchoscopy, and esophagoscopy
HBeAb	hepatitis Be antibody (antigen)
HBED	hydroxybenzylethylene-diamine diacetic acid
HbF	fetal hemoglobin
HBF	hepatic blood flow
HBGA	had it before, got it again
HBGM	home blood glucose monitoring
HBH	Health Belief Model
HBHC	hospital based home care
HBI	Harvey-Bradshaw Index
	hemibody irradiation
HBID	hereditary benign intraepithelial dyskeratosis
HBIG	hepatitis B immune globulin
Hb Kansas	mutant hemoglobin with a low affinity for oxygen
HBLs	hemangioblastomas
HBLV	B-lymphotropic virus human
HBM	Health Belief Model
	human bone marrow
	human breast milk
HBNK	heparin-binding neurotrophic factor
hBNP	human B-type natriuretic peptide (nesiritide [Natrecor])
HBO	hit by owner (Veterinary slang)
	hyperbaric oxygen (HBO_2 preferred)
HBO_2	hyperbaric oxygen
HbO_2	hemoglobin, oxygenated
	hyperbaric oxygen (HBO_2 preferred)
HBOC	hemoglobin-based oxygen carrier
	hereditary breast and ovarian cancer
HBOT	hyperbaric oxygen treatment/therapy (HBO_2T preferred)
HBO_2T	hyperbaric oxygen treatment
HBP	hand breast pump
	high blood pressure
HBPM	home blood pressure monitoring
HBR	half-body radiation
HBr	hydrobromide
HBRT	horseback riding therapy
HBS	Health Behavior Scale
	human body shape
HbS	sickle cell hemoglobin
HBsAg	hepatitis B surface antigen
HbSC	sickle cell hemoglobin C
HBSS	Hank balanced salt solution
HbSS	sickle cell anemia
HBT	hydrogen breath test
	hypertrophy of the base of the tongue
HBV	hepatitis B vaccine

H

hepatitis B virus
honey-bee venom

HBVig hepatitis B virus immune globulin

HBVP high biological value protein

HBW high birth weight

H/BW heart-to-body weight (ratio)

HBEX home-based exercise

HC hair count
hairy cell
handicapped
head circumference
healthy controls
heart catheterization
heel cords
Hickman catheter
home care
hot compress
housecall
Huntington chorea
hydrocephalus
hydrocortisone

4-HC 4-hydroperoxycyclo-phosphamide

H & C hot and cold

HCA health care aide
heterocyclic antidepressant
hypercalcemia
hypothermic circulatory arrest

HCAO hepatitis C-associated osteosclerosis

H-CAP altretamine (hexamethyl-melamine), cyclophosphamide, doxorubicin (Adriamycin), and cisplatin (Platinol)

HCB hexachlorobenzene

HCBR human carbonyl reductase

HCC Hearing Coordination Center
hepatocellular carcinoma
Hürthle cell carcinoma

HCCL heavily calcified coronary lesions

HCD herniate cervical disk
hydrocolloid dressing

HCFA Health Care Financing Administration

HCFC hydrochlorofluorocarbon

HCFU 1-hexylcarbamoyl-5-fluorouracil (Camofur)

hCG human chorionic gonadotropin

HCH hexachlorocyclohexane
hygroscopic condenser humidifier

HCI home care instructions

HCL hairy cell leukemia

HCl hydrochloric acid (when it appears separately [not as part of a drug name])
hydrochloride (when part of a drug name, as in thiamine HCl [thiamine hydrochloride])

HCLF high carbohydrate, low fiber (diet)

HCLs hard contact lenses

HCLV hairy cell leukemia variant

HCM health care maintenance
heterogeneous cation-exchange membrane
hypercalcemia of malignancy
hypertrophic cardiomyopathy

HCMV human cytomegalovirus

HCO_3 bicarbonate

HCP handicapped
healthcare provider
hearing conservation programs
hereditary coporphyria
hexachlorophene
home chemotherapy program
hospital chemistry profile
hydrocephalus

HCPCS HCFA (Health Care Financing Administration) Common Procedural Coding System

HCQ hydroxychloroquine (Plaquenil)

HCR health care review

hCRF human corticotrophin-releasing factor (Xerecept)

HCS heel-cord stretches
human chorionic somatomammotropin
hypercoagulable states

17-HCS 17-hydroxycorticosteroids

HCSE horse chestnut seed extract

HCSS hypersensitive carotid sinus syndrome

HCT head computerized (axial) tomography
hematopoietic cell transplantation
hematocrit
histamine challenge test
human chorionic thyrotropin
hydrochlorothiazide (this is a dangerous abbreviation)
hydrocortisone

HCTU home cervical traction unit

HCTZ hydrochlorothiazide (this is a dangerous abbreviation)

HCV hepatitis C vaccine
hepatitis C virus

HCVD hypertensive cardiovascular disease

HCWs healthcare workers

HCY homocysteine

HCYS homocysteine

HD haloperidol decanoate
Hansen disease
hearing distance
heart disease
Heller-Dor (procedure)
heloma durum
hemodialysis
herniated disk
high definition
high dose
hip disarticulation

Hirschsprung disease
Hodgkin disease
hospital day
hospital discharge
house dust
Huntington disease

HDA heteroduplex analysis
high-dose arm

HDAC histone deacetylase

HD-AC high-dose cytarabine

HDAC2 histone deacetylase 2

HD-ara-C high-dose cytarabine (ara-C)

HDBQ Hilton Drinking Behavior Questionnaire

HD-Bu high-dose busulfan

HDC habilitative day care
high-dose chemotherapy
histamine dihydrochloride

HDC-ASCS high-dose chemotherapy with autologous stem cell support

HDCC high-dose combination chemotherapy

HD-CPA high-dose cyclophosphamide

HDCPT high-dose cyclophosphamide therapy

HDC-SCR high-dose chemotherapy with stem-cell rescue

HDCT high-dose chemotherapy

HDCV rabies virus vaccine, human diploid (human diploid cell vaccine)

HDE Humanitarian Device Exemption (FDA)

H/D-Ex hydrogen/deuterium amide exchange

HDF hemodiafiltration

HDG hydrogel (dressing)

HDGC hereditary diffuse gastric cancer

HDH high-density humidity

HDI high-definition image

HDIs histone deacetylase inhibitors

HDK high-dose ketoconazole

HDL high-density lipoprotein

HDL-C high-density lipoprotein cholesterol

HDLW hearing distance for watch to be heard in left ear

HDM home-delivered meals
house dust mite

HDMEC human dermal microvascular endothelial cells

HDMP high-dose methylprednisolone

HD-MTX high-dose methotrexate

HD-MTX-CF high-dose methotrexate and leucovorin (citrovorum factor)

HD-MTX/LV high-dose methotrexate and leucovorin

HDN hemolytic disease of the newborn
heparin dosing nomogram
high-density nebulizer

HDNS Hodgkin disease, nodular sclerosis

HDP high-density polyethylene
hydroxymethyline diphosphonate

HDPA high-dose pulse administration

HDPAA heparin-dependent platelet-associated antibody

HDPC hand piece

HDPE high-density polyethylene

HDR heparin dose response
high-dose rituximab
husband to delivery room

HDRA histoculture drug response assay

HDRB high-dose rate brachytherapy

HDRS Hamilton Depression Rating Scale

HDRW hearing distance for watch to be heard in right ear

HDS Hamilton Depression (Rating) Scale
herniated disk syndrome

HDSCR health deviation self-care requisite

HDT habilitative day treatment
hearing distraction test

HDU hemodialysis unit
high-dependency unit (an intensive care unit)

HDV hepatitis D virus

HDW hearing distance (with) watch

HDYF how do you feel

HE hard events
hard exudate
health educator
hepatic encephalopathy

H&E hematoxylin and eosin
hemorrhage and exudate
heredity and environment

HEA health

HEAR hospital emergency ambulance radio

HEAT human erythrocyte agglutination test

HEB hydrophilic emollient base

HEC Health Education Center

HeCOG Hellenic Cooperative Oncology Group

HEDIS Health Employer Data and Information Set

HEENT head, eyes, ears, nose, and throat

HeFH heterozygous familial hypercholesterolemia

HEI Health Eating Index (US Department of Agriculture)

HEICS Hospital Emergency Incident Command System

HEK human embryonic kidney

HEL *Helicobacter pylori* vaccine
human embryonic lung

HeLa Helen Lake (tumor cells)

HELLP Syndrome hemolysis, elevated liver enzymes, and low platelet count

HEM hematology
hypertensive emergency

HEMA hydroxyethylmethacrylate

HEMI hemiplegia

Hem/Onc	Hematology/Oncology
HEMOSID	hemosiderin
HEMPAS	hereditary erythrocytic multinuclearity with positive acidified serum test
HEMS	helicopter emergency medical services
HEN	hemorrhages, exudates, and nicking
	home enteral nutrition
He-Ne	helium-neon
HEP	hemoglobin electrophoresis
	hemorrhage, exudates, and papilledemaa
	heparin
	hepatic
	hepatoerythropoietic porphyria
	hepatoma
	histamine equivalent prick
	home exercise program
HEPA	hamster egg penetration assay
	high-efficiency particulate air (filter)
hep cap	heparin cap
HER2	human epidermal growth factor 2
HERP	human exposure (dose)/ rodent potency (dose)
HES	hetastarch (hydroxyethyl starch; Hespan)
	hypereosinophilic syndrome
HEs	hypertensive emergencies
hES	human embryonic stem
hESCs	human embryonic stem cells
20-HETE	20-hydroxyeico-satetraenoic acid
HETF	home enteral tube feeding
HEV	hepatitis E vaccine
	hepatitis E virus
	high-endothelial venule
Hex	altretamine (hexamethylmelamine; Hexalen)
Hexa-CAF	altretamine (hexamethylmelamine), cyclophosphamide, methotrexate (amethopterin), and fluorouracil
HF	Hageman factor
	hard feces
	hay fever
	head of fetus
	heart failure
	high frequency
	Hispanic female
	hot flashes
	house formula
HFA	health facility administrator
	high-functioning autism
	hydrofluoroalkane-134a
HFAS	hereditary flat adenoma syndrome
HFB	high-frequency band
HFC	hydrofluorocarbon
HFCB	horizontal flow clean bench
HFCC	high-frequency chest compression
HFD	high-fiber diet
	high-forceps delivery
	high-frequency discharges
HFE	hemochromatosis gene
hFH	heterozygous familial hypercholesterolemia
HFHD	high-flux hemodialysis
HFHL	high-frequence hearing loss
HFI	hereditary fructose intolerance
HFIP	hexafluoro-isopropranolol
HFJV	high-frequency jet ventilation
H flu	*Haemophilus influenzae*
HFM	hand-foot-and-mouth (disease) (often caused by coxsackievirus A16)
	hemifacial microsomia
HFMD	hand-foot-and-mouth disease (often caused by coxsackievirus A16)
HFO	high-frequency oscillation
HFOV	high-frequency oscillatory ventilation
HFP	hepatic function panel (see page 318)
	Hoffa fat pad
HFPPV	high-frequency positive pressure ventilation
HFR	hemorrhagic fever with renal syndrome vaccine
HFRS	hemorrhagic fever with renal syndrome
HFRT	hyperfractionated radiotherapy
HFS	hand-foot skin (reaction)
	hand-foot syndrome
	hemifacial spasm
	hot flash score
HFSH	human follicle-stimulating hormone
HFST	hearing-for-speech test
HFUPR	hourly fetal urine production rate
HFV	high-frequency ventilation
	high-fruit/vegetable (diet)
HFX RT	hyperfractionated radiation therapy
HG	handgrasp
	handgrip
	Harris-Galante (cups used in hip replacements; types I or II)
	hemoglobin
	hyperemesis gravidarum
Hg	mercury
HGA	high-grade astrocytomas
Hgb	hemoglobin
Hgb ELECT	hemoglobin electrophoresis
Hgb F	fetal hemoglobin
Hgb S	sickle cell hemoglobin
HGD	high grade dysplasia
HGE	human granulocytic ehrlichiosis
HGES	handgrasp equal and strong
HGF	hepatocyte growth factor
	hereditary gingival fibromatosis
HGG	high-grade glioma
	human gamma globulin

HGH	human growth hormone
HGI	Human Genome Initiative
HGM	home glucose monitoring
HGN	hypogastric nerve
HGNT	high-grade neuroendocrine tumors
HGO	hepatic glucose output
	hip guidance orthosis
HGP	Human Genome Project
HGPIN	high-grade prostatic intraepithelial neoplasia
HGPRT	hypoxanthine-guanine phosphoribosyl-transferase
HGS	hand-grip strength
	human genome sequence
HGSIL	high-grade squamous intraepithelial lesion
HGV	hepatitis G vaccine
	hepatitis G virus
HH	hard of hearing
	head hood
	heart healthy
	hereditary hemochromatosis
	hiatal hernia
	home health
	homonymous hemiopia
	household
	hyperhidrosis
	hyperhomocystinemia
	hypogonadotropic hypogonadism
	hypoeninemic hypoaldosteronism
H/H	hemoglobin/hematocrit
H&H	hemoglobin and hematocrit
HHA	health hazard appraisal
	hereditary hemolytic anemia
	home health agency
	home health aid
HH Assist	hand-held assist
HHC	home health care
HHCA	home health care agency
	hypothermic hypokalemic cardioplegic arrest
HHcy	hyperhomocystinemia
HHD	Doctor of Holistic Health
	hand-held dynamometer
	home hemodialysis
	household distance (physical therapy goal of mobility)
	hypertensive heart disease
HHFM	high-humidity face mask
HHH	hypermethionemia, hyperammonemia, and homocitrolinemia (syndrome)
HHHQ	Health Habits and History Questionnaire (Block-National Cancer Institute)
HHIE-S	hearing handicap inventory for the elderly-short form
HHM	high-humidity mask
	humoral hypercalcemia of malignancy
HHN	hand-held nebulizer
HHNC	hyperosmolar hyperglycemic nonketotic coma
HHNK	hyperglycemic hyperosmolar nonketotic (coma)
HHNS	hyperosmolar-hyperglycemic nonketotic syndrome
HHPPS	home health prospective payment system
HHRG	Home Health Resource Group (reimbursement categories for home health)
HHS	Health and Human Service (US Department of)
	Hypothenar Hammer syndrome
HHT	hereditary hemorrhagic telangiectasis
HHTC	high-humidity trach collar
HHTM	high-humidity trach mask
HHTS	high-humidity tracheostomy shield
HHV-8	human herpesvirus 8
HI	*Haemophilus influenzae*
	head injury
	health insurance
	hearing impaired
	hemagglutination inhibition
	homicidal ideation
	hospital insurance
	human insulin
	hypomelanosis of Ito
	hypopnea index
	hypoxic-ischemic
Hi5	HIV positive ("V" being Roman numeral for 5) (slang)
HIA	hemagglutination inhibition antibody
HIAA	hydroxyindoleacetic acid
5-HIAA	5-hydroxyindoleacetic acid
HIAP	human intracisternal A-type particle
HIB	*Haemophilus influenzae* type b (vaccine)
HIB_{cn}	*haemophilus influenzae* type b conjugate vaccine
HIBGIA	had it before, got it again (slang)
HIB_{HbOC}	*haemophilus influenzae* type b vaccine, HbOC conjugate vaccine
$HIB_{PRP\text{-}D}$	*haemophilus influenzae* type b vaccine, PRP-D conjugate vaccine
$HIB_{PRP\text{-}OMP}$	*haemophilus influenzae* type b vaccine, PRP-OMP conjugate vaccine
$HIB_{PRP\text{-}T}$	*haemophilus influenzae* type b vaccine, PRP-T conjugate vaccine
HIB_{ps}	*haemophilus influenzae* type b polysaccharide vaccine
HIC	Human Investigation Committee
	Humphriss immediate contrast (astigmatism test)

hi-cal high caloric
HICF high-information-content fingerprinting
HICPAC Hospital Infection Control Practices Advisory Committee (Centers for Disease Control and Prevention guidelines)
HID headache, insomnia, and depression
herniated intervertebral disk
HIDA hepato-iminodiacetic acid (lidofenin)
HiDAC high-dose cytarabine (ara-C)
HIDS hyperimmunoglobulinemia D syndrome
HIE hyperimmunoglobulinemia E
hypoxic-ischemic encephalopathy
HIF *Haemophilus influenzae*
higher integrative functions
hypoxia-inducible factor
HIFU high-intensity focused ultrasonography
HIHA high impulsiveness, high anxiety
HIHARS hyperventilation-induced high-amplitude rhythmic slowing
HII hepatic-iron index
HIIC heated intraoperative intraperitoneal chemotherapy
HIL hypoxic-ischemic lesion
HILA high impulsiveness, low anxiety
HILIC hydrophilic interaction chromatography
HILP hyperthermic isolated limb perfusion
HIM health information management
hexyl-insulin monoconjugate
HIN *haemophilus influenzae* nontypable strain(s) vaccine
HINI hypoxic-ischemic neuronal injury
HINN Hospital-issued Notice of Noncoverage
HIO health insuring organization
hepatic iron overload
HIP health insurance plan
HIPA heparin-induced platelet aggregation
HIPAA Health Insurance Portability and Accountability Act of 1996
HIPC hormone-independent prostate cancer
HIPPS Health Insurance Prospective Payment System
hi-pro high-protein
HIR head injury routine
HIS Hanover Intensive Score
Health Intention Scale
high-intermittent suction
histidine
Home Incapacity Scale
hospital (healthcare) information system
HISMS How I See Myself Scale
HISTO histoplasmin skin test
histoplasmosis
HIT heparin-induced thrombocytopenia
histamine-inhalation test
home infusion therapy
HITS high-intensity transient signals
HITTS heparin-induced thrombotic thrombocytopenia syndrome
HIU head injury unit
HIV human immunodeficiency virus
human immunodeficiency virus vaccine
HIV-1 human immunodeficiency virus type 1
HIV-2 human immunodeficiency virus type 2
HIVAN human immunodeficiency virus-associated nephropathy
HIVAT home intravenous antibiotic therapy
HIVD herniated intervertebral disk
HIV-D human immunodeficiency virus-related dementia
hi-vit high-vitamin
HIVMP high-dose intravenous methylprednisolone
HIVN human immunodeficiency virus nephropathy
HJB Howell-Jolly bodies
HJR hepatojugular reflux
HK hand-to-knee
heel-to-knee
hexokinase
hK6 human kallikrein 6
HKAFO hip-knee-ankle-foot orthosis
HKAO hip-knee-ankle orthosis
HKD hyperkinetic disorder
HKMN Hickman (catheter)
HKO hip-knee orthosis
HKS heel-knee-shin (test)
HKT heterotopic kidney transplant
HL hairline
half-life
hallux limitus
haloperidol
harelip
hearing level
hearing loss
heavy lifting
hemilaryngectomy
heparin lock
hepatic lipase
Hickman line
Hodgkin lymphoma
hyperlipidemia
H&L heart and lung
HLA human leukocyte antigen
human lymphocyte antigen
HLADR human leukocyte antigen, type DR

HLA negative	heart, lungs, and abdomen negative
HLB	head, limbs, and body
HLD	haloperidol decanoate (Haldol)
	herniated lumbar disk
	high-level disinfection
	high-lipid disorder
HLDP	hypoglossia-limb deficiency phenotype
HLES	hypertensive lower esophageal sphincter
HLGR	high-level gentamicin resistance
HLGT	high-level group term
HLH	helix-loop-helix
	hemophagocytic lymphohistiocytosis
	human luteinizing hormone
HLHS	hypoplastic left-heart syndrome
HLI	head lice infestation
HLK	heart, liver, and kidneys
HLM	heart-lung machine
	hemosiderin-laden macrophages
HLOS	hypertensive lower oesophageal sphincter (United Kingdom and other countries)
HLP	hyperlipoproteinemia
hLS	human lung surfactant
HLT	heart-lung transplantation (transplant)
	high-level term
HLV	herpes-like virus
	hypoplastic left ventricle
HM	hand motion
	head movement
	heart murmur
	heavily muscled
	heloma molle
	Hispanic male
	Holter monitor
	home
	human milk
	human semisynthetic insulin
	humidity mask
HMA	hemorrhages and microaneurysms
	heteroduplex mobility assay
HMB	beta-hydroxy-beta methylbutyrate (a leucine metabolite)
	homatropine methylbromide
	hypersensitivity to mosquito bites
HMBA	hexamethylene bisacetamide
HMD	hyaline membrane disease
HMDP	hydroxymethyline diphosphonate
HME	heat and moisture exchanger
	heat, massage, and exercise
	hereditary multiple exostoses
	home medical equipment
	human monocytic ehrlichiosis
HMEF	heat moisture exchanging filter
HMETSC	heavy metal screen
HMF	human milk fortifier
HMG	human menopausal gonadotropin
HMGB1	high-mobility group box 1 (chromosomal protein)
HMG CoA	hydroxymethyl glutaryl coenzyme A
HMI	healed myocardial infarction
	history of medical illness
HMIS	hospital medical information system
HMK	homemaking
HM & LP	hand motion and light perception
HMM	altretamine (hexamethyl-melamine; Hexalen)
HMO	Health Maintenance Organization
	human milk oligosaccharides
	hypothetical mean organism
HMP	health maintenance plan
	hereditary metabolic profile
	hexose monophosphate
	hot moist packs
HMPAO	hexylmethylpropylene amineoxine
HMPC	Committee on Herbal Medicinal Products (EMEA)
HMPV	human metapneumovirus
HMR	histocytic medullary reticulosis
	Hoechst Marion Roussel
^{1}H-MRS	proton magnetic resonance spectroscopy
HMS	Hunter-MacDonald syndrome
	hyper-reactive malarial splenomegaly
	hypodermic morphine sulfate (this is a dangerous abbreviation)
HMS®	medrysone
hMSCs	human mesenchymal stem cells
HMSN I	hereditary motor and sensory neuropathy type I
HMSR	high medical-social risk
HMSS	hyperactive malarial splenomegaly syndrome
HMV	home mechanical ventilation
HMWCK	high-molecular weight cytokeratin
HMWK	high-molecular weight kininogen
HMX	heat massage exercise
HN	head and neck
	head nurse
	high nitrogen
	home nursing
H&N	head and neck
HN2	mechlorethamine HCl (Mustargen)
H1N1	Spanish influenza virus
H2N2	Asian influenza virus
H3N2	Hong Kong influenza virus
H5N1	avian influenza A virus
HNC	head and neck cancer
	Holistic Nurse, Certified
	human neutrophil collagenase
	hyperosmolar nonketotic coma
HNCa	head and neck cancer

Abbreviation	Meaning
HNCCG	Head and Neck Cancer Cooperative Group
HNE	human neutrophil elastase
HNI	hospitalization not indicated
HNKDC	hyperosomolar nonketotic diabetic coma
HNKDS	hyperosmolar nonketotic diabetic state
HNLN	hospitalization no longer necessary
HNMM	mucosal melanomas of the head and neck
^{1}H-NMR	proton nuclear magnetic resonance (spectroscopy)
HNN	hybrid neural network
HNP	herniated nucleus pulposus
HNPCC	heredity nonpolyposis colorectal cancer
HNPP	hereditary neuropathy with liability to pressure palsies
HNRNA	heterogeneous nuclear ribonucleic acid
HNS	0.45% sodium chloride injection (half-normal saline)
	head and neck surgery
	head, neck, and shaft
HNSCC	squamous cell carcinoma of the head and neck
HNSN	home, no services needed
HNT	hantaan (hantavirus) vaccine
HNV	has not voided
HNWG	has not worn glasses
HO	hand orthosis
	heme oxygenase
	Hemotology-Oncology
	heterotropic ossification
	hip orthosis
	house officer
H/O	history of
+HO	hemoccult positive
H_2O	water
H_2O_2	hydrogen peroxide
HOA	hip osteoarthritis
	hypertropic osteoarthropathy
HOB	head of bed
HOB UPSOB	head of bed up for shortness of breath
HOC	Health Officer Certificate
HOCM	high-osmolality contrast media
	hypertrophic obstructive cardiomyopathy
HOD	heroin overdose
HOG	halothane, oxygen, and gas (nitrous oxide)
	Hoosier Oncology Group
HOH	hand-over-hand (rehabilitation term)
	hard of hearing
HOI	hospital onset of infection
HOM	high-osmolar contrast media
HOMA	homeostatic assessment model algorithm (index)
	homeostatic model assessment
HOME	Home Observation for Measurement of the Environment
HONC	Hooked on Nicotine Checklist
	hyperosmolar, nonketotic coma
HONK	hyperosmolar nonketotic (coma)
HOP	hourly output
HOPI	history of present illness
Hopkins-25	Hopkins Symptom Checklist-25
HOR	higher-order repeat
HORF	high-output renal failure
HORS	Hemiballism/Hemichorea Outcome Rating Score
HOS	Health Outcomes Survey
	hybrid orthosis system
HOSP	hospital
	hospitalization
HOT	home oxygen therapy
HOTV	letter symbols used in pediatric visual acuity testing
HOVT	letter symbols used in pediatric visual acuity testing
Ho:YAG	holmium: yttrium-aluminum-garnet
HP	hard palate
	Harvard pump
	Helicobacter pylori
	hemipelvectomy
	hemiplegia
	herbal products
	high-protein (supplement)
	home program
	hot packs
	house physician
	hydrogen peroxide
	hydrophilic petrolatum
	hypertrophic pachymeningitis
Hp	*Helicobacter pylori*
H&P	history and physical
HPA	hybridization protection assay
	hypothalamic-pituitary-adrenal (axis)
HPAE-PAD	high-pH anion exchange chromatography coupled with pulsed amperometric detection
HPAI	highly pathogenic avian influenza A virus
HPAT	home parenteral antibiotic therapy
HPB	Health Protection Branch (the Canadian equivalent of the U.S. Food and Drug Administration)
HPC	hemangiopericytoma
	hereditary prostate cancer
	history of present condition (complaint)
HPCE	high-performance capillary electrophoresis

HPD	hearing protection device high-protein diet home peritoneal dialysis hours post dose
HpD	hematoporphyrin derivative
HP&D	hemoprofile and differential
HPDP	health promotion and disease prevention
HPE	hemorrhage, papilledema, exudate history and physical examination holoprosencephaly
HPET	*Helicobacter pylori* eradication therapy
HPF	high-power field
HPFH	hereditary persistence of fetal hemoglobin
HPG	human pituitary gonadotropin
2hPG	2-hour post-challenge glucose
HPH	Hashimoto-Pritzker histiocytosis
HPI	history of present illness
HPIP	history, physical, impression, and plan
HPK	hyperkeratosis
HPL	human placenta lactogen hyperlipidemia hyperplexia
HPLC	high-performance (pressure) liquid chromatography
HPM	hemiplegic migraine
HPMC	high-performance membrane chromatography hydroxypropyl methylcellulose
HPMG	hard palate mucosal graft
HPN	home parenteral nutrition
HPNI	hemodialysis prognostic nutrition index
HPNS	high-pressure nervous syndrome
HPO	hydrophilic ointment hypertrophic pulmonary osteoarthropathy
HPOA	hypertrophic pulmonary osteoarthropathy
2HPP	2-hour postprandial (blood sugar)
2HPPBS	2-hour postprandial blood sugar
HPPM	hyperplastic persistent pupillary membrane
hPRL	prolactin, human
HPS	hantavirus pulmonary syndrome hepatopulmonary syndrome *Helicobacter pylori* serology hypertrophic pyloric stenosis
HpSA	*Helicobacter pylori* stool antigen
HPT	heparin protamine titration histamine provocation test home pregnancy test hyperparathyroidism
9HPT	9-hole Peg Test
HPTD	highly permeable transparent dressing
hPTH	human parathyroid hormone I_{34} (teriparatide)
HPTM	home prothrombin time monitoring
HPTX	hemopneumothorax
HPV	human papilloma virus human papilloma virus vaccine human parvovirus
H pylori	*Helicobacter pylori*
HPZ	high-pressure zone
HQC	hydroquinone cream
HQL	health-related quality of life
HR	hallux rigidus Harrington rod hazard ratio health related heart rate hemorrhagic retinopathy histamine release hospital record hour
Hr 0	zero hour (when treatment starts)
Hr -2	minus two hours (two hours prior to treatment)
H & R	hysterectomy and radiation
HRA	high-right atrium histamine-releasing activity
H2RA	histamine$_2$-receptor antagonist
HRC	Human Rights Committee
HRCT	high-resolution computed tomography
HRD	hazard ratios of death human retroviral disease hypertension renal disease hypoparathyroidism, retardation, and dysmorphism (syndrome)
HRE	high-resolution electrocardiography
HRECG	high-resolution electrocardiography
HRF	Harris return flow health-related facility histamine-releasing factor hypertensive renal failure hypoxic respiratory failure
HRI	HMG-CoA (3-hydroxy-3-methylglutaryl-coenzyme A) reductase inhibitors
HRIF	histamine inhibitory releasing factor
HRIG	human rabies immune globulin
HRL	head rotated left
HRLA	human reovirus-like agent
HRLM	high-resolution light microscopy
hRLX-2	synthetic human relaxin
HRMPC	hormone-refractory metastatic prostate cancer
HRMS	high-resolution mass spectrometry

HRNB	Halstead-Reitan Neuropsychological Battery
HROs	high-reliability organizations
HRP	high-risk pregnancy
	horseradish peroxidase
HRP-2	histidine-rich protein-2
HRPC	hormone-refractory prostate cancer
HRQL	health-related quality of life
HRQOL	health-related quality of life
HRR	head rotated right
HRRC	Human Research Review Committee
HRS	Haw River syndrome
	hepatorenal syndrome
	Hodgkin-Reed-Sternberg (cells)
	hours
HRSD	Hamilton Rating Scale for Depression
HRSEM	high-resolution scanning electron microscopy
HRST	heat, reddening, swelling, or tenderness
	heavy-resistance strength training
HRT	heart rate
	heart rate turbulence
	Heidelberg retina tomograph
	heparin-response test
	high-risk transfer
	hormone replacement therapy
	hyperfractioned radiotherapy
HRU	health resource utilization
HRV	heart rate variability
	heterogeneous resistance to vancomycin
HS	bedtime
	half-strength
	hamstrings
	hamstring sets
	handsewn (suture)
	Harmonic scalpel
	Hartman solution (lactated Ringers)
	heart size
	heart sounds
	heavy smoker
	heel spur
	heel stick
	hereditary spherocytosis
	herpes simplex
	hidradenitis suppurativa
	high school
	hippocampal sclerosis
	Hurler syndrome
H → S	heel-to-shin
H&S	hearing and speech
	hemorrhage and shock
	hysterectomy and sterilization
HSA	Health Services Administration (Administrator)
	Health Systems Agency
	human serum albumin
	hypersomnia-sleep apnea
HSAN	hereditary sensory and autonomic neuropathy (types I-IV)
HSB	husband
HSBS	evening blood sugar
HSBG	heel-stick blood gas
HSC	hematopoietic stem cell
HSCL	Hopkins Symptom-Check List
HSCR	Hirschsprung disease
hs-CRP	high-sensitivity C-reactive protein
HSCSS	hypersensitive carotid sinus syndrome
HSCT	hematopoietic stem cell transplant
HSD	Honestly Significant Difference (test) (Turkey)
	hypoactive sexual desire (disorder)
HSDD	hypoactive sexual desire disorder
HSE	herpes simplex encephalitis
	human skin equivalent
	hypertonic saline-epinephrine
HSEES	Hazardous Substances Emergency Events Surveillance
HSES	hemorrhagic shock and encephalopathy
HSG	herpes simplex genitalis
	hysterosalpingogram
HSGYV	heat, steam, gum, yawn, and Valsalva maneuver (for otitis media)
H-SIL	high-grade squamous intraepithelial lesions
HSJ	hepatic schistosomiasis japonica
HSK	herpes simplex keratitis
HSL	herpes simplex labialis
	hormone-sensitive lipase
HSM	hepatosplenomegaly
	holosystolic murmur
HSN	Hansen-Street nail
	heart sounds normal
	hereditary sensory neuropathy
HSOs	health services organizations
HSP	heat shock protein
	Henoch-Schönlein purpura
	hereditary spastic paraplegia
	hypersensitivity pneumonitis
	hysterosalpingography
HSPC	hydrogenated soy phosphatidyl choline
HSPE	high-strength pancreatic enzymes
HSQ	Health Status Questionnaire
HSR	heated serum reagin
	hypersensitivity reaction
	hypofractionated stereotactic radiotherapy
HSS	half-strength saline (0.45% Sodium Chloride)

hypertonic saline solution (3%, 5% or 7.5% sodium chloride injection) (This is a dangerous abbreviation)

HSSE — high soap-suds enema

HS-tk — herpes simplex thymidine kinase

hsUHR-OCT — high-speed ultra-high-resolution optical coherence tomography

HSV — herpes simplex virus
: highly selective vagotomy

HSV-1 — herpes simplex virus type 1
: herpes simplex virus type 1 vaccine

HSV$_2$ — herpes simplex virus type 2 vaccine

HSV$_{12}$ — herpes simplex virus types 1, 2 vaccine

HSV-2 — herpes simplex virus type 2

HSVE — herpes simplex virus encephalitis

HT — hammertoe
: head trauma
: healing time
: hearing test
: heart
: heart transplant
: height
: heparin trap (hep-trap; heparin lock; a venous access device)
: high temperature
: hormonotherapy
: Hubbard tank
: hypermetropia
: hyperopia
: hypertension
: hyperthermia
: hyperthyroid

H/T — heel and toe (walking)

H&T — hospitalization and treatment

H(T) — intermittent hypertropia

HT-1 — hereditary tyrosinemia type 1

5-HT$_1$ — serotonin (5-hydroxytryptamine)

HTA — Health Technology Assessment (Program)
: hydrothermal ablation
: hypertension (French)

ht. aer. — heated aerosol

HTAT — human tetanus antitoxin

HTB — hot tub bath

HTC — heated-tracheostomy collar
: high-throughput (protein) crystallization
: hypertensive crisis

HTDS — high-throughput drug screening

HTE — highly-treatment experienced (patients)

hTERT — human telomerase reverse transcriptase

HTF — house tube feeding

HTGL — hepatic triglyceride lipase

HTK — heel-to-knee (test)

HTL — hearing threshold level
: honey-thick liquid (diet consistency)
: human T-cell leukemia
: human thymic leukemia

HTLV III — human T-cell lymphotrophic virus type III

HTM — *Haemophilus* test medium
: high threshold mechanoceptors
: human tropomyosin

HTML — hypertext markup language

HTN — hypertension

HTO — high tibial osteotomy

HTP — House-Tree-Person-test

5-HTP — serotonin (5-hydroxytryptophan)

HTR — hard tissue replacement

hTRT — human telomerase reverse transcriptase

HTS — head traumatic syndrome
: heel-to-shin (test)
: Hematest(r) stools
: high-throughput screening

HTSCA — human tumor stem cell assay

HtSDS — height standard deviation score

H-TSH — human thyroid-stimulating hormone

HTT — hand thrust test
: hyalinizing trabecular tumor

HTV — herpes-type virus

HTVD — hypertensive vascular disease

HTX — hemothorax

HTx — heart transplant

HU — head unit
: Hounsfield units
: hydroxyurea
: hypertensive urgencies

Hu — Hounsfield units

HUAEC — human umbilical endothelial cells

HUCB — human umbilical cord blood

HUD — humanitarian use device (FDA designation)

HUH — Humana Hospital

HUI — Health Utilities Index

HUI2 — Health Utilities Index Mark 2

HUI3 — Health Utilities Index Mark 3

HUIFM — human leukocyte interferon meloy

HUK — human urinary kallikrein

HUM — heat, ultrasound, and massage

HUM 70/30 — human insulin, regular 30 units/mL with human insulin isophane suspension 70 units/mL (Humulin® 70/30 insulin)

HUMARA — human androgen receptor assay

HUM L — human insulin zinc suspension (Humulin® L Insulin)

HUM N — human insulin isophane suspension (Humulin® N Insulin)

HUM R — human insulin, regular (Humulin® R Insulin)

HUR — hydroxyurea

HUS	head ultrasound
	hemolytic uremic syndrome
	husband
husb	husband
HUT	head-upright tilt (test)
	hyperplasia of usual type
HUTT	head-up tilt-table testing
HUVEC	human umbilical vein endothelial cells
HV	hallux valgus
	Hantavirus
	has voided
	healthy volunteers
	Hemovac®
	hepatic vein
	herpesvirus
	home visit
	hypervariable
H&V	hemigastrecotomy and vagotomy
HVII	hypervariable segment II
HVA	homovanillic acid
HVD	hypertensive vascular disease
HVDO	hypovitaminosis D osteopathy
HVE	high-voltage electrophoresis
HVES	high-voltage electrical stimulation
HVF	Humphrey visual field
HVFD	homonymous visual field defects
HVGS	high-voltage galvanic stimulation
HVI	hollow viscus injury
HVL	half-value layer
	hippocampal volume loss
HVOD	hepatic veno-occlusive disease
HVOO	hepatic venous outflow obstruction
HVPC	high-voltage pulsed current
HVPG	hepatic venous pressure gradient
HYPT	hyperventilation provocation test
HVR	hypoxic ventilatory response
HVS	hyperventilation syndrome
HVS-TK	herpes simplex virus thymidine kinase
HW	hemiwalker
	heparin well
	homework
	housewife
HWB	hot water bottle
HWFE	housewife
HWG	has worn glasses
HWH	halfway house
HWP	hot wet pack
HWPG	has worn prescription glasses
Hx	history
	hospitalization
HXM	altretamine (hexamethylmelamine; Hexalen)
Hx & Px	history and physical (examination)
Hy	hypermetropia
HyCoSy	hysterosalpingo-contrast sonography
HYDRO	hydronephrosis
	hydrotherapy
HYG	hygiene
HYPER	above
	higher than
Hyper Al	hyperalimentation
Hyper K	hyperkalemia
HYPER T & A	hypertrophic tonsils and adenoids
HYPO	below
	hypodermic injection
	lower than
Hypo K	hypokalemia
hypopit	hypopituitarism
HYs	healthy years of life
Hyst	hysterectomy
Hz	Hertz
HZ	herpes zoster
HZD	herpes zoster dermatitis
HZO	herpes zoster ophthalmicus
HZV	herpes zoster virus

I

I — impression
incisal
incontinent
independent
initial
inspiration
intact (bag of waters)
intermediate
iris
one

I_2 — iodine

I^{131} — radioactive iodine

I-3+7 — idarubicin and cytarabine

IA — ideational apraxia
idiopathic anaphylaxis
incidental appendectomy
incurred accidentally
indigenous Australian(s)
intra-amniotic
intra-arterial
invasive aspergillosis

I & A — irrigation and aspiration

IAA — ileoanal anastomosis
insulin autoantibodies
interrupted aortic arch
intra-abdominal abscess
intra-abdominal adiposity
intra-arterial angiography

IAAA — inflammatory abdominal aortic aneurysms

IAAT — intra-abdominal adipose tissue

IAB — incomplete abortion
induced abortion
intermittent androgen blockade

IABC — intra-aortic balloon counterpulsation

IABCP — intra-aortic balloon counterpulsation

IABP — intra-aortic balloon pump
intra-arterial blood pressure

IAC — internal auditory canal
intra-arterial chemotherapy
isolated adrenal cell

IACC — intra-arterial cytoreductive chemotherapy

IAC-CPR — interposed abdominal compressions—cardiopulmonary resuscitation

IACG — intermittent angle-closure glaucoma

IACNS — isolated angiitis of central nervous system

IACP — intra-aortic counterpulsation

IAD — implantable atrial defibrillator
intermittent androgen deprivation
intractable atopic dermatitis
intraoperative autologous (blood) donation

IADHS — inappropriate antidiuretic hormone syndrome

IADL — Instrumental Activities of Daily Living

IA DSA — intra-arterial digital subtraction arteriography

IAEA — International Atomic Energy Agency

IAET — International Association for Enterostomal Therapy (Standards of Care Dermal Wounds: Pressure Ulcers)—see WOCN

IAF — intra-abdominal fat

IAG — indolyl-3-acryloylglycine

IAGT — indirect antiglobulin test

IAHA — immune adherence hemagglutination

IAHC — intra-arterial hepatic chemotherapy

IAHD — idiopathic acquired hemolytic disease

IAI — intra-abdominal infection
intra-abdominal injury
intra-amniotic infection

IALD — instrumental activities of daily living

IAM — internal auditory meatus

IAN — indinavir (Crixivan) associated nephrolithiasis
inferior alveolar nerve
intern's admission note

IAO — immediately after onset

IAP — independent adjudicating panel
intermittent acute porphyria
intra-abdominal pressure
intracarotid amobarbital procedure

IAPP — islet amyloid polypeptide

IAQ — indoor air quality

IARC — International Agency for Research on Cancer

IART — intra-atrial reentrant tachycardia

IAS — idiopathic ankylosing spondylitis
intermittent androgen suppression
internal anal sphincter
Interpersonal Adjective Scales

IASD — interatrial septal defect

IAT — immunoaugmentive therapy
indirect antiglobulin test
intracarotid amobarbital test
intraoperative autologous transfusion

IATT — intra-arterial thrombolytic therapy

IAV — infraclavicular axillary vein
intermittent assist ventilation

IAVC — intrinsic atrioventricular conduction

IB — ileal bypass
insulin-receptor binding test
isolation bed
investigator's brochure

IB1A — interferon beta-1a (Avonex)

IBAM — idiopathic bile acid malabsorption

IBBB — intra-blood-brain barrier

IBBBB incomplete bilateral bundle branch block
IBC Institutional Biosafety Committee
invasive bladder cancer
iron binding capacity
IBCLC International Board-Certified Lactation Consultant
IBD infectious bursal disease
inflammatory bowel disease
isosulfan blue dye
IBDQ Inflammatory Bowel Disease Questionnaire
IBE individual bioequivalence
IBG iliac bone graft
IBI intermittent bladder irrigation
ibid at the same place
IBILI indirect bilirubin
IB-IVUS integrated backscatter intravascular ultrasound
IBM ideal body mass
inclusion body myositis
IBMI initial body mass index
IBMIR instant blood-mediated inflammatory reaction
IBMTR International Bone Marrow Transplant Registry
IBNR incurred but not reported
IBOW intact bag of waters
IBP ibuprofen
intrableb pigmentation
IBPB interscalene brachial plexus block
IBPS Insall-Burstein posterior stabilizer
IBR immediate breast reconstruction
infectious bovine rhinotracheitis
IBRS Inpatient Behavior Rating Scale
IBS irritable bowel syndrome
IBS-C irritable bowel syndrome, constipation-predominant
IBS-D Irritable Bowel Syndrome–Diarrhea Type
IBT ink blot test (Rorschach test)
interblinking time
immune-based therapy
IBTR intrabreast-tumor recurrence
ipsilateral breast tumor recurrence
IBU ibuprofen
IBW ideal body weight
IC between meals
iliac crest
immune complex
immunocompromised
incipient cataract (grade 1+ to 4+)
incomplete
indirect calorimetry
indirect Coombs (test)
individual counseling
informed consent
inspiratory capacity
intensive care
intercostal
intercourse
intermediate care
intermittent catheterization
intermittent claudication
interstitial changes
interstitial cystitis
intracerebral
intracranial
intraincisional
ion chromatography
irritable colon
I/C imipenem-cilastatin (Primaxin)
IC_{50} half maximal inhibitory concentration
ICA ileocolic anastomosis
intermediate care area
internal carotid artery
intracranial abscess
intracranial aneurysm
islet-cell antibody
ICa calcium, ionized
ICAAC Interscience Conference on Antimicrobial Agents and Chemotherapy
ICAD intracranial atherosclerotic disease
ICAM intracellular adhesion molecule
ICAM-1 intercellular adhesion molecule-1
ICAMA Interstate Compact on Adoption and Medical Assistance
ICAO internal carotid artery occlusion
ICAS intermediate coronary artery syndrome
ICAT infant cardiac arrest tray
isotope-coded affinity tag
ICB intracranial bleeding
ICBG iliac crest bone graft
ICBT intercostobronchial trunk
ICC idiopathic chronic cough
immunocytochemistry
Indian childhood cirrhosis
Infection Control Committee
interstitial cells of Cajal
intracluster correlation coefficient
intraclass correlation coefficient
invasive cervical carcinoma
islet cell carcinoma
ICCD intensified charge-coupled device
ICCE intracapsular cataract extraction
ICC-MY myenteric interstitial cells of Cajal
ICCU intensive coronary care unit
intermediate coronary care unit
ICD implantable cardioverter defibrillator
indigocarmine dye
informed consent document
instantaneous cardiac death

intercusp distance (dental)
isocitrate dehydrogenase
irritant contact dermatitis

ICDA International Classification of Disease, Adapted

ICDB incomplete database

ICDC implantable cardioverter defibrillator catheter

ICD 9 CM International Statistical Classification of Diseases, 9th Revision, Clinical Modification

ICD-10 International Classification of Diseases and Related Health Problems, 10th revision

ICD-10-PCS International Statistical Classification of Diseases, 10th Revision, Procedure Coding Classification System

ICDO International Classification of Diseases for Oncology

ICDSC Intensive Care Delirium Screening Checklist

ICE ice, compression, and elevation
ifosfamide, carboplatin, and etoposide
Immigration and Customs Enforcement
individual career exploration
interleukin-1 alpha converting enzyme
interleukin-1 beta converting enzyme
intracardiac echocardiography

+ ice add ice

ICECI International Classification of External Causes of Injuries

ICER incremental cost-effectiveness ratio

ICES ice, compression, elevation, and support

ICF intermediate care facility
intracellular fluid

ICFDH International Classification of Functioning, Disability, and Health

ICG impedance cardiography
indocyanine green

ICGA indocyanine green angiography

ICH immunocompromised host
International Conference on Harmonization (of Technical Requirements for Registration of Pharmaceuticals for Human Use)
intracerebral hemorrhage
intracranial hemorrhage

ICHD-II International Classification of Headache Disorders, 2nd Edition

ICHI International Classification of Health Interventions

ICHT immuno-chemotherapy

ICI intracranial injury

ICIQ-SF International Consultation on Incontinence Questionnaire

ICISG International Cancer Information Service Group

ICIT intensified conventional insulin therapy

ICL intracorneal lens
isocitrate lyase

ICLE intracapsular lens extraction

ICM intercostal margin
intercostal muscle
ischemic cardiomyopathy

ICN infection control nurse
intensive care nursery

ICN2 neonatal intensive care unit level II

ICP inductively coupled plasma
intercostal position (for chest lead)
intracranial pressure
intrahepatic cholestasis of pregnancy

ICPC International Classification of Primary Care
Interstate Compact on the Placement of Children

ICPC-2 International Classification of Primary Care, 2nd revision

ICP-MS inductively-coupled plasma—mass spectrometer

ICP-OES inductively-coupled plasma—optical emission spectrometry

ICPP intubated continuous positive pressure

ICR intercaudate nucleus ratio
intercostal retractions
intrastromal corneal ring

ICRC International Committee of the Red Cross

ICRF-159 razoxane

ICRP International Commission on Radiological Protection

ICRS intrastromal corneal ring segments

ICS ileocecal sphincter
inhaled corticosteroid(s)
intercostal space

ICSC idiopathic central serous choroidopathy

ICSH interstitial cell-stimulating hormone

ICSI intracytoplasmic sperm injection

ICSR Individual Case Safety Reports
intercostal space retractions

ICT icterus
indirect Coombs test
inflammation of connective tissue
intensive conventional therapy
intermittent cervical traction
intracranial tumor
intracutaneous test
islet cell transplant

ICTP	C-terminal telopeptide of type I collagen
ICTX	intermittent cervical traction
ICU	intensive care unit
	intermediate care unit
ICV	intracerebroventricular
ICVH	ischemic cerebrovascular headache
ICW	in connection with
	intact canal wall
	intercellular water
ID	identification
	identify
	idiotype
	ifosfamide, mesna uroprotection, and doxorubicin
	immunodiffusion
	induction delivery
	infectious disease (physician or department)
	initial diagnosis
	initial dose
	intellectual disability
	internal derangement
	intradermal
	iron deficiency
id	the same
I & D	incision and debridement
	incision and drainage
	irrigation and debridement
IDA	idarubicin (Idamycin)
	iron deficiency anemia
IDAM	infant of drug abusing mother
IDB	incomplete database
IDC	idiopathic dilated cardiomyopathy
	invasive ductal cancer
IDCF	immunodiffusion complement fixation
IDCM	idiopathic dilated cardiomyopathy
IDD	insulin-dependent diabetes
	intervertebral disk disease
	iodine-deficiency disorders
I/DD	intellectual and developmental disabilities
IDDD	Interview for Deterioration in Daily Life in Dementia
IDDM	insulin-dependent diabetes mellitus
IDDS	implantable drug delivery system
	intrathecal drug delivery systems
IDE	Investigational Device Exemption
IDEA	Individuals with Disabilities Education Act
IDET	intradiskal electrothermal therapy
IDFC	immature dead female child
ID-GDM	insulin-dependent gestational diabetes mellitus
IDH	isocitric dehydrogenase
IDI	Interpersonal Dependency Inventory
	intrathecal drug infusion
IDIS	Iowa Drug Information System
IDK	internal derangement of knee
IDL	intermediate-density lipoprotein
	ischemic digital loss
IDLH	immediately dangerous to life or health
IDM	infant of a diabetic mother
IDMC	immature dead male child
	Independent Data Monitoring Committee
IDMP	International Drug Monitoring Program
IDMS	isotope dilution mass spectrometry
IDNA	iron-deficient, not anemic
ID-NAT	individual donation nucleic acid (amplification) testing
IDO	idiopathic detrusor overactivity
IDP	initiate discharge planning
	inosine diphosphate
IDPN	intradialytic parenteral nutrition
IDR	idarubicin (Zavedos)
	idiosyncratic drug reaction
	intradermal reaction
IDS	infectious disease service
	integrated delivery system
	intradermal smears
IDSA	Infectious Disease Society of America (guidelines)
IDT	intensive diabetes treatment
	interdisciplinary team
	intradermal test
IDTF	independent diagnostic testing facility
IDTP	immunodiffusion tube precipitin
IDU	idoxuridine
	infectious disease unit
	injecting drug user
IDV	indinavir (Crixivan)
	intermittent demand ventilation
IDVC	indwelling venous catheter
IE	ifosfamide, and etoposide with mesna
	immunoelectrophoresis
	induced emesis
	infectious enteritis
	infective endocarditis
	inner ear
	internal/external (rotation)
	international unit (European abbreviation)
I & E	ingress and egress (tubes)
	internal and external
i.e.	that is
IEC	independent ethics committee
	inpatient exercise center
	intradiskal electrothermal coagulation
IED	immune-enhancing diet

	improvised explosive device
	intermittent explosive disorder
IEED	involuntary emotional expression disorder
IEEG	intracranial electroencephalogram
IEF	isoelectric focusing
IEH	involuntary emergency hospitalization
IEI	idiopathic environmental intolerance
IEL	internal elastic lamina
	intestinal-intraepithelial lymphocyte
IELT	Intravaginal Ejaculatory Latency Time
IEM	immune electron microscopy
	inborn errors of metabolism
iEMG	integrated electromyography
IEMR	integrated electronic medical records
IEN	intraepithelial neoplasia
IEP	idiopathic eosinophilic pneumonia
	immunoelectrophoresis
	Individualized Education Plan
IEPA	immunoelectrophoresis analysis
I:E ratio	inspiratory to expiratory time ratio
IES	Impact of Event Scale
IET	infantile estropia
IF	idiopathic flushing
	ifosfamide (Ifex)
	immunofluorescence
	impaired fecundity
	index finger
	injury factor
	interferon
	interfrontal
	intermaxillary fixation
	internal fixation
	intrinsic factor
	involved field (radiotherapy)
IFA	immunofluorescent assay
	imported fire ants
	indirect fluorescent antibody
	iron and folic acid
IFAT	immunofluorescence antibody test (technique)
IFC	interferential current
	intravital flow cytometry
IFE	immunofixation electrophoresis
	in-flight emergency
IFG	impaired fasting glucose
IFI	invasive fungal infection
IFIS	intraoperative floppy-iris syndrome
IFL	indolent follicular lymphoma
	irinotecan, fluorouracil, and leucovorin
IFM	Intergroupe Francophone du Myélome (myeloma French-speaking group)
	internal fetal monitoring
IFN	interferon
IFN α-1	interferon alfa-1
IFNB	interferon beta-1 b (Betaseron)
IFO	ifosfamide (Ifex)
	in front of
iFOBT	immunochemical fecal occult blood tests
IFOP	infrared fiber-optic probe
IFOS	ifosfamide (Ifex)
IFP	inflammatory fibroid polyps
IFPMA	International Federation of Pharmaceutical Manufacturers Associations
IFRT	involved-field radiotherapy
IFSAC	Inventory of Functional Status After Childbirth
IFSE	internal fetal scalp electrode
IFSP	individualized family service plan
IgA	immunoglobulin A
IGCS	inpatient geriatric consultation services
IgD	immunoglobulin D
IGDE	idiopathic gait disorders of the elderly
IGDM	infant of gestational diabetic mother
IGE	idiopathic generalized epilepsy
IgE	immunoglobulin E
IGF-1	insulin-like growth factor 1
IGFA	indocyanine-green fundus angiography
IGFBP-3	insulin-like growth factor-binding protein 3
IGF1R	insulin-like growth factor 1 receptor
IgG	immunoglobulin G
IGHL	inferior glenohumeral ligament
IGI	image guided implantology
IGIM	immune globulin intramuscular
IGIV	immune globulin intravenous
IgM	immunoglobulin M
IGP	interstitial glycoprotein
IGR	intrauterine growth retardation
IGRT	image-guided radiation therapy
IGT	impaired glucose tolerance
IGTN	impaired glucose tolerance and neuropathy
	ingrown toenail
IH	indirect hemagglutination
	infectious hepatitis
	inguinal hernia
	inhaled (this is a dangerous abbreviation)
	in-house
IHA	immune hemolytic anemia
	indirect hemagglutination
	infusion hepatic arteriography
	intrahepatic arterial
IHC	idiopathic hypercalciuria
	immobilization hypercalcemia
	immunohistochemistry

I

	inner hair cell (in cochlea)
IHD	intermittent hemodialysis
	intraheptic duct (ule)
	ischemic heart disease
IHDN	integrated health delivery network
IHES	idiopathic hypereosinophilic syndrome
IHGK	immortalized human gingival keratinocytes
IHH	idiopathic hypogonadotrophic hypogonadism
IHHE	infantile hepatic hemangioendothelioma
IHI	Institute for Healthcare Improvement
IHO	idiopathic hypertrophic osteoarthropathy
IHP	idiopathic hypertrophic pachymeningitis
	idiopathic hypoparathyroidism
	inferior hypogastric plexus
	isolated hepatic perfusion
IHPH	intrahepatic portal hypertension
IHPS	infantile hypertrophic pyloric stenosis
IHR	inguinal hernia repair
	intrinsic heart rate
IHS	Indian Health Service
	integrated healthcare system
	International Headache Society (criteria)
	Idiopathic Headache Score
IHs	iris hamartomas
IHSA	iodinated human serum albumin
IHSS	idiopathic hypertrophic subaortic stenosis
	in-home supportive services
IHT	insulin hypoglycemia test
IHU	inpatient hospice unit
IHW	inner-heel wedge
II	internal iliac (artery)
IIA	internal iliac artery
IICP	increased intracranial pressure
IICU	infant intensive care unit
IID	infectious intestinal disease
IIDD	idiopathic inflammatory demyelinating diseases
IIEF	International Index of Erectile Function
IIF	indirect immunofluorescence
IIH	idiopathic infantile hypercalcemia
	idiopathic intracranial hypertension
	iodine-induced hyperthyroidism
IIHT	iodide-induced hyperthyroidism
IIM	idiopathic inflammatory myopathies
	intracortical interaction mapping
IINB	iliohypogastric ilioinguinal nerve block
IIP	idiopathic interstitial pneumonitis
IIPF	idiopathic interstitial pulmonary fibrosis
IIQ	Incontinence Impact Questionnaire
IIS	immunization information system
IJ	ileojejunal
	internal jugular
I&J	insight and judgment
IJC	internal jugular catheter
IJD	inflammatory joint disease
IJO	idiopathic juvenile osteoporosis
IJP	internal jugular pressure
IJR	idiojunctional rhythm
IJT	idiojunctional tachycardia
IJV	internal jugular vein
IK	immobilized knee
	interstitial keratitis
IKDC	International Knee Documentation Committee (evaluation; score; form)
IL	immature lungs
	interleukin (1, 2, etc.)
	intralesional
	Intralipid®
IL-2	aldesleukin (Proleukin; interleukin-2)
IL-11	oprelvekin (Neumega; interleukin-11)
ILA	inferior lateral angle
	insulin-like activity
ILAEC	Intersocietal Commission for Accreditation of Echocardiography Laboratories
ILB	incidental Lewy body
ILBBB	incomplete left bundle branch block
ILBW	infant, low birth weight (less than 2,500 g)
ILC	interstitial laser coagulation
	invasive lobular cancer
ILCOR	International Liaison Committee on Resuscitation
ILD	immature lung disease
	indentation load deflection
	interlaminar distance in flexion
	intermediate density lipoproteins
	interstitial lung disease
	ischemic leg disease
ILE	infantile lobar emphysema
	involutional lateral entropion
ILF	indicated low forceps
ILFC	immature living female child
ILHP	ipsilateral hemidiaphragmatic paresis
ILI	influenza-like illness
	isolated limb infusion
ILM	internal limiting membrane
ILMC	immature living male child
ILMI	inferolateral myocardial infarct
ILP	independent living program
	interstitial laser photocoagulation
	isolated limb perfusion

ILQTS idiopathic long QT (interval) syndrome
ILR implantable loop recorder
ILS increased life span
intralabyrinthine schwannomas
ILT interstitial laser therapy
ILVEN inflammatory linear verrucal epidermal nevus
IM ice massage
imatinib mesylate (Gleevec) (This is a very dangerous abbreviation)
infectious mononucleosis
intermetatarsal
internal margin (for radiotherapy)
internal medicine
intramedullary
intramuscular
IMA inferior mesenteric artery
internal mammary artery
IMAC ifosfamide, mesna uroprotection, doxorubicin (Adriamycin), and cisplatin
immobilized metal affinity chromatography
IMAE internal maxillary artery embolization
IMAG internal mammary artery graft
IMARD immunomodulating antirheumatic drugs
IMAT intensity-modulated arc therapy
IMB intermenstrual bleeding
IMBP immobilized mismatch binding protein
IMC intermittent catheterization
intramedullary catheter
IMCI Integrated Management of Childhood Illness
IMCU intermediate care unit
IMDs inherited metabolic disorders
IME important medical event
independent medical examination (evaluation)
isometric exercise
IMF idiopathic myelofibrosis
ifosfamide, mesna uroprotection, methotrexate, and fluorouracil
immobilization mandibular fracture
inframammary fold
intermaxillary fixation
IMG internal medicine group
IMGU insulin-mediated glucose uptake
IMH idiopathic myocardial hypertrophy
intramural hematoma
IMH indirect microhemagglutination (test)
IMI imipramine
impending myocardial infarction
inferior myocardial infarction
intramuscular injection
^{131}I-MIBG iodine^{131}-metaiodobenzyl-guanidine (iobenguane ^{131}I)
IMIG intramuscular immunoglobulin
IMLC incomplete mitral leaflet closure
IMM immunizations
IMN idiopathic membranous nephropathy
immune modulating nutrition (immunonutrition)
internal mammary (lymph) node
intramedullary nail
IMP impacted
important
impression
improved
inosine monophoshate
IMPX impaction
IMQ Infant/Child Monitoring Questionnaires
IMR infant mortality rate
IMRA immunoradiometric assay
iMRI intraoperative magnetic resonance imaging
IMRS intensity-modulated radiosurgery
IMRT intensity-modulated radiation therapy
IMS immunosuppressants
incurred in military service
involuntary movements
ion mobility spectrometry
IMSS Mexican Institute for Social Security (*Instituto Mexicano del Seguro Social*)
IMT inspiratory muscle training
intimal medial thickness
IMU intermediate medicine unit
IMV inferior mesenteric vein
intermittent mandatory ventilation
intermittent mechanical ventilation
IMVP-16 ifosfamide, mesna uroprotection, methotrexate, and etoposide
IN insulin
intranasal (this is a dangerous abbreviation as it can be read as IV [intravenous] or IM [intramuscular]; use nasally or intranasal)
In indium
in. inch
INAD in no apparent distress
Investigational New Animal Drug
INB intercostal nerve blockade
INC incisal
incision
incomplete
incontinent
increase
inside-the-needle catheter
INCC Institut National du Cancer du Canada

I

INCMNSZ	Instituto Nacional de Ciencias Médicas y Nutrición (Mexico)
Inc Spir	incentive spirometer
INCSs	intranasal corticosteroids
IND	incision and drainage indinavir (Crixivan) induced Investigational New Drug (application)
INDA	Investigational New Drug Application
INDIGO	interstitial laser ablation of the prostate
INDM	infant of nondiabetic mother
INDO	indomethacin
^{111}In-DTPA	indium pentetate
INE	infantile necrotizing encephalomyelopathy
INEX	inexperienced
INF	infant infarction infected infection inferior influenza virus vaccine, not otherwise specified information infused infusion intravenous nutritional fluid
INF_a	influenza virus, attenuated live vaccine
INFas	influenza virus attenuated live vaccine, intranasal
INFC	infected infection
INFi	influenza virus inactivated vaccine
INFs	influenza virus vaccine, split viron
INFs-AB3	influenza virus inactivated vaccine, split virion, types A and B, trivalent
INF_w	influenza virus vaccine, whole viron
ING	inguinal
✓ing	checking
INH	inhalation isoniazid (isonicotinic acid hydrazide)
INI	intranuclear inclusion
inj	injection injury
INK	injury not known
INN	International Nonproprietary Name
INO	inhaled nitrous oxide internuclear ophthalmoplegia
INOP	internodal ophthalmoplegia
iNOS	inducible nitric oxide synthase
inpt	inpatient
INQ	inferior nasal quadrant
INR	international normalized ratio (for anticoagulant monitoring)
INS	idiopathic nephrotic syndrome inspection insurance intranasal corticosteroids (steroids)
in situ	in the natural or normal place
INSS	International Neuroblastoma Staging System
INST	instrumental delivery
INT	intermittent needle therapy internal
Int mon	internal monitor
INTERP	interpretation
Int Med	internal medicine
intol	intolerance
int-rot	internal rotation
int trx	intermittent traction
intub	intubation
INV	Invirase (saquinavir, hard gel cap)
inver	inversion
INVOS	in vivo optical spectroscopy
IO	inferior oblique initial opening intestinal obstruction intraocular pressure intra-Ommaya intraoperative intraosseous
I&O	intake and output
IOA	intact on admission
IOC	intern on call intraoperative cholangiogram
IOCG	intraoperative cholangiogram
IOD	implant-supported overdenture interorbital distance
IODM	infant of diabetic mother
IOF	intraocular fluid
IOFB	intraocular foreign body
IOFNA	intraoperative fine needle aspiration
IOH	idiopathic orthostatic hypotension
IO-HDRBT	intraoperative high-dose-rate brachytherapy
IOI	idiopathic orbital inflammation intraosseous infusion
IOL	induction of labor intraocular lens intraocular lymphoma
IOLI	intraocular lens implantation
IOLM	intraoperative lymphatic mapping
IOM	Institute of Medicine
ION	ischemic optic neuropathy
IONIS	indirect optic nerve injury syndrome
IONTO	iontophoresis
IOOA	inferior oblique overaction
IOP	intensive outpatient program intraocular pressure intraosseous puncture

IOR ideas of reference
immature oocyte retrieval
inferior oblique recession
IO-RB intraocular retinoblastoma
IORT intraoperative radiation therapy
IOS intraoperative sonography
IOSH Institute for Occupational Safety and Health
IOT intraocular tension
IOTEE intraoperative transesophageal echocardiography
IOTT intensification-of-treatment trigger (criteria)
IOUS intraocular ultrasound
IOV initial office visit
IP ice pack
incubation period
individualized plan
Infrapatellar
inpatient
in plaster
interpersonal (therapy)
interphalangeal
interstitial pneumonia
intestinal permeability
intraperitoneal
invasive procedures
inverted (inverting) papilloma
I/P iris/pupil
IP3 inositol triphosphate
IPA independent practice association
interpleural analgesia
invasive pulmonary aspergillosis
isopropyl alcohol
IPAA ileo-pouch anal anastamosis
IPAH idiopathic pulmonary arterial hypertension
IPAP inspiratory positive airway pressure
IPB infrapopliteal bypass
IPC indirect pulp cavity
intermittent pneumatic compression (boots)
intraperitoneal chemotherapy
IPCD idiopathic paroxysmal cerebral dysrhythmia
infantile polycystic disease
IPCK infantile polycystic kidney (disease)
IPCT intraperitoneal chemotherapy
IPD idiopathic Parkinson disease
immediate pigment darkening
inflammatory pelvic disease
intermittent peritoneal dialysis
interpupillary distance
interspinous process decompression
invasive pneumococcal disease
IPEX immune dysregulation, polyendocrinopathy, enteropathy, X-linked (syndrome)
IPF idiopathic pulmonary fibrosis
inpatient psychiatric facility
interstitial pulmonary fibrosis
IPFD intrapartum fetal distress
IPG immobilized pH gradient
impedance plethysmography
implantable pulse generator
individually polymerized grass
IPH idiopathic pulmonary hemosiderosis
interphalangeal
intraparenchymal hemorrhage
intraperitoneal hemorrhage
IPHC intraperitoneal hyperthermic chemotherapy
IPHEP independent progressive home exercise program
IPHP intraperitoneal hyperthermic chemotherapy
IPI International Prognostic Index
IPJ interphalangeal joint
IPK intractable plantar keratosis
IPL intense pulsed light
IPM intranodal-palisaded myofibroblastoma
intrauterine pressure monitor
interventional pain management
IPMI inferoposterior myocardial infarct
IPMN intraductal papillary mucinous neoplasm
IPN infantile periarteritis nodosa
intern's progress note
interstitial pneumonia
IPOF immediate postoperative fitting
IPOM intraperitoneal onlay mesh
IPOP immediate postoperative prosthesis
IPP inflatable penile prosthesis
intrapleual pressure
intravesical protrusion of the prostate
isolated pelvic perfusion
IPPA inspection, palpation, percussion, and auscultation
IPPB intermittent positive-pressure breathing
IP-PDT intraperitoneal photodynamic therapy
IPPE initial preventive physical examination
IPPF immediate postoperative prosthetic fitting
IPPI interruption of pregnancy for psychiatric indication
IPPV intermittent positive pressure ventilation
IPS idiopathic pneumonia syndrome
infundibular pulmonic stenosis
initial prognostic score
intermittent photic stimulation
intraparietal sulcus
IPSCs islet-producing stem cells

IPSF immediate postsurgical fitting
IPSID immunoproliferative small intestinal disease
IPSP inhibitory postsynaptic potential
IPSS inferior petrosal sinus sampling
I-PSS International Prostate Symptom Score
IPST intraprocedural stent thrombosis
I PSY intermediate psychiatry
IPT intended primary treatment
intermittent pelvic traction
iPTH parathyroid hormone by radioimmunoassay
IPTX intermittent pelvic traction
IPV inactivated poliovirus vaccine
intimate partner violence
IPVC interpolated premature ventricular contraction
IPW interphalangeal width
IQ intelligence quotient
IQR interquartile range
intraquartile range (statistical term)
IQWiG Leiter des Institus für Qualität and Wirtschaftlichkeit im Gesundheitswesen (Institute for Quality and Economy in Healthcare)
IR immediate-release (tablets)
immunoreactive
inferior rectus
infrared
insulin resistance
internal reduction
internal resistance
internal rotation
intraoral radiography (dental)
I&R insertion and removal
IRA infarct-related artery
IRAAF intraoperative radiofrequency ablation for chronic atrial fibrillation
IRA-EEA ileorectal anastomoses with end-to-end anastomosis
IRAP interleukin-1 receptor antagonist protein
IRB Institutional Review Board
IRBBB incomplete right bundle branch block
IRBC immature red blood cell
irradiated red blood cells
iRBCs *Plasmodium falciparum*-infected red blood cells
IRBP implantable rotary blood pump
interphotoreceptor retinoid-binding protein
IRC indirect radionuclide cystography
infrared coagulation
Institutional Review Committee (Board)
IRCU intensive respiratory care unit
IRD immune renal disease(s)
IRDA intermittent rhythmic delta activity
IRDM insulin-requiring diabetes mellitus
insulin-resistant diabetes mellitus
IR-DRGs International Refined Diagnosis Related Groups
IRDS idiopathic respiratory distress syndrome
infant respiratory distress syndrome
IRE internal rotation in extension
IRED infrared-emission detection
IRF impaired renal function
inpatient rehabilitation facilities
internal rotation in flexion
IRH intraretinal hemorrhage
IRI immunoreactive insulin
irinotecan (Camptosar)
ischemic reperfusion injury
IRIV immunopotentiating reconstituted influenza virosomes
IRM magnetic resonance imaging (French)
IRMA immediate response mobile analysis (blood analysis system)
immunoradiometric assay
intraretinal microvascular abnormalities
IRMS isotope-ratio mass spectrometry
IRN iterated rippled noise
IRNS intercostal repetitive nerve stimulation
IROS ipsilateral routing of signals
IROX irinotecan and oxaliplatin
IRP intellectual property rights
IRR infrared radiation
intrarenal reflux
irregular rate and rhythm
IRRC Institutional Research Review Committee
irreg irregular
IRR HYDRO irreversible hydrocolloid
IRRs incidence rate ratios
IRS Information and Referral Society
insulin receptor substrate
insulin-resistance syndrome
IRSB intravenous regional sympathetic block
IRSG Intergroup Rhabdomyosarcoma Study Group
IRT immunoreactive trypsin
incident response team
IRV inspiratory reserve volume
inverse ratio ventilation
IS incentive spirometer
induced sputum
Information Services (Department)

	in situ
	intercostal space
	inventory of systems
	ipecac syrup
I-S	Ionescu-Shiley (prosthetic heart valve)
I & S	intact and symmetrical
I/S	instruct/supervise
I2S	iduronate-2-sulfatase
ISA	ileosigmoid anastomosis
	Incest Survivors Anonymous
	intrinsic sympathomimetic activity
ISAAC	International Study of Asthma and Allergies in Childhood (questionnaire; protocol)
ISADH	inappropriate secretion of antidiuretic hormone
ISAM	infant of substance abusing mother
ISB	incentive spirometry breathing
ISBN	International Standard Book Number
ISBP	interscalen brachial plexus
ISC	carcinoma *in situ* (also CIS)
	indwelling subclavian catheter
	infant servo-control
	infant skin control
	intermittent self-catheterization
	intermittent straight catheterization
	isolette servo-control
ISCM	intramedullary spinal cord metastases
I/SCN	urinary iodine/thiocyanate ratio
ISCOM	immunostimulating complex
ISCP	infection surveillance and control program
ISCs	irreversible sickle cells
ISCU	infant special care unit
ISD	inhibited sexual desire
	initial sleep disturbance
	intrinsic (urethral) sphincter deficiency
	isosorbide dinitrate (Isordol)
ISDN	isosorbide dinitrate (Isordol)
ISE	internal scalp electrode
	ion-sensitive electrode
ISEL	*in situ* end labeling
ISF	interstitial fluid
ISFET	ion-selective field effect transistor
ISG	immune serum globulin (immune globulin)
ISH	isolated systolic hypertension
ISHH	*in situ* hybridization histochemistry
ISHLT	International Society for Heart and Lung Transplantation
ISHT	isolated systolic hypertension
ISI	Insulin Sensitivity Index
	International Sensitivity Index
ISK	isokinetic
ISMA	infantile spinal muscular atrophy
ISMN	isosorbide mononitrate
ISMO®	isosorbide mononitrate
ISMP	Institute for Safe Medication Practices
ISNA	iron-sufficient, not anemic
ISO	International Organization for Standardization
	isodose
	isolette
	isoproterenol
ISOE	isoetharine
ISOF	isoflurane (Florane)
ISOK	isokinetic
ISOM	isometric
ISOs	isoenzymes
ISP	Individual Service Plan
	inferior spermatic plexus
	interspace
ISPP	individualized sleep promotion plan
ISQ	as before; continue on (*in status quo*)
ISR	injection site reaction
	in situ reconstruction
	in-stent restenosis
	integrated secretory response
ISRCTN	International Standard Randomized Controlled Trial Number
ISS	idiopathic short stature
	Individual Self-Rating Scale
	Injury Severity Score
	irritable stomach syndrome
	Integrated Summary of Safety
IS10S	10% invert sugar in 0.9% sodium chloride (saline) injection
ISSHL	idiopathic sudden sensorineural hearing loss
ISSP	Infant Support Services Program
ISSSTE	The Institute of Social Security and Services for Civil Servants (*Instituto de Seguridad y Servicios Sociales de los Trabajadores del Estado*) (Mexico)
IST	immunosuppressive therapy
	inappropriate sinus tachycardia
	injection sclerotherapy
	insulin sensitivity test
	insulin shock therapy
ISU	intermediate surgical unit
ISW	interstitial water
IS10W	10% invert sugar injection (in water)
ISWI	incisional surgical wound infection
IT	iliotibial
	incentive therapy
	individual therapy
	inferior-temporal
	inferior turbinate
	information technology

I

	Information Technology (Department)
	Inhalation Therapist
	inhalation therapy
	inspiratory time
	intensive therapy
	intermittent traction
	interpreted
	intertrochanteric
	intertuberous
	intrathecal (dangerous abbreviation)
	intratracheal (dangerous, could be interupted as intrathecal)
	intratumoral
	intratympanic (this is a dangerous abbreviation that could be interpreted as intrathecal)
ITA	individual treatment assessment
	inferior temporal artery
	itasetron
ITAG	internal thoracic artery graft
ITAL	intrathoracic artificial lung
ITB	iliotibial band
	intrathecal baclofen
ITBC	intraluminal typical bronchial carcinoid
ITBS	iliotibial band syndrome
	Iowa Tests of Basic Skills
ITC	Incontinence Treatment Center
	in-the-canal (hearing aid)
	isothermal titration calorimetry
ITCP	idiopathic thrombocytopenic purpura
ITCU	intensive thoracic cardiovascular unit
ITD	impedance threshold device
ITE	insufficient therapeutic effect
	in-the-ear (hearing aid)
ITF	inpatient treatment facility
ITFF	intertrochanteric femoral fracture
ITGV	intrathoracic gas volume
ITM	Institute of Tropical Medicine, (Antwerp, Belgium)
ITMTX	intrathecal methotrexate
ITN	irinotecan (Camptosar)
ITNs	insecticide treated nets
ITOC	intratracheal oxygen catheter
ITOP	intentional termination of pregnancy
ITOU	intensive therapy observation unit
ITP	idiopathic thrombocytopenic purpura
	immune thrombocytopenia
	immune thrombocytopenic purpura
	interim treatment plan
ITPA	Illinois Test of Psycholinguistic Ability
ITQ	inferior temporal quadrant
ITR	isotretinoin (Accutane)
ITRA	itraconazole (Sporanox)
ITS	intelligent testing strategies
	internal transcribed spacer
	iontophoretic transdermal system
	isometric trunk stabilization
ITSCU	infant-toddler special care unit
ITT	identical twins (raised) together
	incremental treadmill test
	insulin tolerance test
	intention-to-treat (analysis)
ITU	infant-toddler unit
	intensive therapy unit
	intensive treatment unit
ITVAD	indwelling transcutaneous vascular access device
ITX	immunotoxin(s)
ITx	intestinal transplantation
ITZ	itraconazole (Sporanox)
IU	international unit (this is a dangerous abbreviation as it is read as intravenous; use "units")
IUBT	intrauterine blood transfusion
IUC	intrauterine catheter
IUCD	intrauterine contraceptive device
IUD	intrauterine death
	intrauterine device
IUDE	intrauterine drug exposure
	intravenous drug exposure
IUDR	idoxuridine (Herplex)
IUFB	intrauterine foreign body
IUFD	intrauterine fetal death (demise)
	intrauterine fetal distress
IUFT	intrauterine fetal transfusion
IUGR	intrauterine growth retardation (restriction)
IUI	intrauterine insemination
IULN	institutional upper limit of normal
IUMR	intrauterine myelomeningocele repair
IUP	intrauterine pregnancy
IUPB	infected units per billion
IUPC	intrauterine pressure catheter
IUPD	intrauterine pregnancy delivered
IUP,TBCS	intrauterine pregnancy, term birth, cesarean section
IUP,TBLC	intrauterine pregnancy, term birth, living child
IUR	intrauterine retardation
IUS	intrauterine system
IUT	intersection-union test
	intrauterine transfusion
IUTD	immunizations up to date
IV	four
	interview
	intravenous (i.v.)
	intravertebral
	invasive
	inversion
	symbol for class 4 controlled substances
IVA	Intervir-A

I

IVAD implantable venous access device
implantable vascular access device

IVBAT intravascular bronchoalveolar tumor

IVC inferior vena cava
inspiratory vital capacity
intravenous chemotherapy
intravenous cholangiogram
intraventricular catheter
intraventricular conduction

IVCCM in-vivo corneal confocal microscopy

IVCD intraventricular conduction defect (delay)

IVCF inferior vena cava filter

IVCI intravenous continuous infusion

IVCP inferior vena cava pressure

IVCS intravenous conscious sedation

IVCV inferior venacavography

IVD instrumental vaginal delivery
intervertebral disk
intravenous drip
in vitro diagnostic
ischemic vascular dementia

IVDA intravenous drug abuse

IVDK Information Network of Departments of Dermatology (Göttingen University) (http://www.ivdk.org)

IVDMIAs in vitro diagnostic multivariate index assays

IVDSA intravenous digital subtraction angiography

IVDU intravenous drug user

IVET in vivo expression technology

IVF intervertebral foramina
intravenous fluid(s)
in vitro fertilization

IVFA intravenous fluorescein angiography

IVFE intravenous fat emulsion

IVF-ET in vitro fertilization-embryo transfer

IVFT intravenous fetal transfusion

IVGG intravenous gamma globulin

IVGTT intravenous glucose tolerance test

IVH intravenous hyperalimentation
intraventricular hemorrhage

IVID intravenous iron dextran (INFeD; DexFerrum)

IVIG intravenous immunoglobulin

IVJC intervertebral joint complex

IVK intravitreal injection of triamcinolone acetonide (Kenalog) (also IVTA)

IVL intravascular lymphomatosis
intravenous lock

IVLBW infant of very low birth weight (less than 1,500 g)

IVMP intravenously administered methylprednisolone

IVNC isolated ventricular noncompaction

IVO intraoral vertical osteotomy

IVOX intravascular oxygenator (oxygenation)

IVP intravenous push (this is a dangerous meaning as it is read as intravenous pyelogram)
intravenous pyelogram

IVPB intravenous piggyback

IVPF isovolume pressure flow

IVPU intravenous push

IVR idioventricular rhythm
interactive voice-response (system)
intravaginal ring
intravenous retrograde
intravenous rider (this is a dangerous abbreviation as it has been read as IVP-intravenous push)
isovolumic relaxation (time)

IVRA intravenous regional anesthesia

IVRAP intravenous retrograde access port

IVRG intravenous retrograde

IV-RNV intravenous radionuclide venography

IVRO intraoral vertical ramus osteotomy

IVRS interactive voice response system

IVRT isovolumic relation time

IVS intraventricular septum
irritable voiding syndrome

IVSD intraventricular septal defect

IVSE interventricular septal excursion

IVSO intraoral vertical segmental osteotomy

IVSS intravenous Soluset®

IVST interventricular septum thickness

IVT intravenous transfusion
intraventricular

IVTA intravitreal injection of triamcinolone acetonide

IVTTT intravenous tolbutamide tolerance test

IVU intravenous urography (urogram)

IVUC intravenous ultrasound catheter

IVUS intravascular ultrasound

IW inspiratory wheeze

IWD individual with a disability

IWI inferior wall infarction

IWL insensible water loss
involuntary weight loss

IWMI inferior wall myocardial infarct

IWML idiopathic white matter lesion

IWT ice-water test
impacted wisdom teeth

Ixa ixabepilone

I

J

J — Jaeger measure of near vision with 20/20 about equal to J1
jejunostomy
Jewish
joint
joule
juice
J 1-16 — Jaeger near acuity notation (1 to 16 scale)
JA — joint aspiration
Jack — jackknife position
JAFAR — Juvenile Arthritis Functional Assessment Report
JAMA — *Journal of the American Medical Association*
JAMG — juvenile autoimmune myasthenia gravis
JAN — Japanese Accepted Name
JAR — junior assistant resident
JARAN — junior assistant resident admission note
JBE — Japanese B encephalitis
JBS — Johanson Blizzard syndrome
JC — junior clinicians (medical students)
JCA — juvenile chronic arthritis
JCAHO — Joint Commission on Accreditation of Healthcare Organizations
JCC — Jackson cross cylinder (astigmatism test)
JCO — Journal of Clinical Oncology
JCOG — Japanese Clinical Oncology Group
JCQ — Job Content Questionnaire
JD — Doctor of Jurisprudence (a law degree)
jaundice
JDG — jugulodigastric
JDLR — Just doesn't look right (something is wrong, but no diagnosis has been made yet) (slang)
JDM — juvenile diabetes mellitus
JDMS — juvenile dermatomyositis
JE — Japanese encephalitis
JEB — junctional escape beat
JEJ — jejunum
JEN — Japanese encephalitis vaccine
JER — junctional escape rhythm
JET — jejunal extension tube
junctional ectopic tachycardia
JEV — Japanese encephalitis virus
JF — joint fluid
JFS — Jewish Family Service
JGCT — juvenile granulosa cell tumor
JGI — jejunogastric intussusception
JHR — Jarisch-Herxheimer reaction
JI — jejunoileal
JIA — juvenile idiopathic arthritis
JIB — jejunoileal bypass
JIS — juvenile idiopathic scoliosis
JJ — jaw jerk
J & J — Johnson & Johnson Health Care Systems, Inc.
JLD — just like dad; an explanation for a child's unusual facial features (slang)
JLIS — Jessner lymphocytic infiltration of the skin
JLO — Judgment of Line Orientation (test)
JLP — juvenile laryngeal papillomatosis
JM-9 — iproplatin
JME — juvenile myoclonic epilepsy
JMI — Jones Medical Inc.
JMML — juvenile myelomonocytic leukemia
JMS — junior medical student
JNA — juvenile nasopharyngeal angiofibroma
JNB — jaundice of newborn
JNCL — juvenile-onset neuronal ceroid lipofuscinosis
JND — just noticeable difference
JNR — Just not right (something is wrong, but no diagnosis has been made yet) (slang)
JNT — joint
JNVD — jugular neck vein distention
JODM — juvenile-onset diabetes mellitus
JOF — juvenile ossifying fibroma
JOMAC — judgment, orientation, memory, abstraction, and calculation
JOMACI — judgment, orientation, memory, abstraction, and calculation intact
JOR — jaw-opening reflex
JORRP — juvenile-onset recurrent respiratory papillomatosis
JP — Jackson-Pratt (drain)
Jobst pump
joint protection
JPA — joint position awareness
juvenile pilocytic astrocytoma
JPB — junctional premature beats
JP BS — Jackson-Pratt to bulb suction
JPC — junctional premature contraction
JPOF — juvenile psammomatoid ossifying fibroma
JPS — joint position sense
JPT — Japanese from Tokyo (populations included in HapMap - see HapMap)
JR — junctional rhythm
JRA — juvenile rheumatoid arthritis
JRAN — junior resident admission note
Jr BF — junior baby food

JRC	joint replacement center
JSF	Japanese spotted fever
JSRV	jaagziekte sheep retrovirus
JSW	joint space width
JT	jejunostomy tube joint junctional tachycardia
JTF	jejunostomy tube feeding
JTH	Jebsen Test of Hand (Function)
JTJ	jaw-to-jaw (position)
JTP	joint projection
JTPS	juvenile tropical pancreatitis syndrome
J-Tube	jejunostomy tube
JUV	juvenile
JV	jugular vein
JVC	jugular venous catheter
JVD	jugular venous distention
JVI	jugular-valve incompetencce
JVP	jugular venous pressure jugular venous pulsation jugular venous pulse
JVPT	jugular venous pulse tracing
JW	Jehovah's Witness
Jx	joint
JXG	juvenile xanthogranuloma

K

K	cornea kelvin ketamine (Ketalar, Vitamin K, Special K, and Super K) kilodalton Kosher potassium thousand vitamin K
K′	knee
K^+	potassium
K_1	phytonadione (AquaMETHYTON)
K_2	menatetrenone
K_3	menadione
K_4	menadiol sodium diphosphate
17K	17-ketosteroids
510(k)	Medical Device Premarket Notification
KA	kainic acid kala-azar keratoacanthoma ketoacidosis
Ka	first order absorption constant in $hr.^{-1}$
KAB	knowledge, attitude, and behavior
K-ABC	Kaufman Assessment Battery for Children
KABINS	knowledge, attitude, behavior, and improvement in nutritional status
KACT	kaolin-activated clotting time
KAFO	knee-ankle-foot orthosis
KAO	knee-ankle orthosis
KAS	Katz Adjustment Scale
KASH	knowledge, abilities, skills, and habits
kat	katal
K-A units	King-Armstrong units
KB	ketone bodies knee-bearing
Kb	kilobase (genetics; 1,000 base pairs)
KBD	Kashin-Beck disease
KC	kangaroo care keratoconjunctivitis keratoconus kinship care knees-to-chest Korean conflict
kcal	kilocalorie
KCCQ	Kansas City Cardiomyopathy Questionnaire
KCCT	kaolin cephalin clotting time
KChIPs	potassium channel-interacting proteins
kCi	kilocurie

KCl potassium chloride
KCO potassium channel opener
KCS keratoconjunctivitis sicca
KCZ ketoconazole (Nizoral)
KD Kawasaki disease
Keto Diastix®
ketogenic diet
kidney donors
knee disarticulation
knowledge deficit
kd kilodalton
KDA known drug allergies
kDa kilodalton
KDC® brand name of infant warmer
KDQ Kidney Disease Questionnaire
KDU Kidney Dialysis Unit
KE first order elimination rate constant in $hr.^{-1}$
KED Kendrick extrication device
k_{el} elimination rate constant
KET ketamine (Ketalar)
ketoconazole (Nizoral)
ketones
KETO ketoconazole (Nizoral)
17 Keto 17 ketosteroids
keV kilo-electron volts
KEVD Krupin eye valve with disc
KF kidney function
KFA kinetic fibrinogen assay
KFAB kidney-fixing antibodies
KFAO knee-foot-ankle orthosis
KFD Kyasanur Forrest disease
KFE knee flexion and extension
KFR Kayser-Fleischer ring
KFS Klippel-Feil syndrome
kg kilogram (1 kg = 2.2 pounds)
K-G Kimray-Greenfield (filter)
KGD ketogenic diet
KGF keratinocyte growth factor
KGC Keflin, gentamicin, and carbenicillin
17-KGS 17-ketogenic steroids
KGy kiloGray
K24H potassium, urine 24-hour
KHF Korean hemorrhagic fever
KHQ King's Health Questionnaire
kHz kilohertz
KI karyopyknotic index
knee immobilizer
potassium iodide
KID keratitis, ichthyosis, and deafness (syndrome)
kidney
kilo kilogram
thousand
KIN kinetic
KISS saturated solution of potassium iodide

K

KIT Kahn Intelligence Test
a cytokine receptor expressed on the surface of hematopoietic stem cells as well as other cell types (also known as C-kit receptor and CD117)
KIU kallikrein inhibitor units
KJ kilojoule
knee jerk
KJR knee-jerk reflex
KK knee kick
knock-knee
KKS kallikrein-kinin system
K & L Kellgren and Lawrence (scale for osteoarthritis assessment)
KLB klebsiella vaccine
KL-BET Kleihauer-Betke
Kleb *Klebsiella*
KLH keyhole limpet hemocyanin
K-Lor® potassium chloride tablets
KLS kidneys, liver, and spleen
Kleine-Levin syndrome
KM kanamycin
KMC kangaroo-mother care
$KMnO_4$ potassium permanganate
KMO Kaiser-Meyer-Olkin (measure of statistical sampling adequacy)
KMV killed measles vaccine
KN knee
KNO keep needle open
KNSA Kron Nutritive Sucking Apparatus
KO keep open
knee orthosis
knocked out
KOH potassium hydroxide
KOL key opinion leader
KOR keep open rate
KOSCHI King Outcome Scale for Closed Head Injury
KP hot pack
keratoprecipitate
kinetic perimetry
kPa kilopascal
KPD kidney paired donation
KPE Kelman phacoemulsification
KPM kilopounds per minute
KPS Karnofsky performance status (scores) (scale)
KQI key quality indicators
Kr krypton
K-rod Küntscher rod
KS Kawasaki syndrome
Kaposi sarcoma
kidney stone
Klinefelter syndrome
17-KS 17-ketogenic steroids
17-ketosteroids
KSA knowledge, skills, and abilities

K-SADS	Kiddie Schedule for Affective Disorders and Schizophrenia
KSE	knee sling exercises
KSHV	Kaposi sarcoma-associated herpesvirus
KS/OI	Kaposi sarcoma and opportunistic infections
KSP	Karolinska Scales of Personality
KSR	potassium chloride sustained release (tablets)
KSS	Kearns-Sayre syndrome
KSW	knife stab wound
KT	kidney transplant
	kinesiotherapy
	known to
KTC	knee-to-chest
KTP	potassium-titanyl-phosphate (laser)
KTS	Klippel-Trenaunay syndrome
KTU	kidney transplant unit
	known to us
KTx	kidney transplantation
KTZ	ketoconazole (Nizoral)
KUB	kidney(s), ureter(s), and bladder
	kidney ultrasound biopsy
KUS	kidney(s), ureter(s), and spleen
KV	kilovolt
KVAs	vitamin k antagonists
KVO	keep vein open
KVP	kilovolt peak
KW	Keith-Wagener (ophthalmoscopic finding, graded I-IV)
	Kimmelstiel-Wilson
KWB	Keith, Wagener, Barker
KWIC	keywork in context
K-wire	Kirschner wire

L

L	fifty
	Laribacter
	left (this is a dangerous abbreviation; spell out "left" to avoid surgical errors)
	lente insulin (this is a dangerous abbreviation, since there is also a Lantus insulin available)
	levorotatory
	lingual
	Listeria
	liter (1 L = 1,000 mL = 1 quart plus about 2 ounces)
	liver
	lumbar
	lung
l	levorotatory
L′	lumbar
Ⓛ	left (this is a dangerous abbreviation; spell out "left" to avoid surgical errors)
$L_1...L_5$	lumbar nerve 1 through 5
	lumbar vertebra 1 through 5
L1-2	lumbar spine, between first and second vertebrae (the disk space)
LA	language age
	laryngeal amyloid
	latex agglutination
	Latin American
	left arm
	left atrial
	left atrium
	leukoaraiosis (a radiologic finding)
	light adaptation
	linguoaxial
	linoleic acid
	lives alone
	local anesthesia
	long acting
	lupus anticoagulant
L + A	light and accommodation
	living and active
LAA	large artery atherosclerosis
	left atrium and its appendage
LAAM	levomethadyl acetate (L-alpha acetylmeth-adol, Orlaam)
LAAs	leukemia-associated antigens
LAB	laboratory
	left abdomen (LAb)
LABA	laser-assisted balloon angioplasty
	long-acting beta-2 agonist
LABBB	left anterior bundle branch block
LABC	locally advanced breast cancer

LABD	linear immunoglobulin A bullous dermatosis
LABR	laparoscopic-assisted bowel resection
LAC	laceration
	lactobacillus acidophilus vaccine
	laparoscopic-assisted colectomy
	left antecubital
	left atrial catheter
	locally advanced cancer
	long arm cast
	lupus anticoagulant
LAc	Licensed Acupuncturist
LACC	locally advanced cervical carcinoma
LACI	lacunar circulation infarct
	lipoprotein-associated coagulation inhibitor
LACS	laser-assisted capsular shrinkage
LACT-ART	lactate arterial
LAD	laser anesthesia device
	left anterior descending
	left atrial dimension
	left axis deviation
	leukocyte adhesion deficiency
	ligament augmentation device
LADA	left anterior descending (coronary) artery
LADCA	left anterior descending coronary artery
LADD	left anterior descending diagonal
LAD-MIN	left axis deviation minimal
LADPG	laparoscopically assisted distal partial gastrectomy
LAE	left atrial enlargement
	long above elbow
LAEC	locally advanced esophageal cancer
LAF	laminar air flow
	Latin-American female
	low animal fat
	lymphocyte-activating factor
LAFB	left anterior fascicular block
LAFF	lateral arm free flap
LAFM	locally acquired *Plasmodium falciparum* malaria
LAFR	laminar airflow room
LAG	lymphangiogram
LAGB	laparoscopic-adjustable gastric banding
LAH	left anterior hemiblock
	left atrial hypertrophy
LAHB	left anterior hemiblock
LAHNC	locally advanced (squamous cell) head and neck cancer
LAI	left atrial isomerism
LAIC	left anterior interior chain (of muscles)
LAIT	latex agglutination inhibition test
LAIV	live, attenuated influenza vaccine
LAK	lymphokine-activated killer
LAL	left axillary line
	limulus amebocyte lysate
LALLS	low-angle laser light scattering
LALT	larynx-associated lymphoid tissue
	low-air loss therapy (mattress)
LAM	lactational anovulatory method (birth control)
	laminectomy
	laminogram
	laparoscopic-assisted myomectomy
	laser-assisted myringotomy
	Latin-American male
	lymphangioleiomyomatosis
lam✓	laminectomy check
LAMA	laser-assisted microanastomosis
LAMB	mucocutaneous lentigines, atrial myxoma, and blue nevus (syndrome)
L-AMB	liposomal amphotericin B
LAMMA	laser microprobe mass analysis
LAN	lymphadenopathy
LANC	long arm navicular cast
LA-NSCLC	locally-advanced nonsmall-cell lung cancer
LAO	left anterior oblique
	long-acting opioid(s)
LAP	laparoscopy
	laparotomy
	left abdominal pain
	left atrial pressure
	leucine amino peptidase
	leukocyte alkaline phosphatase
	lower abdominal pain
LAPA	locally-advanced pancreatic adenocarcinoma
lap-appy	laparoscopic appendectomy
LAPC	locally advanced pancreatic cancer
	locally-advanced prostate cancer
lap chole	laparoscopic cholecystectomy
LAPMS	long arm posterior molded splint
LAPW	left atrial posterior wall
LAQ	long arc quad
LAR	laryngeal adductor reflex
	left arm, reclining
	long-acting release
	low anterior resection
LARC	Locally-advanced rectal cancer
LARM	left arm
LARS	laparoscopic antireflux surgery
LARSI	lumbar anterior-root stimulator implants
LAS	lactic acidosis syndrome
	laxative abuse syndrome
	left arm, sitting
	leucine acetylsalicylate

long arm splint
low-amplitude signal
lymphadenopathy syndrome
lymphangioscintigraphy
lysine acetylsalicylate

LASA Linear Analogue Self-Assessment (scales)
lipid-associated sialic acid

LASCC locally advanced squamous cell carcinoma

LASEC left atrial spontaneous echo contrast

LASER light amplification by stimulated emission of radiation

LASGB laparoscopic-adjustable silicone gastric banding

LASIK laser *in situ* keratomileusis

L-ASP asparaginase (Elspar)

LAST left anterior small thoracotomy

LASW Licensed Advanced Social Worker

LAT lateral
latex agglutination test
left anterior thigh
lidocaine, epinephrine, (Adrenalin) and tetracaine

LATCH literature attached to chart

lat.men. lateral meniscectomy

LATS long-acting thyroid stimulator

LAUP laser-assisted uvula-palatoplasty

LAV left atrial volume
live attenuated flavivirus
lymphadenopathy associated virus

LAVA laser-assisted vasal anastomosis

LAVH laparoscopically assisted vaginal hysterectomy

LAVHLSO laparoscopically assisted vaginal hysterectomy, left salpingo-oophorectomy

LAVHRSO laparoscopically assisted vaginal hysterectomy, right salpingo-oophorectomy

LAVM laparoscopic-assisted vaginal myomectomy

LAW left atrial wall

LAWER life-terminating acts without the explicit request

LAX laxative

LAZ length-for-age Z-score

LB large bowel
lateral bend
left breast
left buttock
live births
low back
lung biopsy
lymphoid body

lb pound (1 lb = 0.454 Kg)

L&B left and below

LB3 colonoscope

4LB four-layer bandages

LBA laser balloon angioplasty
lower-body adiposity
lymphocyte blastogenesis assay

LBB left breast biopsy
long-back board

LBBB left bundle branch block

LBBx left breast biopsy

LBC liquid-based cytology

LBCD left border of cardiac dullness

L/B/Cr electrolytes, blood urea nitrogen, and serum creatinine (see page 318)

LBD large bile duct
left border dullness
left brain-damaged
Lewy body dementia
ligand-binding domain
low back disability
low bone density

LBE long below elbow

LBG Landry-Guillain-Barré (syndrome)

LBH length, breadth, and height

LBI Lewy body-like inclusions
low back injury

LBM last bowel movement
lean body mass
loose bowel movement

LBMI last body mass index

LBNA lysis bladder neck adhesions

LBNP lower-body negative pressure

LBO large bowel obstruction

LBOTC laryngeal and base-of-tongue carcinomas

LBP low back pain
low blood pressure

LBQC large base quad cane

LBRF louse-borne relapsing fever

LBS low back syndrome
pounds

LBT low back tenderness
low back trouble

LBV left brachial vein
Lewy body variant
low biological value

LBVO left brachial vein occlusion

LBW lean body weight
low birth weight (less than 2,500 g)

LBWI low birth weight infant

LC Lactation Consultant
Laënnec cirrhosis
laparoscopic cholecystectomy
lethal concentration
left circumflex
leisure counseling
level of consciousness
levocarnitine (Carnitor)
living children
low calorie

	lung cancer
L & C	lids and conjunctivae
3LC	triple-lumen catheter
LC50	median lethal concentration
LCA	Leber congenital amaurosis
	left circumflex artery
	left coronary artery
	leukocyte common antigen
	life cycle assessment
	light contact assist
LCAD	long-chain acyl-coenzyme A dehydrogenase
LCAH	life-care at home
LCAL	large-cell anaplastic lymphoma
LCaP	localized prostate cancer
LCAR	L-carnitine
LCAT	lecithin cholesterol acyltransferase
LCB	left costal border
LCC	left cranial-caudal (mammogram view)
LCCA	left circumflex coronary artery
	left common carotid artery
	leukocytoclastic angiitis
LCCE	Lamaze-Certified Childbirth Educator
LCCS	low cervical cesarean section
LCD	coal tar solution (*liquor carbonis detergens*)
	lattice corneal dystrophy
	localized collagen dystrophy
	low-calcium diet
LCDC	Laboratory Centre for Disease Control (Canada)
LCDCP	low-contact dynamic compression plate
LCDE	laparoscopic common duct exploration
LCDs	local coverage determinations
LCE	laparoscopic cholecystectomy
	left carotid endarterectomy
	leukocyte esterase
LC-EI-MS	liquid chromatography-electron impact-mass spectrometry
LCF	late clinical failure
	left circumflex
LCFA	long-chain fatty acid
LCFM	left circumflex marginal
LCGU	local cerebral glucose utilization
LCH	Langerhans cell histiocytosis
	local city hospital
LCINS	lung cancer in never-smokers
LCIS	lobular cancer *in situ*
LCL	lateral collateral ligament
	localized cutaneous leishmaniasis
LCLC	large-cell lung carcinoma
LCM	laser-capture microdissection
	left costal margin
	lower costal margin
	lymphocytic choriomeningitis
LCMI	left ventricular mass index
LC-MS-MS	liquid chromatography coupled to tandem mass spectrometry
LCN	lidocaine
LCNB	large-core needle biopsy
LCNEC	large-cell neuroendocrine carcinoma
LCO	low cardiac output
LCP	Leishmaniasis Control Program
	long, closed, posterior (cervix)
LCPD	Legg-Calvé-Perthes disease
LCPUFAs	long-chain polyunsaturated fatty acids
LCR	cerebrospinal fluid (French)
	late cortical response
	late cutaneous reaction
	ligase chain reaction
	locus control region
LCRS	Living Conditions Rating Scale
LCS	Leydig cell stimulation
	lids, conjunctiva, and sclera
	low constant suction
	low continuous suction
	Lung Cancer Subscale
LCSG	left cardiac sympathetic ganglionectomy
	lost child support group
LCSS	Lung Cancer Symptom Score
LCSW	Licensed Clinical Social Worker
	low continuous wall suction
LCT	long-chain triglyceride
	low cervical transverse
	lymphocytotoxicity
LCTA	lungs clear to auscultation
LCTCS	low cervical transverse cesarean section
LCTD	low-calcium test diet
LCV	leucovorin
	leukocytoclastic vasculitis
	low cervical vertical
LCX	left circumflex coronary artery
LD	lactic dehydrogenase (formerly LDH)
	laser Doppler
	last dose
	latissimus dorsi
	learning disability
	learning disorder
	left deltoid
	Legionnaires disease
	lethal dose
	levodopa
	Licensed Dietician
	liver disease
	living donor
	loading dose
	long dwell

	low density
	low dosage
	Lyme disease
L&D	labor and deliver
L/D	labor and delivery
	light to dark (ratio)
LD-1	lactic dehydrogenase 1
LD-5	lactic dehydrogenase 5
LD_{50}	median lethal dose
LDA	laser-Doppler anemometry
	linear discriminant analysis
	low density areas
	low-dose arm
LDB	Legionnaires disease bacterium
LDCOC	low-dose combination oral contraceptive
LD-CT	low-dose (spiral) computed tomography
LDD	laser disk decompression
	Lee and Desu D (test)
	light-dark discrimination
	lumbar disk disease
LDDS	local dentist
LDEA	left deviation of electrical axis
LDEI	large-dose extended-interval (dosing)
LDF	laser-Doppler flowmetry
LDH	lactic dehydrogenase
LDIH	left direct inguinal hernia
LDIR	low-dose of ionizing radiation
LDI-TOF-MS	laser desorption/ionization time-of-flight-mass spectrometer
LDK	low-dose ketoconazole
LDL	limitation of daily life
	low-density lipoprotein
LDL-C	low-density lipoprotein cholesterol
LDLT	living donor liver transplantation
LDM	lorazepam, dexamethasone, and metoclopramide
	low-dose metronomic (chemotherapy)
LDMRT	low-dose mediastinal radiation therapy
LDN	laparoscopic donor nephrectomy
	Licensed Dietitian Nutritionist
	living-donor nephrectomy
LDNF	lung-derived neurotrophic factor
LDO	Licensed Dispensing Optician
l-dopa	levodopa
LDP	laparoscopic distal pancreatectomy
LD-PCR	limiting dilution polymerase chain reaction
LDPM	laser Doppler perfusion monitoring
LDR	labor, delivery, and recovery
	length-to-diameter ratio
	long-duration response
LDR/P	labor, delivery, recovery, and postpartum
LDS	Language Development Survey
LDT	left dorsotransverse
LD-T	lactic dehydrogenase total
LDUB	long double upright brace
LDUH	low-dose unfractionated heparin
LDV	laser-Doppler velocimetry
LE	labor epidural
	lateral epicondylitis (tennis elbow)
	left ear
	left eye
	lens extraction
	leptin
	limbic encephalitis
	live embryo
	local excision
	lower extremities
	lupus erythematosus
LEA	lower extremity amputation
	lumbar epidural anesthesia
LEAD	lower extremity arterial disease
LEAP	Lower Extremity Amputation Prevention (program)
LEB	lumbar epidural block
LEC	lens epithelial cell
	low-emetogenic chemotherapy
LECBD	laparoscopic exploration of the common bile duct
LE-CEMRA	lower extremity contrast-enhanced magnetic resonance angiography
LED	liposomal encapsulated doxorubicin (Doxil)
	lowest effective dose
	lupus erythematosus disseminatus
LEE	lower extremity edema
LEEP	loop electrosurgical excision procedure
LEF	lower extremity fracture
LEH	liposome-encapsulated hemoglobin
LEHPZ	lower esophageal high pressure zone
LEJ	ligation of the esophagogastric junction
LEL	low-energy laser
LELs	lymphoepithelial lesions
LEM	lateral eye movements
	light electron microscope
LEMS	Lambert-Eaton myasthenic syndrome
LENT-SOMA	Late Effect of Normal Tissue—Subjective Objective Management Analytic (toxicity table)
LEP	leptospirosis
	limited English proficiency
	liposome-encapsulated paclitaxel
	lower esophageal pressure
LEP 2	leptospirosis 2
LE prep	lupus erythematosus preparation
L-ERX	leukoerythroblastic reaction
LES	local excitatory state
	lower esophageal sphincter

	lumbar epidural steroids
	lupus erythematosus systemic
LESEP	lower extremity somatosensory evoked potential
LESG	Late Effects Study Group
LESI	lumbar epidural steroid injection
LESP	lower esophageal sphincter pressure
LET	lateral elbow tendinopathy
	left esotropia
	leukocyte esterase test
	lidocaine, epinephrine and tetracaine gel
	linear energy transfer
	lupus erythematosus tumidus
LEU	leucine
LEV	levamisole (Ergamisol)
	levator muscle
LEVA	levamisole (Ergamisol)
LeY	Lewis Y (antigen)
LF	laparoscopic fundoplications
	Lassa fever
	left foot
	left frontal
	little finger
	living female
	long finger
	low fat
	low forceps
	low frequency
	lymphatic filariasis
LFA	left femoral artery
	left forearm
	left fronto-anterior
	leukocyte function-associated antigen
	low-friction arthroplasty
	lymphocyte function-associated antigen
LFA-1	leukocyte function-associated antigen-1
LFB	low-frequency band
LFC	lateral femoral condyle
	living female child
	low-fat and cholesterol
LFCS	low-flap cesarean section
LFD	lactose-free diet
	low-fat diet
	low-fiber diet
	low-forceps delivery
	lunate fossa depression
LFGNR	lactose fermenting gram-negative rod
LFI	local-field irradiation
LFL	left frontolateral
LFM	lateral force microscopy
LFP	left frontoposterior
LFS	leukemia-free survival
	Li-Fraumeni syndrome
	liver function series
LFT	latex flocculation test
	left fronto-transverse
	liver function tests
	low-flap transverse
LFU	limit flocculation unit
	lost to follow-up
LG	large
	laryngectomy
	left gluteal
	linguogingival
	lymphography
L-G	Lich-Gregoire (ureteroneocystostomy)
LGA	large for gestational age
	left gastric artery
	localized granuloma annulare
LGBP/LC	laparoscopic gastric bypass with simultaneous cholecystectomy
LGBT	lesbian, gay, bisexual, and transsexual
LGFD	looks good from doorway (patient who complains but looks fine) (slang)
LGG	low-grade gliomas
L-GG	*Lactobacillus rhamnosus* strain GG
LGI	lower gastrointestinal (series)
LGIOS	low-grade intraosseous-type osteosarcoma
LGL	large granular lymphocyte
	low-grade lymphoma(s)
	Lown-Ganong-Levine (syndrome)
LGLS	Lown-Ganong-Levine syndrome
LGM	left gluteus medius (maximus)
LGMD21	limb-girdle muscular dystrophy type 21
LGN	lateral geniculate leaflet
	lobular glomerulonephritis
LGNET	low grade neuroendocrine carcinoma
LG-NHL	low-grade non-Hodgkin lymphoma
LGS	Lennox-Gastaut syndrome
	low-Gomco suction
LGSIL	low-grade squamous intraepithelial lesion
LGV	lymphogranuloma venerum
LH	learning handicap
	left hand
	left hemisphere
	left hyperphoria
	luteinizing hormone
	lymphoid hyperplasia
LHA	left hepatic artery
LHB	long head of the biceps
LHC	left heart catheterization
LHCJ	left heart catheterization, Judkins approach
LHD	left-hand dominant
LHF	left heart failure
LHG	left hand grip
LHH	left homonymous hemianopsia
LHI	Labor Health Institute

LHL	left hemisphere lesions left hepatic lobe
LHON	Leber hereditary optic neuropathy
LHP	left hemiparesis
LHR	legal health record leukocyte histamine release
LHRH	luteinizing hormone-releasing hormone
LHRH-A	luteinizing hormone-releasing hormone analogue
LHRT	leukocyte histamine release test
LHS	left hand side long-handled sponge
LHSH	long-handled shoe horn
LHT	left hypertropia
LI	lactose intolerance lamellar ichthyosis large intestine laser iridotomy learning impaired linguoincisal liver involvement
Li	lithium
LIA	laser interference acuity left iliac artery
LIB	left in bottle local in breast
LIC	left iliac crest left internal carotid leisure interest class
LICA	left internal carotid artery
LICD	lower intestinal Crohn disease
LICM	left intercostal margin
Li_2CO_3	lithium carbonate
LICS	left intercostal space
LID	levodopa-induced dyskinesia
Lido	lidocaine
LIF	laser-induced fluorescence left iliac fossa left index finger leukemia-inhibiting factor liver (migration) inhibitory factor
LIFE	laser-induced fluorescence emission lung imaging fluorescence endoscopy
LIG	ligament lymphocyte immune globulin
LIGHTS	phototherapy lights
LIH	laparoscopic inguinal herniorrhaphy left inguinal hernia
LIHA	low impulsiveness, high anxiety
LIID	latanoprost-induced iris darkening
LIJ	left internal jugular
LILA	low impulsiveness, low anxiety
LILT	low-intensity laser therapy
LIM	limited toxicology screening
LIMA	left internal mammary artery (graft)
LIMS	laboratory information management system(s)
LIN	liquid nitrogen lobular intraepithelial neoplasia
LINAC	linear accelerator
LINCL	late-infantile neuronal ceroid lipofuscinosis
LINDI	lithium-induced nephrogenic diabetes insipidus
LING	lingual
LIO	laser-indirect ophthalmoscope left inferior oblique (muscle)
LIOU	laparoscopic intraoperative ultrasound
LIP	lithium-induced polydipsia lymphocytic interstitial pneumonia
LIPV	left inferior pulmonary vein
LIQ	liquid liquor lower inner quadrant
LIR	left iliac region left inferior rectus
LIR-1	leucocyte immunoglobulin-like receptor-1
LIS	late-onset idiopathic scoliosis lateral internal sphincterotomy left intercostal space locked-in syndrome low intermittent suction lung injury score
LISS	low ionic strength saline
LISW	Licensed Independent Social Worker
LIT	literature liver injury test low-intensity (resistance) training
LITA	left internal thoracic artery
LITH	lithotomy
LITHO	lithotripsy
LITT	laser-induced thermotherapy
LIV	left innominate vein
L-IVP	limited intravenous pyelogram
LIVB	live birth
LIVC	left inferior vena cava
LIVPRO	liver profile (see page 318)
LIWS	low intermittent wall suction
LJ	left jugular lockable joints
LJL	lateral joint line
LJM	limited joint mobility
LK	lamellar keratoplasty left kidney
LKA	Lazare-Klerman-Armour (Personality Inventory)
LKM-3	liver-kidney microsomal antibodies type 3
LKS	Landau-Kleffner syndrome liver, kidneys, spleen
LKSB	liver, kidneys, spleen, and bladder

L

LKSNP	liver, kidneys, and spleen not palpable
LL	large lymphocyte
	left lateral
	left leg
	left lower
	left lung
	lepromatous leprosy
	lid lag
	long leg (brace or cast)
	lower lid
	lower limb
	lower lip
	lower lobe
	lumbar laminectomy
	lumbar length
	lymphocytic leukemia
	lymphoblastic lymphoma
L&L	lids and lashes
LL2	limb lead two
LLA	lids, lashes, and adnexa
	limulus lysate assay
LLAs	lipid-lowering agents
LLAT	left lateral
LLB	last living breath
	left lateral bending
	left lateral border
	long leg brace
LLC	laparoscopic laser cholecystectomy
	Lewis lung carcinoma
	limited liability corporation
	long leg cast
LLBCD	left lower border of cardiac dullness
LLCH	localized Langerhans' cell histiocytosis
LLD	late-life depressions
	left lateral decubitus
	left length discrepancy
	leg length differential
LLE	left lower extremity
	little league elbow
LLETZ	large-loop excision of the transformation zone
LLFG	long leg fiberglas (cast)
LLG	left lateral gaze
LL-GXT	low-level graded exercise test
LLI	leg-length inequality
LLINs	long-lasting insecticidal (bed) nets
LLL	left lower lid
	left lower lobe (lung)
LLLE	lower lid, left eye
LLLNR	left lower lobe, no rales
LLLT	low-level laser therapy
LLN	lower limit of normal
LLO	Legionella-like organism
LLOD	lower lid, right eye
	lower limit of detection
LLOS	lower lid, left eye
LLP	Limited Liability Partnership
	long leg plaster
LLPDD	late luteal phase dysphoric disorder
LLPS	low-load prolonged stress
LLQ	left lower quadrant (abdomen)
	lower limit of quantitation
LLR	left lateral rectus
LLRE	lower lid, right eye
LLS	lazy leukocyte syndrome
LLSB	left lower sternal border
LLSD	laser light scattering detector
LLT	left lateral thigh
	lowest level term
LLWC	long leg walking cast
LLX	left lower extremity
LM	landmarks
	left main
	lentigo maligna
	light microscopy
	linguomesial
	living male
	lung metastases
	lymphatic malformation
L/M	liters per minute
LMA	laryngeal mask airway
	left mentoanterior
	liver membrane autoantibody
LMAM	left message on answering machine
LMB	Laurence-Moon-Biedl syndrome
	left main bronchus
LMC	living male child
LMCA	left main coronary artery
	left middle cerebral artery
LMCAT	left middle cerebral artery thrombosis
LMCL	left midclavicular line
LMD	Langer mesomelic dysplasia
	local medical doctor
	low molecular weight dextran
LME	left mediolateral episiotomy
LMEE	left middle ear exploration
LMF	left middle finger
	melphalan (L-PAM), methotrexate, and fluorouracil
LMFT	Licensed Marriage and Family Therapist
LMHC	Licensed Mental Health Counselor
LMI	large multivalent immunogen
L/min	liters per minute
LML	left medial lateral
	left middle lobe
LMLE	left mediolateral episiotomy
LMLO	left medial-lateral oblique (mammogram view)
LMM	lentigo maligna melanoma
LMN	letter of medical necessity
	lower motor neuron
LMNL	lower motor neuron lesion

LMOR	left message on recorder
LMP	last menstrual period
	left mentoposterior
	low malignant potential
LMP1	latent membrane protein 1
LMPC	laser microdissection and pressure catapulting
LMR	left medial rectus
LMRM	left modified radical mastectomy
LMRP	Local Medical Review Policy
LMS	lateral medullary syndrome
	leiomyosarcomas
LMT	lateral meniscus tear
	left main trunk
	left mentotransverse
	Licensed Massage Therapist
	light moving touch
LMW	low molecular weight
LMWD	low molecular weight dextran
LMWH	low molecular weight heparins
LMX-4®	4% lidocaine topical cream
LN	latent nystagmus
	left nostril (nare)
	lymph nodes
LN_2	liquid nitrogen
LNA	alpha-linolenic acid
LNB	lymph node biopsy
LNC	Legal Nurse Consultant
LNCaP	lymph node carcinoma of the prostate
LNCC	Legal Nurse Consultant, Certified
LNCs	lymph node cells
LND	light-near dissociation
	living non-directed (donors)
	lonidamine
	lymph node dissection
LNE	lymph node enlargement
	lymph node excision
LNF	laparoscopic Nissen fundoplication
LNG	levonorgestrel
LNM	Lansinoh for Nursing Mothers (ointment used for sore nipples)
	lymph node metastases
LNMC	lymph node mononuclear cells
LNMP	last normal menstrual period
LNNB	Luria-Nebraska Neuropsychological Battery
LNS	lymph node sampling
LNT	late neurological toxicity
LNU	laparoscopic nephroureterectomy
	learned nonuse (splint)
LO	lateral oblique (x-ray view)
	linguo-occlusal
	lumbar orthosis
5-LO	5-lipoxygenase
LOA	late-onset agammaglobulinemia
	leave of absence
	left occiput anterior
	long-acting opioid
	looseness of associations
	lysis of adhesions
LOAD	late-onset Alzheimer disease
LOAEL	lowest observed adverse effect level
LOB	loss of balance
LOC	laxative of choice
	level of care
	level of comfort
	level of concern
	level of consciousness
	local
	loss of consciousness
LOCF	last observation carried forward (used for inputting data missing due to dropouts in longitudinal clinical trials)
LOCM	low-osmolality contrast media
LOD	limit of detection
	line of duty
	log of odds
LOE	lack of efficacy
	left otitis externa
LOEL	lowest-observed-effect level
LOF	leaking of fluids
	leave on floor
LOFD	low-outlet forceps delivery
LOG	Logmar chart
log	logarithm any base
$\log_{10}$	logarithm base 10
$\log_2$	logarithm base 2
$\log_e$	logarithm base 3 (natural)
logMAR	logarithm of the minimum angle of resolution
LOH	loss of heterozygosity
LOHF	late-onset hepatic failure
LOHP	oxaliplatin (Eloxatin)
LOIH	left oblique inguinal hernia
LOI	level of injury
	Leyton Obsessional Inventory
	loss of imprinting
LOINC	Logical Observation Identifier Names and Codes
LOL	laughing out loud
	left occipitolateral
	little old lady
LOLINAD	little old lady in no apparent distress
LOM	left otitis media
	limitation of motion
	little old man
	loss of motion
	low-osmolar (contrast) media
LOMSA	left otitis media, suppurative, acute
LOMSC	left otitis media, suppurative, chronic
LoNa	low sodium
LOO	length of operation
LOOCV	leave-one-out cross-validation
LOP	laparoscopic orchiopexy

	leave on pass
	left occiput posterior
	level of pain
LOQ	limit(s) of quantitation
	lower outer quadrant
LOR	loss of resistance
LORS-I	Level of Rehabilitation Scale-I
LOS	length of stay
	loss of sight
	lower oesophageal sphincter (United Kingdom and other countries)
	low-output syndrome
lo-SES	lower socioeconomic status
LOT	left occiput transverse
	Licensed Occupational Therapist
LOV	loss of vision
LOVA	loss of visual acuity
LOX	lipid oxidation
LOZ	lozenge
LP	lamina propria
	laparoscopic pyeloplasty
	lash ptosis
	Licensed Psychologist
	light perception
	linguopulpal
	lipid panel (see page 298)
	lipoprotein
	low protein
	lumbar puncture
L/P	lactate-pyruvate ratio
	lidocaine and prilocaine
LP5	Life-Pak 5
LPA	left pulmonary artery
Lp(a)	lipoprotein (a)
LPA%	left pulmonary artery oxygen saturation
L-PAM	melphalan (Alkeran)
LPC	laser photocoagulation
	Licensed Professional Counselor
LPCC	Licensed Professional Certified Counselor
LPC-L	lymphoplasmacytoid lymphoma
LPcP	light perception with projection
LPD	leiomyomatosis peritonealis disseminata
	low-potassium dextran
	low-protein diet
	luteal phase defect
	luteal phase deficiency
	lymphoproliferative disease
LPDA	left posterior descending artery
LPEP	left pre-ejection period
LPF	late parasitological failure
	liver plasma flow
	low-power field
	lymphocytosis-promoting factor
LPFB	left posterior fascicular block
LPFL	lateral patellofemoral ligament
LPH	left posterior hemiblock
	lumbar puncture headache
LPHB	left posterior hemiblock
LPI	laser peripheral iridectomy
	last patient in
	leukotriene pathway inhibitor
LPICA	left posterior internal carotid artery
LPIH	left-posterior-inferior hemiblock
LPL	laparoscopic pelvic lymphadenectomy
	left posterolateral
	lipoprotein lipase
	lymphoplasmacytic lymphoma
LPLC	low-pressure liquid chromatography
LPLND	laparoscopic pelvic lymph node dissection
LPM	latent primary malignancy
	liters per minute
LPME	liquid-phase microextraction
LPN	laparoscopic partial nephrectomy
	Licensed Practical Nurse
LPO	left posterior oblique
	light perception only
LPPC	leukocyte-poor packed cells
LPPH	late postpartum hemorrhage
LPR	laryngopharyngeal reflux
	leprosy (Hansen disease) vaccine
LPS	last Pap smear
	latency to persistent sleep
	lipopolysaccharide
LPSDT	laryngopharyngeal sensory discrimination testing
LP SHUNT	lumboperitoneal shunt
LPsP	light perception without projection
LPT	leptospirosis (Leptospira-*Leptospires* sp.) vaccine
	Licensed Physical Therapist
	low-pain threshold
LPTN	Licensed Psychiatric Technical Nurse
LPV	left portal vein
	left pulmonary vein
	lopinavir (Kaletra)
LPV/r	lopinavir and ritonavir
LPZ	lateral peripheral zone (prostate needle biopsy location)
LQTS	long QT (interval) syndrome
LR	labor room
	lactated Ringer (injection)
	laser resection
	lateral rectus
	late relapse
	left-right
	light reflex
	likelihood ratios
	local recurrence
L&R	left and right

L → R left to right
LR1A labor room 1A
LRA left radial artery
left renal artery
LRC locoregional control
lower rib cage
LRCP Licentiate of the Royal College of Physicians
LRCS Licentiate of the Royal College of Surgeons
LRD limb reduction defects
living-related donor
living renal donor
LRDT living-related donor transplant
LRE localization-related epilepsy
LREH low-renin essential hypertension
LRF left rectus femoris
left ring finger
local-regional failure
L&R gtt Levophed and Regitine drip (infusion)
LRHT living-related hepatic transplantation
LRI lower respiratory infection
LRLT living-related liver transplantation
LRM left radical mastectomy
local regional metastases
LRMP last regular menstrual period
LRN laparoscopic radical nephrectomy
LRND left radical neck dissection
LRO long-range objective
Lrot left rotation
LRP laparoscopic radical prostatectomy
lung-resistance protein
LRQ lower right quadrant
LROU lateral rectus, both eyes
LRR light reflection rheography
locoregional recurrences
LRRT locoregional radiotherapy
LRS lactated Ringer solution
lumbosacral radicular syndrome
LRT likelihood ratio test
living renal transplant
local radiation therapy
lower respiratory tract
LRTD living relative transplant donor
LRTI ligament reconstruction with tendon interposition
lower respiratory tract infection
LRV left renal vein
log reduction value
LRW LAL (*Limulus* amebocyte lysate) reagent water
LRYGB laparoscopic Roux-en-Y gastric bypass
LRZ lorazepam (Ativan)
LS left side
legally separated
Leigh syndrome
liver scan
liver-spleen
loose stool
low salt
lumbosacral
lung sounds
L/S lecithin-sphingomyelin ratio
L&S ligation and stripping
liver and spleen
L5-S1 lumbar fifth vertebra to sacral first vertebra (where the lumbar and sacral spines join)
LSA left sacrum anterior
lipid-bound sialic acid
lymphosarcoma
LSAs low-sedating antihistamines
LSB left scapular border
left sternal border
local standby
lumbar spinal block
lumbar sympathetic block
LS BPS laparoscopic bilateral partial salpingectomy
LSC laser-scanning cytometry
last sexual contact
late systolic click
least significant change
left subclavian (artery) (vein)
leukemia stem cells
lichen simplex chronicus
liquid scintillation counting
LSCA left scapuloanterior
LSCC laryngeal squamous cell carcinoma
LSCCB limited-state small-cell cancer of the bladder
LSCM laser-scanning confocal microscopy
LSCP left scapuloposterior
LSCS lower segment cesarean section
LSD least significant difference
low-salt diet
lumbosacral derangement
lysergide
LSE local side effects
LSed level of sedation
LSF low-saturated fat
LSFA low-saturated fatty acid (diet)
LSH laparoscopic supracervical hysterectomy
leishmaniasis vaccine
LSI levonorgestrel subdermal implant
L-SIL low-grade squamous intraepithelial lesions
LSK liver, spleen, and kidneys
LSKM liver-spleen-kidney-megalgia
LSL left sacrolateral
left short leg (brace)
LSLF low sodium, low fat (diet)
LSM laser scanning microscope

L

	late systolic murmur
	least squares mean
	limited sampling model
	liver, spleen masses
LSMFT	liposclerosing myxofibrous tumor
LSMT	life-sustaining medical treatment
LSO	left salpingo-oophorectomy
	left superior oblique
	lumbosacral orthosis
LSP	left sacrum posterior
	liver-specific (membrane) lipoprotein
L–Spar	Elspar (asparaginase)
L-spine	lumbar spine
LSQ	Life Situation Questionnaire
LSR	laser skin resurfacing
	left superior rectus
L/S ratio	lecithin/sphingomyelin ratio
LSS	limb-sparing surgery
	liver-spleen scan
	lumbar spinal stenosis
LSSS	large, simple safety study
	Liverpool Seizure Severity Scale
LST	left sacrum transverse
LSTAT	life support for trauma and transport
LSTC	laparoscopic tubal coagulation
LSTL	laparoscopic tubal ligation
LSTM	lean soft tissue mass
L's & T's	lines and tubes
LSU	life support unit
LSV	left subclavian vein
	lesser saphenous vein
LSVC	left superior vena cava
LSW	left-side weakness
	Licensed Social Worker
LT	laboratory technician
	left
	left thigh
	left triceps
	leukotrienes
	Levin tube
	light
	light touch
	low transverse
	lumbar traction
	lung transplantation
	lunotriquetral
	lymphotoxin
L&T	lettuce and tomato
LT3	liothyronine sodium (Cytomel)
LT4	levothyroxine
LTA	laryngotracheal applicator
	laryngeal tracheal anesthesia
	lateral thoracic arteries
	local tracheal anesthesia
LTAC	long-term acute care
LTACHs	long-term acute care hospitals
LTAS	left transatrial septal
LTB	laparoscopic tubal banding
	laryngotracheobronchitis
LTB_4	leukotriene B_4
LTBI	latent tuberculosis infection
LTC	Lapra-Ty (suture) clip
	left to count
	long-term care
	long thick closed
LTC_4	leukotriene C_4
LTC-101	long-term care form-101
LTCBDE	laparoscopic transcystic common bile duct exploration
LTCCS	low-transverse cervical cesarean section
LTCF	long-term care facility
LTCH	long-term care hospital (average length of stay greater than 25 days)
LTC-IC	long-term culture-initiating cells
LTCR	long-term complete remission(s)
LTCS	low-transverse cesarean section
LTD	largest tumor dimension
	leg transfer device
	line, tube, and drain (incident)
	lipid tear deficiency
	long-term depression
	long-term disability
LTD_4	leukotriene D_4
LTE	less than effective
LTE_4	leukotriene E_4
LTED	long-term estrogen deprivation
LTF	lost to follow-up
LTFU	long-term follow-up
LTG	lamotrigine (Lamictal)
	long-term goal
	low-tension glaucoma
LTGA	left transposition of great artery
LTH	left total hip (arthroplasty)
	luteotropic hormone
LTK	laser thermal keratoplasty
	left total knee (arthroplasty)
LTL	laparoscopic tubal ligation
	left temporal lobectomy
LTM	long-term memory
	long-term monitoring
LTNPs	long-term nonprogressors (AIDS patients)
LTOT	long-term oxygen therapy
LTP	laser trabeculoplasty
	lateral tibial plateau
	lateral trochanteric pain
	long-term plan
	long-term potentiation
LTPA	leisure-time physical activity
LTR	long terminal repeats
	lower trunk rotation
LTRA	leukotriene receptor antagonist
LTS	laparoscopic tubal sterilization
	laryngotracheal stenosis

	long-term survivors
LTT	lactose tolerance test
	lymphocyte transformation test
LTUI	low transverse uterine incision
LTV	long-term variability
	long-term ventilation
	Luche tumor virus
LTV+	long-term variability– average to moderate
LTV 0	long-term variability–absent
LTVC	long-term venous catheter
LTWN	long-term low-level white noise
LTx	liver transplant
	lung transplantation
LTZ	letrozole (Femara)
LU	left upper
	left ureteral
	living unit
	Lutheran
L & U	lower and upper
LUA	left upper arm
LUD	left uterine displacement
LUE	left upper extremity
Lues I	primary syphilis
Lues II	secondary syphilis
Lues III	tertiary syphilis
LUFF	lateral upper arm free flap (reconstruction of pharyngeal defect)
LUL	left upper lid
	left upper lobe (lung)
LUM	laparoscopic-ultraminilaparotomic myomectomy
LUNA	laparoscopic uterosacral nerve ablation
LUOB	left upper outer buttock
LUOQ	left upper outer quadrant
LUQ	left upper quadrant
LURD	living-unrelated donor
LUS	laparoscopic ultrasonography
	lower uterine segment
LUSB	left upper scapular border
	left upper sternal border
LUST	lower uterine segment transverse
LUT	lower urinary tract
LUTD	lower urinary tract dysfunction
LUTS	lower urinary tract symptoms
LUTT	lower urinary tract tumor
LuTX	lung transplantation
LUW	lungworm vaccine
LUX	left upper extremity
LV	leave
	left ventricle
	leucovorin
	live virus
LVA	left ventricular aneurysm
LVAS	large vestibular aqueduct syndrome
LVC	laser vision correction
	low-viscosity cement
	low-vision clinic
LVAD	left ventricular assist device
LV Angio	left ventricular angiogram
L-VAM	leuprolide acetate, vinblastine, doxorubicin (Adriamycin), and mitomycin
LVAS	left ventricular assist system
LVAT	left ventricular activation time
LVBP	left ventricle bypass pump
LVD	left ventricular dimension
	left ventricular dysfunction
LVDd	left ventricular end-diastolic diameter
LVDP	left ventricular diastolic pressure
LVDs	left ventricular systolic diameter
LVDT	linear variable differential transformer
LVDV	left ventricular diastolic volume
LVE	left ventricular enlargement
LVEDD	left ventricular end-diastolic diameter
LVEDP	left ventricular end diastolic pressure
LVEDV	left ventricular end-diastolic volume
LVEF	left ventricular ejection fraction
LVEP	left ventricular end pressure
LVESD	left ventricular end-systolic dimension
LVESV	left-ventricular end-systolic volumes
LVESVI	left ventricular end-systolic volume index
LVET	left ventricular ejection time
LVF	left ventricular failure
	left visual field
LVFP	left ventricular filling pressure
LVFU	leucovorin and fluorouracil
LVFWR	left ventricular free wall rupture
LVG	left ventrogluteal
LVH	left ventricular hypertrophy
LVHR	laparoscopic ventral hernia repair
LVID	left ventricular internal diameter
LVIDd	left ventricle internal diameter at end-diastole
LVIDs	left ventricle internal dimension systole
LVL	large volume leukapheresis
	left vastus lateralis
LVM	left ventricular mass
LVMI	left ventricular mass index
LVMM	left ventricular muscle mass
LVN	Licensed Visiting Nurse
	Licensed Vocational Nurse
LVO	left ventricular opacification
	left ventricular output
	left ventricular overactivity
LVOT	left ventricular outflow tract
LVOTO	left ventricular outflow tract obstruction

LVP	large volume parenteral
	left ventricular pressure
LVPW	left ventricular posterior wall
LVR	leucovorin
LVRS	lung-volume reduction surgery
LVRT	liver-volume replaced by tumor
LVS	laryngeal videostroboscopy
	left ventricular strain
LVS EMI	left ventricular subendocardial myocardial ischemia
LVSD	left ventricular systolic dysfunction
LVSF	left ventricular systolic function
LVSI	lymph-vascular space invasion (involvement)
LVSP	left ventricular systolic pressure
LVSW	left ventricular stroke work
LVSWI	left ventricular stroke work index
LVT	levetiracetam (Keppra)
LVV	left ventricular volume
	live varicella vaccine
LVW	left ventricular wall
LVWI	left ventricular work index
LVWMA	left ventricular wall motion abnormality
LVWMI	left ventricular wall motion index
LVWT	left ventricular wall thickness
LW	lacerating wound
	living will
L & W	Lee and White (coagulation)
	living and well
LWAQ	Living with Asthma Questionnaire
LWCT	Lee-White clotting time
LWBS	left without being seen
LWC	leave without consent
LWCT	left without completing treatment
LWD	Leri-Weill dyschondrosteosis
LWDC	Leri-Weill dyschondrosteosis
LWOP	leave without pay
LWOT	left without treatment
LWP	large whirlpool
LX	larynx local irradiation
	lower extremity
LXC	laxative of choice
LXT	left exotropia
LYCD	live-yeast cell derivative
LYEL	lost-years of expected life
LYG	lymphomatoid granulomatosis
LYM	Lyme disease vaccine
	lymphocytes
lymphs	lymphocytes
LYS	large yellow soft (stools)
	life-year saved (cost of)
	lysine
lytes	electrolytes (Na, K, Cl, etc.)
	electrolyte panel (see page 318)
LZ	landing zone
LZP	lorazepam (Ativan)

M

M	male
	manual
	marital
	married
	masked (audiology)
	mass
	medial
	memory
	mesial
	meta
	meter (m)
	mild
	million
	minimum
	molar
	Monday
	monocytes
	mother
	mouth
	M sign—patient just utters "Mmmm" (slang)
	murmur
	muscle
	Mycobacterium
	Mycoplasma
	myopia
	myopic
	thousand
Ⓜ	murmur
M_1	first mitral sound
M1	left mastoid
	tropicamide 1% ophthalmic solution (Mydriacyl)
M1 to M7	categories of acute nonlymphoblastic leukemia
M_2	second mitral sound
m^2	square meters (body surface)
M2	right mastoid
M-2	vincristine, carmustine, cyclophosphamide, melphalan, and prednisone
M_3	third mitral sound
M-3	medical student 3rd year
3M	mitomycin, mitoxantrone, and methotrexate
M-3+7	mitoxantrone and cytarabine
M-4	medical student 4th year
M200	volociximab
MA	machine
	Master of Arts
	mean arterial (blood pressure)
	medical assistance
	medical authorization

megestrol acetate
menstrual age
mental age
meter angle
Mexican American
microalbuminuria
metabolic acidosis
microaneurysms
Miller-Abbott (tube)
milliamps
monoclonal antibodies
motorcycle accident

M/A mood and/or affect

MA-1 Bennett volume ventilator

MAA macroaggregates of albumin
Marketing Authorization Application (European Union)

MAARI medically attended acute respiratory illness

MAAS Motor Activity Assessment Scale

MAB Massachusetts Biologic Laboratories
maximum androgen blockade

Mab monoclonal antibody

MABC Movement Assessment Battery for Children

MABM mandibular alveolar bone mass

MABP mean arterial blood pressure

MAC Macintosh laryngoscope blade
macrocytic erythrocytes
macrophage
macula
maximal allowable concentration
medial arterial calcification
membrane attack complex
Mental Adjustment to Cancer (scale)
methotrexate, dactinomycin (Actinomycin D), and cyclophosphamide
microcystic adnexal carcinoma
mid-arm circumference
minimum alveolar concentration
monitored anesthesia care
multi-access catheter
Mycobacterium avium complex

MACC methotrexate, doxorubicin, (Adriamycin) cyclophosphamide, and lomustine (Cee Nu)

MACCC Master Arts, Certified Clinical Competence

MACE major adverse cardiac (cardiovascular) event(s)
Malon antegrade continence (colonic) enema

MACI Master of Arts in Clinical Investigation

MACOP-B methotrexate, doxorubicin, (Adriamycin) cyclophosphamide, vincristine (Oncovin), prednisone, and bleomycin with leucovorin rescue

MACRO macrocytes

MACS magnetic activated cell sorting

MACs malignancy-associated changes

MACTAR McMaster-Toronto Arthritis Patient Reference (Disability Questionnaire)

MAD major affective disorder
mandibular advancement device
mind altering drugs
moderate atopic dermatitis

MADD Mothers Against Drunk Driving
multiple acyl-CoA dehydrogenase deficiency

MADL mobility activities of daily living

MADRS Montgomery-Åsburg Depression Rating Scale

MAE medical air evacuation
moves all extremities

MAES moves all extremities slowly

MAEEW moves all extremities equally well

MAEW moves all extremities well

MAF malignant ascites fluid
metabolic activity factor
Mexican-American female

MAFAs movement-associated fetal (heart rate) accelerations

MAFO molded ankle/foot orthosis

MAFP maternal alpha-fetoprotein

MAG magnesium (Mg)
medication administration guideline (record)

mag cit magnesium citrate

MAGIC mouth and genital ulcers with inflamed cartilage (syndrome)

MAGP meatal advancement glandulophaleoplasty

mag sulf magnesium sulfate

MAHA macroangiopathic hemolytic anemia

MAHS malignancy-associated hemophagocytic syndrome

MAI maximal aggregation index
Medication Appropriateness Index
minor acute illness
multiphoton autofluorescence imaging
Mycobacterium avium-intracellulare

MAID mesna, doxorubicin (Adriamycin), ifosfamide, and dacarbazine
monofocal acute inflammatory demyelinating (lesions)

MAIR metabolic acidosis-induced retinopathy

MAL malaria vaccine

M

	malignant
	methyl aminolevulinate
	midaxillary line
	Motor Activity Log
MALDI	matrix-assisted laser desorption ionization
MALDI-TOFMS	matrix-assisted laser desorption ionization-time-of-flight mass spectrometry
MALG	Minnesota antilymphoblast globulin
malig	malignant
M alpha (1)	alpha (1)-microglobulin
MALT	mucosa-associated lymphoid tissue
MALToma	lymphoma of mucosa-associated lymphoid tissue
MAM	mammogram
	Mexican-American male
	monitored administration of medication
MAMC	mid-arm muscle circumference
Mammo	mammography
MAMP	milliampere
m-AMSA	amsacrine
MAMTT	minimal active muscle tendon tension
MAN	malignancy associated neutropenia
	massive aspiration of newborn
MAND	McCarron Assessment of Neuromuscular Development
Mand	mandibular
MANE	Morrow Assessment of Nausea and Emesis
MANIP	manipulation
MANOVA	multivariate analysis of variance
MAO	maximum acid output
	methylaminolevulinate
MAO-A	monoamine oxidase type A
MAO-B	monoamine oxidase type B
MAOI	monoamine oxidase inhibitor
MAOP	Mid-Atlantic Oncology Program
MAP	magnesium, ammonium, and phosphate (Struvite stones)
	malignant atrophic papulosis
	mean airway pressure
	mean arterial pressure
	Medical Assistance Program
	megaloblastic anemia of pregnancy
	Miller Assessment for Preschoolers (test for developmental delays)
	mitogen-activated protein
	mitomycin, doxorubicin (Adriamycin), and cisplatin (Platinol)
	morning after pill (oral contraceptives)
	muscle-action potential
	Mycobacterium avium subspecies *paratuberculosis*
	MYH (MutY homolog) - associated polyposis
MAPC	multipotent adult progenitor cell
MA-PD	Medicare Part C prescription drug plan
MAPI	Millon Adolescent Personality Inventory
MAPS	Make a Picture Story
MAR	marital
	medication administration record
	melanoma-associated retinopathy
	mineral apposition rates
MARE	manual active-resistive exercise
MARSA	methicillin-aminoglycoside-resistant *Staphylococcus aureus*
MARV	Marburg virus
MAS	macrophage activation syndrome
	McClune-Albright syndrome
	meconium aspiration syndrome
	Memory Assessment Scale
	minimum-access surgery
	mobile arm support
	Modified Ashworth Scale
mAs	milliampere seconds
MASA	mutant allele-specific amplification
MASDA^{SM}	Multiple-Allele-Specific Diagnostic Assay
MASER	microwave amplification (application) by stimulated emission of radiation
MASH	mobile Army surgical hospital
MASHPOT	mashed potatoes
MAST	mastectomy
	medical antishock trousers
	Michigan Alcoholism Screening Test
	military antishock trousers
MAT	manual arts therapy
	maternal
	maternity
	mature
	medication administration team
	metabolic activation therapy
	microscopic agglutination test
	Miller-Abbott tube
	Miller Analogies Test
	multifocal atrial tachycardia
MATHS	muscle pain, allergy, tachycardia and tiredness, and headache syndrome
MATTB	Manufacturers Assistance and Technical Training Branch (FDA)
MAU	microalbuminuria
MAUDE	Manufacturer and User Facility Device Experience (FDA)
MAVR	mitral and aortic valve replacement
MAWL	maximum acceptable weight of lift
max	maxillary
	maximal
MAX A	maximum assistance (assist)

MAXCONT maximum contrast method
MAxL midaxillary line
MAYO mayonnaise
MB buccal margin
mandible
Mallory body
Medical Board
medulloblastoma
mesiobuccal
methylene blue
myocardial bands
M/B mother/baby
MBA Master of Business Administration
Mini Battery of Achievement
M-BACOD methotrexate (high-dose), bleomycin, doxorubicin (Adriamycin), cyclophosphamide, vincristine (Oncovin), and dexamethasone with leucovorin rescue
2-MBAD 2-methylbutyryl-CoA dehydrogenase
MBC male breast cancer
maximum bladder capacity
maximum breathing capacity
metastatic breast cancer
methotrexate, bleomycin, and cisplatin
minimal bactericidal concentration
MB-CK a creatinine kinase isoenzyme
MBD metabolic bone disease
metastatic bone disease
methyl-binding domain
methylene blue dye
minimal brain damage
minimal brain dysfunction
MBE may be elevated
medium below elbow
MBF meat-base formula
myocardial blood flow
MBFC medial brachial fascial compartment
MBEST modulus blipped echo-planar single-pulse technique
MBHI Millon Behavioral Health Inventory
MBI Maslach Burnout Inventory
methylene blue installation
Modified Barthel Index
molecular breast imaging
MBL mannose-binding lectin
menstrual blood loss
metallo-beta-lactamases
MBL-D mannan-binding lectin deficiency
MBM mind-body medicine
mother's breast milk
MBNW multiple-breath nitrogen washout
MBO malignant bowel obstruction
mesiobuccal occulsion
MBOT mucinous borderline ovarian tumors
MBP malignant brachial plexopathy
mannan-binding protein
mannose-binding protein
mechanical bowel preparation
medullary bone pain
mesiobuccopulpal
myelin basic protein
MBq megabecquerels
MBR major breakpoint region
Medical Birth Registry
MBS modified barium swallow
MBT maternal blood type
2-mercaptobenzothiazole
multiple blunt trauma
MBTS modified Blalock-Taussig shunt
MC male child
medium-chain (triglycerides)
metacarpal
metatarso - cuneiform
microcalcifications (breast)
mini-laparotomy cholecystectomy
mitoxantrone and cytarabine
mitral commissurotomy
mixed cellularity
molluscum contagiosum
monocomponent highly purified pork insulin
Moraxella catarrhalis
mouth care
multicenter (study)
myocarditis
m + c morphine and cocaine
MC3 third metacarpal
MCA Medicines Control Agency (United Kingdom)
megestrol, cyclophosphamide, and doxorubicin (Adriamycin)
metacarpal amputation
micrometastases clonogenic assay
middle cerebral aneurysm
middle cerebral artery
monoclonal antibodies
motorcycle accident
multichannel analyzer
multiple congenital anomalies
2-MCA 2-methyl citric acid
MCAD medium-chain acyl-CoA dehydrogenase
MCAF monocyte chemoattractant and activity factor
MCAO middle cerebral artery occlusion
MCAP middle cerebral artery pressure
McAS McCune-Albright syndrome
MCAT Medical College Admission Test
MCB Medicines Control Board (United Kingdom's equivalent to the United States Food and Drug Administration)
midcycle bleeding

middle chamber bubbling
MCBDD National Center on Birth Defects and Developmental Disabilities
McB pt McBurney point
MCBS Medicare Current Beneficiary Survey
MCC meningococcal serogroup C conjugate
Merkel cell carcinoma
microcrystalline cellulose
midstream clean-catch
MCCU mobile coronary care unit
MCD malformation of cortical development
mean cell diameter
Medicaid
minimal-change disease
multicystic dysplasia
MCDK multicystic dysplasia of the kidney
MCDT mast cell degranulation test
MCE major coronary event
myocardial contrast echocardiography
MCF multicentric foci
MCFA medium-chain fatty acid
mcg microgram (1,000 mcg = 1 milligram) (do not hand write µg, as it is mistakenly read as milligram [mg])
MCG magnetocardiogram
magnetocardiography
MCGN minimal-change glomerular nephritis
MCH mean corpuscular hemoglobin
microfibrillar collagen hemostat
muscle contraction headache
MCHC mean corpuscular hemoglobin concentration
MCHL medial head of the coracohumeral ligament
MCI mild cognitive impairment
mCi millicurie
MCID minimum clinically important difference(s)
mckat microkatal (1 millionth [10^{-6}] of a katal)
MCL mantle cell lymphoma
maximum comfort level
medial collateral ligament
midclavicular line
midcostal line
modified chest lead
most comfortable level
mcL microliter (1/1,000 of an mL)
MCLL most comfortable listening level
MCLNS mucocutaneous lymph node syndrome
MCMI Millon Clinical Multiaxial Inventory
mcmol micromoles (one millionth [10^{-6}] of a mole)
MCN minimal change nephropathy
MCNS minimal change nephrotic syndrome
MCO managed care organization
mupirocin calcium ointment (Bactroban Nasal)
Mco2 carbon dioxide excretion
MCP mean carotid pressure
metacarpophalangeal joint
metoclopramide (Reglan)
monocyte chemotactic protein
MCR Medicare
metabolic clearance rate
minor cluster region
myocardial revascularization
MC=R moderately constricted and equally reactive
MCRC metastatic colorectal cancer
MCS manufacturer cannot supply
maternal cigarette smoking
mental component summary
microculture and sensitivity
minimally conscious state
moderate constant suction
motor cortex stimulation
multiple chemical sensitivity
myocardial contractile state
MCs mast cells
MCSA minimal cross-sectional area
M-CSF macrophage colony-stimulating factor
MC-SR moderately constricted and slightly reactive
MCT manual cervical traction
mean circulation time
medial canthal tendon
medium chain triglyceride
medullary carcinoma of the thyroid
microwave coagulation therapy
multislice computed tomography
MCTC metrizamide computed tomography cisternogram
MCTD mixed connective tissue disease
MCTZ methyclothiazide (Enduron)
MCU micturating cystourethrogram
MCUG micturating cystourethrogram
MCV mean corpuscular volume
measles-containing vaccine
microvolt
MCV4 meningococcal conjugate vaccine
MCVRI minimal coronary vascular resistance index
MCYLS marginal cost per year of life saved
MD macula degeneration
maintenance dialysis
maintenance dose
major depression
mammary dysplasia
manic depression
mean deviation
medical doctor
mediodorsal

Menière disease
mental deficiency
mesiodistal
microdialysis
movement disorder
multiple dose
muscular dystrophy
myocardial damage

MD-50® diatrizoate sodium injection 50%

MDA malondialdehyde
manual dilation of the anus
mass drug administrations (diethylcarbamazine plus albendazole to stop transmission of filariasis)
Medical Devises Agency (United Kingdom)
methylenedioxyamphetamine
micrometastases detection assay
motor discriminative acuity
Multichannel Discrete Analyzer

MDAC multiple-dose activated charcoal

MDACC MD Anderson Cancer Center

MDA LDL malondialdehydeconjugated low-density lipoprotein

MDASI MD Anderson Symptom Inventory

MDASI-BT MD Anderson Symptom Inventory-Brain Tumor Module

MDC Major Diagnostic Category
medial dorsal cutaneous (nerve)

MDCM mildly dilated congestive cardiomyopathy

MDCT multidetector computed tomography

MDCTA multidetector computed tomographic angiography

MDD major depressive disorder
manic-depressive disorder
Medical Device Directive (EU)

MDE major depressive episode

MDF myocardial depressant factor

MDG4 Millennium Development Goal 4

MDGF macrophage-derived growth factor

MDGs Millennium Development Goals

MDI manic-depressive illness
mental developmental index
metered-dose inhaler
methylenedioxyindenes
multi-directional instability
multiple daily injection
multiple dosage insulin

MDIA Mental Development Index, Adjusted

MDII multiple daily insulin injection

MDIS metered-dose inhaler-spacer (device)

MDiv Master of Divinity

MDL microdirect laryngoscopy

MDM mid-diastolic murmur
minor determinant mix (of penicillin)

MDMA methylenedioxy-methamphetamine (ecstasy)

MDNT midnight

MDO mentally disordered offender

MDOT modified directly observed therapy

MDP methylene diphosphonate

MDPH Michigan Department of Public Health

MDPI maximum daily permissible intake

MDR Medical Device Reporting (regulation)
minimum daily requirement
multidrug resistance

MD=R moderately dilated and equally reactive

MDR-1 multidrug resistance gene

MDRD Modification of Diet in Renal Disease

MDRE multiple-drug-resistant enterococci

MDREF multidrug resistant enteric fever

MDRO multidrug resistant organism

MDRS I/P Mattis Dementia Rating Scale-Initiation/Perseveration subscale

MDRSP multidrug resistant *Streptococcus pneumoniae*

MDRT multiple-drug rescue therapy

MDRTB multidrug resistant tuberculosis

MDS maternal deprivation syndrome
Miller-Dieker syndrome
Minimum Data Set
myelodysplastic syndromes

MD-SR moderately dilated and slightly reactive

MDTS® Metered Dose Transdermal Spray system

MDSU medical day stay unit

MDT maggot debridement therapy
Mechanical Diagnostic Therapist
motion detection threshold
multidisciplinary team
multidrug therapy

MDTM multidisciplinary team meeting

MDTP multidisciplinary treatment plan

MDU maintenance dialysis unit
microvascular Doppler ultrasonography

MDUO myocardial disease of unknown origin

MDV Marek disease virus
multiple dose vial

MDY month, date, and year

ME macular edema
manic episode
medical events
medical evidence
medical examiner
mestranol
Methodist

M

middle ear
myalgic encephalomyelitis

M/E metabolic/endocrine
monitor and evaluate
myeloid-erythroid (ratio)

M&E Mecholyl and Eserine
mucositis and enteritis

MEA microwave endometrial ablation
measles virus vaccine

MEA-I multiple endocrine adenomatosis type I

MEB Medical Evaluation Board
methylene blue

MEC meconium
medical eligibility criteria
middle ear canal(s)
mitoxantrone, etoposide, and cytarabine
moderately emetogenic chemotherapy

MeCCNU semustine

MECG maternal electrocardiogram

MECH mechanical

mech soft mechanical soft

MeCP semustine (methyl CCNU) cyclophosphamide, and prednisone

MECs measured environmental concentrations

MED male erectile dysfunction
maximal (maximum) economic dose
medial
median erythrocyte diameter
medical
medication
medicine
medium
medulloblastoma
minimal erythema dose
minimum effective dose
multiple epiphyseal dysplasia

MEd Master of Education

MEDAC multiple endocrine deficiency Addison disease (autoimmune) candidiasis

MEDCO Medcosonolator

MedDRA Medical Dictionary for Regulatory Activities

MEDEX medication administration record

MED-LARS Medical Literature Analysis and Retrieval System

MEDLINE National Library of Medicine medical database

MED NEC medically necessary

MedPAC Medicare Payment Advisory Commission

MedPAR Medicare Provider Analysis Review File

MEDS medications

MEE maintenance energy expenditure
measured energy expenditure
middle ear effusion

MEE/OC middle ear exploration with ossicular chain reconstruction

MEF maximum expired flow rate
middle ear fluid

MEFR mid expiratory flow rate

MEFV maximum expiratory flow-volume

MEG magnetoencephalogram
magnetoencephalography

Meg-CSF megakaryocytic colony-stimulating factor

MEGX monoethylglycinexylidide

MeHg methylmercury

MEI magnetic endoscope imaging
medical economic index

MEIA microparticle enzyme immunoassay

MEKC micellar electrokinetic chromatography

MEL maximum exposure limit
melatonin

MELAS mitochondrial encephalomyopathy with lactic acidosis, and stroke-like episodes (syndrome)

MEL B melarsoprol (Arsobal)

MELD Model for End-Stage Liver Disease (score)

MEM memory
monocular estimate method (near retinoscopy)

MEMB modified eosin-methylene blue (agar)

MEMG masseter (muscle) electromyographic (events)

MEN medically-enhanced normality
meningeal
meninges
meningitis
meningococcal (*Neisseria meningitidis*) (serogroups unspecified) vaccine

MEN (II) multiple endocrine neoplasia (type II)

$\text{MEN}_{\text{cn-AC}}$ meningococcal (*Neisseria meningitidis*) serogroups A, C conjugate vaccine

$\text{MEN}_{\text{cn-B}}$ meningococcal (*Neisseria meningitidis*) serogroup B conjugate vaccine

MEN_{ps} meningococcal (*Neisseria meningitidis*) polysaccharide vaccine, not otherwise specified

$\text{MEN}_{\text{ps-ACYW}}$ meningococcal (*Neisseria meningitidis*) serogroups A, C, Y, W-135 polysaccharide vaccine

$\text{MEN}_{\text{ps-B}}$ meningococcal (*Neisseria meningitidis*) serogroup B polysaccharide vaccine

MENS	microcurrent electrical neuromuscular stimulation
	mini-electrical nerve stimulator
MEO	malignant external otitis
	Medical Examiner's Office
MeOH	methyl alcohol
MEOS	microsomal ethanol oxidizing system
MEP	maximal expiratory pressure
	meperidine (Demerol)
	motor-evoked potential
	multimodality-evoked potential
MEPA	Medication Error Prevention Analysis (FDA)
MEPS	Medical Expenditure Panel Survey
mEq	milliequivalent
mEq/24 H	millequivalents per 24 hours
mEq/L	milliequivalents per liter
MER	medical evidence of record
	methanol-extracted residue (of phenol-treated BCG)
	milk ejection reflex
M/E ratio	myeloid/erythroid ratio
MERRF	myoclonic epilepsy and ragged red fibers
MERS-TM	Medical Event Reporting System - Transfusion Medicine
MES	maximal electroshock
	mesial
	myoelectric signals
MESA	microsurgical epididymal sperm aspiration
MESCC	metastatic epidural spinal cord compression
MeSH	Medical Subject Headings of the National Library of Medicine
MESS	Mangled Extremity Severe Score
MEST	mesodermal specific transcript (gene)
MET	medical emergency team
	medical emergency treatment
	metabolic
	metamyelocytes
	metastasis
	metronidazole
meT	methyltestosterone
META	metamyelocytes
METH	methamphetamine
	methicillin
MetHb	methemoglobin
	methemoglobinemia
methyl CCNU	semustine
methyl G	mitroguazone dihydrochloride (Zyrkamine)
methyl GAG	mitroguazone dihydrochloride (Zyrkamine)
METS	metabolic equivalents (multiples of resting oxygen uptake)
	metastases
MetS	metabolic syndrome
METT	maximum exercise tolerance test
MEV	million electron volts
MEWDS	multifocal evanescent white dot syndrome
MEX	Mexican
MF	Malassezia folliculitis
	Malassezia furfur
	masculinity/femininity
	meat-free
	median frequency (anesthesia-depth monitor)
	mesial facial
	methotrexate and fluorouracil
	midcavity forceps
	middle finger
	midforceps
	mother and father
	mycosis fungoides
	myelofibrosis
	myocardial fibrosis
M/F	male-female ratio
M & F	male and female
	mother and father
MFA	malaise, fatigue, and anorexia
MFAT	multifocal atrial tachycardia
MFB	metallic foreign body
	multiple-frequency bioimpedance
MFC	medial femoral condyle
MfC	*Medicines for Children*
MFCU	Medicaid Fraud Control Unit
MFD	Memory for Designs
	midforceps delivery
	milk-free diet
	multiple fractions per day
MFEM	maximal forced expiratory maneuver
mfERG	multifocal electroretinography
MFFT	Matching Familiar Figures Test
MFH	malignant fibrous histiocytoma
MFI	mean fluorescent intensity
	Multidimensional Fatigue Inventory
M-FISH	multicolor fluorescence in situ hybridization
MFM	maternal fetal medicine
	multifidus muscle
MFNS	mometasone furoate nasal spray (Nasonex)
MFPS	myofascial pain syndrome
MFR	mid-forceps rotation
	myofascial release
MFS	Marfan syndrome
	maternal-fetal surgery
	Medicare Fee Schedule
	metastases free survival
	Miller-Fisher syndrome
	mitral first sound
	monofixation syndrome

MFT muscle function test
MFU medical follow-up
MFVNS middle fossa vestibular nerve section
MFVPT Motor Free Visual Perception Test
MFVR minimal forearm vascular resistance
MG mammography
Marcus Gunn
Michaelis-Gutmann (bodies)
milligram (mg)
myasthenia gravis
mg milligram (1,000 mg = 1 gram)
Mg magnesium
mG milligauss
μg microgram (1/1000 of a milligram) (This is a dangerous abbreviation when handwritten, as it is read as mg. Use mcg)
M&G myringotomy and grommets
mg% milligrams per 100 milliliters
MGBG mitoguazone (Zyrkamine)
MGCT malignant glandular cell tumor
MGD mammography-detected (breast cancer)
meibomian gland dysfunction
MGd motexafin gadolinium (Xcytrin)
MGDF megakaryocyte growth and development factor
mg/dl milligrams per 100 milliliters
MGF macrophage growth factor
mast cell growth factor
maternal grandfather
MGG May-Grünwald-Giemsa (stain)
MGGM maternal great grandmother
MGHL middle glenohumeral ligament
MGIT mycobacteria growth indicator (incubator) tube
mg/kg milligram per kilogram
mg/kg/d milligram per kilogram per day
mg/kg/hr milligram per kilogram per hour
MGM maternal grandmother
milligram (mg is correct)
MGMA Medical Group Management Association
MGN membranous glomerulonephritis
MGO methylglyoxal
MgO magnesium oxide
MG/OL molecular genetics/oncology laboratory
MGP Marcus Gunn pupil
medical group practice
MGPS Multi-item Gamma Poisson Shrinker
MGR murmurs, gallops, or rubs
MGS magnetic guidance system
malignant glandular schwannoma
$MgSO_4$ magnesium sulfate (Epsom salt) (this is dangerous terminology as it can be interpreted as morphine sulfate)
MGT management
mgtt minidrop (60 minidrops = 1 mL)
MGUS monoclonal gammopathy of undetermined significance
MGW multiple gunshot wound
MGW enema magnesium sulfate, glycerin, and water enema
M-GXT multistage graded exercise test
mGy milligray (radiation unit)
MH macular hemorrhage
macular hole
malignant hyperthermia
marital history
medical history
menstrual history
mental health
moist heat
MHA Mental Health Assistant
methotrexate, hydrocortisone, and cytarabine (ara-C)
microangiopathic hemolytic anemia
microhemagglutination
migraine headache
MHA-TP microhemagglutination-*Treponema pallidum*
MHB maximum hospital benefits
MHb methemoglobin
MHBSS modified Hank balanced salt solution
MHC major histocompatibility complex
mental health center (clinic)
mental health counselor
M/hct microhematocrit
MHD 10-hydroxycarbazepine (oxcarbazepine metabolite)
maintenance hemodialysis
maximum heart distance (radiation therapy)
mHg millimeters of mercury
MHH mental health hold
MHI Mental Health Index (information)
MHL maximum heart length (radiation therapy)
mesenchymal hamartoma of the liver
MHIP mental health inpatient
MHLW Ministry of Health, Labor, and Welfare (Japan)
MH/MR mental health and mental retardation
MHN massive hepatic necrosis
MHO medical house officer
MHP moist heat packs
MHRA Medicines and Healthcare Products Regulatory Agency (United Kingdom)
MHRI Mental Health Research Institute
MHS major histocompatibility system
malignant hyperthermia susceptible
monomethyl hydrogen sulfate

	multihospital system
MHsFHF	malarial hepatitis-simulating fulminant-hepatic failure
MHSI	medical hyperspectral imaging
MHT	malignant hypertension
	mental health team
	Mental Health Technician
MHTAP	microhemagglutination assay for antibody to *Treponema pallidum*
MHV	mechanical heart valves
	middle hepatic vein
MHW	medial heel wedge
	mental health worker
MHX	methohexital sodium
MHx	medical history
MHxR	medical history review
MHz	megahertz
MI	membrane intact
	mental illness
	mental institution
	mesial incisal
	mitral insufficiency
	myocardial infarction
MIA	medically indigent adult
	minimally-invasive anesthesia
	missing in action
MIBE	measles inclusion body encephalitis
MIBI	technetium Tc99m sestamibi (a myocardial perfusion agent; Cardiolite)
MIBG	iobenguane sulfate I 123 (meta-iodobenzyl guanidine I 123)
MIBK	methylisobutylketone
MIC	maternal and infant care
	methacholine inhalation challenge
	medical intensive care
	microscope
	microcytic erythrocytes
	minimum inhibitory concentration
MICA	mentally ill, chemical abuser
MICAR	Mortality Medical Indexing, Classification, and Retrieval
MICE	mesna, ifosfamide, carboplatin, and etoposide
MICN	Mobile Intensive Care Nurse
MICR	methacholine inhalation challenge response
MICRO	microcytes
MICROG	microgram
microV	microvolt
MICS	minimally invasive cardiac surgery
MICU	medical intensive care unit
	mobile intensive care unit
MID	mesioincisodistal
	microvillus inclusion disease
	minimal ineffective dose
	multi-infarct dementia
MIDAS	migraine disability assessment scale
MIDCAB	minimally invasive direct coronary artery bypass
MIDD	maternally inherited diabetes and deafness
MID EPIS	midline episiotomy
MIDI	myocardial infarction during intercourse
Mid I	middle insomnia
MIE	maximim inspiratory effort
	meconium ileus equivalent (cystic fibrosis)
	medical improvement expected
MIEI	medication-induced esophageal injury
MIF	Merthiolate, iodine, and formalin
	mifepristone (RU 486; Mifeprex)
	migration inhibitory factor
MIFR	midinspiratory flow rate
MIF 50% VC	midinspiratory flow at 50% of vital capacity
MIG	measles immune globulin
MIGET	multiple inert gas elimination technique
MIH	medication-induced headache
	migraine with interparoxysmal headache
	myointimal hyperplasia
MII	multichannel intraluminal impedance
MIL	military
	mesial incisal lingual (surface)
	mother-in-law
MIMCU	medical intermediate care unit
MIN	mammary intraepithelial neoplasia
	melanocytic intraepidermal neoplasia
	mineral
	minimum
	minor
	minute (min)
MIN A	minimal assistance (assist)
MIME	mitoguazone, ifosfamide, methotrexate, and etoposide with mesna
MINE	Medical Information Network of Europe
	mesna, ifosfamide, mitoxantrone (Novantrone), and etoposide
	medical improvement not expected
MINI	Mini International Neuropsychiatric Interview
MIO	minimum identifiable odor
	monocular indirect ophthalmoscopy
MIP	macrophage inflammatory protein
	maximum inspiratory pressure
	maximum-intensity projection (radiology)
	mean intrathoracic pressure
	mean intravascular pressure
	medical improvement possible

	metacarpointerphalangeal
	Michigan Biologic Products Institute
MIPP	maximum-intensity pixel projection (images for MRI)
MIRD	medical internal radiation dose
MIRP	myocardial infarction rehabilitation program
MIRS	Medical Improvement Review Standard
MIRU-VNTR	mycobacterial interspersed repetitive units containing variable number of tandem repeats
MIS	management information systems
	melanoma *in situ*
	minimally invasive surgery
	mitral insufficiency
	moderate intermittent suction
MISA	mentally ill and substance abusing
MISC	miscarriage
	miscellaneous
M Isch	myocardial ischemia
MISH	multiple *in situ* hybridization
MISO	misonidazole
MISS	minimally invasive spine surgery
	Modified Injury Severity Score (Scale)
	Mothers in Sympathy and Support
MIT	meconium in trachea
	miracidia immobilization test
	mono-iodotyrosine
	multiple injection therapy (of insulin)
MITO-C	mitomycin (Mutamycin)
MITOX	mitoxantrone (Novantrone)
MITT	modified intent-to-treat
MIU	million international units
	minor injury unit
mIU	milli-international unit (one-thousandth of an International unit)
MIVA	mivacurium (Mivacron)
MIVE	maximum isometric voluntary extension
MIVF	maximum isometric voluntary flexion
MIW	mental inquest warrant
mix mon	mixed monitor
MJ	marijuana
	megajoule
MJD	Machado-Joseph Disease
MJL	medial joint line
MJS	medial joint space
MJT	Mead Johnson tube
μkat	microkatal (micro-moles/sec)
MKAB	may keep at bedside
MKB	married, keeping baby
MK-CSF	megakaryocyte colony-stimulating factor
MKI	mitotic-karyorrhectic index
MKM	Mehrkoordinaten Manipulator
	microgram per kilogram per minute
ML	malignant lymphoma
	mediolateral
	middle lobe
	midline
	mucosal leishmaniasis
mL	milliliter (1,000 mL = 1 liter)
M/L	monocyte to lymphocyte (ratio)
	mother-in-law
MLA	medical laboratory assay
	mento-laeva anterior
MLAC	minimum local analgesic concentration
MLAP	mean left atrial pressure
MLB	microlaryngoscopy and bronchoscopy
	microlaryngobronchoscopy
MLBW	moderately low birth weight
MLC	metastatic liver cancer
	minimal lethal concentration
	mixed lymphocyte culture
	multilevel care
	multilumen catheter
	myelomonocytic leukemia, chronic
MLD	manual lymph drainage
	masking level difference
	melioidosis (*Pseudomonas pseudomallei*) vaccine
	metachromatic leukodystrophy
	microlumbar diskectomy
	microsurgical lumbar diskectomy
	minimal lethal dose
	minimal luminal diameter
MLDA	Mutational Load Distribution Analysis
MLDT	Manual Lymph Drainage Therapist
MLE	maximum likelihood estimation
	midline (medial) episiotomy
MLEE	multilocus enzyme electrophoresis
MLF	median longitudinal fasciculus
MLHFQ	Minnesota Living With Heart Failure Questionnaire
MLN	manifest latent nystagmus
	mediastinal lymph node
	melanoma vaccine
	mesenteric lymph node
MLNS	minimal lesions nephrotic syndrome
	mucocutaneous lymph node syndrome (Kawasaki syndrome)
MLO	medial-lateral oblique (mammogram view)
	mesiolinguo-occlusal (dental)
MLP	mento-laeva posterior
	mesiolinguopulpal
	midlevel provider
MLPA	multiple ligation probe amplification

MLPJ mechanical loosening of prosthetic joint
MLPN Medical Licensed Practical Nurse
MLPP maximum loose-packed position
MLPs mid-level providers
MLR middle latency response
mixed lymphocyte reaction
multiple logistic regression
MLRA multiple linear-regression analysis
MLS macrolides, lincosamides, and streptogramins
Maroteaux-Lamy syndrome
maximum likelihood score
mediastinal B-cell lymphoma with sclerosis
MLST multi-locus sequence typing
MLT melatonin
mento-laeva transversa
MLU mean length of utterance
MLV monitored live voice
MLWHF Minnesota Living with Heart Failure (questionnaire)
MM major medical (insurance)
malignant melanoma
malignant mesothelioma
Marshall-Marchetti
medial malleolus
medication management
member months
meningococcic meningitis
mercaptopurine and methotrexate
methadone maintenance
micrometastases
millimeter (mm)
mismatch (ing)
mist mask
morbidity and mortality
motor meal
mucous membrane
multiple myeloma
muscle movement
muscularis mucosae
myelomeningocele
mM. millimole (mmol)
mm millimeter
M&M milk and molasses
morbidity and mortality
MMA maxillomandibular advancement
methylmalonic acid
methylmethacrylate
middle meningeal artery
MMC migrating motor complex
mitomycin (mitomycin C)
myelomeningocele
myoelectrical migrating complex
MMCT mitomycin C trabeculectomy
MMD malignant metastatic disease
moyamoya disease
mucus membranes dry
myotonic muscular dystrophy
MME membrane metalloendopeptidase
MMECT multiple monitor electroconvulsive therapy
MMEFR maximal mid-expiratory flow rate
MMF maxillomandibular fixation
mean maximum flow
mismatch field
mycophenolate mofetil (CellCept)
MMFR maximal mid-expiratory flow rate
MMG mammography
mechanomyography
mm Hg millimeters of mercury
MMI maximal medical improvement
MMK Marshall-Marchetti-Krantz (cystourethropexy)
MML minimal masking level (audiology)
MMM metastatic malignant melanoma
mitoxantrone, methotrexate, and mitomycin
mucous membrane moist
myelofibrosis with myeloid metaplasia
mMMSE modified version of the mini mental status examination
MMMT malignant mixed mesodermal tumor
metastatic mixed müllerian tumor
MMN mismatch negativity
multifocal motor neuropathy
multiple micronutrients
MMOA maxillary mandibular odontectomy alveolectomy
mmol millimole
μmol micromole
MMORPGs massively multiplayer online role-playing games
MMP matrix metalloproteinase
mitochondrial myopathy
mucous membrane pemphigoid
multiple medical problems
multiplexed molecular profiling (system)
MMP-8 metalloproteinase-8
MMPI matrix metalloproteinase inhibitor
Minnesota Multiphasic Personality Inventory
MMPI-A Minnesota Multiphasic Personality Inventory - Adolescent version
MMPI-D Minnesota Multiphasic Personality Inventory-Depression Scale
6-MMPR 6-methylmercaptopurine riboside
MMPs membership medical practices
MMR measles, mumps, and rubella
menometrohaggia
midline malignant reticulosis
mild mental retardation
mismatch repair

MMRISK a skin cancer mnemonic; **m**oles that are atypical, **m**oles that are many in number, **r**ed hair or freckles, **i**nability to tan, **s**unburn, **k**indred
MMRM Mixed-effects Models Repeated Measures (analysis)
MMRS Metropolitan Medical Response System
MMR-VAR measles virus, mumps virus, rubella virus, and varicella virus vaccine
MMS Medication Management Standards
Mini-Mental State (examination)
Mohs micrographic surgery
MMSE Mini-Mental State Examination
MMT malignant mesenchymal tumors
manual muscle test
meal-tolerance test
medial meniscal tear
methadone maintenance treatment
Mini Mental Test
mixed müllerian tumors
MMTP Methadone Maintenance Treatment Program
MMTV malignant mesothelioma of the tunica vaginalis
monomorphic ventricular tachycardia
mouse mammary tumor virus
MMV mandatory minute volume
MMWR *Morbidity and Mortality Weekly Report*
MMx multimatrix; a tablet formulation designed to begin dissolution in the terminal ileum
MN Master's Degree in Nursing
midnight
mononuclear
Mn manganese
M&N morning and night
Mydriacyl and Neo-Synephrine
MNC monomicrobial necrotizing cellulitis
mononuclear leukocytes
MNCV motor nerve conduction velocity
MND minor neurological dysfunction
modified neck dissection
motor neuron disease
MNF myelinated nerve fibers
MNG multinodular goiter
MNGIE mitochondrial neurogasterointestinal encephalomyopathy (syndrome)
MNM mononeuritis multiplex
MNMCB motor neuropathy with multifocal conduction block
MNNB Monas-Nitz Neuropsychological Battery
MnP2 mandibular second premolar
MNPRT mixed neutron and photon radiotherapy
MNR marrow neutrophil reserve
MNS mean nocturnal saturation
MNSc Master of Nursing Science
MnSOD manganese superoxide dismutase
Mn SSEPS median-nerve somatosensory-evoked potentials
MNTB medial nucleus of the trapezoid body
MNX meniscectomy
MNZ metronidazole (Flagyl)
MO medial oblique (x-ray view)
menhaden oil
mesio-occlusal
mineral oil
month (mo)
months old
morbidly obese
mother
myositis ossificans
Mo molybdenum
M/O morning of
MOA mechanism of action
metronidazole, omeprazole, and amoxicillin
MoAb monoclonal antibody
MOAHI mixed obstructive apnea and hypopnea index
MOAS Modified Overt Aggression Scale
MOB medical office building
mobility
mobilization
mother of baby
MOB-PT mitomycin, vincristine (Oncovin), bleomycin, and cisplatin (Platinol)
MOC medial olivocochlear
Medical Officer on Call
metronidazole, omeprazole, and clarithromycin
mother of child
MOCI Maudsley Obsessive-Compulsive Inventory
MOD maturity onset diabetes
medical officer of the day
mesio-occlusodistal
moderate
mode of death
moment of death
multiorgan dysfunction
MOD A moderate assistance (assist)
MODEMS Musculoskeletal Outcomes Data Evaluation and Management Scale
MOD I modified independent (for example, a patient who is independent, but requires a walker)
MODM mature-onset diabetes mellitus
MODS microscopic-observation drug-susceptibility (assay)

	multiple-organ dysfunction syndrome (score)
MODY	maturity-onset diabetes of youth
MOE	movement of extremities
MOEMs	micro-opto-electro-mechanical systems
MOF	mesial occlusal facial
	methotrexate, vincristine (Oncovin), and fluorouracil
	methoxyflurane (Penthrane)
	multiple-organ failure
MOFS	multiple-organ failure syndrome
MOG	myelin oligodendrocyte glycoprotein
MOH	medication overuse headache
	Ministry of Health
MoH	Ministry of Health (Canada)
Mohs	Mohs technique; serial excision and microscopic examination of skin cancers
MOI	mechanism of injury
	multiplicity of infection
MoICU	mobile intensive care unit
MOID	Mammalian Orthologous Intron Database
MOJAC	mood orientation, judgement, affect, and content
MOL	method of limits
MOM	metal-on-metal (arthroplasty)
	milk of magnesia
	mother
	mucoid otitis media
MoM	multiples of the median
MOMP	major outer membrane protein
MON	maximum observation nursery
	monitor
MONO	infectious mononucleosis
	monocyte
	monospot
mono, di	monochorionic, diamniotic
mono, mono	monochorionic, monoamniotic
MOP	medical outpatient
8 MOP	methoxsalen (Oxsorlen)
MOPD II	Majewski osteodysplastic primordial dwarfism type II
MOPP	mechlorethamine, vincristine (Oncovin), procarbazine, and prednisone
MOPV	monovalent oral poliovirus vaccine
mOPV1	monovalent oral type 1 poliovirus vaccine
MOR	morphine (This is a dangerous abbreviation)
	mortality odds ratio
mOR	matched odds ratio
MOS	Medical Outcome Study
	mirror optical system
	months
mOS	median overall survival
MOSES	Multidimensional Observational Scale for Elderly Subjects
MOSF	multiple-organ system failure
MOSFET	metal oxide semiconductor field-effect transistor (dosimeter)
MOS sf-20	Medical Outcomes Study, short form 20 items
MOS sf-36	Medical Outcomes Study, short form, 36 items
mOsm	milliosmole
mOsmol	milliosmole
MOT	motility examination
MOTA	Method Other Than Acceleration
MOTS	mucosal oral therapeutic system
MOTT	mycobacteria other than tubercle
MOU	medical oncology unit
	memorandum of understanding
MOUS	multiple occurrences of unexplained symptoms
MOV	minimum obstructive volume
	multiple oral vitamin
MOW	Meals on Wheels
MP	malignant pyoderma
	melphalan and prednisone
	menstrual period
	mercaptopurine (Purinethol)
	metacarpal phalangeal joint
	methylprednisolone
	mitoxantrone and prednisone
	moist park
	monitor pattern
	monophasic
	motor potential
	mouthpiece
	muscularis propria
	myocardial perfusion
M:P	milk to plasma ratio (related to breast feeding concentrations of drug)
M & P	Millipore and phase
4 MP	methylpyrazole (fomepizole; Antizol)
6-MP	mercaptopurine (Purenthol)
MPA	main pulmonary artery
	Medical Products Agency (Sweden)
	medroxyprogesterone acetate
MPa	megapascal
MPAC	Memorial Pain Assessment Card
MPA/E_2C	medroxyprogesterone acetate; estradiol cypionate (Lunelle)
MPAP	mean pulmonary artery pressure
MPAQ	McGill Pain Assessment Questionnaire
MPAS	Masters of Physician Assistant Studies
MPB	male-pattern baldness
	mephobarbital
MPBFV	mean pulmonary-blood-flow velocity

MPBNS modified Peyronie bladder neck suspension
MPC meperidine, promethazine, and chlorpromazine
mucopurulent cervicitis
MPCC Medical Policy Coordinating Committee
MPCN microscopically positive and culturally negative
M-PCR multiplex polymerase chain reaction
MPCU medical progressive care unit
MPD maximum permissable dose
methylphenidate (Ritalin)
moisture permeable dressing
multiple personality disorder
myeloproliferative disorder
myofascial pain dysfunction (syndrome)
mPD minimal peripheral dose
MPE malignant pleural effusion
massive pulmonary embolism
mean prediction error
multiphoton excitation
myxopapillary ependymoma
MPEC multipolar electrocoagulation
MPEG methoxypolyethylene glycol
MPF methotrexate, cisplatin (Platinol), and fluorouracil
methylparaben free
MPFL medial patellofemoral ligament
m-PFL methotrexate, cisplatin (Platinol), fluorouracil, and leucovorin
MPGN membranoproliferative glomerulonephritis
MPH massive pulmonary hemorrhage
Master of Public Health
methylphenidate (Ritalin)
miles per hour
MPHD multiple pituitary hormone deficiencies
MPI manufacturer's package insert
master patient index
Maudsley Personality Inventory
milk-product intolerance
myocardial perfusion imaging
MPIF-1 myeloid progenitor inhibitory factor-1
MPJ metacarpophalangeal joint
MPK milligram per kilogram
MPL maximum permissable level
mesiopulpolingual
MPL® monophosphoryl lipid A
MPLC medium pressure liquid chromatography
MPM malignant peritoneal mesothelioma
malignant pleural mesothelioma
Mortality Prediction Model
MPN monthly progress note
most probable number
multiple primary neoplasms
MP-NAT minipool nucleic acid (amplification) testing
MPNST malignant peripheral nerve sheath tumor
MPO male-pattern obesity
myeloperoxidase
MPOA medial preoptic area
MPOD macular pigment optical density
MPP massive periretinal proliferation
maximum pressure picture
MPP multiple presentation phenotype
MPQ McGill Pain Questionnaire
MPPT methylprednisolone pulse therapy
MPR massive periretinal retraction
medication possession ratio
multiplanar reconstruction
MPS Maternal Perinatal Scale
mean particle size
mononuclear phagocyte system
mucopolysaccharidosis
multiphasic screening
MPS-1 mucopolysaccharidosis I
MPS-II mucopolysaccharidosis II (Hunter syndrome)
MPSS massively parallel signature sequencing
methylprednisolone sodium succinate
MPSV4 meningococcal polysaccharide vaccine
MPT melphalan, prednisone, and thalidomide
multiple parameter telemetry
MPTRD motor, pain, touch, and reflex deficit
MPU maternal pediatric unit
MPV mean platelet volume
MPZ midperipheral zone (prostate needle biopsy location)
MQ mefloquine (Lariam)
memory quotient
MQOL McGill Quality of Life Questionnaire
MR Maddox rod
magnetic resonance
manifest refraction
may repeat
mean ranking
measles-rubella
medial rectus
medical record
mental retardation
milliroentgen
mitral regurgitation
moderate resistance
M&R measure and record
MR × 1 may repeat times one (once)
MRA magnetic resonance angiography

main renal artery
medical record administrator
medical research associate
midright atrium
multivariate regression analysis

mrad millirad

MRAN medical resident admitting note

MRAP mean right atrial pressure

MRAS main renal artery stenosis

MRC Master of Rehabilitation Counseling

MRCA magnetic resonance coronary angiography

MRCC metastatic renal cell carcinoma

MRCP magnetic resonance cholangiopancreatography
Member of the Royal College of Physicians
mental retardation, cerebral palsy

MRCPs movement-related cortical potentials

MRCS Member of the Royal College of Surgeons

MRD margin reflex distance
Medical Records Department
Minimal Record of Disability
minimal residual disease

MRDD maximum recommended daily dose
Mental Retardation and Development Disabilities
mentally retarded and developmentally disabled

MRDM malnutrition-related diabetes mellitus

MRDSA magnetic resonance digital subtraction angiography

MRE magnetic resonance elastography
manual resistance exercise
most recent episode

MRFC mouse rosette-forming cells

MR FIT Multiple Risk Factor Intervention Trial

MRG mortality reference group
murmurs, rubs, and gallops

MRH Maddox rod hyperphoria
multicentric reticulohistiocytoses

MRHD maximum recommended human dose

MRHT modified rhyme hearing test

MRI magnetic resonance imaging

M & R I & O measure and record input and output

MRK Merck & Co., Inc.

MRKH Mayer-Rokitansky-Kuster-Hauser (syndrome)

MRL minimal response level
moderate rubra lochia

MRLVD maximum residue limits of veterinary drugs

MRLT mesalamine-related lung toxicity

MRM modified radical mastectomy

MRN magnetic resonance neurography
malignant renal neoplasm
medical record number
medical resident's note

mRNA messenger ribonucleic acid

MRO multidrug resistant organism(s)

MROU medial rectus, both eyes

MRP multidrug resistance-associated protein

MP-RAGE magnetization prepared rapid acquisition gradient-echo

MRPN medical resident progress note

MRPs medication-related problems

MRR medical record review
Medication Reconciliation Record

MRS magnetic resonance spectroscopy
Melkersson Rosenthal Syndrome
mental retardation syndrome
methicillin-resistant *Staphylococcus aureus*

MRSA methicillin-resistant *Staphylococcus aureus*

MRSE methicillin-resistant *Staphylococcus epidermidis*

MRSI magnetic resonance spectroscopic imaging

MRSS methicillin-resistant *Staphylococcus* species
modified Rodnan skin-thickness score

MRT magnetic resonance tomography
malignant rhabdoid tumor
mean response time
modified rhyme test

MRTA magnetic resonance tomographic angiography

MRTI magnetic resonance thermal imaging

MRU medical resource utilization

MRV magnetic resonance venography

MRV(r) mixed respiratory vaccine

MRX *Moraxella catarrhalis* vaccine

MR × 1 may repeat once

MS mass spectroscopy
Master of Science
median sternotomy
medical student
mental status
milk shake
milliseconds
minimal support
mitral sounds
mitral stenosis
moderately susceptible
morning stiffness
morphine sulfate (This is a dangerous abbreviation)
motile sperm
motility study
motion sickness

M

	multiple sclerosis
	muscle spasm
	muscle strength
	musculoskeletal
M & S	microculture and sensitivity
3MS	Modified Mini-Mental Status (examination)
MS III	third-year medical student
MSA	Medical Savings Accounts
	membrane-stabilizing activity
	methane sulfonic acid
	metropolitan statistical area
	microsomal autoantibodies
	multiple system atrophy
MSAF	meconium-stained amniotic fluid
MSAFP	maternal serum alpha-fetoprotein
MSAP	mean systemic arterial pressure
MSAS	Mandel Social Adjustment Scale
MSAS-SF	Memorial Symptom Assessment Scale–short form
MSB	mainstem bronchus
MSBOS	maximum surgical blood order schedule
MSBP	Munchausen syndrome by proxy
MSC	major symptom complex
	Medical Service Corps
	mesenchymal stromal cells
	midsystolic click
	MS Contin®
MSCA	McCarthy Scales of Children's Abilities
MSCC	malignant spinal cord compression
	metastatic spinal cord compression
	midstream clean-catch (urine culture)
MSCCC	Master Sciences, Certified Clinical Competence
MSCR-AMMS	microbial surface component reacting with adhesive matrix molecules
MSCs	mesenchymal stem cells
MSCT	multislice computed tomography
MSCU	medical special care unit
MSCWP	musculoskeletal chest wall pain
MSD	male sexual dysfunction
	microsurgical diskectomy
	midsleep disturbance
	musculoskeletal disorder
MSDBP	mean sitting diastolic blood pressure
MSDS	material safety data sheet
MSE	mean squared error
	Mental Status Examination
msec	milliseconds
MSEL	myasthenic syndrome of Eaton-Lambert
MSER	mean systolic ejection rate
	Mental Status Examination Record
MSF	meconium-stained fluid
	Médicins Sans Frontières (Doctors Without Borders)
	Mediterranean spotted fever
	megakaryocyte stimulating factor
MSG	massage
	methysergide (Sansert)
	monosodium glutamate
MSGT	malignant salivary gland tumor
MSH	melanocyte-stimulating hormone
MSHA	mannose-sensitive hemagglutinin
MSI	magnetic source imaging
	mass sociogenic illness
	microsatellite instability
	multiple subcortical infarction
	musculoskeletal impairment
MSIA	mass spectrometric immunoassay
MSIR®	morphine sulfate immediate release tablets
MSIS	Multiple Severity of Illness System
MSK	medullary sponge kidney
	musculoskeletal
MSKCC	Memorial Sloan-Kettering Cancer Center
MSL	midsternal line
	multiple symmetrical lipomatosis
MSLT	multiple sleep latency test
MSM	magnetic starch microspheres
	men who have sex with men
	methsuximide (Celontin)
	methylsulfonylmethane
	midsystolic murmur
MSN	Master of Science in Nursing
MSNA	muscle sympathetic nerve activity
MSO	managed services organization
	mentally stable and oriented
	mental status, oriented
	most significant other
MSO_4	morphine sulfate (this is a dangerous abbreviation)
MSOD	multisystem organ dysfunction
MSOF	multisystem organ failure
MSP	Medoff sliding plate
MS-PCR	methylation-specific polymerase chain reaction
MSPN	medical student progress notes
MSPU	medical short procedure unit
MSQ	Mental Status Questionnaire
	meters squared
MSR	muscle stretch reflexes
MSRPP	Multidimensional Scale for Rating Psychiatric Patients
MSS	Marital Satisfaction Scale
	maternal serum screening
	mean sac size
	microsatellite stable
	minor surgery suite

M

MSSA methicillin-susceptible *Staphylococcus aureus*
MSS-CR mean sac size and crown-rump length
MSSO Maintenance and Support Services Organization
MSSP Maternal Support Services Program
MSSU midstream specimen of urine
MST maladies sexuellement transmissibles (French for sexually transmitted diseases)
mean survival time
median survival time
mental stress test
modified Schirmer test
multiple subpial transection
MSTA® mumps skin test antigen
MSTI multiple soft tissue injuries
MSTS American Musculoskeletal Tumor Society (functional rating system)
MSU maple-syrup urine
midstream urine
monosodium urate
MSUD maple-syrup urine disease
MSUS musculoskeletal ultrasound
MSUs midstream specimens of urine
mSv millisievert (radiation unit)
MSW Master of Social Work
multiple stab wounds
MT empty
macular target
maggot therapy
maintenance therapy
malaria therapy
malignant teratoma
Medical Technologist
metatarsal
middle turbinate
monitor technician
mucosal thickening
muscles and tendons
muscle tone
music therapy (Therapist)
myringotomy tube(s)
M/T masses of tenderness
myringotomy with tubes
M & T *Monilia* and *Trichomonas*
muscles and tendons
myringotomy and tubes
MTA Medical Technical Assistant
metatarsal adduction
mineral trioxide aggregate
multi-targeted antifolate (pemetrexed disodium [Alimta])
4-MTA 4-methylthioamphetamine
MTAD tympanic membrane of the right ear
MT/AK music therapy/ audiokinetics
MTAS tympanic membrane of the left ear
MTAU tympanic membranes of both ears
MTB *Mycobacterium tuberculosis*
MTBC Music Therapist-Board Certified
MTBE methyl tert-butyl ether
MTBI mild traumatic brain injury
MTC magnetization transfer contrast (radiology)
medullary thyroid carcinoma
metoclopramide
mitomycin (Mutamycin)
MTCSA mid-thigh muscle cross-sectional area
MTCT mother-to-child transmission
MTD maximum tolerated dose
metastatic trophoblastic disease
methadone
Monroe tidal drainage
Mycobacterium tuberculosis direct (test)
MTDDA Minnesota Test for Differential Diagnosis of Aphasia
MTDI maximum tolerable daily intake
MTDT *Mycobacterium* tuberculosis direct test
MTE multiple trace elements
MTE-4® trace metal elements injection (there is also a #5, #6, and #7)
MTET modified treadmill exercise testing
MTF male-to-female (transmission)
medical treatment facility
MTG middle temporal gyrus (gyri)
midthigh girth
MTHFR methylene tetrahydrofolate reductase
MTI magnetization transfer imaging
malignant teratoma intermediate
MTJ midtarsal joint
MTL medial temporal lobe
mediastinal tuberculous lymphadenitis
Metropolitan Life (Insurance Company) Table (for desirable weight)
MTLE medial (mesial) temporal-lobe epilepsy
MTLV midtidal lung volume
MTM medication therapy management
modified Thayer-Martin medium
mouth-to-mouth (resuscitation)
MTNX methylnaltrexone
mTOR mammalian target of rapamycin
MTP master treatment plan
medial tibial plateau
medical termination of pregnancy
metatarsophalangeal
microsomal triglyceride transfer protein
MTPJ metatarsophalangeal joint

M

MTR	mother
MTR-$\overline{O}$	no masses, tenderness, or rebound
MTRS	Licensed Master Therapeutic Recreation Specialist
MTS	mesial temporal sclerosis
	Muir-Torre syndrome
MTST	maximal treadmill stress test
MTT	mamillothalamic tract
	mean transit time
	methylthiotetrazole
MTU	malignant teratoma undifferentiated
	methylthiouracil
MTWA	microvolt T-wave alternans
MTX	methotrexate
MTZ	mirtazapine (Remeron)
	mitoxantrone (Novantrone)
MU	million units
	Murphy unit
mU	milliunits
MUA	manipulation under anesthesia
MUAC	middle upper arm circumference
MUAP	motor unit action potential
MUD	matched-unrelated donor
MUDDLES	miosis, urination, diarrhea, diaphoresis, lacrimation, excitation of central nervous system, and salivation (effects of cholinesterase inhibitors)
MUDPILES	*m*ethanol, metformin; *u*remia; *d*iabetic ketoacidosis; *p*henformin, paraldehyde; *i*ron, *i*soniazid, ibuprofen; *l*actic acidosis; *e*thanol, ethylene glycol; and *s*alicylates, sepsis (causes of metabolic acidosis)
MUE	medication use evaluation
MUFA	monounsaturated fatty acid
MUG	microgram (mcg is preferred)
MUGA	multigated (radionuclide) angiogram
	multiple gated acquisition (scan)
MUGX	multiple gated acquisition exercise
MUI	mixed urinary incontinence
MULE	microcomputer upper limb exerciser
MULTIP	multipara
MuLV	murine leukemia virus
MUM	mumps virus vaccine
MUNE	motor unit estimates
MUNSH	Memorial University of Newfoundland Scale of Happiness
MUO	metastasis of unknown origin
MUPAT	multiple-site perineal applicator technique
MUPS	melanoma of unknown primary site
MUSE®	Medicated Urethral System for Erection (alprostadil urethral suppository)
mus-lig	musculoligamentous
MUU	mouse uterine units
MV	manual ventilation
	mechanical ventilation
	millivolts
	minute volume
	mitoxantrone and etoposide (VePesid)
	mitral valve
	mixed venous
	multivesicular
MVA	malignant vertricular arrhythmias
	manual vacuum aspiration
	mitral valve area
	modified vaccinia ankara
	motor vehicle accident
M-VAC	methotrexate, vinblastine doxorubicin (Adriamycin), and cisplatin
MVB	methotrexate and vinblastine
	mixed venous blood
MVC	maximal voluntary contraction
	motor vehicle collision (crash)
MVc	mitral valve closure
MV-CBCT	meta-voltage cone-beam computed tomography
MVD	microvascular decompression
	microvessel density
	mitral valve disease
	multivessel disease
MVE	mitral valve (leaflet) excursion
	Murray Valley encephalitis
MV Grad	mitral valve gradient
MVI	malignant vascular injury
	multiple vitamin injection
MVI®	brand name for parenteral multivitamins
MVI 12®	brand name for parenteral multivitamins
MVIC	maximum voluntary isometric contractions
MVID	microvillus inclusion disease
MVO	mixed venous oxygen saturation
MVO$_2$	myocardial oxygen consumption
MVP	mean venous pressure
	mitomycin, vinblastine, and cisplatin (Platinol)
	mitral valve prolapse
MVPA	moderate-to-vigorous physical activity
MVPP	mechlorethamine, vinblastine, procarbazine, and prednisone
MVPS	mitral valve prolapse syndrome
MVR	massive vitreous retraction
	micro-vitreoretinal (blade)
	mitral valve regurgitation
	mitral valve replacement
MVRI	mixed vaccine respiratory infections
MVS	mitral valve stenosis
	motor, vascular, and sensory

	Multichannel Verification System
MVT	movement
	multiform ventricular tachycardia
	multivitamin
MVU	Montevideo units
MVV	maximum ventilatory volume
	maximum voluntary ventilation
	mixed vespid venom
6-MW	6-minute walk (test)
12-MW	12-minute walk (test)
MWA	migraine with aura
MWB	minimal weight bearing
MWC	major wound complications
MWCO	molecular weight cutoff
MWD	maximum walking distance
	microwave diathermy
6-MWD	6-minute walking distance
M-W-F	Monday-Wednesday-Friday
MWI	Medical Walk-In (Clinic)
MWOA	migraine without aura
MWS	Mickety-Wilson syndrome
MWT	maintenance of wakefulness test
	Mallory-Weiss tear
	malpositioned wisdom teeth
	maximal walking time
6-MWT	6-minute walk test
MWTP	municipal wastewater treatment plants
Mx	mammography
	manifest refraction
	mastectomy
	maxilla
	movement
	myringotomy
My	myopia
MYD	mydriatic
myelo	myelocytes
	myelogram
MyG	myasthenia gravis
MYOP	myopia
MYR	myringotomy
MYS	medium yellow soft (stools)
MZ	monozygotic
M/Z	mass/charge
MZL	marginal zone lymphocyte
MZT	monozygotic twins

N

N	nausea
	negative
	Negro
	Neisseria
	nerve
	neutrophil
	never
	newton
	night
	nipple
	nitrogen
	no
	nodes
	nonalcoholic
	none
	normal
	North (as in the location 2N, would be second floor, North wing)
	not
	notified
	noun
	NPH insulin
	size of sample
N1	study night 1
N I . . . . N XII	first through twelfth cranial nerves
O.1 N	tenth-normal
N_2	nitrogen
N 2.5	phenylephrine HCl 2.5% ophthalmic solution (Neo-Synephrine)
n-3	omega-3
5′-N	5′-nucleotidase
N-9	nonoxynol 9
NA	Narcotics Anonymous
	Native American
	Negro adult
	new admission
	nicotinic acid
	nonalcoholic
	norethindrone acetate
	normal axis
	not admitted
	not applicable
	not available
	nurse aide
	nurse's aid
	Nurse Anesthetist
	nursing assistant
Na	sodium
Na^+	sodium
N & A	normal and active
NAA	*N*-acetylaspartate
	National Average Allowance (federal physician office visit cost guide)

N

	neutron activation analysis no apparent abnormalities nucleic acid amplification
NAAA	neo-adjuvant androgen ablation
NAAC	no apparent anesthesia complications
NAA/Cr	N-acetylaspartate/creatine ratio
NAAD	neoadjuvant androgen deprivation (therapy)
NAAT	nucleic acid amplification techniques (testing)
NAATPT	not available at the present time
NAB	not at bedside
NABS	normoactive bowel sounds
NAbs	neutralizing antibodies
NABT	normal-appearing brain tissue
NABTC	North American Brain Tumor Consortium
NABX	needle aspiration biopsy
NAC	acetylcysteine (N-acetylcysteine; Mucomyst) neoadjuvant chemotherapy nipple-areola complex no acute changes no anesthesia complications
NACD	no anatomical cause of death
NaCIO	sodium hypochlorite
NaCl	sodium chloride (salt)
NaCMC	sodium carboxymethyl cellulose
NACS	Neurologic and Adaptive Capacity Score
NACT	neoadjuvant chemotherapy
NAD	nicotinamide adenine dinucleotide no active disease no acute distress no apparent distress no appreciable disease normal axis deviation nothing abnormal detected
NADA	New Animal Drug Application
NADase	nicotinamide adenine dinucleotide glycohydrolase
NADE	New Animal Drug Evaluation
NADPH	nicotinamide adenine dinucleotide phosphate
NADSIC	no apparent disease seen in chest
NaE	exchangeable sodium
NAEPP	National Asthma Education and Prevention Program (guidelines)
NAF	nafcillin Native-American female Negro adult female normal adult female Notice of Adverse Findings (FDA post-audit letter)
NaF	sodium fluoride
NaFeEDTA	sodium iron (III) ethylenediaminetetraacetic acid (sodium iron edetic acid)
NAFLD	nonalcoholic fatty liver disease
NAG	N-acetyl-beta-d-glucosaminidase narrow angle glaucoma
$NaHCO_3$	sodium bicarbonate
NAHI	nonaccidental head injury
NAI	no action indicated no acute inflammation nonaccidental injury Nuremberg Aging Inventory
NaI	sodium iodide
NAION	nonarteritic anterior ischemic optic neuropathy
NAIT	neonatal alloimmune thrombocytopenia
NAL	nasal angiocentric lymphoma
NAM	nail-apparatus melanoma Native-American male no abnormal masses normal adult male
NAMCS	National Ambulatory Medical Care Survey
nAMD	neovascular age-related macular degeneration
NANB	non-A, non-B (hepatitis) (hepatitis C)
NANBH	non-A, non-B hepatitis (hepatitis C)
NANC	nonadrenergic, noncholinergic
NANDA	North American Nursing Diagnosis Association (taxonomy)
NaNP	sodium nitroprusside (Nipride)
NANSAIDs	nonaspirin, nonsteroidal anti-inflammatory drugs
NANT	New Approaches to Neuroblastoma Therapy (consortium)
NaOCl	sodium hypochlorite
NaOH	sodium hydroxide
NAP	narrative, assessment, and plan nosocomial acquired pneumonia
NAPA	N-acetyl procainamide
NAPD	no active pulmonary disease
Na Pent	Pentothal Sodium
NAR	nasal airflow resistance no action required no adverse reaction nonambulatory restraint not at risk nursing assessment record
NARC	narcotic(s)
NaRI	noradrenaline reuptake inhibitor
NARP	neuropathy, (neurogenic muscle weakness) ataxia and retinitis pigmentosa (syndrome)
NART	National Adult Reading Test (United Kingdom)
NAS	nasal neonatal abstinence syndrome no abnormality seen no added salt

N

NASBA	nucleic-acid sequencing based amplification
NaSCN	sodium thiocyanate
NASH	nonalcoholic steatohepatitis
NAS-NRC	National Academy of Sciences – National Research Council
NaSSA	noradrenergic and specific serotonergic antidepresssant
NASTT	nonspecific abnormality of ST segment and T wave
NAT	N-acetyltransferase
	no action taken
	no acute trauma
	nonaccidental trauma
	nonspecific abnormality of T wave
	nucleic acid test (testing)
Na^{99m} TcO_4^-	sodium pertechnetate Tc 99m
NAUC	normalized area under the curve
NAUTI	nosocomially-associated urinary tract infections
NAW	nasal antral window
NAWM	normal-appearing white matter
NB	nail bed
	needle biopsy
	neuroblastomas
	newborn
	nitrogen balance
	note well
NB-BAL	nonbronchoscopic-bronchoalveolar lavage
NBC	newborn center
	nonbed care
	nuclear, biological, and chemical
NBCCS	nevoid basal-cell carcinoma syndrome
NBD	neurologic bladder dysfunction
	no brain damage
NBF	not breast fed
NBH	new bag (bottle) hung
NBHH	newborn helpful hints
NBI	no bone injury
NBICU	newborn intensive care unit
nBiPAP	nasal bilevel (biphasic) positive airway pressure
NBIs	nosocomial bloodstream infections
NBL/OM	neuroblastoma and opsoclonus-myoclonus
NBM	no bowel movement
	normal bone marrow
	normal bowel movement
	nothing by mouth
NBN	newborn nursery
NBP	needle biopsy of prostate
	no bone pathology
NBQC	narrow base quad cane
NBR	no blood return
NBRM	negative binomial regression model
NBS	newborn screen (serum thyroxine and phenylketonuria)
	Nijmegen breakage syndrome
	no bacteria seen
	normal bowel sounds
NBT	nitroblue tetrazolium reduction (tests)
	normal breast tissue
NBTE	nonbacterial thrombotic endocarditis
NBTNF	newborn, term, normal female
NBTNM	newborn, term, normal, male
NBW	normal birth weight (2,500–3,999 g)
NC	nasal cannula
	Negro child
	neurologic check
	no change
	no charge
	no complaints
	noncontributory
	normocephalic
	nose clamp
	nose clips
	not classified
	not completed
	not cultured
9 NC	rubitecan (9-nitrocamptothecin; Orathecin)
NCA	neurocirculatory asthenia
	no congenital abnormalities
N/CAN	nasal cannula
NCAP	nasal continuous airway pressure
	noncalcified coronary artery plaque
NCAS	zinostatin (neocarzinostatin)
NC/AT	normocephalic atraumatic
NCB	natural childbirth
	no code blue
NCBI	National Center for Biotechnology Information (NIH)
NCC	neurocysticercosis
	no concentrated carbohydrates
	nursing care card
NCCAM	National Center for Complementary and Alternative Medicine (NIH)
NCCDPHP	National Center for Chronic Disease and Prevention and Health Promotion (CDC)
NCCI	National Correct Coding Initiative
NCCLS	National Committee for Clinical Laboratory Standards
NCCN	National Comprehensive Cancer Network
NCCP	noncardiac chest pain
NCCT	noncontrast computed tomography
NCCTG	North Central Cancer Treatment Group
NCCU	neurosurgical continuous care unit
NCD	National Coverage Determination (Manual)

Abbreviation	Meaning
	neck-capsule distance
	no congenital deformities
	normal childhood diseases
	not considered disabling
	not considered disqualifying
	Nursing-Care Dependency (scale)
NCDB	National Cancer Data Base
NCDR	new case-detection rate
NCDs	national coverage determinations
NCE	new chemical entity
NCEH	National Center for Environmental Health (CDC)
NCEP	National Cholesterol Education Program
NCF	neurocognitive function
	neutrophilic chemotactic factor
	no cold fluids
NC=F	noncompleter=failure
NCHGR	National Center for Human Genome Research (NIH)
NCHS	National Center for Health Statistics
NCICB	National Cancer Institute Center for Bioinformatics
NCI	National Cancer Institute
NCICB	National Cancer Institute Center for Bioinformatics
NCIC	National Cancer Institute of Canada
NCI-CTC	National Cancer Institute Common Toxicity Criteria
NCIC-CTG	National Cancer Institute of Canada Clinical Trials Group
NCID	National Center for Infectious Diseases (CDC)
NCIE	nonbullous congenital ichthyosiform erythroderma
NCIPC	National Center for Injury Prevention and Control (CDC)
NCIS	National Coroners Information System (Australia)
	nursing care information sheet
NCIT	Nursing Care Intervention Tool
NCJ	needle catheter jejunostomy
NCL	neuronal ceroid lipofuscinosis
	no cautionary labels
	nuclear cardiology laboratory
NCKX	sodium-calcium-potassium exchanger
NCLD	neonatal chronic lung disease
NCM	nailfold capillary microscope
	nonclinical manager
NCNC	normochromic, normocytic
NCNR	National Center for Nursing Research (NIH)
NCO	no complaints offered
	noncommissioned officer
NCOG	North California Oncology Group
NCP	no caffeine or pepper
	nursing care plan
NCPAP	nasal continuous positive airway pressure
NCPB	neurolytic celiac plexus block
NCPE	noncardiogenic pulmonary edema
NcpPCu	nonceruloplasmin plasma copper
NCPR	no cardiopulmonary resuscitation
NCQA	National Commission for Quality Assurance
NCR	no carbon (paper) required (treated paper which produces a copy of what was written on the paper above)
nCR	nodular complete response
NCRA	National Cancer Registrars Association
NCRC	nonchild-resistant container
NCRI	National Cancer Research Institute (United Kingdom)
NCRR	National Center for Research Resources (NIH)
NCS	nerve conduction studies
	no concentrated sweets
	noncontact supervision
	not clinically significant
	Nutcracker syndrome
	zinostatin (neocarzinostatin)
NCSE	nonconvulsive status epilepticus
NCSN	National Certified School Nurse
NCT	neoadjuvant chemotherapy
	neutron capture therapy
	noncontact tonometry
	number connection test
	Nursing Care Technician
NCTR	National Center for Toxicological Research
NCV	nerve conduction velocity
	nuclear venogram
NCVHS	National Committee on Vital and Health Statistics
NCX	sodium-calcium exchanger
ND	Doctor of Naturopathy (Naturopathic Physician)
	nasal deformity
	nasal discharge
	nasoduodenal
	natural death
	neck dissection
	neonatal death
	neurological development
	neurotic depression
	Newcastle disease
	no data
	no disease
	nondisabling
	nondistended
	none detectable
	normal delivery
	normal development

	nose drops
	not detected
	not diagnosed
	not done
	nothing done
	Nursing Doctorate
N&D	nodular and diffuse
Nd	neodymium
NDA	New Drug Application
	no data available
	no demonstrable antibodies
	no detectable activity
NDC	National Drug Code
	nondigestible carbohydrates
NDD	no dialysis days
NDE	near-death experience
NDEA	no deviation of electrical axis
NDF	neutral density filter (test)
	no disease found
NDGA	nordihydroguaiaretic acid
NDI	National Death Index
	nephrogenic diabetes insipidus
NDIR	nondispersive infrared
NDIRS	nondispersive infrared spectrometer
NDM	neonatal diabetes mellitus
NDMS	National Disaster Medical System
Nd/NT	nondistended, nontender
NDO	neurogenic detrusor overactivity
NDP	nedaplatin
	net dietary protein
	Nurse Discharge Planner
NDPH	new daily persistent headache
NDR	neurotic depressive reaction
	normal detrusor reflex
NDRI	norepinephrine and dopamine reuptake inhibitor
NDS	Neurologic Disability Score
	neuropathy disability score
	New Drug Submission
NDSC	nasal dermoid sinus cyst
NDSO	nasolacrimal drainage system obstruction
NDST	neurodevelopmental screening test
NDT	nasal duodenostomy tube
	Neurocognitive Driving Test
	neurodevelopmental techniques
	neurodevelopmental treatment
	noise detection threshold
NDV	Newcastle disease virus
Nd:YAG	neodymium:yttrium-aluminum-garnet (laser)
Nd:YLF	neodymium: yttrium-lithium-fluoride (laser)
NE	nasoenteric
	nausea and emesis
	nephropathica epidemica
	neurological examination
	never exposed
	no effect
	no enlargement
	norethindrone
	norepinephrine
	not elevated
	not estimable
	not examined
NEAA	nonessential amino acids
NEAC	norethindrone acetate
NEAD	nonepileptic attack disorder
NEAT	nonexercise activity thermogenesis
NEB	hand-held nebulizer
NEC	necrotizing entercolitis
	noise equivalent counts
	nonesterified cholesterol
	not elsewhere classified
NECT	nonenhanced computed tomography (scan)
NED	neuroendocrine differentiation
	no evidence of disease
NEDSS	National Electronic Disease Surveillance System
NEE	neonatal epileptic encephalopathy
NEEG	normal electroencephalogram
NEEP	negative end-expiratory pressure
NEF	negative expiratory force
NEFA	nonesterified fatty acid(s)
NEFG	normal external female genitalia
NEFT	nasoenteric feeding tube
NEG	negative
	neglect
NEI	National Eye Institute (NIH)
NEJM	*New England Journal of Medicine*
NEM	neurotrophic enhancing molecule
	no evidence of malignancy
	nucleoside excision mutation
NEMD	nonexudative macular degeneration
	nonspecific esophageal motility disorder
NENT	nasal endotracheal tube
NEO	necrotizing external otitis
NEOH	neonatal high risk
NEOM	neonatal medium risk
NEP	needle-exchange program
	neutral endopeptidase
	no evidence of pathology
NEPD	no evidence of pulmonary disease
NEPHRO	nephrogram
NEPPK	nonepidermolytic palmoplantar keratoderma
NEQAS	National External Quality Assurance Scheme (United Kingdom)
NER	no evidence of recurrence
NERD	no evidence of recurrent disease
	nonerosive reflux disease
NES	nonepileptic seizure
	nonstandard electrolyte solution
	not elsewhere specified

NESP	novel erythropoiesis stimulating protein (darbepoetin [Aranesp])
NESTT	nonhazardous explosives for security training and testing
NET	choroidal or subretinal neovascularization
	Internet
	naso-endotracheal tube
	neuroectodermal tumor
	neuroendocrine tumors
NETA	norethindrone acetate (Aygestin)
NETSS	National Electronic Telecommunications System for Surveillance
NETT	nasal endotracheal tube
NETZ	needle (diathermy) excision of the transformation zone
NEVA	nocturnal electrobioimpedance volumetric assessment (penile measurement)
NEX	nose-to-ear-to-xiphoid
	number of excitations (radiology)
NEXUS	National Emergency X-Radiography Utilization Study (criteria)
NF	National Formulary
	necrotizing fasciitis
	Negro female
	neurofibromatosis
	night frequency (of voiding)
	nodular fasciitis
	none found
	nonfasting
	not found
	nursed fair
	nursing facility
Nf	*Naegleria fowleri*
NF1	neurofibromatosis type 1
NF2	neurofibromatous type 2
NF90	nuclear factor 90
NFA	Nerve Fiber Analyzer®
NFALO	Nerve Fiber Analyzer laser oththalmoscope
NFAP	nursing facility-acquired pneumonia
NFAR	no further action required
NFCS	Neonatal Facial Coding System
NFD	nephrogenic fibrosing dermopathy
	no family doctor
NFFD	not fit for duty
NFI	nerve-function impairment
	no-fault insurance
	no further information
	normal female infant
NFL	nerve fiber layer
	Novantrone (mitoxantrone), fluorouracil, and leucovorin
NFLX	norfloxacin (Noroxin)
NFP	natural family planning
	no family physician
	not-for-profit
	not for publication
NFPA	nonfluent progressive aphasia
NFT	no further treatment
NFTD	normal full-term delivery
NFTE	not found this examination
NFTs	neurofibrillary tangles
	neurologic function tests
NFTSD	normal full-term spontaneous delivery
NFTT	nonorganic failure to thrive
NFV	nelfinavir (Viracept)
NFW	nursed fairly well
NG	nanogram (ng) (10^{-9} gram)
	nasogastric
	night guard
	nitroglycerin
	no growth
	norgestrel
ng	nanogram
NGAL	neutrophil gelatinase-associated lipocalin
NGB	neurogenic bladder
NGF	nerve growth factor
n giv	not given
NGJ	nasogastro-jejunostomy
NGM	norgestimate
NGMAST	*Neisseria gonorrhoeae* multi-antigen sequence typing
NGO	nongovernmental organization
NGOs	nongovernmental organizations
NGR	nasogastric (tube) replacement
NGRI	not guilty by reason of insanity
NGSF	nothing grown so far
NGT	nasogastric tube
	normal glucose tolerance
NGTD	no growth to date
NgTD	negative to date
NGU	nongonococcal urethritis
NH	normal-hearing
	nursing home
$-NH_2$	amine
NH_4^+	ammonium
NHA	no histologic abnormalities
NHANES III	third National Health and Nutrition Examination Survey
NHB	nonheart-beating (donor)
NHBD	nonheart-beating donor
NHC	neighborhood health center
	neonatal hypocalcemia
	nursing home care
NH_3	ammonia
NH_4Cl	ammonium chloride
NHCU	nursing home care unit
NHD	nocturnal hemodialysis
	normal hair distribution
NHE	sodium/hydrogen exchanger
NHEJ	nonhomologous end-joining

NHGRI National Human Genome Research Institute (NIH)
NHIS National Health Interview Survey
NHL nodular histiocytic lymphoma
non-Hodgkin lymphomas
nHL normalized hearing level
NHLBI National Heart, Lung, and Blood Institute (NIH)
NHLPP hereditary neuropathy with liability for pressure palsy
NHM no heroic measures
NHO notify house officer
NHP Nottingham Health Profile
nursing home placement
NHPs natural health products
NHPT nine-hole peg test
NHS National Health Service (UK)
NHSP Newborn Hearing Screening Program
NHT neoadjuvant hormonal therapy
nursing home transfer
NHTR nonhemolytic transfusion reaction
NHTSA National Highway Traffic Safety Administration
NHW nonhealing wound
NI neurological improvement
no improvement
no information
none indicated
not identified
not isolated
NIA National Institute on Aging (NIH)
no information available
NIAAA National Institute on Alcohol Abuse and Alcoholism (NIH)
NIADDK National Institute of Arthritis, Diabetes, and Digestive and Kidney Diseases (NIH)
NIAID National Institute of Allergy and Infectious Diseases (NIH)
NIAL not in active labor
NIAMS National Institute of Arthritis and Musculoskeletal and Skin Diseases (NIH)
NIA-RI National Institute on Aging–Reagan Institute
NIBP noninvasive blood pressure
NIBPM noninvasive blood pressure measurement
NIC Nursing Intervention Classification
NICC neonatal intensive care center
noninfectious chronic cystitis
NICE National Institute for Clinical Excellence (United Kingdom)
new, interesting, and challenging experiences
NICHD National Institute of Child Health and Human Development (NIH)
NICO neuralgia-inducing cavitational osteonecrosis
noninvasive cardiac output (monitor)
NICS noninvasive carotid studies
NICU neonatal intensive care unit
neurosurgical intensive care unit
NID no identifiable disease
not in distress
NIDA National Institute of Drug Abuse (NIH)
NIDA five National Institute on Drug Abuse screen for cannabinoids, cocaine metabolite, amphetamine/methamphetamine, opiates, and phencyclidine
NIDCD National Institute of Deafness and other Communication Disorders (NIH)
NIDCR National Institute of Dental and Craniofacial Research (NIH)
NIDD noninsulin-dependent diabetes
NIDDK National Institute of Diabetes and Digestive and Kidney Diseases (NIH)
NIDDM noninsulin-dependent diabetes mellitus
NIDR National Institute of Dental Research (NIH)
NIEHS National Institute of Environmental Health Sciences (NIH)
NIF negative inspiratory force
neutrophil inhibitory factor
not in file
NIFS noninvasive flow studies
NIG NSAIA (nonsteroidal anti-inflamatory agent) induced gastropathy
NIGMS National Institute of General Medical Sciences (NIH)
NIH National Institutes of Health
NIHD noise-induced hearing damage
NIHL noise-induced hearing loss
NIHSS National Institutes of Health Stroke Scale
NIID neuronal intranuclear inclusion disease
NIL not in labor
NIM nerve integrity monitor
NIMAs noninherited maternal antigens
NIMH National Institute of Mental Health (NIH)
NIMHDIS National Institute for Mental Health Diagnostic Interview Schedule (NIH)
NIMR National Institute of Medical Research (United Kingdom)
NINDS National Institute of Neurological Disorders and Stroke (NIH)

NINR National Institute for Nursing Research (NIH)
NINU neuro intermediate nursing unit
NINVS noninvasive neurovascular studies
NIOPCs no intraoperative complications
NIOSH National Institute of Occupational Safety and Health (Centers for Disease Control and Prevention)
NIP catnip
National Immunization Program
no infection present
no inflammation present
NIPAs noninherited paternal antigens
NIPD nocturnal intermittent peritoneal dialysis
NIPPV noninvasive positive-pressure ventilation
NIPS Neonatal Infant Pain Scale
NIP/S noninvasive programming stimulation
NIPSV noninvasive pressure support ventilation
NIR near infrared
nitroprusside-induced relaxation
NIRCA nonisotopic RNase cleavage assay
NIRS near infrared spectroscopy
NIS sodium iodide symporter (protein)
NISH nonradioactive *in situ* hybridization
NISS New Injury Severity Score
NISs no-impact sports
NIST National Institute of Standards and Technology
NISV nonionic surfactant vesicle
NITD neuroleptic-induced tardive dyskinesia'
Nitro nitroglycerin (this is a dangerous abbreviation)
sodium nitroprusside (this is a dangerous abbreviation)
NIV noninvasive ventilation
NIVLS noninvasive vascular laboratory studies
NIVs nutrient intake values
NJ nasojejunal
NJT nasojejunal tube
NK natural killer (cells)
not known
NK_1 neurokinin 1
NKA no known allergies
nkat nanokatal (nanomole/sec)
NKB no known basis
not keeping baby
neurokinin B
NKC nonketotic coma
NKD no known diseases
NKDA no known drug allergies
NKFA no known food allergies
NKH nonketotic hyperglycemia
NKHA nonketotic hyperosmolar acidosis
NKHHC nonketotic hyperglycemic-hyperosmolar coma
NKHOC nonketotic hyperosmolar coma
NKHS nonketotic hyperosmolar syndrome
NKMA no known medication (medical) allergies
NKT natural-killer T (cells)
NL nasolacrimal
nonlatex
normal
normal libido
nL nanoliter (if nL was used in the clinical setting it would be dangerous as it could be seen or heard as mL)
NLB needle liver biopsy
NLC nocturnal leg cramps
NLC & C normal libido, coitus, and climax
NLD nasolacrimal duct
necrobiosis lipoidica diabeticorum
no local doctor
NLDO nasolacrimal duct obstruction
NLE neonatal lupus erythematosus
nursing late entry
NLEA Nutrition Labeling and Education Act of 1990
NLF nasolabial fold
nelfinavir (Viracept)
NLFGNR nonlactose fermenting gram-negative rod
NLM National Library of Medicine
no limitation of motion
NLMC nocturnal leg muscle cramp
NLN National League for Nursing
no longer needed
NLNAC National League for Nursing Accrediting Commission
NLO nasolacrimal occlusion
NLP natural language processing
nodular liquifying panniculitis
no light perception
NLPHL nodular lymphocyte-predominant Hodgkin lymphoma
NLS neonatal lupus syndrome
NLs neuroimmunophilin ligands
NLT not later than
not less than
NLV nelfinavir (Viracept)
NM nanometer (nm) (10^{-9} meters)
Negro male
neoplastic meningitis
neuromuscular
neuronal microdysgenesis
nodular melanoma
nonmalignant

	not measurable
	not measured
	not mentioned
	nuclear medicine
	nurse manager
N & M	nerves and muscles
	night and morning
NMB	neuromuscular blockade
NMBA	neuromuscular blocking agent
NMBS	nuclear medicine bone scan
NMC	no malignant cells
NMD	Doctor of Naturopathic Medicine
	neuromuscular disorders
	neuronal migration disorders
	Normosol M and 5% Dextrose®
NMDA	*N*-methyl-D-aspartate
NMDP	National Marrow Donor Pool
NME	new molecular entity
NMES	neuromuscular electrical stimulation
NMF	neuromuscular facilitation
NMH	neurally mediated hypotension
NMHH	no medical health history
NMI	no manifest improvement
	no mental illness
	no middle initial
	no more information
	normal male infant
NMJ	neuromuscular junction
NML	normal
NMKB	not married, keeping baby
NMM	nodular malignant melanoma
NMN	no middle name
NMNKB	not married, not keeping baby
NMO	neuromyelitis optica (Devic syndrome)
nmol	nanomole (one billionth [10^{-9}] of a mole)
NMOH	no medical ocular history
NMP	normal menstrual period
NMPPAS	non-resonant multiphoton photoacoustic spectroscopy
NMR	nuclear magnetic resonance (same as magnetic resonance imaging)
NMRS	nuclear magnetic resonance spectroscopy
NMRT (R)	Nuclear Medicine Radiologic Technologist (Registered)
NMS	neonatal morphine solution
	neuroleptic malignant syndrome
NMSC	nonmelanoma skin cancer
NMSE	normalized mean square root
NMSIDS	near-miss sudden infant death syndrome
NMT	nebulized mist treatment
	no more than
NMTB	neuromuscular transmission blockade
NMTCB	Nuclear Medicine Technology Certification Board
NMT(R)	Nuclear Medicine Technologist Registered
NMU	nitrosomethylurea
NN	narrative notes
	Navajo neuropathy
	neonatal
	neural network
	normal nursery
	nurses' notes
N/N	negative/negative
NNB	normal newborn
	number-needed-to-benefit
NNBC	node-negative breast cancer
NND	neonatal death
	number needed to detain
NNDSS	National Notifiable Diseases Surveillance System
NNE	neonatal necrotizing enterocolitis
NNH	number needed to harm
NNIS	National Nosocomial Infections Surveillance
NNM	Nicolle-Novy-MacNeal (media)
NNL	no new laboratory (test orders)
NNN	normal newborn nursery
NNO	no new orders
NNP	Neonatal Nurse Practitioner
	non-nociceptive pain
N:NPK	grams of nitrogen to non-protein kilocalories
NNR	not necessary to return
NNRTI	non-nucleoside reverse transcriptase inhibitor
NNS	neonatal screen (hematocrit, total bilirubin, and total protein)
	nicotine nasal spray
	non-nutritive sucking
	number needed to screen
NNT	number needed to treat
NNTB	number needed to treat to benefit
NNTB/NNTH	number needed to treat, benefit-to-harm ratio
NNTH	number needed to treat to harm
NNU	net nitrogen utilization
NNWT	noncontact normothermic wound therapy
NO	nasal oxygen
	nitric oxide
	nitroglycerin ointment
	none obtained
	nonobese
	number (no.)
	nursing office
NO_2	nitrogen dioxide
N_2O	nitrous oxide
NOA	nonobstructive azoospermia

N

NOAA	National Oceanic and Atmospheric Administration
NOAE	nonoccupational asbestos exposures
NOAEL	no observed adverse effect level
N_2O:O_2	nitrous oxide to oxygen ratio
NOC	nonorgan-confined
	Nursing Outcome Classification
noc.	night
noct	nocturnal
NOD	nonobese diabetic
	notice of disagreement
	notify of death
NOE	naso-orbitoethmoid
NOED	no observed effect dose
NOEL	no observable effect level
NOF	National Osteoporosis Foundation (treatment criteria)
	nonossifying fibroma
NOFT	nonorganic failure to thrive
NOFTT	nonorganic failure to thrive
NOGM	nonoxidative glucose metabolism
NOH	neurogenic orthostatic hypotension
NOI	nature of illness
NOK	next of kin
NOL	not on label
NOM	nonoperative management
	nonsuppurative otitis media
NOMI	nonocclusive mesenteric infarction
NOMID	neonatal-onset multisystem inflammatory disease
NOMS	not on my shift
NO/N_2	nitric oxide; nitrogen
NONMEM	nonlinear mixed-effects model (modeling)
non pal	not palpable
NonPARs	Nonparticipating Physicians (Medicare)
non-REM	nonrapid eye movement (sleep)
non rep	do not repeat
NON VIZ	not visualized
NOOB	not out of bed
NOP	not on patient
NOR	norethynodrel
	normal
	nortriptyline
NOR-EPI	norepinephrine (Levophed)
norm	normal
NOS	neonatal opium solution (diluted deodorized tincture of opium)
	new-onset seizures
	nitric oxide synthase
	no organisms seen
	not on staff
	not otherwise specified
NOS3	nitric oxide synthase, type 3
NOSI	nitric oxide synthase inhibitors
NOSIE	Nurse's Observation Scale (Schedule) for Inpatient Evaluation
NOSPECS	categories for classifying eye changes in Graves ophthalmopathy: **n**o signs or symptoms, **o**nly signs, **s**oft tissue involvement with symptoms and signs, **p**roptosis, **e**xtraocular muscle involvement, **c**orneal involvement, and **s**ight loss (visual acuity)
NOT	nocturnal oxygen therapy
NOTT	nocturnal oxygen therapy trial
NOU	not on unit
NOV	Novartis
NoV	Norovirus
NOV 70/30	human insulin, regular 30 units/mL with human insulin isophane suspension 70 units/mL (Novolin 70/30)
NOV L	human insulin zinc suspension (Novolin L)
NOV N	human insulin isophane suspension (Novolin N)
NOV R	human insulin regular (Novolin R)
NP	nasal polyps
	nasal prongs
	nasopharyngeal
	near point
	neuropathic pain
	neurophysin
	neuropsychiatric
	neutrogenic precautions
	newly presented
	nonpalpable
	no pain
	not performed
	not pregnant
	not present
	nuclear pharmacist
	nuclear pharmacy
	nursed poorly
	nurse practitioner
NPA	nasal pharyngeal airway
	nasopharyngeal aspirate
	near point of accommodation
	no previous admission
NPAT	nonparoxysmal atrial tachycardia
NPBC	node-positive breast cancer
NPBCC	nonpigmented basal cell carcinoma
NPC	nasopharyngeal carcinoma
	near-point convergence
	Niemann-Pick disease Type C (sphingomyelin lipidosis)
	nodal premature contractions
	nonpatient contact
	nonproductive cough
	nonprotein calorie
	no prenatal care

N

no previous complaint(s)

NP-C Nurse Practitioner, Certified

NPCC nonprotein carbohydrate calories

NPCPAP nasopharyngeal continuous positive airway pressure

NPD narcissistic personality disorder
Niemann-Pick disease
nonpolarized (contact) dermoscopy
nonprescription drugs
no pathological diagnosis

NPDL nodular poorly differentiated lymphocytic

NPDR nonproliferative diabetic retinopathy

NPE neurogenic pulmonary edema
neuropsychologic examination
no palpable enlargement
normal pelvic examination

NPEM nocturnal penile erection monitoring

NPF nasopharyngeal fiberscope
no predisposing factor

N-PFMSO$_4$ nebulized preservative-free morphine sulfate (This is a dangerous abbreviation)

NPFS nonpenetrating filtering surgery

NPG nonpregnant
normal-pressure glaucoma

NPH isophane insulin (neutral protamine Hagedorn)
no previous history
normal-pressure hydrocephalus

NPhx nasopharynx

NPI National Provider Identifier
Neuropsychiatric Inventory
no present illness
Nottingham Prognostic Index

NPIS Numeric Pain Intensity Scale

NPJT nonparoxysmal junctional tachycardia

NPL insulin lispro protamine suspension

component neural protamine lispro (insulin)

NPLSM neoplasm

NPK nonprotein kilocalories

NPM nothing per mouth

NPN nonprotein nitrogen

NPNC no prenatal care

NPNT nonpalpable, nontender

n.p.o. nothing by mouth

NPOC nonpurgeable organic carbon

NPOD Neuropsychiatric Officer of the Day

NPP nonphysician practitioner
normal postpartum
Nurse Practitioner, Psychiatric

NPPE negative-pressure pulmonary edema

NPPI nonpeptidic protease inhibitor

NPPNG nonpenicillinase-producing *Neisseria gonorrhoeae*

NPPV noninvasive positive-pressure ventilation

NPR normal pulse rate
nothing per rectum

NPRL normal pupillary reaction to light

NPRM Notice of Proposed Rulemaking

NPRS numerical pain rating scale

NPS nasopharyngoscopy
National Pharmaceutical Stockpile
neuropsychiatric symptoms
new patient set-up

NPSA nonphysician surgical assistant

NPSD nonpotassium-sparing diuretics

NPSF National Patient Safety Foundation

NPSG National Patient Safety Goal
nocturnal polysomnography

NPSLE neuropsychiatric systemic lupus erythematosus

NPT near-patient tests
neopyrithiamin hydrochloride
nocturnal penile tumescence
no prior tracings
normal pressure and temperature

NPU net protein utilization

NPV negative predictive value
nothing per vagina

NPWT negative pressure wound therapy

NPY neuropeptide Y

NPZ neuropsychologic text z

NQECN nonqueratinizing epidermoid carcinoma

NQMI non-Q wave myocardial infarction

NQR not quite right (slang)

NQT narrow QRS complex tachycardia

NQW non-Q-wave

NQWMI non-Q wave myocardial infarction

NR do not repeat
newly reformulated
none reported
nonreactive
nonrebreathing
nonresponder
no refills
no report
no response
no return
normal range
normal reaction
not reached
not reacting
not remarkable
not resolved
number

NRAF nonrheumatic atrial fibrillation

NRB Noninstitutional Review Board
nonrebreather (oxygen mask)

NRBC normal red blood cell
nucleated red blood cell

NRBS nonrebreathing system

NRC National Research Council
normal retinal correspondence

	Nuclear Regulatory Commission
NREH	normal renin essential hypertension
NREM	nonrapid eye movement
NREMS	nonrapid eye movement sleep
NREMT-P	National Registry of Emergency Medical Technicians–Paramedic level
NRF	normal renal function
NRFHT	nonreasurring fetal heart rate
NRI	nerve root involvement
	nerve root irritation
	no recent illnesses
	norepinephrine reuptake inhibitor
NRL	natural rubber latex
N-RLX	nonrelaxed
NRM	nonrebreathing mask
	no regular medicines
	normal range of motion
	normal retinal movement
NRN	no return necessary
NRNST	nonreassuring-nonstress test
NRO	neurology
NROM	normal range of motion
NRP	neonatal resuscitation program
	nonreassuring patterns
NRPR	nonbreathing pressure relieving
NRR	net reproduction rate
NRS	Neurobehavioral Rating Scale
NRSs	nonrandomized studies
NRT	neuromuscular reeducation techniques
	nicotine-replacement therapy
NRTI	nucleoside reverse transcriptase inhibitor
NRTs	nitron radical traps
NS	nephrotic syndrome
	neurological signs
	neurosurgery
	never-smokers
	nipple stimulation
	nodular sclerosis
	no-show
	nonsmoker
	normal saline solution (0.9% sodium chloride solution)
	normospermic
	no sample
	not seen
	not significant
	nuclear sclerosis
	nursing service
	nutritive sucking
	nylon suture
NSA	neck-shaft angle
	normal serum albumin (albumin, human)
	no salt added
	no significant abnormalities
	number of signals averaged (radiology)
NSAA	nonsteroidal antiandrogen
NSABP	National Surgical Adjuvant Breast Project
NSAD	no signs of acute disease
NSAIA	nonsteroidal anti-inflammatory agent
NSAID	nonsteroidal anti-inflammatory drug
NSAP	nonspecific abdominal pain
NSBGP	nonspecific bowel gas pattern
NSC	neural stem cells
	no significant change
	nonservice-connected
NSCC	nonsmall cell carcinoma
NSCD	nonservice-connected disability
NSCFPT	no significant change from previous tracing
NSCIDRC	National Spinal Cord Injury Data Research Center
NSCLC	nonsmall-cell–lung cancer
NSCST	nipple stimulation contraction stress test
NSD	nasal septal deviation
	nominal standard dose
	nonstructural deterioration
	normal spontaneous delivery
	no significant disease (difference, defect, deviation)
NSDA	nonsteroid dependent asthmatic
NSDU	neonatal stepdown unit
NSE	neuron-specific enolase
	normal saline enema (0.9% sodium chloride)
N s E	nausea without emesis
NSEACS	non-ST-elevation acute coronary syndromes
NSF	nephrogenic systemic fibrosis
	no significant findings
NSFTD	normal spontaneous full-term delivery
NSG	nursing
NSGCT	nonseminomatous germ-cell tumors
NSGCTT	nonseminomatous germ-cell tumor of the testis
NSGI	nonspecific genital infection
NSGT	nonseminomatous germ-cell tumor
NSHC	no-self-harm contract
NSHD	nodular sclerosing Hodgkin disease
NSHL	nonsyndromic hearing loss
NSI	needlestick injury
	negative self-image
	no signs of infection
	no signs of inflammation
NSICU	neurosurgery intensive care unit
NSILA	nonsuppressible insulin-like activity
NSIP	nonspecific interstitial pneumonia
NSLRP	nerve-sparing laparoscopic radical prostatectomy

NSMMVT nonsustained monomorphic ventricular tachycardia
NSN Neo-Synephrine
nephrotoxic serum nephritis
NSNSAIDs nonselective nonsteroidal anti-inflammatory drugs
NSO Neosporin® ointment
NSOM near field scanning optical microscope
NSOP no soft organs palpable
NSP neck and shoulder pain
NSPs needle and syringe exchange programs
nonstarch polysaccharides
NSPVT nonsustained polymorphic ventricular tachycardia
NSR nasoseptal repair
nonspecific reaction
normal sinus rhythm
not seen regularly
NSRP nerve-sparing radical prostatectomy
NSS nephron-sparing surgery
neurological signs stable
neuropathy symptom score
normal size and shape
not statistically significant
nutritional support service
sodium chloride 0.9% (normal saline solution)
1/2 NSS sodium chloride 0.45% (1/2 normal saline solution)
NSSC normal size, shape and consistency (uterus)
NSSL normal size, shape, and location
NSSP normal size, shape, and position
NSSTT nonspecific ST and T-wave
NSST-TWCs nonspecific ST-T wave changes
NST nonmyeloablative stem-cell transplant
Nonsense Syllable Test
nonstress test
normal sphincter tone
not sooner than
nutritional support team
NSTD nonsexually transmitted disease
NSTE non-ST segment elevation
NSTE-ACS non-ST-elevation acute coronary syndrome
NSTEMI non-ST-segment elevation myocardial infarction
NSTGCT nonseminomatous testicular germ cell tumor
NSTI necrotizing soft-tissue infection
NSTT nonseminomatous testicular tumors
NSU neurosurgical unit
nonspecific urethritis
NSV nonspecific vaginitis
NSVD nonstructural valve deterioration
normal spontaneous vaginal delivery
NSVT nonsustained ventricular tachycardia
NSX neurosurgical examination
NSY nursery
NT nasotracheal
next time
Nordic Track®
normal temperature
normotensive
nortriptyline
not tender
not tested
nourishment taken
numbness and tingling
nursing technician
N&T nose and throat
numbness and tingling
N Tachy nodal tachycardia
NT-ANP N-terminal atrial natriuretic peptide
NTBR not to be resuscitated
NTC neurotrauma center
NTCS no tumor cells seen
NTD negative to date
neural-tube defects
nitroblue tetrazolium dye (test)
NTE neutral thermal environment
not to exceed
NTED neonatal toxic-shock-syndrome-like exanthematous disease
NTF neurotrophic factor
normal throat flora
NTG nitroglycerin
nontoxic goiter
nontreatment group
normal tension glaucoma
NTGO nitroglycerin ointment
NTI narrow therapeutic index
no treatment indicated
NTIS National Technical Information Service (U.S. Department of Commerce)
NTL nectar-thick liquid (diet consistency)
nortriptyline (Aventyl; Pamelor)
no time limit
NTLE neocortical temporal-lobe epilepsy
NTM nocturnal tumescence monitor
nontuberculous mycobacterium
NTMB nontuberculous myobacteria
NTMI nontransmural myocardial infarction
NTND not tender, not distended
NTP narcotic treatment program
National Toxicology Program
Nitropaste® (nitroglycerin ointment)
nonthrombocytopenic preterm (infant)
normal temperature and pressure

	sodium nitroprusside
NTPD	nocturnal tidal peritoneal dialysis
NTPR	National Transplantation Pregnancy Registry
NT-proBNP	N-terminal pro-brain natriuretic peptide
NTS	nasotracheal suction
	nicotine transdermal system
	nontyphoidal salmonellae
	nucleus tractus solitarii
NTSCI	nontraumatic spinal cord injury
NTT	nasotracheal tube
	near-total thyroidectomy
	nonthrombocytopenic term (infant)
	nontreponemal test
NTTP	no tenderness to palpation
NTU	nephelometric turbidity units
NTX	naltrexone (ReVia)
	neurotoxicity
Ntx	N-telopeptide
NTZ	nitazoxanide (Alinia)
NTZ Long-acting®	oxymetazoline nasal spray
NU	name unknown
NUD	nonulcer dyspepsia
NUG	necrotizing ulcerative gingivitis
nullip	nullipara
NUN	nonurea nitrogen
NV	naked vision
	nausea and vomiting
	near vision
	negative variation
	neovascularization
	neurovascular
	new vessel
	next visit
	nonvenereal
	nonveteran
	normal value
	not vaccinated
	not verified
N&V	nausea and vomiting
NVA	near visual acuity
NVAF	nonvalvular atrial fibrillation
NVB	Navelbine (vinorelbine tartrate)
	neurovascular bundle
NVBo	oral vinorelbine
NVC	neurovascular checks
nvCJD	new-variant Creutzfeldt-Jakob disease
NVD	nausea, vomiting, and diarrhea
	neck vein distention
	neovascularization of the (optic) disc
	neurovesicle dysfunction
	normal vaginal delivery
	no venereal disease
	no venous distention
	nonvalvular disease
NVDC	nausea, vomiting, diarrhea, and constipation
NVE	native
	native valve endocarditis
	neovascularization elsewhere
NVG	neovascular glaucoma
	neoviridogrisein
NVI	neovascularization of the iris
NVL	neurovascular laboratory
NVLD	nonverbal learning disability
NVM	neovascular membrane
NVP	nausea and vomiting of pregnancy
	nevirapine (Viramune)
NVS	neurological vital signs
	neurovascular status
NVSS	normal variant short stature
NW	naked weight
	nasal wash
	normal weight
	not weighed
NWB	nonweight bearing
NWBL	nonweight bearing, left
NWBR	nonweight bearing, right
NWC	number of words chosen
NWD	neuroleptic withdrawal
	normal well developed
NWS	New World screwworm (*Cochliomyia hominivorax* [Coquerel])
NWTS	National Wilms Tumor Study (rating scale)
NWTSG	National Wilms Tumor Study Group
Nx	nephrectomy
	next
NX211	liposomal lurtotecan
NXG	necrobiotic xanthogranuloma
NXY-059	disufenton sodium (Cerovive)
NYB	New York Blood Center
NYD	not yet diagnosed
NYHA	New York Heart Association (classification of heart disease)
NYST	nystagmus
NZ	enzyme

N

O

O eye
objective findings
obvious
occlusal
often
open
oral
ortho
O sign; a patient whose mouth is open when unconscious (slang)
other
oxygen
pint
zero

ō negative
no
none
pint
without

O+ blood type O positive (O positive is preferred)

O− blood type O negative (O negative is preferred)

Ⓞ orally (by mouth)

$_1O_2$ singlet oxygen

O_2 both eyes
oxygen

O_2^- superoxide

O_3 ozone

O157 *Escherichia coli* O157

OA occipital artery
occipitoatlantal
occiput anterior
old age
on admission
on arrival
ophthalmic artery
oral airway
oral alimentation
osteoarthritis
ovarian ablation
Overeaters Anonymous

O/A on or about

O & A observation and assessment
odontectomy and alveoloplasty

OAA Old Age Assistance

OAA/S Observer's Assessment of Alertness/Sedation

OAB overactive bladder

OAC omeprazole, amoxicillin, and clarithromycin
oral anticoagulant(s)
overaction

OAD obliterative airway disease
obstructive airway disease
occlusive arterial disease
overall diameter

OAE otoacoustic emissions

OAF oral anal fistula
osteoclast activating factor

OAG open angle glaucoma

OAM omeprazole, amoxicillin, and metronidazole

OAMER over-active milk ejection reflex

OA/OS ovarian ablation/suppression

OAP old age pension
over-anxious patient

OAR Ottawa Ankle Rules

OARs organs at risk (from radiation therapy)

OAS Older Adult Services
oral allergy syndrome
organic anxiety syndrome
outpatient assessment service
overall survival
Overt Aggression Scale

OASDHI Old Age, Survivors, Disability, and Health Insurance

OASI Old Age and Survivors Insurance

OASIS Outcomes and Assessment Information Set

OASO overactive superior oblique

OASR overactive superior rectus

OASS Overt Agitation Severity Scale

OAT oligoasthenoteratozoospermia
oral anticoagulant therapy
ornithine aminotransferase

OATP organic anion-transporting polypeptide

OATS osteochondral autograft transfer system

OAV oculoauriculovertebral (dysplasia)

OAW oral airway

OB obese
obesity
obstetrics
occult blood
osteoblast

OBA office-based anesthesia
Office of Biotechnology Activities (NIH)

OB-A obstetrics-aborted

OBD obscure digestive bleeding
optimal biologic dose

OB-Del obstetrics-delivered

OBE out-of-body experience

OBE-CALP placebo capsule or tablet

OBF ocular blood flow

OBG obstetrics and gynecology

Ob-Gyn obstetrics and gynecology

Obj	objective
obl	oblique
OB marg	obtuse marginal
OB-ND	obstetrics-not delivered
OBP	office blood pressure
OBR	optimized background regimen
OBRR	obstetric recovery room
OBS	observed
	obstetrical service
	organic brain syndrome
OBT	obtained
OBTM	omeprazole, bismuth subcitrate, tetracycline, and metronidazole
OBUS	obstetrical ultrasound
OBW	open bed warmer
OC	observed cases
	obstetrical conjugate
	occlusal curvature (dental)
	office call
	on call
	only child
	open cholecystectomy
	open colectomy
	open crib
	optical chromatography
	oral care
	oral contraceptive
	osteocalcin
	osteoclast
	ovarian cancer
	OxyContin (oxycodone)
O & C	onset and course
OCA	oculocutaneous albinism
	open care area
	oral contraceptive agent
OCAD	occlusive carotid artery disease
OCB	obstructive chronic bronchitis
OCBZ	oxcarbazepine(Trileptal)
OCC	occasionally
	occlusal
	old chart called
OCCC	open chest cardiac compression
	ovarian clear cell carcinoma
occl	occlusion
OCCM	open chest cardiac massage
OCC PR	open chest cardiopulmonary resuscitation
OCC Th	occupational therapy
Occup Rx	occupational therapy
OCD	obsessive-compulsive disorder
	osteochondritis dissecans
OCE	outpatient code editor
OCG	oral cholecystogram
OCI	Obsessive-Compulsive Inventory
OCJ	osteochondral junction
OCL®	oral colonic lavage
OCME	Office of the Chief Medical Examiner
OCN	obsessive-compulsive neurosis
	Oncology Certified Nurse
OCNS	Obsessive-Compulsive Neurosis Scale
O-CNV	occult choroidal neovascularization
OCOR	on-call to operating room
OCP	ocular cicatricial pemphigoid
	oral contraceptive pills
	ova, cysts, parasites
OCR	oculocephalic reflex
	optical character recognition
OCS	Obsessive-Compulsive Scale
	Office of Child Services (government agency)
	oral cancer screening
11-OCS	11-oxycorticosteroid
OCT	octreotide (Sandostatin)
	optical coherence tomograph (tomography)
	oral cavity tumors
	ornithine carbamyl transferase
	oxytocin challenge test
OCU	observation care unit
OCVM	occult cerebrovascular malformations
OCX	oral cancer examination
OD	Doctor of Optometry
	Officer-of-the-Day
	oligodendroglial
	once daily (this is a dangerous abbreviation as it is read as right eye; use "once daily")
	on duty
	optic disc
	oral-duodenal
	outdoor
	outside diameter
	ovarian dysgerminoma
	overdose
	right eye
Δ OD 450	deviation of optical density at 450
ODA	occipitodextra anterior
	once-daily aminoglycoside
	osmotic driving agent
ODAC	Oncologic Drugs Advisory Committee (of the US Food and Drug Administration)
	on-demand analgesia computer
ODAT	one day at a time
ODC	oral disease control
	ornithine decarboxylase
	outpatient diagnostic center
ODCH	ordinary diseases of childhood
ODCs	ozone-depleting chemicals
ODD	oculodentodigital (dysplasia)
	oppositional defiance disorder
OD'd	overdosed
ODE	optic disc edema

O

ODECL open-door expansile cervical laminoplasty
ODed overdosed
ODI Oswestry Disability Index
  oxygen desaturation index
ODM occlusion dose monitor
  ophthalmodynamometry
ODMP on-going data management plan
ODN optokinetic nystagmus
ODP occipitodextra posterior
  offspring of diabetic parents
OD/P right eye patched
ODQ on direct questioning
ODS Office of Drug Safety (FDA)
  organized delivery system
  osmotic demyelination syndrome
ODSS Office of Disability Support Services
ODSU oncology day stay unit
  One-Day Surgery Unit
ODT occipitodextra transerve
  optical Doppler tomography
  orally disintegrating tablet
ODTS organic dust toxic syndrome
OE on examination
  orthopedic examination
  otitis externa
O-E standard observed minus expected
O&E observation and examination
OEC outer ear canal
OECD Organization for Economic Cooperation and Development
OECs olfactory ensheathing cells
OEI opioid escalation index
O_2EI oxygen extraction index
OEL occupational exposure level
OENT oral endotracheal tube
OEP Office of Emergency Preparedness
  oil of evening primrose (evening primrose oil)
OEPA vincristine (Oncovin), etoposide, prednisone, and doxorubicin (Adriamycin)
OER oxygen extraction ratios
O_2ER oxygen extraction ratio
OERR order entry/results-reports (Veterans Administration's physician computer order entry system)
OET oral esophageal tube
OETT oral endotracheal tube
OF occipital-frontal
  optic fundi
  osteitis fibrosa
  outlet forceps (delivery)
OFC occipital-frontal circumference
  orbitofacial cleft
  osteitis fibrosa cystica
OFF shoes off during weighing
OFFD organ-failure-free days
OFG orofacial granulomatosis
OFI other febrile illness
OFLOX ofloxacin (Floxin)
OFLX ofloxacin (Floxin)
OFM open-face mask
  oral focal mucinosis
OFNE oxygenated fluorocarbon nutrient emulsion
OFPF optic fundi and peripheral fields
OFR oxygen-free radicals
OFRs ocular following responses
OFS osteoplastic frontal sinusotomy
OFTT organic failure to thrive
OG Obstetrics-Gynecology
  orogastric (feeding)
  outcome goal (long-term goal)
OGC oculogyric crisis
OGCT ovarian germ cell tumor
OGD oesophagogastro-duodenoscopy (United Kingdom and other countries)
  Office of Generic Drugs (of the Food and Drug Administration)
OGIB obscure gastrointestinal bleeding
OGNP Obstetric-Gynecology Nurse Practitioner
OGT orogastric tube
OGTT oral glucose tolerance test
OH occupational history
  ocular history
  ocular hypertension
  on hand
  open-heart
  oral hygiene
  orthostatic hypotension
  outside hospital
−OH hydroxyl
17-OH 17-hydroxycorticosteroids
OHA oral hypoglycemic agents
OHC outer hair cell (in cochlea)
OH Cbl hydroxycobalamine
17-OHCS 17-hydroxycorticosteroids
OHD hydroxy vitamin D
  organic heart disease
25(OH)D 25-hydroxyvitamin D
25(OH)D_3 25-hydroxyvitamin D (calcifediol, Calderol)
OHF old healed fracture
  Omsk hemorrhagic fever
  overhead frame
OHFA hydroxy fatty acid
OHFT overhead frame and trapeze
OHG oral hypoglycemic
OHI oral hygiene instructions
  other health impairment
OHIAA hydroxyindolacetic acid
OHL oral hairy leukoplakia

7-OHMTX 7-hydroxymethotrexate
OHNS Otolaryngology, Head, and Neck Surgery (Dept.)
OHP obese hypertensive patient
oxygen under hyperbaric pressure
17 OHP 17-hydroxyprogesterone
OHRP Office for Human Research Protections (Department of Health Human Services)
open-heart rehabilitation program
OHR-QOL oral health-related quality of life
OHRR open-heart recovery room
OHS obesity hypoventilation syndrome
occupational health service
ocular histoplasmosis syndrome
ocular hypoperfusion syndrome
open-heart surgery
OHSS ovarian hyperstimulation syndrome
OHT ocular hypertension
overhead trapeze
OHTN ocular hypertension
OHTx orthotopic heart transplantation
OI opportunistic infection
osteogenesis imperfecta
otitis interna
OIC opioid-induced constipation
OICD occupational irritant contact dermatitis
OIF oil-immersion field
OIG Office of the Inspector General
OIH orthoiodohippurate
OIHA orthoiodohippuric acid
OI&I occupational injury and illness
OIM optical immunoassay
OINT ointment
OIR oxygen-induced retinopathy
OIRDA occipital intermittent rhythmical delta activity
OIS ocular ischemic syndrome
optical intrinsic signal (imaging)
optimum information size
OIs opportunistic infections
OIT ovarian immature teratoma
OIU optical internal urethrotomy
OJ orange juice (this is a dangerous abbreviation as it is read as OS, left eye)
orthoplast jacket
OK all right
approved
correct
OKAN optokinetic after nystagmus
OKC odontogenic keratocyst
open kinetic chain
OKN optokinetic nystagmus
OKT Ortho Kung T-cell, designation for a series of antigens
OL left eye
open label (study)
OLA occiput left anterior
occipitolaevoanterior
OLAP online analytical processing
OLB open-liver biopsy
open-lung biopsy
OLBPQ Oswestry Low Back Pain Questionnaire
OLC ouabain-like compound
OLD obstructive lung disease
OLE olive leaf extract
OLF ouabain-like factor
OLM ocular larva migrans
ophthalmic laser microendoscope
OLNM occult lymph node metastases
OLP oral lichen planus
OLR optic labyrinthine righting
otology, laryngology, and rhinology
OLRM ordinary linear regression model
OLS ordinary least squares
ouabain-like substance
OLT occipitolaevoposterior
orthotopic liver transplantation
OLTP online transaction processing
OLTx orthotopic liver transplantation
OLV one-lung ventilation
OLZ olanzapine (Zyprexa)
OM every morning (this is a dangerous abbreviation)
obtuse marginal
ocular melanoma
oral motor
oral mucositis
organomegaly
osteomalacia
osteomyelitis
otitis media
O_2M oxygen mask
OM_1 first obtuse marginal (branch)
OM_2 second obtuse marginal (branch)
OMA older maternal age
OMAC otitis media, acute, catarrhal
OMAS Olerud-Molander Ankle Score
otitis media, acute, suppurating
OMB obtuse marginal branch
Office of Management and Budget
OMB_1 first obtuse marginal branch (of the circumflex coronary artery)
OMB_2 second obtuse marginal branch (of the circumflex coronary artery)
OMC open mitral commissuortomy
ostiomeatal complex
OMCA otitis media, catarrhalis, acute
OMCC otitis media, catarrhalis, chronic
OMD organic mental disorder
OME Office of Medical Examiner
otitis media with effusion
7-OMEN menogaril

OMFS oral and maxillofacial surgery
OMG ocular myasthenia gravis
OMI old myocardial infarct
OMIEI oral medication induced esophageal injury
OMP oculomotor (third nerve) palsy
open mediastinal biopsy
OMPA otitis media, purulent, acute
OMPC otitis media, purulent, chronic
OMR operative mortality rate
OMS oral morphine sulfate
organic mental syndrome
organic mood syndrome
OMSA otitis media secretory (or suppurative) acute
OMSC otitis media secretory (or suppurative) chronic
OMT oral mucosal transudate
Osteopathic manipulative technique (treatment)
OMVC open mitral valve commissurotomy
OMVD optimized microvessel density (analysis)
OMVI operating motor vehicle intoxicated
ON every night (this is a dangerous abbreviation)
optic nerve
optic neurophathy
oronasal
Ortho-Novum®
overnight
ONB olfactory neuroblastoma
ONC Orthopedic Nurse, Certified
over-the-needle catheter
vincristine (Oncovin)
OND Office of New Drugs (FDA)
ondansetron (Zofran)
other neurologic disorder(s)
ONH optic nerve head
optic nerve hypoplasia
ONJ osteonecrosis of the jaw
ONM ocular neuromyotonia
ON RR overnight recovery room
ONS Office for National Statistics (United Kingdom)
ONSD optic nerve sheath decompression
ONSF optic nerve sheath fenestration
ONTD open neural tube defect(s)
ONTR orders not to resuscitate
OO ophthalmic ointment
oral order
out of
o/o on account of
O&O off and on
OOB out of bed
OOBL out of bilirubin light
OOBBRP out of bed with bathroom privileges
OOC onset of contractions
out of cast
out of control
OO Con out of control
OOD outer orbital diameter
out of doors
OO-EMG electromyographic recording of the orbicularis oculi muscles
OOF out of facility
OOH out of hospital
OOH&NS ophthalmology, otorhinolaryngology, and head and neck surgery
OOI out of isolette
OOL onset of labor
OOLR ophthalmology, otology, laryngology, and rhinology
OOM onset of menarche
OOP out of pelvis
out of plaster
out on pass
OOPD Office of Orphan Product Development (FDA)
OOPS out of program status
OOR out of room
OORW out of radiant warmer
OOS out of sequence
out of specification (deviation from standard)
out of splint
out of stock
OOT out of town
OOW out of wedlock
out of work
OP oblique presentation
occiput posterior
open
operation
organophosphorous
oropharynx
oscillatory potentials
osteoporosis
outpatient
overpressure
O&P ova and parasites (stool examination)
OPA Office of the Public Advocate (guardians)
oral pharyngeal airway
outpatient anesthesia
OPAC opacity (opacification)
OPAT outpatient parenteral antibiotic therapy
OPB outpatient basis
OPC operable pancreatic carcinoma
oropharyngeal candidiasis
outpatient care
outpatient catheterization
outpatient clinic
OPCA olivopontocerebellar atrophy

O

OPCAB off-pump coronary artery bypass (grafting)
op cit in the work cited
OPCs oligodendrocyte precursor cells
OPCS-4 Classification of Surgical Operations and Procedures (4th revision)
OPCx oligodendrocyte progenitor cells
OPD oropharyngeal dysphagia
Orphan Products Development (office of)
outpatient department
O′p′-DDD mitotane (Lysodren)
OPDRA Office of Postmarketing Drug Risk Assessment (FDA) (name changed to Office of Drug Safety [ODS])
OPDUR on-line prospective drug utilization review
OPE oral peripheral examination
outpatient evaluation
OPEN vincristine (Oncovin), prednisone, etoposide, and mitoxantrone (Novantrone)
OPERA outpatient endometrial resection/ablation
OPG ocular plethysmography
orthopantomogram (dental)
osteoprotegerin
OPIDP organophosphate-induced delayed polyneuropathy
OPK ovulation predictor kit
OPKA opsonophagocytic killing assay
OPL oral premalignant lesion
other party liability
OPLC optimum performance liquid chromatography
OPLL ossification of the posterior longitudinal ligament
OPM occult primary malignancy
oral and pharyngeal mucositis
OPMD oculopharyngeal muscular dystrophy
OPN open partial nephrectomy
osteopontin
OPO organ procurement organizations
overnight pulse oximetry
OPOC oral pharynx, oral cavity
OPP opposite
OPPG oculopneumoplethysmography
OPPOS opposition
OPPS Outpatient Prospective Payment System
OPQRST onset, provocation, quality, radiation, severity, and time (an EMT mnemonic used in initial patient questioning)
OPRDU outpatient renal dialysis unit
OPRT orotate phosphoribosyl transferase
OPS Objective Pain Scores
operations
orange palpebral spots
Orpington prognostic scale
orthogonal polarization spectral (imaging)
outpatient surgery
overnight polysomnography
OPSI overwhelming postsplenectomy infection
OPSU oblique partial sit-up
outpatient surgical unit
O PSY open psychiatry
OPT optimal pharmacological therapy
optimum
outpatient treatment
OPT c CA Ohio pediatric tent with compressed air
OPT c O_2 Ohio pediatric tent with oxygen
OPTN Organ Procurement and Transplantation Network
OPT-NSC outpatient treatment, nonservice-connected
OPT-SC outpatient treatment, service-connected
OPTX occult pneumothorax
OPV oral polio vaccine
outpatient visit
OR odds ratio
oil retention
open reduction
operating room
Orthodox
own recognizance
ORA occiput right anterior
ORC outpatient rehabilitation centers
ORCH orchiectomy
ORD orderly
OREF open reduction, external fixation
ORF open reading frame
OR&F open reduction and fixation
ORIF open reduction internal fixation
ORL oblique retinacular ligament
otorhinolaryngology (otology, rhinology and laryngology)
ORMF open reduction metallic fixation
ORN operating room nurse
osteoradionecrosis
OROS ostomotic release oral system
ORP occiput right posterior
open radical prostatectomy
ORR overall response rate
ORS oculorespiratory syndrome
olfactory reference syndrome
oral rehydration salts
ORSA oxacillin-resistant *Staphylococcus aureus*
ORT oestrogen (estrogen)-replacement therapy (United Kingdom and elsewhere)

O

	operating room technician
	oral rehydration therapy
	Registered Occupational Therapist
OR X1	oriented to time
OR X2	oriented to time and place
OR X3	oriented to time, place, and person
OR X4	oriented to time, place, person, and objects (watch, pen, book)
OS	left eye
	mouth (this is a dangerous abbreviation as it is read as left eye)
	occipitosacral
	oligospermic
	opening snap
	open surgery
	ophthalmic solution (this is a dangerous abbreviation as it is read as left eye)
	oral surgery
	Osgood-Schlatter (disease)
	osmium
	osteosarcoma
	overall survival
OSA	obstructive sleep apnea
	off-site anesthesia
	online sexual activities
	osteosarcoma
OSA/HS	obstructive sleep apnea/ hypopnea syndrome
OSAS	obstructive sleep apnea syndrome
OSC	oral self-care
OSCAR	On-line Survey Certification and Reporting
OSCC	oral squamous cell carcinoma
OSCE	Objective Structured Clinical Examination
OSD	one-stop dispensing (United Kingdom)
	Osgood-Schlatter disease
	overseas duty
	overside drainage
OSE	ovarian surface epithelium
OSESC	opening-snap ejection systolic click
OSFM	oral saliva fertility monitoring
OSFT	outstretched fingertips
OSG	osteosonogram (osteosonogrammetry)
OSH	outside hospital
OSHA	Occupational Safety & Health Administration
O sign	a patient whose mouth is open when unconscious (slang)
OSM S	osmolarity serum
OSM U	osmolarity urine
OSN	off-service note
OSP	outside pass
OS/P	left eye patched
OSR	open septorhinoplasty
	open sigmoid resection
OSS	osseous
	over-shoulder strap
OSSI	orthognathic surgery simulating instrument
OSSN	ocular surface squamous neoplasia
OST	occipitosubtemporal
	optimal sampling theory
	osteogenic sarcoma
OT	occiput transverse
	Occupational Therapist
	occupational therapy
	old tuberculin
	on-treatment
	oral transmucosal
	orotracheal
	outlier threshold
	oxytocin (Pitocin)
O/T	oral temperature
OTA	open to air
OTC	occult tumor cell
	ornithine transcarbamoylase
	Orthopedic Technician, Certified
	over-the-counter (sold without prescription)
	oxytetracycline
OTCD	ornithine-transcarbamylase deficiency
OTD	optimal therapeutic dose
	organ tolerance dose
	out-the-door
OTE	(McMaster) Overall Treatment Evaluation
OTFC	oral transmucosal fentanyl citrate (Fentanyl Oralet; Actiq)
OTH	other
OTHS	occupational therapy home service
OTIS	Organization of Teratology Information Services
OTJ	on-the-job (injury; training)
OTO	one-time only
	otolaryngology
	otology
OTPT	oral triphasic tablets (contraceptive)
OTR	Occupational Therapist, Registered
OTRL	Occupational Therapist, Registered Licensed
OT/RT	occupational therapy/recreational therapy
OTS	orotracheal suction
OTT	oral transit time
	orotracheal tube
OTW	off-the-wall
OU	each eye
OUES	oxygen uptake efficiency slope
OULQ	outer upper left quadrant
OU/P	both eyes patched
OURQ	outer upper right quadrant

OUS	obstetric ultrasound
OV	office visit
	ovary
	ovum
OVAL	ovalocytes
OvCa	ovarian cancer
OVD	occlusal vertical dimension
	ophthalmic viscosurgical device
OVF	Octopus® visual field
OVLT	organum vasculosum of lamina terminalis
OVR	Office of Vocational Rehabilitation
OVS	obstructive voiding symptoms (syndrome)
OW	once weekly (this is a dangerous abbreviation)
	open wound
	oral warts
	outer wall
	out of wedlock
	ova weight
	overweight
O/W	oil in water (emulsion)
	otherwise
OWL	out of wedlock
OWNK	out of wedlock, not keeping (baby)
OWR	Osler-Weber-Rendu (disease)
OWT	zero work tolerance
OX	oximeter
O×1	oriented to time
O×2	oriented to time and place
O×3	oriented to time, place, and person
O×4	oriented to time, place, person, and objects (watch, pen, book)
OXA	oxacillinase
	oxaliplatin (Eloxatin)
OXC	oxcarbazepine (Trileptal)
Oxi	oximeter (oximetry)
Ox-LDL	oxidized low-density lipoprotein
OXPHOS	oxidative phosphorylation
OxPt	oxaliplatin (Eloxatin)
OXM	pulse oximeter
OXT	oxytocin (Pitocin)
Oxy-5®	benzoyl peroxide
OxyIR®	oxycodone immediate release capsules
OXZ	oxazepam (Serax)
OZ	optical zone
	ounce

P

P	Lasix (furosemide) as in vitamin P (slang)
	para
	peripheral
	phosphorus
	pint
	plan
	Plasmodium
	poor
	protein
	Protestant
	pulse
	pupil
P	statistical probability value
$\overline{p}$	after
/P	partial lower denture
P/	partial upper denture
P1	pilocarpine 1% ophthalmic solution
	postnatal day 1
	first phalanx
P_2	pulmonic second heart sound
P2	middle phalanx
	postnatal day 2
P3	distal phalanx
P20	Ocusert® P20
^{32}P	radioactive phosphorus
P40	Ocusert® P40
P53	tumor suppressive gene
PA	panic attack
	paranoid
	peanut allergy
	periapical (x-ray)
	pernicious anemia
	phenol alcohol
	physical activity
	Physician Assistant
	pineapple
	platelet aggregometry
	posterior-anterior (posteroanterior) (x-ray)
	premature adrenarche
	presents again
	primary aldosteronism
	prior approval
	professional association (similar to a corporation)
	Pseudomonas aeruginosa
	psychiatric aide
	psychoanalysis
	pulmonary artery
Pa	pascal
P&A	percussion and auscultation
	phenol and alcohol

position and alignment

$P_2 > A_2$ pulmonic second heart sound greater than aortic second heart sound

PAA pulmonary artery aneurysm

PAAA para-anastomotic aneurysm of the aorta

PAAD persistently and acutely disabled

PAB premature atrial beat
pulmonary artery banding

PABA aminobenzoic acid (para-aminobenzoic acid)

PABD preoperative autologous blood donation

PAC cisplatin (Platinol), doxorubicin (Adriamycin), and cylcophosphamide
phenacemide
Physical Assessment Center
Physician Assistant, Certified
picture archiving communication (system)
Port-a-cath®
premature atrial contraction
prophylactic anticonvulsants
pulmonary artery catheter

PA-C Physician Assistant, Certified

PACATH pulmonary artery catheter

PACE population-adjusted clinical epidemiology
Programs of All-Inclusive Care for the Elderly

PACG primary angle-closure glaucoma

PACH pipers to after coming head

PACI partial anterior cerebral infarct

$PACO_2$ partial pressure (tension) of carbon dioxide, alveolar

$PaCO_2$ partial pressure (tension) of carbon dioxide, artery

PACS picture archiving and communications systems

PACT prism and alternate cover test
Program of Assertive Community Treatment

PAC-V cisplatin (Platinol), doxorubicin (Adriamycin), and cyclophosphamide

PACU postanesthesia care unit

PAD pelvic adhesive disease
peripheral artery disease
persistently and acutely disabled
pharmacologic atrial defibrillator
physician-assisted death
preliminary anatomic diagnosis
preoperative autologous donation
primary affective disorder
pulmonary artery diastolic

PADCAB perfusion-assisted direct coronary artery bypass

PADP pulmonary arterial diastolic pressure
pulmonary artery diastolic pressure

PADS Post Anesthesia Discharge Scoring System

PADT primary androgen deprivation therapy

PAE percutaneous angiographic embolization
postanoxic encephalopathy
postantibiotic effect
pre-admission evaluation
progressive assistive exercise

PAEDP pulmonary artery and end-diastole pressure

PAEE physical activity energy expenditure

PAEF primary aortoenteric fistula

PAF paroxysmal atrial fibrillation
platelet-activating factor
population attributable fraction

PA&F percussion, auscultation, and fremitus

PAFE postantifungal effect

PAGA premature appropriate for gestational age

PAGE polyacrylamide gel electrophoresis

PAH para-aminohippurate
partial abdominal hysterectomy
phenylalanine hydroxylase
polycyclic aromatic hydrocarbons
polynuclear aromatic hydrocarbon
predicted adult height
primary adrenal hyperplasia
pulmonary arterial hypertension

PAHO Pan American Health Organization

PAI penetrating abdominal injury
plasminogen activator inhibitor
platelet accumulation index

PAIDS pediatric acquired immunodeficiency syndrome

PAIgG platelet-associated immunoglobulin G

PAIR Puncture, Aspiration, Injection, Reaspiration (technique)

PAIS Psychological Adjustment to Illness Scale

PAIVMs passive accessory intervertebral movements

PAIVS pulmonary atresia with intact ventricular septum

PAK p21-activated kinase
pancreas and kidney

PAL physical activity levels
posterior axillary line
posteroanterior and lateral
pyothorax-associated lymphoma

PALA N-phosphoacetate-L aspartate

Pa Line pulmonary artery line

PALN para-aortic lymph node

PALP palpation

P

PALS	pediatric advanced life support
	periarterial lymphatic sheath
PAM	partial allosteric modulators
	Payment Accuracy Measurement
	potential acuity meter
	primary acquired melanosis
	primary amebic meningoencephalitis
	protein A mimetic
2-PAM	pralidoxime (Protopam)
PAMP	pulmonary arterial (artery) mean pressure
PAN	pancreas
	pancreatic
	pancuronium (Pavulon)
	panoral x-ray examination
	periodic alternating nystagmus
	polyacrylonitrile (filter)
	polyarteritis nodosa
	polyomavirus-associated nephropathy
pANCA	perinuclear antineutrophil cytoplasmic antibody
PANDAS	pediatric autoimmune neuropsychiatric disorders associated with streptococcal infections
PANENDO	panendoscopy
PANESS	physical and neurological examination for soft signs
PanIN-1	pancreatic intraepithelial neoplasm (low grade); there is a 1A and 1B
PanIN-2	pancreatic intraepithelial neoplasm (moderate grade)
PanIN-3	pancreatic intraepithelial neoplasm (high grade)
PANP	pelvic autonomic nerve preservation
PANSS	Positive and Negative Syndrome Scale
PANSS-EC	Positive and Negative Symptoms of Schizophrenia-Excited Component
PAO	peak acid output
	peripheral arterial occlusion
PAO_2	alveolar oxygen pressure (tension)
PaO_2	arterial oxygen pressure (tension)
PAOD	peripheral arterial occlusive disease
PAOP	pulmonary artery occlusion pressure
PAP	passive-aggressive personality
	patient assistance program
	peroxidase-anti-peroxidase
	pokeweed antiviral protein
	positive airway pressure
	primary atypical pneumonia
	prostatic acid phosphatase
	pulmonary alveolar proteinosis
	pulmonary artery pressure
PAPAW	pushrim-activated power-assisted wheelchair
PAPm	mean pulmonary artery pressure
PAPS	primary antiphospholipid syndrome
Pap smear	Papanicolaou smear
PA/PS	pulmonary atresia/pulmonary stenosis
PAPVC	partial anomalous pulmonary venous connection
PAPVR	partial anomalous pulmonary venous return
PAQLQ	Pediatric Asthma Quality of Life Questionnaire
PAR	parafin
	parainfluenza (paramyxovirus) vaccine
	parallel
	participating (physician)
	perennial allergic rhinitis
	platelet aggregate ratio
	population attributable risks
	possible allergic reaction
	postanesthetic recovery
	procedures, alternatives, and risks
	pulmonary arteriolar resistance
PAR1	pseudoautosomal region 1
PARA	number of pregnancies producing viable offspring
	paraplegic
	parathyroid
PARA 1	having borne one child
Paraflu	Parainfluenza
PARC	perennial allergic rhinoconjunctivitis
PAROM	passive assistance range of motion
PARQ	procedures, risks, alternatives and questions
PARR	plasma aldosterone/renin activity ratio
	postanesthesia recovery room
PARS	postanesthesia recovery score
PARs	participating physicians (Medicare)
PART	para-aortic radiotherapy
PARU	postanesthetic recovery unit
PAS	aminosalicylic acid (para-aminosalicylic acid)
	perinatal arterial stroke
	periodic acid-Schiff (reagent)
	peripheral anterior synechia
	physician-assisted suicide
	pneumatic antiembolic stocking
	postanesthesia score
	postanesthetic shivering
	premature auricular systole
	Professional Activities Study
	pulmonary artery stenosis
	pulsatile antiembolism system (stockings)
PA-S	Physician Assistant, Student
PASA	aminosalicylic acid (para-aminosalicylic acid)
	proximal articular set angle

PAS-ADD Psychiatric Assessment Schedule for Adults with Developmental Disability
PASARR Preadmission Screening Assessment and Annual Resident Review
PASAT Paced Auditory Serial Addition Test
PA/S/D pulmonary artery systolic/diastolic
PASE pacing atrial stress echocardiography
Physical Activity Scale for the Elderly
Pas Ex passive exercise
PASG pneumatic antishock garment
PASI Psoriasis Area and Severity Index
PASI 75 at least 75% improvement in psoriasis area and severity index
PASK peripheral anterior stromal keratopathy
PASP pulmonary artery systolic pressure
PASS Pain Anxiety Symptoms Scale
PAT Paddington alcohol test
paroxysmal atrial tachycardia
passive alloimmune thrombocytopenia
patella
patient
percent acceleration time
peripheral arterial tone
platelet aggregation test
preadmission testing
pregnancy at term
process analytical technology
PATB pes anserinus tendonitis/bursitis
PATH Physicians at Teaching Hospitals (Medicare Audit)
pituitary adrenotropic hormone
pathology
PATP preadmission testing program
PATS payment at time of service
PAV Pavulon (pancuronium bromide)
pre-admission visit (hospice care initial home visit)
PAVe procarbazine, melphalan (Alkeran), and vinblastine (Velban)
PAVF pulmonary arteriovenous fistula
PAVM pulmonary arteriovenous malformation
PAVNRT paroxysmal atrial ventricular nodal re-entrant tachycardia
PAWP pulmonary artery wedge pressure
PAX periapical x-ray
PB barometric pressure
British Pharmacopeia
parafin bath
phenylbutyrate
piggyback
powder board
power building
premature beat
Presbyterian
protein-bound
Prussian blue
pudendal block
pyridostigmine bromide (Mestinon)
Pb lead
phenobarbital
p/b postburn
P&B pain and burning
Papanicolaou and breast (examinations)
phenobarbital and belladonna
PBA percutaneous bladder aspiration
pseudobulbar affect
PBAC Pharmaceutical Benefits Advisory Committee
PBAL protected bronchoalveolar lavage
PbB whole blood lead
PBC point of basal convergence
prebed care
primary biliary cirrhosis
PBCC pigmented basal cell carcinoma
PBD percutaneous biliary drainage
postburn day
proliferative breast disease
PBDE poly brominated diphenyl ether (flame retardant)
PBDs psychotic and behavioral disturbances
PBE partial breech extraction
population bioequivalence
power building exercise
PBF peripheral blood film
placental blood flow
pulmonary blood flow
PBFS penile blood flow study
PBG porphobilinogen
pressure breathing for G protection
pupillary block glaucoma
PBGD porphobilinogen deaminase
PBI partial breast irradiation
protein-bound iodine
PBK pseudophakic bullous keratopathy
PBL peripheral blood lymphocyte
primary breast lymphoma
primary brain lymphoma
problem-based learning
PBLC premature birth live child
PB-LC-EI-MS particle beam liquid chromatography-electron impact-mass spectrometry
PBM pancreaticobiliary maljunction
pharmacy benefit management (manager)
PBMA polybutylmethacrylate
PBMC peripheral blood mononuclear cell
PBMNC peripheral blood mononuclear cell

P

PBN polymyxin B sulfate, bacitracin, and neomycin
PB:ND problem: nursing diagnosis
PBNS percutaneous bladder neck stabilization
PBO placebo
PBP penicillin-binding protein
phantom breast pain
protein-bound polysaccharide
PBPC peripheral blood progenitor cell
PBPCT peripheral blood progenitor cell transplantation
PBPI penile-brachial pulse index
PBPK physiologically based pharmacokinetic
PBPs penicillin-binding proteins
PBS Pharmaceutical Benefit Scheme (lists all of the subsidized medicines available from the Australian Government)
phosphate-buffered saline
prune-belly syndrome
PBSC peripheral blood stem cells
PBT primary brain tumor
PBT_4 protein-bound thyroxine
$PbtO_2$ brain tissue partial pressure of oxygen
PBV percutaneous balloon valvuloplasty
PBZ phenoxybenzamine (Dibenzyline)
phenylbutazone
pyribenzamine
ΦBZ phenylbutazone
PC after meals (*p.c.* preferred)
cisplatin (Platinol) and cyclophosphamide
packed cells
paclitaxel; carboplatin
palliative care
pancreatic carcinoma
pathologic consultation
photocoagulation
placebo-controlled (study)
platelet concentrate
Pneumocystis carinii
poor condition
politically correct
popliteal cyst
posterior canals (vestibular)
posterior chamber
prednicarbate
premature contractions
present complaint
productive cough
professional corporation
psychiatric counselor
pubococcygeus (muscle)
p.c. after meals
PCA passive cutaneous anaphylaxis
patient care assistant (aide)
patient-controlled analgesia
penicillamine (Cuprimine)
pill count adherence
porous coated anatomic (joint replacement)
postcardiac arrest
postciliary artery
postconceptional age
posterior cerebral artery
posterior communicating artery
procainamide
procoagulation activity
prostate cancer
PCa prostate cancer
PCAC Physical Care Assessment Center
P-CAC preparative continuous annular chromatography
PCAD posterior circulation arterial dissection
PCASSO patient-centered access to secure systems online
PCB pancuronium bromide
para cervical block
placebo
postcoital bleeding
prepared childbirth
procarbazine (Matulane)
Pseudomonas cepacia bacteremia
PCBH personal care boarding home
PCBMN palmar cutaneous branch of the median nerve
PCBs polychlorinated biphenyls
PCBUN palmar cutaneous branch of the ulnar nerve
PCC patient care coordinator
petrous carotid canal
pheochromocytoma
pneumatosis cystoides coli
poison control center
precipitated calcium carbonate
progressive cardiac care
PCCC pediatric critical care center
PCCI penetrating craniocerebral injuries
PCCM primary care case management
pulmonary and critical care medicine
PCCP percutaneous compression plate
PCCU postcoronary care unit
PCD pacer-cardioverter-defibrillator
paroxysmal cerebral dysrhythmia
plasma cell dyscrasias
polarized contact dermoscopy
postmortem cesarean delivery
primary ciliary dyskinesia
programmed cell death
PCDAI Pediatric Crohn Disease Activity Index
PCE physical capacities evaluation

P

	potentially compensable event
	pseudophakic corneal edema
PCE®	erythromycin particles in tablets
PCEA	patient-controlled epidural analgesia
PCEAO	postcarotid endarterectomy airway obstruction
PCEC	purified chick embryo cell (culture)
PCECV	purified chick embryo cell vaccine
PCF	pharyngeal conjunctival fever
PCFL	primary cutaneous follicular lymphoma
PCFT	platelet complement fixation test
PCG	phonocardiogram
	plasma cell granuloma
	primary congenital glaucoma
	pubococcygeus (muscle)
PCGG	percutaneous coagulation of gasserian ganglion
PCGLV	poorly contractile globular left ventricle
PCG/Ts	Primary Care Groups and Trusts
PCH	paroxysmal cold hemoglobinuria
	periocular capillary hemangioma
	personal care home
PCHI	permanent childhood hearing impairment
PCHL	permanent childhood hearing loss
PC&HS	after meals and at bedtime
PCI	percutaneous coronary intervention
	pneumatosis cystoides intestinalis
	prophylactic cranial irradiation
PCINA	patient-controlled intranasal analgesia
PCIOL	posterior chamber intraocular lens
PC-IRV	pressure-controlled inverse-ratio ventilation
PCI-S	percutaneous coronary intervention with stenting
PCKD	polycystic kidney disease
PCL	pacing cycle length
	plasma cell leukemia
	posterior chamber lens
	posterior cruciate ligament
	proximal collateral ligament
PCLD	polycystic liver disease
PCLI	plasma cell labeling index
PCLN	psychiatric consultation liaison nurse
PCLR	paid claims loss ratio
PCLS	precision-cut lung slices
PCM	paracoccidioidomycosis
	pharmaceutical case management
	primary cutaneous melanoma
	protein-calorie malnutrition
	pubococcygeal muscle
PC-MRI	phase-contrast magnetic resonance imaging
PCMX	chloroxylenol
PCMZL	primary cutaneous marginal zone B-cell lymphoma
PCN	penicillin
	percutaneous nephrostomy
	primary care nursing
PCNA	patient care nursing assistant
	proliferating cell nuclear antigen
PCNL	percutaneous nephrostolithotomy
PCNs	posterior cervical nodes
PCNSL	primary central nervous system lymphoma
PCNT	percutaneous nephrostomy tube
PCO	patient complains of
	polycystic ovary
	posterior capsular opacification
PCO_2	partial pressure (tension) of carbon dioxide, artery
PCOD	polycystic ovarian disease
PCOE	prescriber (physician) computer order entry
P COMM A	posterior communicating artery
PCOS	polycystic ovary syndrome
PCP	Palliative Care Program
	pancytopenia
	patient care plan
	phencyclidine (phenylcyclohexyl piperidine)
	Pneumocystis carinii (jirovecii) pneumonia
	primary care person
	primary care physician
	primary care provider
	prochlorperazine (Compazine)
	pulmonary capillary pressure
PCPC	Pediatric Cerebral Performance Category (Scale)
PCPs	personal care products
PCR	patient care report
	percutaneous coronary revascularization
	polymerase chain reaction
	protein catabolic rate
PCr	plasma creatinine
pCR	pathological complete response
PCRA	pure red-cell aplasia
PCR/PSA	polymerase chain reaction analysis of prostate-specific antigen
PCS	patient care system
	patient-controlled sedation
	personal care service
	photon correlation spectroscopy
	physical component summary
	portable cervical spine
	portacaval shunt
	postconcussion syndrome
P c/s	primary cesarean section
PCSM	prostate cancer-specific mortality

PC-SPES an herbal refined powder preparation of eight medicinal plants

PCT parasite-clearance time
percent
photochemical treatment
poker chip tool (for rating pain)
porphyria cutanea tarda
postcoital test
posterior chest tube
Primary Care Trust (United Kingdom)
primary chemotherapy
progesterone challenge test

PCTA percutaneous transluminal angioplasty

PCTS patient-controlled transdermal system

PCU palliative care unit
primary care unit
progressive care unit
protective care unit

PCV packed cell volume
polycythemia vera
pressure-controlled ventilation
procarbazine, lomustine (CCNU [Cee Nu]), and vincristine

PCV 7 pneumococcal 7-valent conjugate vaccine (Prevnar)

PCV 23 pneumococcal vaccine polyvalent (Pneumovax 23; Pnu-Imune 23)

PCVC percutaneous central venous catheter

PCWP pulmonary capillary wedge pressure

PCX paracervical

PCXR portable chest radiograph

PCZ procarbazine (Matulane)
prochlorperazine (Compazine)

PD interpupillary distance
Paget disease
pancreaticoduodenectomy
panic disorder
Parkinson disease
patient detected
penile sclerosis
percutaneous drain
peritoneal dialysis
personality disorder
pharmacodynamics
pocket depth (dental)
poorly differentiated
post dates
postural drainage
pressure dressing
prism diopter
probing depth (dental)
progressive disease
pupillary distance

P/D packs per day (cigarettes)

2PD two point discriminatory test

^{103}Pd palladium 103

PDA pancreatic ductal adenocarcinoma
parenteral drug abuser
patent ductus arteriosus
pathological demand avoidance (syndrome)
personal digital assistant
poorly differentiated adenocarcinoma
posterior descending (coronary) artery
property damage accident

PDAD photodiode array detector

PDAF platelet-derived angiogenesis factor

PDAP peritoneal dialysis-associated peritonitis

PDB preperitoneal distention balloon

PDC patient denies complaints
poorly differentiated carcinoma
private diagnostic clinic
property damage collision (crash)
pyruvate dehydogenase complex

PD&C postural drainage and clapping

PDCA Plan-Do-Check-Act (process improvement)

PDD cisplatin (Platinol)
Parkinson disease cases with dementia
pervasive developmental disorder
premenstrual dysphoric disorder
primary degenerative dementia

PDDNOS pervasive developmental disorder, not otherwise specified

PDDs pervasive developmental disorders

PDE paroxysmal dyspnea on exertion
pulsed Doppler echocardiography

PDE4 phosphodiesterase type 4

PDE5 phosphodiesterase type 5

PDEGF platelet-derived epidermal growth factor

PDEIs phosphodiesterase inhibitors (Viagra, Levitra, and Cialis)

PDF Portable Document Format

PDFC premature dead female child

PDGF platelet-derived growth factor

PDGXT predischarge graded exercise test

PDH past dental history
pyruvate dehydrogenase

PDI Pain Disability Index
phasic detrusor instability
psychomotor developmental index

PDIGC patient dismissed in good condition

PDL periodontal ligament
poorly differentiated lymphocytic
postures of daily living
preferred drug list
progressively diffused leukoencephalopathy

pulsed-dye laser
PDL-D poorly differentiated lymphocytic-diffuse
PDL-N poorly differentiated lymphocytic-nodular
PDM primary dermal melanoma
PDMC premature dead male child
PDN Paget disease of the nipple
painful diabetic neuropathy
prednisone
private duty nurse
prosthetic disk nucleus
PDNE poorly differentiated neuroendocrine (carcinoma)
PDOX pegylated doxorubicin
PDP pachydermoperiostosis
peak diastolic pressure
prescription drug plan
PD & P postural drainage and percussion
PDPH postdural puncture headache
PDPM peripapillary detachment in pathologic myopia
PDPT patient-delivered partner therapy
PDQ pretty damn quick (at once)
PDQ-39 Parkinson Disease Questionnaire
PDQ-R Personality Diagnostic Questionnaire-Revised
PDR patients' dining room
Physicians' Desk Reference
point of decreasing response
postdelivery room
proliferative diabetic retinopathy
prospective drug review
PDRcVH proliferative diabetic retinopathy with vitreous hemorrhage
PDRP proliferative diabetic retinopathy
PDRUL palmar distal radioulnar ligament
PDS pain dysfunction syndrome
persistent developmental stuttering
polydioxanone suture
power Doppler sonography
Progressive Deterioration Scale
PDSA Plan, Do, Study, and Act
PDSCC poorly differentiated squamous cell carcinoma
PDSS Postpartum Depression Screening Scale
PDT percutaneous dilatational tracheostomy
photodynamic therapy
postdisaster trauma
PDTC pyrrolidine dithiocarbamate
PDU PCR (polymerase chain reaction)-detectable units
pulsed Doppler ultrasonography
PDUFA Prescription Drug User Fee Act (1992)
PDUR postdialysis urea rebound
prospective drug utilization review
PDW platelet distribution width
PDWHF platelet-derived wound healing factors
PDWI proton-density-weighted image(s)
PDX pyridoxine (vitamin B_6)
PDx principal diagnosis
pDXA peripheral dual energy x-ray absorptiometry
PE cisplatin (Platinol) and etoposide
pedal edema
pelvic examination
pharyngoesophageal
phenytoin equivalent (150 mg of fosphenytoin sodium is equivalent to 100 mg of phenytoin sodium)
physical education (gym)
physical examination
physical exercise
plasma exchange
pleural effusion
pneumatic equalization
polyethylene
preeclampsia
premature ejaculation
pressure equalization
pulmonary edema
pulmonary embolism
P_1E_1® epinephrine 1%, pilocarpine 1% ophthalmic solution
P&E prep and enema
PE24 Preemie Enfamil 24
PEA pelvic examination under anesthesia
phenylethylamine
pre-emptive analgesia
pulseless electrical activity
Peanut primitive neuroectodermal tumor (PNET) (slang)
PEARL physiologic endometrial ablation/resection loop
pupils equal accommodation, reactive to light
pupils equal and reactive to light
PEARLA pupils equal and react to light and accommodation
PEB cisplatin, etoposide, and bleomycin
PEC pectoralis
Physician Emergency Certificate (the 15 day hold certificate used in psychiatric hospitals)
posterior exterior chain (of muscles)
Psychiatric Emergency Clinic
pulmonary ejection click
PECCE planned extracapsular cataract extraction
PECHO prostatic echogram
PECHR peripheral exudative choroidal hemorrhagic retinopathy

P

PECO$_2$	mixed expired carbon dioxide tension
PED	paroxysmal exertion-induced dyskinesia
	pediatrics
	pigment epithelial detachments
PEDD	proton-electron dipole-dipole
PEDI	pediatric evaluation of disability inventory
PEDI-DEG	pediatric deglycerolized red blood cells
PEDs	performance-enhancing drugs
	periodic epileptiform discharges
Peds	pediatrics
PedsQL 4.0	Pediatric Quality of Life Inventory, version 4.0
PEE	punctate epithelial erosion
PEEP	positive end-expiratory pressure
PEF	cisplatin (Platinol), epirubicin, and fluorouracil
	peak expiratory flow
PEFR	peak expiratory flow rate
PEFSR	partial expiratory flow static recoil curve
PEG	pegylated
	percutaneous endoscopic gastrostomy
	pneumoencephalogram
	polyethylene glycol
PEG-ELS	polyethylene glycol and iso-osmolar electrolyte solution
PEGG	Parent Education and Guidance Group
PEG-J	percutaneous endoscopic gastrojejunostomy
PEG-JET	percutaneous endoscopic gastrostomy with jejunal extension tube
PEG-SOD	polyethylene glycol-conjugated superoxide dismutase (pegorgotein)
PEH	paraesophageal hernia
	postexercise hypotension
PEI	cisplatin (Platinol), etoposide, and ifosfamide
	percutaneous ethanol injection
	phosphate excretion index
	physical efficiency index
	polyethylenimine
PEIT	percutaneous ethanol injection therapy
PEJ	percutaneous endoscopic jejunostomy
PEK	punctate epithelial keratopathy
PEL	pelvis
	permissible exposure limits
	primary effusion lymphomas
PELD	percutaneous endoscopic lumbar diskectomy
PELE	postextubation laryngeal edema
PELOD	pediatric logistic organ dysfunction (score)
PELV	pelvimetry
PEM	prescription event monitoring
	protein-energy malnutrition
PEMA	phenylethylmalonamide
PEMS	physical, emotional, mental, and safety
	postexercise muscle soreness
PEN	pancreatic endocrine neoplasm
	parenteral and enteral nutrition
	penicillin
	Pharmacy Equivalent Name
PENS	percutaneous electrical nerve stimulation
	percutaneous epidural nerve stimulator
PEO	progressive external ophthalmoplegia
PEP	patient education program
	pharmacologic erection program
	positive expiratory pressure
	postexposure prophylaxis
	preejection period
	primer extension preamplification
	protein electrophoresis
PEP/ET	pre-ejection period/ ejection time
PEPI	preejection period index
PEPP	payment error prevention program
PER	by
	pediatric emergency room
	pertussis (whooping cough) vaccine, antigens not otherwise unspecified
	protein efficiency ratio
PER$_a$	pertussis, acellular antigen(s), vaccine
PERC	perceptual
	percutaneous
PERF	perfect
	perforation
Peri Care	perineum care
PERIO	periodontal disease
	periodontitis
peri-pads	perineal pads
PERL	pupils equal, reactive to light
PERLA	pupils equally reactive to light and accommodation
per os	by mouth (this is a dangerous abbreviation as it is read as left eye [OS])
PERR	pattern evoked retinal response
PERRL	pupils equal, round, and reactive to light
PERRLA	pupils equal, round, reactive to light and accommodation
PERR-LADC	pupils equal, round, reactive to light and accommodation directly and consensually

PERRRLA	pupils equal, round, regular, react to light and accommodation
PERS	personal emergency response systems
PERT	pancreatic enzyme replacement therapy
	program evaluation and review technique
PERV	porcine endogenous retroviruses
PER$_w$	pertussis, whole-cell antigens, vaccine
PES	paclitaxel-eluting stent
	polyethersulfone
	postextubation stridor
	preexcitation syndrome
	programmed electrical stimulation
	pseudoexfoliation syndrome
PESA	percutaneous epididymal sperm aspiration
peSPL	peak equivalent sound pressure level
PET	poor exercise tolerance
	positron-emission tomography
	preeclamptic toxemia
	pressure equalizing tubes
	problem elicitation technique
PEth	phosphatidyl ethanol
PETN	pentaerythritol tetranitrate
PEX	plasma exchange
	pseudoexfoliation (glaucoma)
PEx	physical examination
PEX# 3	plasma exchange number three
PEY	patient exposure years
PF	patellofemoral
	peak flow
	pemphigus foliaceus
	peripheral fields
	Pharmacopeia Forum
	plantar flexion
	Pontiac fever
	power factor
	preservative free
	prostatic fluid
	pulmonary fibrosis
	push fluids
Pf	*Plasmodium falciparum*
PF3	platelet factor 3
PF4	platelet factor 4
16PF	The Sixteen Personality Factors test
PFA	foscarnet (phosphonoformatic acid) (Foscavir)
	patellofemoral arthritis
	platelet function analysis
	psychological first aid
	pure free acid
PFAA	profunda femoris artery aneurysm
PFAPA	periodic fever, aphthous stomatitis, pharyngitis, and cervical adenitis
PFB	potential for breakdown
	pseudofolliculitis barbae
PFC	patient-focused care
	perfluorochemical
	permanent flexure contracture
	persistent fetal circulation
	prefrontal cortex
	prolonged febrile convulsions
$\overline{P}$ FEEDS	after feedings
PFFD	proximal femoral focal deficiency (defect)
PFFFP	Pall filtered fresh frozen plasma
PFG	patellofemoral grind
	percutaneous fluoroscopic gastrostomy
	proximal femur geometry
	pulsed-field gradient
PFGE	pulsed field gel electrophoresis
PfHRP-2	*Plasmodium falciparum* histidine-rich protein 2
PFHx	positive family history
PFI	pill-free intervals
	progression-free interval
PFIC	progressive familial intrahepatic cholestasis
PFJ	patellofemoral joint
PFJS	patellofemoral joint syndrome
PFL	cisplatin (Platinol), fluorouracil, and leucovorin
	patellofemoral ligament
PFL+IFN	cisplatin (Platinol), fluorouracil, leucovorin, and interferon alfa 2b
PFM	peak flow meter
	permanent first molars
	porcelain fused to metal
	primary fibromyalgia
PFME	pelvic floor muscle exercise
PFN	proximal femoral nail
PFO	patent foramen ovale
PFP	progression free probability
	proinsulin fusion protein
PFPC	Pall filtered packed cells
PFPS	patellofemoral pain syndrome
PFR	parotid flow rate
	peak flow rate
	pelvic floor relaxation
PFRC	plasma-free red cells
PFROM	pain-free range of motion
PFS	patellar femoral syndrome
	patient financial services
	Physician Fee Schedule
	prefilled syringe
	preservative-free solution (system)
	primary fibromyalgia syndrome
	progression-free survival
	prolonged febrile seizure
	pulmonary function studies (study)
PFSH	past, family, and social history (histories)
PFT	parafascicular thalamotomy

P

pulmonary function test
PFTC primary fallopian tube carcinoma
PFU plaque-forming unit
PFW pHisoHex® face wash
PFWB Pall filtered whole blood
  Psychological General Well-Being (index)
PFWT pain-free walking time
PG paclitaxel and gemcitabine
  paged in hospital
  paregoric
  performance goal (short-term goal)
  phosphatidylglycerol
  picogram (pg) (10^{-12} gram)
  placental grade (biophysical profile)
  polygalacturonate
  practice guidelines
  pregnant
  prostaglandin
  pyoderma gangrenosum
PGA prostaglandin A
  prothrombin time, **g**amma-glutamyl transpeptidase activity, and serum **a**polipoprotein AI concentration
PGB pregabalin (Lyrica)
PGBD polyglucosan body disease
PGCG peripheral giant cell granuloma
PGCH postinfantile giant cell hepatitis
PGCR pharyngoglottal closure reflex
PGCs primordial germ cells
PGD pelvic girdle dysfunction
  preimplantation genetic diagnosis
3-PGDH 3-phosphoglyerate-dehdyrogenase
PGE partial generalized epilepsy
  posterior gastroenterostomy
  proximal gastric exclusion
PGE$_1$ alprostadil (prostaglandin E_1)
PGE$_2$ dinoprostone (prostaglandin E_2)
PGED Practice Guideline for Eating Disorders
PGF paternal grandfather
  placental growth factor
PGF$_{2\alpha}$ dinoprost (prostaglandin $F_{2\alpha}$)
PGGF paternal great-grandfather
PGGM paternal great-grandmother
PGH pituitary growth hormones
PGI potassium, glucose, and insulin
PGI$_2$ epoprostenol (Prostacyclin)
PGL persistent generalized lymphadenopathy
  primary gastric lymphoma
PGM paternal grandmother
  phosphoglucomutase
PGP paternal grandparent
Pgp P-glycoprotein
PGR pulse-generated runoff
PgR progesterone receptor
P-graph penile plethysmograph
PGRN Pharmacogenomics Research Network
  progranulin
PGS Persian Gulf syndrome
  posterior glottic stenosis
  purple glove syndrome
PGT play-group therapy
PGTC primary generalized tonic-clonic (seizures)
P±GTC partial seizures with or without generalized tonic-clonic seizures
pGTD persistent gestational trophoblastic disease
PGTP primary glaucoma triple procedure
PG-TXL poly (L-glutamic acid)-paclitaxel
PGU postgonococcal urethritis
PGW person gametocyte week
PGY-1 postgraduate year one (first year resident)
pH hydrogen ion concentration
PH past history
  personal history
  pinhole
  poor health
  pubic hair
  public health
  pulmonary hypertension
P&H physical and history
Ph^1 Philadelphia chromosome
PHA arterial pH
  passive hemagglutinating
  paternal history of alcoholism
  peripheral hyperalimentation
  phenylalanine
  phytohemagglutinin antigen
  postoperative holding area
PHAC Public Health Agency of Canada
PHACO phacoemulsification
PHACO OD phacoemulsification of the right eye
PHACO OS phacoemulsification of the left eye
PHAL peripheral hyperalimentation
PHAR pharmacist
  pharmacy
  pharynx
Pharm Pharmacy
PharmD Doctor of Pharmacy
PHb pyridoxylated hemoglobin
PHC permissive hypercapnia
  posthospital care
  primary health care
  primary hepatocellular carcinoma
PHCA profound hypothermic cardiac arrest
PHD paroxysmal hypnogenic dyskinesia
  Public Health Department
PhD Doctor of Philosophy

	phospholipase D
PHE	periodic health examination
PHEN-FEN	phentermine and fenfluramine
PHEO	pheochromocytoma
PHEP	progressive home exercise program
PHF	paired helical filament
PHG	portal hypertensive gastropathy
PHH	paraesophageal hiatus hernia
	posthemorrhagic hydrocephalus
PHHI	persistent hyperinsulinemic hypoglycemia of infancy
PHI	patient health information
	personal health information
	phosphohexose isomerase
	prehospital index
	protected health information
PHIS	posthead injury syndrome
PHL	permanent hearing loss
	Philadelphia (chromosome)
PHLIS	Public Health Laboratory Information System
PHLS	Public Health Laboratory Service (United Kingdom)
PHM	partial hydatidiform mole
	preventative health maintenance
PHMB	polyhexamethylene biguanine
PHMD	polyhexamethylene (Baquacil, a pool cleaner)
PHN	postherpetic neuralgia
	Public Health Nurse
	Puritan® heated nebulizer
PHNC	public health nurse coordinator
PHNI	pinhole no improvement
PHO	Physician/Hospital Organization
PHOB	phobic anxiety
PHONO	phonophoresis
PHOS	phosphatase
	Phosphate
	Phosphorous
PHP	pooled human plasma
	postheparin plasma
	prepaid health plan
	pseudohypoparathyroidism
	pyridoxalated hemoglobin polyoxyethylene conjugate
PHPPO	Public Health Practice Program Office
PHPT	primary hyperparathyroidism
PHPV	persistent hyperplastic primary vitreous
PHQ-9	Patient Health Questionnaire (9-item depression scale)
PHR	peak heart rate
	personal health record
PhRMA	Pharmaceutical Research and Manufacturers of America
PHRN	Pre-Hospital Registered Nurse
PHS	partial hospitalization program
	Prolene hernia system
	US Public Health Service
PHT	phenytoin (Dilantin)
	portal hypertension
	posterior hyaloidal traction
	postmenopausal hormone therapy
	primary hyperthyroidism
	pulmonary hypertension
PHTC	pulmonary hypertensive crises
PHV	peak height velocity
	pediatric health visit
PHVA	pinhole visual acuity
pHVA	plasma homovanillic acid
PHVD	posthemorrhagic ventricular dilatation
PHx	past history
Phx	pharynx
PHY	physician
PhyO	physician's orders
PI	package insert
	pallidal index
	pancreatic insufficiency
	Pearl Index
	performance improvement
	peripheral iridectomy
	persistent illness
	physically impaired
	plaque index (dental)
	poison ivy
	postincident
	postinfection
	postinjury
	premature infant
	present illness
	principal investigator
	protease inhibitor
	pulmonary infarction
	pulmonic insufficiency
PI-3	parainfluenza 3 virus
P & I	probe and irrigation
PIA	personal injury accident
	polysaccharide intercellular adhesine
PIAF	cisplatin (Platinol), recombinant interferon alpha 2B, doxorubicin (Adriamycin), and fluorouracil
PIAT	Peabody Individual Achievement Test
PIB	partial ileal bypass
	professional information brochure
PiB	Pittsburgh Compound B
PIBD	paucity of interlobular bile ducts
PIBF	progesterone-induced blocking factor
PIC	penicillin-inhibitor combinations
	peripherally inserted catheter
	personal injury collision (crash)
	polysaccharide-iron complex
	postintercourse
PICA	Porch Index of Communicative Ability

posterior inferior cerebellar artery
posterior inferior communicating artery

PICC peripherally inserted central catheter

PICHI pulse-inversion contrast harmonic imaging

PICT pancreatic islet cell transplantation

PICU pediatric intensive care unit
psychiatric intensive care unit

PICVA percutaneous *in situ* coronary venous arterialization

PICVC peripherally inserted central venous catheter

PID pelvic inflammatory disease
primary immunodeficiency
prolapsed intervertebral disk
proportional-integral-derivative (controller)

PIE pulmonary infiltration with eosinophilia
pulmonary interstitial emphysema

PIEE pulsed irrigation for enhanced evacuation

PIF peak inspiratory flow

PIFG poor intrauterine fetal growth

PIFR peak inspiratory flow rate

PIG pertussis immune globulin

PIGD postural instability and gait difficulty (disorder)

PIGI pregnancy-induced glucose intolerance

PIGN postinfectious glomerulonephritis

PIH pregnancy-induced hypertension
preventricular intraventricular hemorrhage
prolactin-inhibiting hormone

PIIID peripheral indwelling intermediate infusion device

PIIIP aminoterminal type three procollagen propeptide

PIIS posterior inferior iliac spine

PIL patient information leaflet
purpose in life

PILO pilocarpine

PIM Program Integrity Manual
pulse-inversion mode (ultrasound)

PIMIA potentiometric ionophore mediated immunoassay

PIMS programmable implantable medication system

PIN pain in the neck (no place for such a term in a written document)
personal identification number
population impact number
posterior interosseous nerve
prostatic intraepithelial neoplasia
provider identification number

PIND progressive intellectual and neurological deterioration

PINP N-terminal propeptide of type I collagen

PINS persons in need of supervision

PIO pemoline (Cylert)

PIO_2 partial pressure of inspired oxygen

PIOK poikilocytosis

PIOL primary intraocular lymphoma

PIOP patient informed of policy

PIP peak inspiratory pressure
postictal psychosis
postinfusion phlebitis
proximal interphalangeal (joint)
pulmonary immaturity of prematurity
pulmonary insufficiency of the premature

PIPB performance index phonetic balance

PI-PB performance intensity-phonemically balanced

PIPIDA N-para-isopropyl-acetanilide-iminodiacetic acid

PIPJ proximal interphalangeal joint

PIPP Premature Infant Pain Profile

PIP/TZ piperacillin-tazobactam (Zosyn)

PIQ Performance Intelligence Quotient (part of Wechsler tests)

PIR pirarubicin

PIS pregnancy interruption service

PISA phase invariant signature algorithm
proximal isovelocity surface area

PIT pancreatic islet transplantation
patellar inhibition test
peak isometric torque
Pitocin (oxytocin)
Pitressin (vasopressin) (this is a dangerous abbreviation as it can be taken for Pitocin)
pituitary
pulsed-inotrope therapy

PITA pain in the ass (slang)

PITP pseudo-idiopathic thrombocytopenic purpura

PITR plasma iron turnover rate

PIV peripheral intravenous

PIV-3 parainfluenza virus type 3

PIVD protruded intervertebral disk

PIVH periventricular-intraventricular hemorrhage

PIVKA proteins induced in vitamin K absence

PIWT partially impacted wisdom teeth

PIXI Peripheral Instantaneous X-ray Imaging (dual-energy x-ray absorptiometry system)

PJ procelin jacket (crown)

PJB premature junctional beat

PJC	premature junctional contractions
PJI	prosthetic joint infection
PJIF	prosthetic joint implant failure
PJP	pneumocystis jirovecii pneumonia
PJRT	permanent form of junctional reciprocating tachycardia
PJS	peritoneojugular shunt
	Peutz-Jeghers syndrome
PJT	paroxysmal junctional tachycardia
PJVT	paroxysmal junctional-ventricular tachycardia
PK	penetrating keratoplasty
	pharmacokinetics
	plasma potassium
	pyruvate kinase
PKB	prone knee bend
PKC	protein kinase C
PKD	paroxysmal kinesigenic dyskinesia
	polycystic kidney disease
PKDL	post-kala-azar dermal leishmaniasis
PKI	public key infrastructure
PKND	paroxysmal nonkinesigenic dyskinesia
PKP	penetrating keratoplasty
PK/PD	pharmacokinetic/ pharmacodynamic
PKR	phased knee rehabilitation
PK Test	Prausnitz-Küstner transfer test
PKU	phenylketonuria
pk yrs	pack-years (smoking one pack of cigarettes a day for one year is termed 1 pack-year of smoking, thus 2 packs a day for 20 years would be 40 pack-years)
PL	light perception
	palmaris longus
	peroneus longus
	pharyngolaryngectomy
	place
	placebo
	plantar
	plethoric (infant color)
	transpulmonary pressure
PLA	placebo
	Plasma-Lyte A
	poly-L-lactic acid (Sculptra)
	posterolateral (coronary) artery
	potentially lethal arrhythmia
	Product License Application
	pulpolinguoaxial
PLAC	placenta
PLAD	proximal left anterior descending (artery)
Plan B®	levonorgestrel (a progestogen emergency contraceptive)
PLAP	placental alkaline phosphatase
PLAT C	platelet concentration
PLAT P	platelet pheresis
PLAX	parasternal long axis
PLB	percutaneous liver biopsy
	phospholamban
	placebo
	posterolateral branch
	pursed-lip breathing
PLBO	placebo
PLC	peripheral lymphocyte count
	permanent legal custodianship
	pityriasis lichenoides chronica
PLCH	pulmonary Langerhans cell histiocytosis
PLD	partial lower denture
	pegylated liposomal doxorubicin
	percutaneous laser diskectomy
PLDD	percutaneous laser disk decompression
PLE	polymorphic light eruption
	polypodium leucotomos extract (natural fern extract)
	protein-losing enteropathy
PLED	periodic lateralizing epileptiform discharge
PLEK	posterior lamellar endothelial keratoplasty
PLEVA	pityriasis lichenoides et varioliformis acuta
PLF	prior level of function
PLFC	premature living female child
PLG	plague (*Yersinia pestis*) (*la Peste*) vaccine
PLH	paroxysmal localized hyperhidrosis
PLIF	posterior lumbar interbody fusion
PLIG	posterior lumbar interbody graft
PLIL	partial laryngectomy with imbrication laryngoplasty
PLK	posterior lamellar keratoplasty
PLL	posterior longitudinal ligament
	prolymphocytic leukemia
PLLA	poly-l-lactic acid (Sculptra)
PLM	partial lateral meniscectomy
	periodic leg movement
	Plasma-Lyte M
	polarized-light microscope
	precise lesion measuring (device)
	product-line manager
PLMC	premature living male child
PLMD	periodic limb movement disorder
PLMS	periodic limb movements during sleep
PMLT	painful legs and moving toes (syndrome)
PLN	pelvic lymph node
	popliteal lymph node
PLND	pelvic lymph node dissection
PLO	pluronic lecithin organogels
PLOF	previous level of functioning
PLOS	postoperative length of stay

Abbreviation	Meaning
PLOSA	physiologic low stress angioplasty
PLP	partial laryngopharyngectomy
	phantom limb pain
	protolipid protein
PLPH	postlumbar puncture headache
PLR	pupillary light reflex
PLRT	postlumpectomy radiotherapy
PLS	Papillon-Lefèvre syndrome
	phantom limb syndrome
	plastic surgery
	point locator stimulator
	Preschool Language Scale
	primary lateral sclerosis
PLs	premalignant lesions
PLSD	protected least significant difference (statistical test)
PLSO	posterior leafspring orthosis
PLST	progressively lowered stress threshold
PLSURG	plastic surgery
PLT	platelet
PLT EST	platelet estimate
PLTF	plaintiff
PLTS	platelets
PLUG	plug the lung until it grows
PLV	partial left ventriculectomy
	posterior left ventricular
PLX	plexus
PLYO	plyometric
PLZF	promyelocytic leukemia zinc finger
PM	afternoon
	evening
	pacemaker
	papillary muscles
	paraspinal mapping
	particulate matter
	petit mal
	physical medicine
	pneumomediastinum
	poliomyelitis
	polymyositis
	poor metabolizers
	postmenopausal
	postmortem
	presents mainly
	pretibial myxedema
	primary motivation
	prostatic massage
	pulpomesial
Pm	*Plasmodium malariae*
PM_{10}	particulate matter less than 10 micrometers diameter
PMA	positive mental attitude
	post-menstrual age
	premarket approval (application) (for medical devices)
	premenstrual asthma
	primary meningococcal arthritis

Abbreviation	Meaning
	Prinzmetal angina
	progress myoclonic ataxia
PMAA	Premarket Approval Application (medical devices)
PMB	polymorphonuclear basophil (leukocytes)
	polymyxin B
	postmenopausal bleeding
PMC	premature mitral closure
	pseudomembranous colitis
PMCP	para-monochlorophenol
	perinatal mortality counseling program
PMCT	perinatal mortality counseling team
	postmortem computed tomography
PMCWR	post-mastectomy chest wall relapse
PMD	perceptual motor development
	primary myocardial disease
	primidone (Mysoline)
	private medical doctor
	progressive muscular dystrophy
PMDD	premenstrual dysphoric disorder
pMDI	pressurized metered-dose inhaler
PM/DM	polymyositis and dermatomyositis
PME	pelvic muscle exercise
	phosphomonoester(s)
	polymorphonuclear esosinophil (leukocytes)
	postmenopausal estrogen
	progressive myoclonus epilepsy
PMEALS	after meals
PMEC	pseudomembranous enterocolitis
PMF	peptide mass fingerprinting
	primary myelofibrosis
	progressive massive fibrosis
	pupils mid-position, fixed
PMH	past medical history
PMHNP	Psychiatric Mental Health Nurse Practitioner
PMHx	past medical history
PMI	Pain Management Index
	past medical illness
	patient medication instructions
	perioperative myocardial injury
	plea of mental incompetence
	point of maximal impulse
	posterior myocardial infarction
PMID	PubMed Unique Identifier (National Library of Medicine)
PML	polymorphonuclear leukocytes
	posterior mitral leaflet
	premature labor
	progressive multifocal leukoencephalopathy
	promyelocytic leukemia
PMLCL	primary mediastinal large-cell lymphoma
PMM	partial medial meniscectomy

PMMA	polymethyl methacrylate
PMMF	pectoralis major myocutaneous flap
PMN	polymodal nociceptors
	polymorphonuclear leukocyte
	Premarket Notification (medical devices)
PMNL	polymorphonuclear leukocyte
PMNN	polymorphonuclear neutrophil
PMNS	postmalarial neurological syndrome
PMO	postmenopausal osteoporosis
	probable medication overuse
pmol	picomole
PMP	pain management program
	previous menstrual period
	psychotropic medication plan
PMPA	tenofovir (Viread)
PMPM	per member, per month
PMPO	postmenopausal palpable ovary
PMPY	per member, per year
PMR	pacemaker rhythm
	percutaneous revascularization
	polymorphic reticulosis
	polymyalgia rheumatica
	premedication regimen
	prior medical record
	progressive muscle relaxation
	proportional mortality ratios
PM&R	physical medicine and rehabilitation
PMRT	postmastectomy radiotherapy
PMS	performance measurement system
	periodic movements of sleep
	poor miserable soul
	postmarketing surveillance
	postmenopausal syndrome
	premenstrual syndrome
	pulse, motor, and sensory
PMSF	phenylmethylsulfonyl fluoride
PMT	pacemaker-mediated tachycardia
	percutaneous mechanical thrombectomy
	point of maximum tenderness
	premenstrual tension
PMTS	premenstrual tension syndrome
PMV	percutaneous mitral (balloon) valvuloplasty
	prolapse of mitral valve
PMW	pacemaker wires
PMZ	postmenopausal zest
PN	parenteral nutrition
	peanut (when testing for an allergy)
	percussion note
	percutaneous nephrosonogram
	percutaneous nephrostomy
	percutaneous nucleotomy
	periarteritis nodosa
	peripheral neuropathy
	plexiform neurofibroma
	pneumonia
	polyarteritis nodosa
	poorly nourished
	positional nystagmus
	postnasal
	postnatal
	practical nurse
	premie nipple
	primary nurse
	progress note
	pyelonephritis
P & N	pins and needles
	psychiatry and neurology
PN_2	partial pressure of nitrogen
PNA	Pediatric Nurse Associate
	pneumonia
	polynitroxyl albumin
PNa	plasma sodium
PNAB	percutaneous needle aspiration biopsy
PNAC	parenteral nutrition associated cholestasis
PNAR	perennial nonallergic rhinitis
PNAS	prudent no added salt
PNB	percutaneous needle biopsy
	popliteal nerve block
	premature newborn
	premature nodal beat
	prostate needle biopsy
PNC	penicillin
	peripheral nerve conduction
	postnecrotic cirrhosis
	premature nodal contraction
	prenatal care
	prenatal course
	Psychiatric Nurse Clinician
PNCV7	pneumococcal 7-valent conjugate vaccine (Prevnar)
PND	paroxysmal nocturnal dyspnea
	pelvic node dissection
	postnasal drip
	pregnancy, not delivered
PNDS	Perioperative Nursing Data Set
	postnasal drip syndrome
PNE	peripheral neuroepithelioma
	primary nocturnal enuresis
PNECs	predicted no effect concentrations
PNES	psychogenic non-epileptic seizures
PNET	primitive neuroectodermal tumors
PNET-MB	primitive neuroectodermal tumors-medulloblastoma
PNEUMO	pneumothorax
PNF	primary nonfunction
	proprioceptive neuromuscular fasciculation (reaction)
PNFA	progressive nonfluent aphasia
PNH	paroxysmal nocturnal hemoglobinuria
	polynitroxyl-hemoglobin

	progressive nodular hyperplasia
PNI	peripheral nerve injury
	Prognostic Nutrition Index
PNKD	paroxysmal nonkinesigenic dyskinesia
PNL	percutaneous nephrolithotomy
	prenatal labs
PNM	primary nodular melanoma
PNMG	persistent neonatal myasthenia gravis
PNMT	phenylethanolamine-N-methyltransferase
PNNP	Perinatal Nurse Practitioner
PNP	peak negative pressure
	Pediatric Nurse Practitioner
	progressive nuclear palsy
	purine nucleoside phosphorylase
PNR	person needed ride (minor ailment but called ambulance instead of taxi) (slang)
	physician's nutritional recommendation
PNRB	partial non-rebreather (oxygen mask)
PNS	partial nonprogressing stroke
	peripheral nerve stimulator
	peripheral nervous system
	practical nursing student
	Pump N' Style (breast pump machine)
PNSP	penicillin-nonsusceptible *Streptococcus pneumoniae*
PNT	percutaneous nephrostomy tube
	percutaneous neuromodulatory therapy
	pneumatic trabeculoplasty
pnthx	pneumothorax
PNTML	pudendal-nerve terminal motor latency
PNU	pneumococcal (*Streptococcus pneumoniae*) vaccine, not otherwise specified
	protein nitrogen units
PNUcn-7	pneumococcal (*Streptococcus pneumoniae*) conjugate vaccine, 7-valent vaccine (Prevnar)
PNUps23	pneumococcal (*Streptococcus pneumoniae*) polysaccharide, 23-valent vaccine (Pneumovax-23; Pnu-Imune-23)
PNV	postoperative nausea and vomiting
	prenatal vitamins
Pnx	pneumonectomy
	pneumothorax
PO	by mouth
	phone order
	postoperative
	Plasmodium ovale
	prophylactic oophorectomy
	punctal occlusion
Po	polonium
P/O	prosthetics and orthotics
P&O	parasites and ova
	prosthetics and orthotics
Po_2	partial pressure (tension) of oxygen, artery
PO_4	phosphate
POA	pancreatic oncofetal antigen
	power of attorney
	present on admission
	present on arrival
	primary optic atrophy
POACH	prednisone, vincristine (Oncovin), doxorubicin (Adriamycin), cyclophosphamide, and cytarabine
POAF	postoperative atrial fibrillation
POAG	primary open-angle glaucoma
POB	phenoxybenzamine (Dibenzyline)
	place of birth
POBA	plain old balloon angioplasty
POBC	primary operable breast cancer
POC	peri-operative chemotherapy
	plans of care
	point-of-care
	position of comfort
	postoperative care
	product of conception
POCD	postoperative cognitive dysfunction
POCT	point-of-care testing (test)
	point-of-care therapy
POD	pacing on demand
	place of death
	Podiatry
	polycystic ovarian disease
	prevention of disability
	progression of disease
POD 1	postoperative day one
PODs	patients' own drugs
PODx	preoperative diagnosis
POE	patient-oriented evidence
	point (portal, port) of entry
	position of ease
	prone on elbows
	provider order entry
POEM	Patient-Oriented Evidence That Matters
POEMS	plasma cell dyscrasia with polyneuropathy, organomegaly, endocrinopathy, monoclonal protein (M-protein), and skin changes
POEx	postoperative exercise
POF	physician's order form
	position of function
	premature ovarian failure
P of I	proof of illness
POG	Pediatric Oncology Group
	Penthrane,® oxygen, and gas (nitrous oxide)

	products of gestation
POGO	percentage of glottic opening
POH	perillyl alcohol
	personal oral hygiene
	presumed ocular histoplasmosis
	progressive osseous heteroplasia
	prone on hands
POHA	preoperative holding area
POHI	physically or otherwise health impaired
POHS	by mouth, at bedtime
	presumed ocular histoplasmosis syndrome
POI	Personal Orientation Inventory
	postoperative ileus
	postoperative instructions
POIB	place outpatient in inpatient bed
POIK	poikilocytosis
POL	physician's office laboratory
	poliovirus vaccine, not otherwise specified
	premature onset of labor
POLS	postoperative length of stay
POLY	polychromic erythrocytes
	polymorphonuclear leukocyte
POLY-CHR	polychromatophilia
POM	pain on motion
	polyoximethylene
	prescription-only medication
POMA	Performance-Oriented Mobility Assessment
POMC	pro-opiomelanocortin
POMP	prednisone, vincristine (Oncovin), methotrexate, and mercaptopurine (Purinthol)
POMR	problem-oriented medical record
POMS	Profile of Mood States
POMS-FI	Fatigue-Inertia Subscale of the Profile of Mood States
PON	paraoxonase (genes)
	postoperative note
PONI	postoperative narcotic infusion
PONV	postoperative nausea and vomiting
POOH	postoperative open heart (surgery)
POOL	premature onset of labor
POP	pain on palpation
	persistent occipitoposterior
	persistent organic pollutants
	plaster of paris
	popiliteal
	posterior oral pharynx
POp	postoperative
POPC	Pediatric Overall Performance Category (scale)
poplit	popliteal
POPS	postoperative pain service
POPs	persistent organic pollutants
	progesterone-only pills
POPTA	passed out prior to arrival
POR	physician of record
	problem-oriented record
PORN	pornography
	progressive outer retinal necrosis
PORP	partial ossicular replacement prosthesis
PORR	postoperative recovery room
PORT	perioperative respiratory therapy
	portable
	postoperative radiotherapy
	postoperative respiratory therapy
POS	parosteal osteosarcoma
	physician's order sheet
	point-of-service
	positive
PoS	plane of surgery
POSHPATE	**p**roblem, **o**nset, associated **s**ymptoms, previous **h**istory, **p**recipitating factors, **a**lleviating/aggravation factors, **t**iming, an **e**tiology (prompts for taking history and chief complaint)
poss	possible
post	posterior
	postmortem examination (autopsy)
PostC	posterior chamber
PostCap	posterior capsule
Post-M	urine specimen after prostate massage
post op	postoperative
Post Sag D	posterior sagittal diameter
post tib	posterial tibial
PostVD	posterior vitreous detachment
POSYC	Pain Observation Scale for Young Children
POT	peak occupancy time
	plans of treatment
	potassium
	potential
	primary orthostatic tremor
POTS	postural orthostatic tachycardia syndrome
POU	placenta, ovaries, and uterus
	point-of-use
POV	privately owned vehicle
POVD	peripheral occlusive vascular disease
POW	Powassan (virus)
	prisoner of war
POWSBP	pulse oximetry waveform systolic blood pressure
POX	pulse oximeter (reading)
PP	near point of accommodation
	pancreatic pseudocyst
	paradoxical pulse
	partial upper and lower dentures
	pedal pulse

	per protocol
	periodontal pockets
	peripheral pulses
	pin prick
	pink puffer (emphysema)
	Planned Parenthood
	plasmapheresis
	plaster of paris
	poor person
	posterior pituitary
	postpartum
	postprandial
	presenting part
	private patient
	prophylactics
	protoporphyria
	proximal phalanx
	psychogenic polydipsia
	pulse pressure
	push pills
P-P	probability-probability (plots)
P&P	pins and plaster
	policy and procedure
PIIIP	aminoterminal type three protocollegan propeptide
PPIX	protoporphyrin nine
PPA	palpation, percussion, and auscultation
	phenylpropanolamine
	phenylpyruvic acid
	postpartum amenorrhea
	Prescription Pricing Authority (United Kingdom)
	primary progressive aphasia
PP&A	palpation, percussion, and auscultation
PPAR	peroxisome-proliferator-activated receptor
$PPAR_g$	peroxisome-proliferator-activated receptor gamma
PPARs	peroxisome proliferator-activated receptors
PPAS	postpolio atrophy syndrome
PPB	parts per billion
	pleuropulmonary blastoma
	positive pressure breathing
	prostate puncture biopsy
PPBE	postpartum breast engorgment
PPBS	postprandial blood sugar
PPBTL	postpartum bilateral tubal ligation
PPC	plaster of paris cast
	positive product control
	primary peritoneal carcinoma
	progressive patient care
PPCD	posterior polymorphous corneal dystrophy
PPCF	plasma prothrombin conversion factor
PPCM	peripartum cardiomyopathy
PPD	packs per day
	para-phenylenediamine (a dye)
	permanent partial disability (rating)
	pinch-point density (histologic)
	posterior polymorphous dystrophy
	postpartum day
	postpartum depression
	probing pocket depth (dental)
	purified protein derivative (of tuberculin)
	pylorus-sparing pancreaticoduodenectomy
P & PD	percussion & postural drainage
PPD-B	purified protein derivative, Battey
PPDR	preproliferative diabetic retinopathy
PPD-S	purified protein derivative, standard
PPE	palmar-plantar erythrodysesthesia (syndrome)
	personal protective equipment
	professional performance evaluation
	pruritic papular eruption
PPES	palmar-plantar erythrodysesthesia syndrome
	pedal pulses equal and strong
PPF	pellagra preventive factor
	plasma protein fraction
PPG	photoplethysmography
	portal pressure gradients
	postprandial glucose
	pylorus-preserving gastrectomy
PPGI	psychophysiologic gastrointestinal (reaction)
PPGSS	papular-purpuric "glove and socks" syndrome
PPH	postpartum hemorrhage
	primary postpartum hemorrhage
	primary pulmonary hypertension
	procedure for prolapse and hemorrhoids
PPHN	persistent pulmonary hypertension of the newborn
PPHTN	portopulmonary hypertension
PPHx	previous psychiatric history
PPIX	protoporphyrin nine
PPI	patient package insert
	permanent pacemaker insertion
	postpacing interval
	prepulse inhibition
	Present Pain Intensity
	proton-pump inhibitor
	Psychopathic Personality Inventory
PPIA	parental presence during induction of anesthesia
PPIVMs	passive physiological intervertebral movements
PPJ	pure pancreatic juice

PPK	population pharmacokinetics
PPL	pars plana lensectomy
Ppl	pleural pressure
PPLO	pleuropneumonia-like organisms
PPLOV	painless progressive loss of vision
PPM	parts per million permanent pacemaker persistent pupillary membrane physician practice management
PPMA	postpoliomyelitis muscular atrophy
PPMS	primary progressive multiple sclerosis psychophysiologic musculoskeletal (reaction)
PPMs	potentially pathogenic microorganisms
PPN	peripheral parenteral nutrition
PPNAD	primary pigmented nodular adrenocortical disease
PPNG	penicillinase-producing *Neisseria gonorrhoeae*
PPO	permanent punctal occlusion preferred provider organization pump-prime only
PPOB	postpartum obstetrics
PPP	patient prepped and positioned pearly penile papules pedal pulse present peripheral pulses palpable (present) platelet-poor plasma postpartum psychosis preferred practice patterns proportional pulse pressure (SBP minus DBP)/SBP protamine paracoagulation phenomenon
PPPBL	peripheral pulses palpable both legs
PPPD	pylorus-preserving pancreatoduodenectomy
PPPG	postprandial plasma glucose
PPPM	Parents' Postoperative Pain Measure per patient, per month
PPPY	per patient, per year
PPQ	Postoperative Pain Questionnaire
PPR	patient progress record
PPr	periodontal prophylactics
PPRC	Physician Payment Review Commission
PPROM	premature rupture of the membranes before 37 weeks gestation
PPS	pentosan polysulfate (Elmiron) peripheral pulmonary stenosis per protocol set postpartum sterilization post-pericardiotomy syndrome postperfusion syndrome postpoliomyelitis syndrome postpump syndrome prospective payment system pulses per second
PPSS	peripheral protein sparing solution
PPT	parts-per-trillion person, place, and time Physical Performance Test posterior pelvic tilt postpartum thyroiditis
PPTg	pedunculopontine tegmental nucleus
PPTL	postpartum tubal ligation
PPTR	pulsed photothermal radiometry
PPU	perforated peptic ulcer
PPV	pars plana vitrectomy patent processus vaginalum percutaneous polymethyl-methacrylate vertebroplasty phakomatosis pigmentovascularis pneumococcal polysaccharide vaccine positive predictive value positive-pressure ventilation
PPVI	percutaneous pulmonary valve implantation
PPVT	Peabody Picture Vocabulary Test
PPVT-R	Peabody Picture Vocabulary Test-Revised
PPW	plantar puncture wound premature P-wave
PPX	paclitaxel poliglumex
PPY	packs per year (cigarettes)
PQ	pronator quadratus
pQCT	peripheral quantitative computed tomography
PQOCN	Psychiatric Questionnaire Obsessive-Compulsive Neurosis
PQoL	perceived quality of life
PQRI	Product Quality Research Initiative
PR	far point of accommodation pack removal panoramic radiography (dental) partial remission partial response patient relations perennial rhinitis per rectum pityriasis rosea premature profile progressive resistance prolonged remission prone Protestant Puerto Rican pulmonic regurgitation pulse rate
P=R	pupils equal in size and reaction
P & R	pelvic and rectal pulse and respiration

PR-2 — Bennett pressure ventilator
PRA — panel reactive antibodies (organ transplants)
percent reactive antibody
plasma renin activity
PRAFO — pressure relief ankle-foot orthosis
PRAMS — Pregnancy Risk Assessment Monitoring System
PRAT — platelet radioactive antiglobulin test
PRBC — packed red blood cells
PRC — packed red cells
peer review committee
People's Republic of China
proximal row carpectomy
PRCA — pure red cell aplasia
PrCa — prostate cancer
PRCC — papillary renal cell carcinoma
PRCT — partial rotator-cuff tear
prospective randomized controlled trial
PRD — polycystic renal disease
Prdx6 — peroxiredoxin 6
PRE — passive resistance exercises
progressive resistive exercise
proton relaxation enhancement
Pred — prednisone
PREG — Pregestimil® (infant formula)
Pre-M — urine specimen before prostate massage
PREMIE — premature infant
Pre-O_2 — preoxygenation
pre-op — before surgery
prep — prepare for surgery
preposition
PRERLA — pupils round, equal, react to light and accommodation
PRES — posterior reversible encephalopathy syndrome
prev — prevent
previous
PRFD — percutaneous radio-frequency denervation
PRFNB — percutaneous radio-frequency facet nerve block
PrFP — pre-exposure prophylaxis
PRG — phleborheogram
PRH — past relevant history
postocclusive reactive hyperemia
preretinal hemorrhage
PRHO — preregistration house officer
PRI — Pain Rating Index
Patient Review Instrument
prim — primary
PRIMIP — primipara (1st pregnancy)
PR interval — part of the electrocardiographic cycle from onset of atrial depolarization on onset of ventricular depolarization
PRISM — Pediatric Risk of Mortality Score
PRIT® — pretargeted radioimmunotherapy
PRK — photorefractive keratectomy
PRL — prolactin
PRLA — pupils react to light and accommodation
PRM — partial rebreathing mask
passive range of motion
phosphoribomutase
photoreceptor membrane
prematurely ruptured membrane
primidone (Mysoline)
PRMF — preretinal macular fibrosis
PRMS — progressive relapsing multiple sclerosis
PRM-SDX — pyrimethamine; sulfadoxine (Fansidar)
PRN — plaque reduction neutralization
p.r.n. — as occasion requires
PRNS — phrenic repetitive nerve stimulation
PRNT — plaque-reduction neutralization test
PRO — Professional Review Organization
proline
pronation
protein
prothrombin
prob — probable
PROCTO — procotoscopic
proctology
PROG — prognathism
prognosis
program
progressive
PROM — passive range of motion
premature rupture of membranes
ProMACE — prednisone, methotrexate, calcium leucovorin, doxorubicin (Adriamycin), cyclophosphamide, and etoposide
PROMM — passive range of motion machine
Promy — promyelocyte
PRO MYELO — promyelocytes
PRON — pronation
PROP — physiologic-reduced oxygen protocol
PROS — prostate
prosthesis
PROT REL — protrusive relationship
prov — provisional
PROVIMI — proteins, vitamins, and minerals
PROX — proximal
PRP — panretinal photocoagulation
patient recovery plan
penicllinase-resistant penicillin
penicillin-resistant pneumococci
pityriasis rubra pilaris
platelet rich plasma

P

	polyribose ribitol phosphate
	poor progression of R wave in precordial leads
	progressive rubella panencephalitis
PrP	prion protein
PRP-D	*Haemophilus influenzae,* type b diphtheria conjugate vaccine
PRPP	5-phosphoribosyl-1-pyrophosphate
PRP-T	polysaccharide tetanus conjugate vaccine
PRRE	pupils round, regular, and equal
PRRERLA	pupils round, regular, equal; react to light and accommodation
PRRs	proportional reporting ratios
PRS	Pain Rating Scale
	photon radiosurgery system
	postradiation sarcoma
	pressure-redistribution surface
	prolonged respiratory support
PRSL	potential renal solute load
PRSP	penicillinase-resistant synthetic penicillins
	penicillin-resistant *Streptococcus pneumoniae*
PRSs	positive rolandic spikes
PRST	Blood Pressure, Heart Rate, Sweating, and Tears (scale to assess analgesic needs)
PRT	pelvic radiation therapy
	protamine response test
PRTCA	percutaneous rotational transluminal coronary angioplasty
PRTH-C	prothrombin time control
PRV	polycythemia rubra vera
PRVEP	pattern reversal visual evoked potentials
PRW	past relevant work
	polymerized ragweed
PRX	panoramic facial x-ray
PRZF	pyrazofurin
PS	paradoxic sleep
	paranoid schizophrenia
	pathologic stage
	patient's serum
	performance status
	peripheral smear
	physical status
	plastic surgery (surgeon)
	polysulfone (filter)
	posterior subcapsular (cataract type)
	posterior synechiae
	posterior synechiotomy
	pressure sore
	pressure support
	protective services
	Proteus syndrome
	pulmonary stenosis
	pyloric stenosis
	pyrimethamine; sulfadoxine (Fansidar)
	serum from pregnant women
P/S	polyunsaturated to saturated fatty acids ratio
P & S	pain and suffering
	paracentesis and suction
	permanent and stationary
PS I	healthy patient with localized pathological process
PS II	a patient with mild to moderate systemic disease
PS III	a patient with severe systemic disease limiting activity but not incapacitating
PS IV	a patient with incapacitating systemic disease
PS V	moribund patient not expected to live
	(These are American Society of Anesthesiologists' physical status patient classifications. Emergency operations are designated by "E" after the classification.)
PSA	polysubstance abuse
	power spectral analysis
	product selection allowed
	prostate-specific antigen
	Pseudomonas aeruginosa
PsA	psoriatic arthritis
PSAB	pretreatment prostate-specific antigen
PSAD	prostate-specific antigen density
PSADT	prostate-specific antigen doubling time
PSAG	*Pseudomonas aeruginosa*
PSARP	posterior sagittal anorectoplasty
PSAV	prostate-specific antigen velocity
PSBO	partial small bowel obstruction
PSC	Pediatric Symptom Checklist
	percutaneous suprapubic cystostomy
	posterior semicircular canal
	posterior subcapsular cataract
	primary sclerosing cholangitis
	pronation spring control
	pubosacrococcygeal (diameter)
PSCA	prostate stem cell antigen
PSCC	posterior subcapsular cataract
PSC Cat	posterior subcapsular cataract
PSCH	peripheral stem cell harvest
PSCP	papillary serous carcinoma of the peritoneum
	posterior subcapsular precipitates
PSCT	peripheral stem cell transplant
PSCU	pediatric special care unit
PSD	partial sleep deprivation
	pattern standard deviation
	pilonidal sinus disease
	poststroke depression

	power spectral density
	psychosomatic disease
PSDA	Patient Self-Determination Act
PSDS	palmar surface desensitization
PSE	photosensitive epilepsy
	portal systemic encephalopathy
	pseudoephedrine
PSF	posterior spinal fusion
PSG	peak systolic gradient
	polysomnogram
	portosystemic gradient
PSGN	poststreptococcal glomerulonephritis
PSH	past surgical history
	postspinal headache
PSHx	past surgical history
PSI	passenger space intrusion (motor vehicle accident)
	Physiologic Stability Index
	pounds per square inch
	prostate seed implant
	punctate subepithelial infiltrate
PSIC	pediatric surgical intensive care
PSIG	pounds per square inch gauge
PSIS	posterior superior iliac spine
PSM	patient self-management
	positive surgical margin
	presystolic murmur
PSMA	personal self-maintenance activities
	progressive spinal muscular atrophy
	prostate-specific membrane antigen
PSMF	protein-sparing modified fasting (Blackburn diet)
PSM-R	Optimism-Pessimism Scale, revised
PSMS	Physical Self Maintenance Scale
PSN	peripheral sensory neuropathy
PSNP	progressive supranuclear palsy
PSO	Patient Safety Officer
	pelvic stabilization orthosis
	physician supplemental order
	Polysporin ointment
	proximal subungual onychomycosis
pSO_2	arterial oxygen saturation
PSOC	Puget Sound Oncology Consortium
P/sore	pressure sore
PSP	pancreatic spasmolytic peptide
	phenolsulfonphthalein
	photostimulable phosphor
	progressive supranuclear palsy
PSPDV	posterior superior pancreaticoduodenal vein
PSR	posthumous sperm retrieval
	Psychiatric Status Rating (scale)
PSRA	pressure sore risk assessment
PSRBOW	premature spontaneous rupture of bag of waters
PSReA	poststreptococcal reactive arthritis
PSRT	photostress recovery test
PSS	painful shoulder syndrome
	pediatric surgical service
	phenotypic-sensitivity scores
	physiologic saline solution (0.9% sodium chloride)
	primary Sjögren syndrome
	progressive systemic sclerosis
PSSP	penicillin-sensitive *Streptococcus pneumoniae*
PST	paroxysmal supraventricular tachycardia
	patient self-testing
	Patient Service Technician
	penicillin skin testing
	platelet survival time
	posterior sub-Tenon (capsule)
	postural stress test
PSTT	placental site trophoblastic tumor
PSU	pseudomonas (*P. aeruginosa*) vaccine
PSUD	psychoactive substance use disorder
PSUR	Periodic Safety Update Reporting (EMEA)
PSV	peak systolic velocity
	persistent sciatic vein(s)
	pressure supported ventilation
PSVT	paroxysmal supraventricular tachycardia
PSW	psychiatric social worker
PSWF	positive sharp wave fibrillations (electromyograph)
PSY	presexual youth
PsyD	psychological distress
PSZ	pseudoseizures
PT	cisplatin (Platinol)
	parathormone
	parathyroid
	paroxysmal tachycardia
	patch test
	patient
	phacotrabeculectomy
	phage type
	phenytoin (Dilantin)
	phototoxicity
	physical therapy
	pine tar
	pint
	posterior tibial
	Preferred Term
	preterm
	pronator teres
	prothrombin time
Pt	platinum
pt	pint (1 pint US = 473 mL; 1 pint UK = 568 mL)
pT	pathologic tumor (various lettered and numbered stages, such as pT1)

P/T	pain and tenderness
	piperacillin/tazobactam (Zosyn®)
	prior to
pT0	No tumor
P1/2T	pressure one-half time
P&T	pain and tenderness
	paracentesis and tubing (of ears)
	peak and trough
	permanent and total
	Pharmacy and Therapeutics (Committee)
PTA	pancreas transplant alone
	patellar tendon autograft
	percutaneous transluminal angioplasty
	Physical Therapist Assistant
	plasma thromboplastin antecedent
	posterior tibial artery
	post-traumatic amnesia
	pretreatment anxiety
	prior to admission
	prior to arrival
	pure-tone average
PTAB	popliteal-tibial artery bypass
PTAS	percutaneous transluminal angioplasty with stent placement
PTB	patellar tendon bearing
	potassium taurine bicarbonate
	prior to birth
	pulmonary tuberculosis
PTBA	percutaneous transluminal balloon angioplasty
PTBD	percutaneous transhepatic biliary drain (drainage)
PTBD-EF	percutaneous transhepatic biliary drainage—enteric feeding
PTBS	post-traumatic brain syndrome
PTB-SC-SP	patellar tendon bearing-supracondylar-suprapatellar
PTC	papillary thyroid carcinoma
	patient to call
	percutaneous transhepatic cholangiography
	Pharmacy and Therapeutics Committee
	plasma thromboplastin components
	post-tetanic count
	premature tricuspid closure
	prior to conception
	pseudotumor cerebri
PT-C	prothrombin time control
PTCA	percutaneous transluminal coronary angioplasty
PTCDLF	pregnancy, term, complicated delivered, living female
PTCDLM	pregnancy, term, complicated delivered, living male
PTCL	peripheral T-cell lymphoma
PTCR	percutaneous transluminal coronary recanalization
PTCRA	percutaneous transluminal coronary rotational atherectomy
PTD	percutaneous transpedicular diskectomy
	period to discharge
	permanent and total disability
	persistent trophoblastic disease
	pharmacy to dose
	pharyngotracheal duct
	preterm delivery
	prior to delivery
PTDM	post-transplant diabetes mellitus
PTDP	permanent transvenous demand pacemaker
PTE	post-traumatic epilepsy
	pretibial edema
	proximal tibial epiphysis
	pulmonary thromboembolectomy
	pulmonary thromboembolism
PTE-4®	trace metal elements injection (there is also a #5 and #6)
PTED	pulmonary thromboembolic disease
PTER	percutaneous transluminal endomyocardial revascularization
PTF	patient transfer form
	Patient Treatment File
	pentoxifylline (Trental)
	post-tetanic facilitation
PTFE	polytetrafluoroethylene
PTFJ	proximal tibiofibular joint
PTG	parathyroid gland
	photoplethysmogram
PTGBD	percutaneous transhepatic gallbladder drainage
PTH	parathyroid hormone
	post-transfusion hepatitis
	prior to hospitalization
PTHC	percutaneous transhepatic cholangiography
PTHrP	parathyroid hormone-related protein
PTHS	post-traumatic hyperirritability syndrome
PTI	pressure-time integral
	prior to induction
PTJV	percutaneous transtracheal jet ventilation
PTK	pancreas-after-kidney (transplantation)
	phototherapeutic keratectomy
PTL	preterm labor
	pudding-thick liquid (diet consistency)
	Sodium Pentothal
PTLD	post-transplantation lymphoproliferative disorder (disease)

PTLR percutaneous transmyocardial laser revascularization
PTM patient monitored
posterior trabecular meshwork
post-translational modification
PTMC percutaneous transvenous mitral commissurotomy
PTMDF pupils, tension, media, disc, and fundus
PTMR percutaneous transmyocardial revascularization
PT-NANB post-transfusion non-A, non-B (hepatitis C)
PTNB preterm newborn
pTNM postsurgical resection-pathologic staging of cancer
PTNS percutaneous tibial nerve stimulation
PTO part-time occlusion (eye patch)
please turn over
proximal tubal obstruction
PTP phonation threshold pressure
posterior tibial pulse
post-transfusion purpura
PTPM post-traumatic progressive myelopathy
PTPN peripheral (vein) total parenteral nutrition
P-to-P point-to-point
PTR paratesticular rhabdomyosarcoma
patella tendon reflex
patient to return
prothrombin time ratio
PT-R prothrombin time ratio
PTRA percutaneous transluminal renal angioplasty
PTR-MS proton transfer reaction mass spectrometry
PTS patellar tendon suspension
Pediatric Trauma Score
permanent threshold shift
post-thrombotic syndrome
prior to surgery
PTSD post-traumatic stress disorder
PTSD-T post-traumatic stress disorder related to the transplant
PTT partial thromboplastin time
pharyngeal transit time
platelet transfusion therapy
posterior tibial tendon
protein truncation testing
pulse transit time
PTT-C partial thromboplastin time control
PTTD posterior tibial tendonitis dysfunction
PTTG pituitary tumor transforming gene
PTTW patient tolerated traction well
PTU pain treatment unit
pregnancy, term, uncomplicated
propylthiouracil
PTUCA percutaneous transluminal ultrasonic coronary angioplasty
PTUDLF pregnancy, term, uncomplicated delivered, living female
PTUDLM pregnancy, term, uncomplicated delivered, living male
PTV patient-triggered ventilation
planning target volume (radiation therapy)
posterior tibial vein
PTWTKG patient's weight in kilograms
PTX paclitaxel (Taxol)
parathyroidectomy
pelvic traction
pentoxifylline (Trental)
phototherapy
pneumothorax
PTX3 pentraxin 3
PTZ pentylenetetrazol
phenothiazine
PU paws up (dead) (Veterinary slang)
pelvic-ureteric
pelviureteral
peptic ulcer
pregnancy urine
P & U Pharmacia & Upjohn Company
PUA pelvic (examination) under anesthesia
PUB pubic
PUBS percutaneous umbilical blood sampling
purple urine bag syndrome
PUC pediatric urine collector
PUD partial upper denture
peptic ulcer disease
percutaneous ureteral dilatation
PUE pyrexia of unknown etiology
PUF pure ultrafiltration
PUFA polyunsaturated fatty acids
PUFFA polyunsaturated free fatty acids
PUJ pelviureteral junction
pul. pulmonary
PULP pulpotomy
Pulse A pulse apical
PULSE OX pulse oximetry
Pulse R pulse radial
PULSES (physical profile) **p**hysical condition, **u**pper limb functions, **l**ower limb functions, **s**ensory components, **e**xcretory functions, and **s**upport factors
PUN plasma urea nitrogen
PUND pregnancy, uterine, not delivered
PUNL percutaneous ultrasonic nephrolithotripsy
PUO pyrexia of unknown origin

PUP	percutaneous ultrasonic pyelolithotomy
	previously untreated patient
PU/PL	partial upper and lower dentures
PUPPP	pruritic urticarial papules and plaque of pregnancy
PURA	pressure-ulcer risk assessment
PUS	percutaneous ureteral stent
	preoperative ultrasound
PUU	Puumala hantavirus
PUV	posterior urethral valves
PUVA	psoralen (methoxsalen) plus ultraviolet light of A wavelength (treatment)
PUW	pick-up walker
PV	papillomavirus
	Parvovirus
	pemphigus vulgaris
	percutaneous vertebroplasty
	per vagina
	plasma volume
	polio vaccine
	polycythemia vera
	popliteal vein
	portal vein
	postoperative vomiting
	postvoiding
	prenatal vitamins
	projectile vomiting
	pulmonary vein
Pv	*Plasmodium vivax*
P & V	peak and valley (this is a dangerous abbreviation, use peak and trough)
	pyloroplasty and vagotomy
PVA	polyethylene vinyl acetate
	polyvinyl alcohol
	Prinzmetal variant angina
PVAD	prolonged venous access devices
PVAM	potential visual acuity meter
PVAN	polyomavirus-associated nephropathy
PVAR	pulmonary vein atrial reversal
PVB	cisplatin, (Platinol) vinblastine, and bleomycin
	paravertebral block
	porcelain veneer bridge
	premature ventricular beat
PVC	paclitaxel, vinblastine, and cisplatin
	polyethylene vacuum cup
	polyvinyl chloride
	porcelain veneer crown
	postvoiding cystogram
	premature ventricular contraction
	pulmonary venous congestion
PVCD	percutaneous vascular closure device
$Pvco_2$	partial pressure (tension) of carbon dioxide, vein
PVD	patient very disturbed
	peripheral vascular disease
	posterior vitreous detachment
	premature ventricular depolarization
PVDA	prednisone, vincristine, daunorubicin, and asparaginase
PVDF	polyvinylidene difluoride
PVE	perivenous encephalomyelitis
	portal vein embolization
	premature ventricular extrasystole
	prosthetic value endocarditis
P vera	polycythemia vera
PVF	peripheral visual field
PVFS	postviral fatigue syndrome
PVGM	perifoveolar vitreoglial membrane
PVH	periventricular hemorrhage
	periventricular hyperintensity
	pulmonary vascular hypertension
PVI	pelvic venous incompetence
	peripheral vascular insufficiency
	portal-vein infusion
	protracted venous infusion
	pulmonary valve insufficiency
	pulmonary vein isolation
PVK	penicillin V potassium
PVL	Panton-Valentine leukocidin
	peripheral vascular laboratory
	periventricular leukomalacia
PVM	paraverteabral muscle
	proteins, vitamins, and minerals
PVMS	paravertebral muscle spasms
PVN	peripheral venous nutrition
PVNS	pigmented villonodular synovitis
PVO	peripheral vascular occlusion
	portal vein occlusion
	pulmonary venous occlusion
PVo	pulmonary valve opening
Pvo_2	partial pressure (tension) of oxygen, vein
	peripheral vascular occlusive disease
PVOD	pulmonary vascular obstructive disease
PVP	cisplatin (Platinol) and etoposide (VePesid)
	penicillin V potassium
	peripheral venous pressure
	Photoselective Vaporization of the Prostate (procedure)
	polyvinylpyrrolidone
	portal venous pressure
	posteroventral pallidotomy
P-VP-B	cisplatin (Platinol), etoposide (VP-16), and bleomycin
PVR	peripheral vascular resistance
	perspective volume rendering
	postvoiding residual
	proliferative vitreoretinopathy
	pulmonary valve replacement
	pulmonary vascular resistance

	pulse-volume recording
PVRI	pulmonary vascular resistance index
PVRQOL	Pediatric Voice-Related Quality-of-Life
PVS	percussion, vibration and suction
	peripheral vascular surgery
	peritoneovenous shunt
	persistent vegetative state
	Plummer-Vinson syndrome
	pubovaginal sling
	pulmonic valve stenosis
PVT	paroxysmal ventricular tachycardia
	physical volume test
	portal vein thrombosis
	previous trouble
	private
	proximal vein thrombosis
PVTT	tumor thrombus in the portal vein
PVV	persistent varicose veins
PW	pacing wires
	patient waiting
	plantar wart
	posterior wall
	pulse width
	puncture wound
P&W	pressures and waves
PWA	persons with AIDS
	P-wave axis
PWACR	Prader-Willi/Angelman critical region
P wave	part of the electrocardio-graphic cycle representing atrial depolarization
PWB	partial weight bearing
	Positive Well-being (scale)
	psychological well-being
PWBL	partial weight bearing, left
PWBR	partial weight bearing, right
PWC	personal watercraft
	physical working capacity
	powered wheelchair
PWCA	personal watercraft accident
PWD	patients with diabetes
	person(s) with a disability
	powder
PWE	people with epilepsy
PWI	pediatric walk-in clinic
	perfusion-weighted (magnetic resonance) imaging
	posterior wall infarct
PWLV	posterior wall of left ventricle
PWM	pokeweed mitogens
PWMI	posterior wall myocardial infarction
PWO	persistent withdrawal occlusion
PWP	pulmonary wedge pressure
PWS	plagiocephaly without synostosis
	port-wine stain
	Prader-Willi syndrome
PWT	pad weight test(s)
	posterior wall thickness
	primary writing tremor
PWTd	posterior wall thickness at end-diastole
PWV	polistes wasp venom
	pulse-wave velocity
Px	physical exam
	pneumothorax
	prognosis
	prophylaxis
PXAT	paroxysmal atrial tachycardia
PXE	pseudoxanthoma elasticum
PXF	pseudoexfoliation
PXL	paclitaxel (Taxol)
PXS	dental prophylaxis (cleaning)
PY	pack-years (see pk yrs)
	person-year
PYAR	person-years at risk
PYE	person-years of exposure
PYHx	packs per year history
PYLL	potential years of life lost
PYP	pyrophosphate
PYP®	technetium Tc 99m pyrophosphate kit
PZ	peripheral zone
PZA	pyrazinamide
	pyrazoloacridine (a drug class of sedative/hypnotics)
PZD	partial zona drilling
	partial zonal dissection
PZI	protamine zinc insulin
PZR	posterior zygomatic root

Q

Q Q sign; a patient whose mouth is open with their tongue hanging out when unconscious (slang)
quadriceps

q every (care must be taken to make sure that the handwritten q is not seen as a 9)

QA quality assurance

QAC before every meal (this is a dangerous abbreviation)

QALE quality-adjusted life expectancy

QALYs quality-adjusted life years

QAM every morning (this is a dangerous abbreviation because the Q can be read as a 9 becoming 9 AM)

QAPI quality assessment and performance improvement

QAS quality-adjusted survival

QATTP quality-adjusted time to progression

QB blood flow

QC quad cane
quality checks
quality control
quick catheter

QCA quantitative coronary angiography

Q compound Chinese cucumber

QCSW Qualified Clinical Social Worker

QCT quantitative computed tomography

QD dialysate flow
every day (this is a dangerous abbreviation as it is read as four times daily-QID; use "once daily")
quinupristin and dalfopristin (Synercid)

QDAM once daily in the morning (this is a dangerous abbreviation)

QDAY every day

QDNs quantum dot nanocrystals

QDPM once daily in the evening (This is a dangerous abbreviation)

QDS United Kingdom abbreviation for four times a day

QE quinidine effect

QED every even day (this is a dangerous abbreviation as it will be read as four times daily-QID)
quick and early diagnosis

QEE quadriceps extension exercise

qEEG quantitative electroencephalography

QEMG quantitative electromyography

QF quadriceps femoris (muscle)

QFB Qu'mico Farmacéutico Bi-logo (Chemist Pharmacist Biologist; Pharmacist in Mexico)

QF-PCR quantitative fluorescence polymerase chain reaction

QFV Q fever (*Coxiella burnetii*) vaccine

QGS quantitative gate SPECT (single photon emission computed tomography)

q4h every four hours

q.h. every hour

qhs once daily at bedtime, each day (this is a dangerous abbreviation as it is read as every hour-QHR or four times daily-QID)

QIAD Quantitative Inventory of Alcohol Disorders

q.i.d. four times daily

QIDM four times daily with meals and at bedtime

QIG quantitative immunoglobulins

QIMT quantitative intima media thickness

QIO Quality Improvement Organization

QIW four times a week (this is a dangerous abbreviation)

QJ quadriceps jerk

QKD interval Korotkoff sounds

QL quality of life

QLI Quality of Life Index

QLS quality of life score

QM every morning (this is a dangerous abbreviation as it will not be understood)

Qmax maximal flow rate

QMB qualified Medicare beneficiary

QMI Q-wave myocardial infarction

QMRP qualified mental retardation professional

QMT quantitative muscle testing

q.n. every night (this is a dangerous abbreviation as it is read as every hour)

q.n.s. quantity not sufficient

qod every other day (this is a dangerous abbreviation as it is read as every day or four times a day-QID)

qoh every other hour (this is a dangerous abbreviation as it is read as every day or four times a day-QID)

qohs every other day at bedtime (this is a dangerous abbreviation as it is read as every hour-QHR or four times daily-QID)

QOL quality of life

QOLIE-31 quality of life in epilepsy

QOM quality of motion

Q

QON every other night (this is a dangerous abbreviation)
QOPI Quality Oncology Practice Initiative (of the American Society of Clinical Oncology)
QPCR quantitative polymerase chain reaction
qpm every evening (this is a dangerous abbreviation as it is seen as 9 pm)
QPOS Quality Point of Service
QP/QS ratio of pulmonary blood to systemic blood flow
qqh every four hours (United Kingdom)
qqs every four hours (United Kingdom)
QR quiet room
QRC qualitative radiocardiography
QRDR quinolone resistance-determining region(s)
QRE quality-related event
QRNG quinolone-resistant *N. gonorrhoeae*
QRS part of electrocardio-graphic wave representing ventricular depolarization
QS every shift
quadriceps set
quadrilateral socket
Quality Services (Department)
sufficient quantity
qs ad a sufficient quantity to make
QSAR quantitative structure-activity relationship
Q sign a patient whose mouth is open with their tongue hanging out when unconscious (slang)
QS&L quarters, subsistence, and laundry
Qs/Qt intrapulmonary shunt fraction
QSP physiological shunt fraction
QSRL Q-switched ruby laser
QT the time between the beginning of the QRS complex and the end of the T-wave
qt quart (US, 1 quart = 2 pints = 946 mL; UK, 1 quart = 1,137 mL)
QTB quadriceps tendon bearing
QTC quantitative tip cultures
QTc the QTc interval is the length of time it takes the electrical system in the heart to repolarize, adjusted for heart rate (normal 350-440 milliseconds)
QTL quantitative trait locus
QTP quetiapine fumarate (Seroquel)
Q-TWiST quality-adjusted time without symptoms (of disease) and toxicity
QTY quantity
QUAD quadrant
quadriceps
quadriplegic
QU quiet
QUART quadrantectomy, axillary dissection, and radiotherapy
QUEST Quality of Upper Extremity Skills Test
QUICKI quantitative insulin sensitivity check index
QUM Quality Use of Medicines (Australia)
QuMA quantitative microsatellite analysis
QUS quantitative (bone) ultrasound
QW every week (this is a dangerous abbreviation)
Q-wave
q4w every 4 weeks (this is a dangerous abbreviation)
QWB Quality of Well-Being (scale)
QWE every weekend (this is a dangerous abbreviation)
QWK once a week (this is a dangerous abbreviation)
Q4wk every four weeks
(this is a dangerous abbreviation)
QWMI Q-wave myocardial infarction

R

R	radial
	rate
	ratio
	reacting
	rectal
	rectum
	regular
	regular insulin
	resistant
	respiration
	reticulocyte
	retinoscopy
	rifampicin [part of tuberculosis regimen, see RHZ(E/S)/HR]
	right (this a dangerous abbreviation; spell out "right" to avoid surgical errors)
	Ritalin (methylphenidate) as in vitamin R
	roentgen
	rub
r	recombinant
®	rectal (rectally, rectum)
	registered trademark
	right (this is a dangerous abbreviation; spell out "right" to avoid surgical errors)
−R	Rinne test, negative
+R	Rinne test, positive
R-2	rohypnol (Roofies) (slang)
RA	radial artery
	radiographic absorptiometry
	rales
	readmission
	renal artery
	repeat action
	retinoic acid
	rheumatoid arthritis
	right arm
	right atrium
	right auricle
	room air
	rotational atherectomy
RAA	renin-angiotensin-aldosterone
	right atrial abnormality
	right atrial appendage
RAAA	ruptured abdominal aortic aneurysm
RAAS	renin-angiotensin-aldosterone system
RAB	rabies vaccine, not otherwise specified
	rice (rice cereal), applesauce, and banana (diet)
RAB_{DEV}	rabies vaccine, duck embryo culture
RAB_{FRhL-2}	rabies vaccine, diploid fetal-rhesus-lung-2 cell line
RABG	room air blood gas
RAB_{HDCV}	rabies vaccine, human diploid cell culture
RABig	rabies immune globulin
RAB_{PCEC}	rabies vaccine, purified chick embryo cell culture
RAC	Recombinant DNA Advisory Committee
	right antecubital
	right atrial catheter
RACCO	right anterior caudocranial oblique
RACT	recalcified whole-blood activated clotting time
RACZ	a procedure of dissolving lumbar scar tissue (epidurolysis)
RAD	ionizing radiation unit
	radical
	radiology
	rapid antigen detection
	reactive airway disease
	reactive attachment disorder
	renal (tubule) assist device
	right axis deviation
RADCA	right anterior descending coronary artery
RADE	reactive airway disease exacerbation
RADISH	rheumatoid arthritis diffuse idiopathic skeletal hyperostosis
RADS	ionizing radiation units
	rapid assay delivery systems
	reactive airway disease syndrome
RADT	rapid antigen detection testing
RAE	right atrial enlargement
RAEB	refractory anemia, erythroblastic
RAEB-T	refractory anemia with excess blasts in transition
RAF	rapid atrial fibrillation
RAFF	rectus abdominis free flap
RAFT	Rehabilitative Addicted Family Treatment
RAG	room air gas
RAH	right atrial hypertrophy
RAHB	right anterior hemiblock
rAHF	antihemophilic factor (recombinant)
RAI	radioactive iodine
	Resident Assessment Instrument
RAID	radioimmunodetection
RAIT	radioimmunotherapy
RAIU	radioactive iodine uptake
RALP	robotic-assisted laparoscopic prostatectomy
RALT	routine admission laboratory tests
RAM	radioactive material
	rapid alternating movements
	rectus abdominis myocutaneous

R

RA/MAC regional anesthesia with monitored anesthesia care
RAMBAs retinoic acid metabolism blocking agents
RAMP® Rapid Analyte Measurement Platform
RAN resident's admission notes
R_2AN second year resident's admission notes
RANKL receptor activator of NFκB ligand
RANTES regulated upon activation, normal T cell expressed and secreted
RANZCOG Fellows of the Royal Australian and New Zealand College of Obstetricians and Gynaecologists
RANZCP Fellows of the Royal Australian and New Zealand College of Psychiatrists
RAO right anterior oblique
rAOM recurrent acute otitis media
RAP renal artery pseudoaneurysm
request for advance payment
right abdominal pain
right atrial pressure
RAPA radial artery pseudoaneurysm
RAQ right anterior quadrant
RAP recurrent abdominal pain
request for anticipated payment
Resident Assessment Protocol (long-term care)
RAPD random amplified polymorphic DNA
relative afferent pupillary defect
RAPs Resident Assessment Protocols
RAR right arm, reclining
RARs retinoic acid receptors
RAS recurrent aphthous stomatitis
renal artery stenosis
renal artery stenting
renin-angiotensin system
reticular activating system
right arm, sitting
RASE rapid-acquisition spin echo
r-ASRM score Revised American Society for Reproductive Medicine (score/staging) (Infertility with endometriosis staging)
RASS Richmond Agitation-Sedation Scale
RAST radioallergosorbent test
RAT right anterior thigh
RA test test for rheumatoid factor
RATG rabbit antithymocyte globulin
RATx radiation therapy
RAU recurrent aphthous ulcers
RAVLT Rey Auditory Verbal Learning Test
R(AW) airway resistance
RB relieved by
retinoblastoma
retrobulbar
right breast
right buttock
R & B right and below
RBA right basilar artery
right brachial artery
risks, benefits, and alternatives (discussion with patient)
RBB right breast biopsy
RBBB right bundle branch block
RBBX right breast biopsy examination
RBC ranitidine bismuth citrate
red blood cell (count)
RBCD right border cardiac dullness
RBCM red blood cell mass
RBC s/f red blood cells spun filtration
RBCV red blood cell volume
RBD REM (rapid eye movement sleep) behavior disorder
right border of dullness
right brain-damaged
RbDe residue-based diagram editor
RBE relative biologic effectiveness
RBF renal blood flow
RBG random blood glucose
RBILD respiratory bronchiolitis-associated interstitial lung disease
RBL Roche Biomedical Laboratory
RBON retrobulbar optic neuritis
RBOW rupture bag of water
RBP recurrent bacterial pneumonia
retinol-binding protein
RBRVS Recourse-Based Relative Value Scale (Medicare)
RBS random blood sugar
redback spider
RBT rational behavior therapy
RBV read-back verbal (order)
right brachial vein
RBVO read-back verbal order
right brachial vein occlusion
RBX ruboxistaurin
RC race
radiocarpal (joint)
Red Cross
report called
retention catheter
retrograde cystogram
retruded contact (position)
right coronary
Roman Catholic
root canal
rotator cuff
R/C reclining chair
R & C reasonable and customary (charges)
RCA radiographic contrast agent
radionuclide cerebral angiogram
right carotid artery

	right coronary artery
	rolling circle amplification
	root cause analysis
RC/AL	residential care, assisted living
RCBF	regional cerebral blood flow
RCC	rape crisis center
	Rathke cleft cyst
	resectable colon cancer
	renal cell carcinoma
	right cranial-caudal (mammogram view)
	Roman Catholic Church
RCCA	right common carotid artery
RCCT	randomized controlled clinical trial
RCD	relative cardiac dullness
RCDAD	recurrent *Clostridium difficile*-associated diarrhea
RCE	right carotid endarterectomy
RCF	Reiter complement fixation
RCF®	enteral nutrition product
RCFA	right common femoral angioplasty
	right common femoral artery
RCFE	residential care facility for the elderly
RCH	residential care home
RCHF	right-sided congestive heart failure
R-CHOP	rituximab (Rituxan), cyclophosphamide, doxorubicin (hydroxydaunorubicin), vincristine (Oncovin), and prednisone
RCIN	radiographic-contrast-media-induced nephropathy
RCIP	rape crisis intervention program
RCL	radial collateral ligament
	range of comfortable loudness
RCM	radiographic contrast media
	restricted cardiomyopathy
	retinal capillary microaneurysm
	right costal margin
RCMAR	Resource Centers for Minority Aging Research (NIH)
RCN	radiocontrast-agent-induced nephrotoxicity
RCO	revoked court order
RCOG	Royal College of Obstetricians and Gynaecologists
RCOT	revoked court-ordered treatment
RCP	respiratory care plan
	retrograde cerebral perfusion
	Royal College of Physicians
RCPM	raven-colored progressive matrices
RCPT	Registered Cardiopulmonary Technician
RCR	replication-competent retrovirus (assay)
	responsible conduct of research
	rotator cuff repair
RCRA	Resource Conservation Recovery Act (U.S. Environmental Protection Agency)
RCS	repeat cesarean section
	reticulum cell sarcoma
	Royal College of Surgeons
RCT	randomized clinical trial
	Registered Care Technologist
	root canal therapy
	Rorschach Content Test
	rotator cuff tear
RCU	respiratory care unit
RCV	red cell volume
	right colic vein
RCVD	received
RCVP	retrograde coronary vein perfusion
	rituximab, cyclophosphamide, vincristine, and prednisolone
RCX	ramus circumflexus
RD	radial deviation
	Raynaud disease
	reaction of degeneration
	reading disability
	reflex decay
	Registered Dietitian
	renal disease
	respiratory disease
	respiratory distress
	restricted duty
	retinal detachment
	Reye disease
	rhabdomyosarcoma
	right deltoid
	ruptured disk
RDA	recommended daily allowance
	Registered Dental Assistant
	representational difference analysis
RDB	randomized double-blind (trial)
RDCS	Registered Diagnostic Cardiac Sonographer
RDD	renal dose dopamine
	Rosai-Dorfman disease
RDE	remote data entry
	respiratory disturbance events
RDEA	right deviation of electrical axis
RDEB	recessive dystrophic epidermolysis bullosa
RDG	right dorsogluteal
RDH	Registered Dental Hygienist
RDI	respiratory disturbance (distress) index
RDIH	right direct inguinal hernia
RDLBBB	rate-dependent left bundle branch block
RDM	right deltoid muscle
RDMS	Registered Diagnostic Medical Sonographer

R

RDMs	reactive drug metabolites
RDOD	retinal detachment, right eye
RDOS	retinal detachment, left eye
RDP	random donor platelets
	right dorsoposterior
RDPE	reticular degeneration of the pigment epithelium
RDS	research diagnostic criteria
	respiratory distress syndrome
RDT	rapid diagnostic test
	regular dialysis (hemodialysis) treatment
RDTD	referral, diagnosis, treatment, and discharge
RDU	recreational drug use
RDVT	recurrent deep vein thrombosis
RDW	red (cell) distribution width
RE	concerning
	Rasmussen encephalitis
	rectal examination
	reflux esophagitis
	regarding
	regional enteritis
	reticuloendothelial
	retinol equivalents
	right ear (this is a dangerous abbreviation as it can be read as right eye)
	right eye (this a dangerous abbreviation as it can be read as right ear)
	rowing ergometer
^{186}Re	rhenium 186
R & E	rest and exercise
	round and equal
R ↑ E	right upper extremity
R ↓ E	right lower extremity
RE✓	recheck
READM	readmission
REAL	Revised European American Lymphoma (classification)
REALM	Rapid Estimation of Adult Literacy in Medicine
REC	gingival recession
	rear-end collision
	recommend
	record
	recovery
	recreation
	recur
RECA	right external carotid artery
RECIST	Response Evaluation Criteria in Solid Tumors (guidelines) CR = complete response PR = partial response PD = progressive disease SD = stable disease
RECT	rectum
REDA	Registered Eating Disorders Associate
REDs	reproductive endocrine diseases
reds	red blood cells
RED SUBS	reducing substances
REE	resting energy expenditure
RE-ED	re-education
R-EEG	resting electroencephalogram
REEGT	Registered Electroencephalogram Technologist
REF	referred
	refused
	renal erythropoietic factor
ref→	refer to
REG	radioencephalogram
	regression analysis
	regular
Reg block	regional block anesthesia
regurg	regurgitation
rehab	rehabilitation
REL	relative
	religion
RELE	resistive exercise, lower extremities
REM	rapid eye movement
	recent event memory
	remarried
	remission
	roentgen equivalent unit
REMI	remifentanil (Ultiva)
REMS	rapid eye movement sleep
REO	respiratory and enteric orphan (viruses)
REP	rapid electrophoresis
	repair
	repeat
	report
REP CK	rapid electrophoresis creatine kinase
REPL	recurrent early pregnancy loss
repol	repolarization
REPS	repetitions
REPT	Registered Evoked Potential Technologist
RER	renal excretion rate
RER+	replication error positive
RES	recurrent erosion syndrome
	resection
	resident
	reticuloendothelial system
RESC	resuscitation
RESP	respirations
	respiratory
REST	restoration
	restriction of environmental stimulation therapy
RET	resistance exercise training
	retention
	reticulocyte
	retina

	retired
	return
	right esotropia
ret detach	retinal detachment
retic	reticulocyte
RETRO	retrograde
RETRX	retractions
REUE	resistive exercise, upper extremities
REV	reverse
	review
	revolutions
RF	radiofrequency
	reduction fixation
	refill; refilled (prescriptions)
	renal failure
	respiratory failure
	restricted fluids
	rheumatic fever
	rheumatoid factor
	ring finger
	right foot
	risk factor
	radiofrequency
R/F	retroflexed
R&F	radiographic and fluoroscopic
RF6	rejection-free survival at 6 months
RFA	radiofrequency ablation
	right femoral artery
	right forearm
	right frontoanterior
rFVIIa	recombinant activated coagulation factor VII (NovoSeven)
RFB	retained foreign body
	radial flow chromatography
	residual functional capacity
RFC	reduced folate carrier
RFCA	radiofrequency catheter ablation
RFD	residue-free diet
RFDT	Reach in Four Directions Test
RFE	return flow enema
RFFF	radial forearm free flap (reconstruction of pharyngeal defect)
RFFIT	rapid fluorescent focus inhibition test
rFVIII FS	antihemophilic factor (recombinant), formulated with sucrose (Kogenate)
RFg	visual fields by Goldmann-type perimeter
rFGF-2	recombinant fibroblast growth factor-2
RFID	radio frequency identification
RFIPC	Rating Form of IBD (inflammatory bowel disease) Patient Concerns
RFL	radionuclide functional lymphoscintigraphy
	right frontolateral
RFLF	retained fetal lung fluid
RFLP	restriction fragment length polymorphism (patterns)
RFM	rifampin (Rifadin)
RFP	Renal function panel (see page 318)
	request for payment
	request for proposal
	right frontoposterior
RFS	rapid frozen section
	recurrence-free survival
	refeeding syndrome
	relapse-free survival
RFT	respiratory function test
	right frontotransverse
	routine fever therapy
RFTA	radiofrequency thermal ablation
RFTC	radiofrequency thermocoagulation
RFUT	radioactive fibrinogen uptake
RFV	reason for visit
	right femoral vein
RFVTR	radiofrequency volumetric tissue reduction
RG	regurgitated (infant feeding)
	right (upper outer) gluteus
R/G	red/green
RGA	right gastroepiploic artery
RGCSE	refractory generalized convulsive status epilepticus
RGEA	right gastroepiploic artery
RGM	rapidly growing *Mycobacteria*
	recurrent glioblastoma multiforme
	right gluteus medius
RGO	reciprocating gait orthosis
RGP	rigid gas-permeable (contact lens)
Rh	Rhesus factor in blood
RH	radical hysterectomy
	reduced haloperidol
	relative humidity
	rest home
	retinal hemorrhage
	right hand
	right hemisphere
	right hyperphoria
	room humidifier
Rh+	Rhesus positive
Rh−	Rhesus negative
RHA	rheumatoid arthritis (therapeutic) vaccine
	right hepatic artery
rHA	recombinant human albumin
RHABDO	rhabdomyolysis
rhAPC	recombinant human activated protein C
RHB	raise head of bed
	right heart border
RH/BSO	radial hysterectomy and bilateral salpingo-oophorectomy
RHC	respiration has ceased
	right heart catheterization

R

	right hemicolectomy
	routine health care
	rural health clinic
RHD	radial head dislocation
	relative hepatic dullness
	rheumatic heart disease
	right-hand dominant
rh-DNase	dornase alfa (Pulmozyme)
rhEPO	recombinant human erythropoietin
RHF	rheumatic fever vaccine
	right heart failure
RHG	right-hand grip
rhGAA	recombinant human lysosomal acid alpha-glucosidase
rhGH	recombinant human growth hormone
r-hGH(m)	mammalian-cell–derived recombinant human growth hormone (Serostim)
RHH	right homonymous hemianopsia
RHIA	Registered Health Information Administrator
RHINO	rhinoplasty
RHIOs	regional health information organizations
RHIT	Registered Health Information Technician
RHL	right hemisphere lesions
	right heptic lobe
rhm	roentgens per hour at one meter
RHO	right heel off
Rho(D)	immune globulin to an Rh-negative woman
RhoGAM®	Rh_O (D) immune globulin
RHP	resting head pressure
rhPDGF	recombinant human platelet-derived growth factor
RHR	resting heart rate
RHS	right-hand side
RHT	regional hyperthermia
	right hypertropia
rHuEPO	recombinant human erythropoietin
rHuKGF	recombinant human keratinocyte growth factor (Palifermin)
Rhupus	coexistence of rheumatoid arthritis and systemic lupus erythematosus
RHV	right hepatic vein
RHW	radiant heat warmer
RHZ(E/S)/HR	a tuberculosis treatment regimen consisting of rifampicin, isoniazid, pyrazinamide, ethambutol, streptomycin, isoniazid, and rifampicin (also see 2EHRZ/6HE)
RI	ramus intermedius (coronary artery)
	refractive index
	Registered Indian (Canada)
	regular insulin
	relapse incidence
	renal insufficiency
	respiratory illness
	retroillumination
	rooming in
RIA	radioimmunoassay
	reversible ischemic attack
RIAC	rapid inflation, asymmetrical compression (device)
RIAT	radioimmune antiglobulin test
RIBA	recombinant immunoblot assay
RIBC	residual infiltrating breast cancer
RIC	reduced intensity conditioning
	right iliac crest
	right internal carotid (artery)
RICA	right internal carotid artery
RICE	rest, ice, compression, and elevation
RICM	right intercostal margin
RICS	right intercostal space
RICU	respiratory intensive care unit
RID	radial immunodiffusion
	ruptured intervertebral disk
RIDL	Release of Insects with a Dominant Lethal (mutations)
RIE	radiation induced emesis
	reactive ion etching
	rocket immunoelectrophoresis
RIF	rifampin
	right iliac fossa
	right index finger
	rigid internal fixation
RIG	rabies immune globulin
RIGS	radioimmunoguided surgery
RIH	right inguinal hernia
RIHP	renal interstitial hydrostatic pressure
RIJ	right internal jugular
RIMA	reversible inhibitor of monoamine oxidase-type A
	right internal mammary anastamosis
	right internal mammary artery
RIN	radiocontrast-induced nephropathy
RIND	reversible ischemic neurologic defect
RINV	radiation-induced nausea and vomiting
RIO	right inferior oblique (muscle)
RIOJ	recurrent intrahepatic obstructive jaundice
R-IOL	remove intraocular lens
RIP	radioimmunoprecipitin test
	rapid infusion pump
	respiratory inductance plethysmograph
	rhythmic inhibitory pattern
RIPA	ristocetin-induced platelet agglutination
RIR	right inferior rectus
RIS	radioimmunoscintigraphy
	responding to internal stimuli

	risperidone (Risperdal)
RISA	radioactive iodinated serum albumin
RiskMAP	risk minimization action plan
RISS	regular insulin sliding scale
RIST	radioimmunosorbent test
RIT	radioimmunotherapy
	ritonavir (Norvir)
	Rorschach Inkblot Test
RITA	right internal thoracic artery
RIVD	ruptured intervertebral disk
RIX	radiation-induced xerostomia
RJ	radial jerk (reflex)
	right jugular
RK	radial keratotomy
	right kidney
RKS	renal kidney stone
RKT	Registered Kinesiotherapist
RL	right lateral
	right leg
	right lower
	right lung
	Ringer lactate
	rotation left
R → L	right to left
RLA	right lower arm
RLB	right lateral bending
	right lateral border
RLBCD	right lower border of cardiac dullness
RLC	Registered Lactation Consultant
	residual lung capacity
RLD	reference listed drug
	related living donor
	remaining life expectancy
	right lateral decubitus
	ruptured lumbar disk
RLDP	right lateral decubital position
RLE	right lower extremity
RLF	retrolental fibroplasia
	right lateral femoral
RLFP	Remaining Lifetime Fracture Probability
RLG	right lateral gaze
RLGS	restriction landmark genomic scanning
RLH	reactive lymphoid hyperplasia
RLL	right liver lobe
	right lower lid
	right lower lobe
RLN	recurrent laryngeal nerve
	regional lymph node(s)
RLND	regional lymph node dissection
RLQ	right lower quadrant
RLQD	right lower quadrant defect
RLR	right lateral rectus
RLRTD	recurrent lower respiratory tract disease
RLS	resonance light scattering
	restless legs syndrome
	Ringer lactate solution
	stammerer who has difficulty in enunciating R, L, and S
RLSB	right lower scapular border
	right lower sternal border
RLT	right lateral thigh
RLTCS	repeat low transverse cesarean section
RLUs	relative light units
RLWD	routine laboratory work done
RLX	raloxifene (Evista)
	right lower extremity
RM	radical mastectomy
	repetitions maximum
	respiratory movement
	risk manager (management)
	risk model
	room
R&M	routine and microscopic
1-RM	single repetition maximum lift
RMA	reduction in metabolic activity
	refused medical assistance
	Registered Medical Assistant
	right mentoanterior
	Rivermead motor assessment
RMB	right main bronchus
RMBPC	Revise Memory and Behavior Problems Checklist
RMCA	right main coronary artery
	right middle cerebral artery
RMCAT	right middle cerebral artery thrombosis
RMCL	right midclavicular line
RMD	recommended maintenance dose
	restrictive myocardial disease
	rippling muscle disease
	risk management database
RMDQ	Roland and Morris disability questionnaire
RME	reasonable maximum exposure
	resting metabolic expenditure
	right mediolateral episiotomy
RMEE	right middle ear exploration
rMET	recombinant methioninase
RMF	right middle finger
RMGIC	resin-modified glass ionomer cement (dental)
RMI	Rivermead Mobility Index
RMK #1	remark number 1
RML	right mediolateral
	right middle lobe
RMLE	right mediolateral episiotomy
RMLO	right medial-lateral oblique (mammogram view)
RMMA	rhythmic masticatory muscle activity
RMO	responsible medical officer

R

rMOG	recombinant myelin oligodendrocyte glycoprotein
RMP	right mentoposterior risk management program
RMR	resting metabolic rate right medial rectus root mean square residue
RMRM	right modified radical mastectomy
RMS	red-man syndrome Rehabilitation Medicine Service repetitive motion syndrome rhabdomyosarcoma Rocky Mountain spotted fever vaccine root-mean-square
RMS®	rectal morphine sulfate (suppository)
RMSB	right middle sternal border
RMSE	root-mean-square error
RMSF	Rocky Mountain spotted fever
RMT	Registered Music Therapist right mentotransverse
RMV	respiratory minute volume
RMW	respiratory muscle weakness
RN	radiation necrosis Registered Nurse right nostril (nare)
Rn	radon
R/N	renew
RNA	radionuclide angiography Restorative Nursing Assistant ribonucleic acid routine nursing assistance
RNAi	deoxyribonucleic acid interference
RN,BC	Registered Nurse, Board Certified (many clinical specialties)
RNC	Registered Nurse, Certified
RNCD	Registered Nurse, Chemical Dependency
RNCNA	Registered Nurse Certified in Nursing Administration
RNCNAA	Registered Nurse Certified in Nursing Administration Advanced
RNCS	Registered Nurse Certified Specialist
RND	radical neck dissection
RNEF	resting (radio-) nuclide ejection fraction
RNF	regular nursing floor
RNFA	registered nurse first assistant
RNFL	retinal nerve fiber layer
RNFLT	retinal nerve fiber layer thickness
RNI	reactive nitrogen intermediates rubella nonimmune
RNLP	Registered Nurse, license pending
RNP	Registered Nurse Practitioner restorative nursing program ribonucleoprotein
RNS	recurrent nephrotic syndrome replacement normal saline (0.9% sodium chloride)
RNST	reactive nonstress test
RNUD	recurrent nonulcer dyspepsia
RNV	radionucleotide ventriculogram
RO	reality orientation relative odds report of reverse osmosis routine order(s) Russian Orthodox
R/O	rule out
ROA	radiographic osteoarthritis right occiput anterior
ROAC	repeated oral doses of activated charcoal
ROAD	reversible obstructive airway disease
ROBE	routine operative breast endoscopy
ROBO	run over by owner (Veterinary slang)
ROC	receiver operating characteristic record of contact resident on call residual organic carbon
ROCF	Rey-Osterrieth complex figure
ROD	rapid opioid detoxification renal osteodystrophy
RODA	rapid opiate detoxification under anesthesia
ROE	report of event right otitis externa
ROF	review of outside films
ROG	rogletimide
ROH	rubbing alcohol
ROI	region of interest (radiology) release of information
ROIDS	hemorrhoids
ROIH	right oblique inguinal hernia
ROJM	range of joint motion
ROL	right occipitolateral
ROLC	roentgenologically occult lung cancer
ROLL	radioguided occult lesion localization
ROM	range of motion rifampicin 600 mg, ofloxacin 400 mg, and minocycline 100 mg right otitis media rupture of membranes
ROMA	representative oligonucleotide microarray analysis
Romb	Romberg
ROMCP	range of motion complete and painfree
ROMI	rule out myocardial infarction
ROMSA	right otitis media, suppurative, acute
ROMSC	right otitis media, suppurative, chronic
ROMWNL	range of motion within normal limits
RON	radiation optic neuropathy
RONTD	risk of neural tube defect
ROP	retinopathy of prematurity

	right occiput posterior
Ropi	ropivacaine (Naropin)
ROPS	roll-over protection structures
ROR	the French acronym for measles-mumps-rubella vaccine
	retinoid-related orphan receptor
	reporting odds ratio
R or L	right or left
ROS	review of systems
	rod outer segments
	rule out sepsis
ROSA	rank-order stability analysis
ROSC	restoration of spontaneous circulation
ROSS	review of signs and symptoms
ROT	remedial occupational therapy
	right occipital transverse
	rotator
ROU	recurrent oral ulcer
ROUL	rouleaux (rouleau)
ROW	rest of (the) week
RP	radial pulse
	radical prostatectomy
	radiopharmaceutical
	Raynaud phenomenon
	responsible party
	resting position
	restorative proctocolectomy
	retinitis pigmentosa
	retrograde pyelogram
	retropubic prostatectomy
	root plane
RPA	radial photon absorptiometry
	recursive partitioning analysis
	Registered Physician's Assistant
	repolarization alternans
	restenosis postangioplasty
	retinitis punctata albescens
	ribonuclease protection assay
	right pulmonary artery
RPAC	Registered Physician's Assistant Certified
RPC	root planing and curettage
RPCDBM	randomized, placebo-controlled, double-blind, multinational (study)
RPCF	Reiter protein complement fixation
RPD	removable partial denture
RPDB	Registered Persons Database (Canada)
RPE	rating of perceived exertion
	retinal pigment epithelium
RPED	retinal pigment epithelium detachment
RPEP	rabies postexposure prophylaxis
	right pre-ejection period
RPF	regional progression-free
	relaxed pelvic floor
	renal plasma flow
	retroperitoneal fibrosis
RPFT	Registered Pulmonary Function Technologist
RPG	retrograde percutaneous gastrostomy
	retrograde pyelogram
RPGN	rapidly progressive glomerulonephritis
RPH	retroperitoneal hemorrhage
RPh	Registered Pharmacist
RPHA	reverse passive hemagglutination
RPI	resting pressure index
	reticulocyte production index
RPICA	right posterior internal carotid artery
RPICCE	round pupil intracapsular cataract extraction
RPL	retroperitoneal lymphadenectomy
RPLC	reversed-phase liquid chromatography
RPLND	retroperitoneal lymph node dissection
RPLS	reversible posterior leukoencephalopathy syndrome
RPM/L	respirations per minute per liter
RPN	renal papillary necrosis
	resident's progress notes
R_2PN	second year resident's progress notes
RPO	right posterior oblique
RPP	radical perineal prostatectomy
	rate-pressure product
	retropubic prostatectomy
RPPS	retropatellar pain syndrome
RPR	rapid plasma reagin (test for syphilis)
	Reiter protein reagin
RPS	rhabdoid predisposition syndrome
RPSGT	Registered Polysomnography Technician
RPT	Registered Physical Therapist
RPTA	Registered Physical Therapist Assistant
RPU	retropubic urethropexy
RPV	right portal vein
	right pulmonary vein
RQ	respiratory quotient
RQLQ	Respiratory Quality of Life Questionnaire
RR	rate ratio(s)
	recovery room
	regular rate
	regular respirations
	relative risk
	respiratory rate
	response rate
	retinal reflex
	rotation right
R/R	rales-rhonchi
R&R	rate and rhythm
	recent and remote
	recession and resection

	resect and recess (muscle surgery)
	rest and recuperation
	remove and replace
RRA	radioreceptor assay
	Registered Record Administrator (for newer title, see RHIA)
	right radial artery
	right renal artery
RRAM	rapid rhythmic alternating movements
RRC	cohort relative risk
RRCT, no(m)	regular rate, clear tones, no murmurs
RRD	removable rigid dressing
	rhegmatogenous retinal detachment
RRE	round, regular, and equal (pupils)
RRED®	Rapid Rare Event Detection
RREF	resting radionuclide ejection fraction
RRI	renal resistive index
RR-IOL	remove and replace intraocular lens
RRM	reduced renal mass
	right radial mastectomy
	risk-reducing mastectomy
RRMS	relapsing-remitting multiple sclerosis
RRNA	Resident Registered Nurse Anesthetist
rRNA	ribosomal ribonucleic acid
RRND	right radical neck dissection
RROM	resistive range of motion
R rot	right rotation
RRP	radical retropubic prostatectomy
	recurrent respiratory papillomatosis
RRR	recovery room routine
	regular rhythm and rate
	relative risk reduction
RRRN	round, regular, and react normally
RRRs̄M	regular rate and rhythm without murmur
RRSO	risk-reducing salpingo-oophorectomy
RRT	Registered Respiratory Therapist
RRU	rapid reintegration unit
RRVO	repair relaxed vaginal outlet
RRVS	recovery room vital signs
RRV-TV	rhesus rotavirus tetravalent (vaccine)
RRW	rales, rhonchi or wheezes
RS	Raynaud syndrome
	rectal swab
	recurrent seizures
	Reed-Sternberg (cell)
	Reiter syndrome
	remote sensing
	reschedule
	restart
	Rett syndrome
	Reye syndrome
	rhythm strip
	right side
	Ringer solution
	rumination syndrome
R/S	reschedule
	rest stress
	rupture spontaneous
R & S	restraint and seclusion
R/S I	resuscitation status one (full resuscitative effort)
R/S II	resuscitation status two (no code, therapeutic measures only)
R/S III	resuscitation status three (no code, comfort measures only)
RSA	radiostereometric analysis
	right sacrum anterior
	right subclavian artery
RSAPE	remitting seronegative arthritis with pitting edema
RSB	right sternal border
RSBI	rapid shallow breathing index
RSBQ	Rett Syndrome Behavior Questionnaire
RSC	right subclavian (artery) (vein)
RScA	right scapuloanterior
RSCL	Rotterdam Symptom Check List
RScP	right scapuloposterior
RSCS	respiratory system compliance score
rscu-PA	recombinant, single-chain, urokinase-type plasminogen activator
RSD	reflex sympathetic dystrophy
	relative standard deviation
RSDS	reflex-sympathetic dystrophy syndrome
RSE	rattlesnake envenomation
	reactive subdural effusion
	refractory status epilepticus
	right sternal edge
RSI	rapid sequence intubation
	repetitive strain (stress) injury
R-SICU	respiratory-surgical intensive care unit
RSL	renal solute load
RSLR	reverse straight leg raise
RSM	remote study monitoring
RSNI	round spermatid nuclear injection
RSO	right salpingooophorectomy
	right superior oblique
rS_{O2}	regional oxygen saturation
RSOC	regular source of care
RSOP	right superior oblique palsy
RSP	rapid straight pacing
	respirable suspended particles
	restriction site polymophism
	right sacroposterior
RS3PE	remitting seronegative symmetrical synovitis with pitting edema
RSR	regular sinus rhythm
	relative survival rate
	right superior rectus

RSRI renal:systemic renin index
RSS reduced space symbologies
representative sample sectioned
Russell-Silver syndrome
RSSE Russian spring-summer encephalitis
RST rapid simple tests
rapid Streptococcal test
right sacrum transverse
RSTs Rodney Smith tubes
RSV respiratory syncytial virus
right subclavian vein
RSVC right superior vena cava
RSV_{IGIV} respiratory syncytial virus immune globulin, intravenous
RSV_{mab} respiratory syncytial virus monoclonal antibody, intramuscular (palivizumab; Synagis)
RSVP rapid serial visual presentation
RSW right-sided weakness
RT radiation therapy
Radiologic Technologist
recreational therapy
rectal temperature
renal transplant
repetition time
resistance training
Respiratory Therapist
reverse transcriptase
right
right thigh
room temperature
R/t related to
RTA ready to administer
renal tubular acidosis
road traffic accident
t-RA tretinoin (*trans*-retinoic acid)
RTAE right atrial enlargement
RTAH right anterior hemiblock
RTAT right anterior thigh
RTB return to baseline
RTC Readiness to Change (questionnaire)
return to clinic
round the clock
RTCA ribavirin
RT3D real-time three-dimensional (echocardiography)
RTER return to emergency room
rt.↑ext. right upper extremity
RTF ready-to-feed
return to flow
RTFS return to flying status
RTH right total hip (arthroplasty)
RTI reproductive tract infection
respiratory tract infection
reverse transcriptase inhibitor
road traffic injuries
RTIS response to internal stimuli
RTK rhabdoid tumor of the kidney
right total knee (arthroplasty)
RTL reactive to light
right temporal lobectomy
RTLF respiratory-tract lining fluids
RTM regression to the mean
routine medical care
RTMCI real-time myocardial contrast perfusion imaging
RTMD right mid-deltoid
rTMS repetitive transcranial magnetic stimulation
RTN renal tubular necrosis
RTNM retreatment staging of cancer
RTO return to office
RTOG Radiation Therapy Oncology Group
RTP renal transplant patient
return to pharmacy
return-to-play
rtPA alteplase (recombinant tissue-type plasminogen activator) (Activase)
RT-PCR reverse transcription polymerase chain reaction
RTPJ right temporoparietal junction
RTR renal transplant recipient(s)
return to room
RT (R) Radiologic Technologist (Registered)
RTRR return to recovery room
RTS radial tunnel syndrome
raised toilet seat
real-time scan
Resolve Through Sharing
return to school
return to sender
Revised Trauma Score
Rothmund-Thomson syndrome
Rubinstein-Taybi syndrome
RTT Respiratory Therapy Technician
RT_3U resin triiodothyronine uptake
RTUS realtime ultrasound
RTV ritonavir (Norvir)
rotavirus vaccine, not otherwise specified
RTV_{rr} rotavirus vaccine, rhesus reassortant
RTW return to ward
return to work
Richard Turner Warwick (urethroplasty)
RTWD return to work determination
RTX resiniferatoxin
RTx radiation therapy
renal transplantation
RU residual urine
resin uptake
retrograde ureterogram
right upper
routine urinalysis
RU 486 mifepristone (Mifeprex)

R

RUA	right upper arm routine urine analysis
RUB	rubella virus vaccine
RUE	right upper extremity
RUG	resource utilization group retrograde urethrogram
RUI	recurring urinary infections
RUL	right upper lid right upper lobe
RUOQ	right upper outer quadrant
rupt.	ruptured
RUQ	right upper quadrant
RUQD	right upper quadrant defect
RURTI	recurrent upper respiratory tract infection
RUS	resonant ultrasound spectroscopy
RUSB	right upper scapular border right upper sternal border
RUT	rapid urease test
RUTF	ready-to-use therapeutic food
RUTI	recurring urinary tract infections
RUV	residual urine volume
RUX	right upper extremity
RV	rectovaginal residual volume respiratory volume retinal vasculitis return visit rhinovirus right ventricle rubella vaccine
RVA	rabies vaccine, adsorbed right ventricular apex right vertebral artery
RVAD	right ventricular assist device
RVCD	right ventricular conduction deficit
RVD	reference vessel diameter regulatory volume decrease relative vertebral density renal vascular disease right ventricular dysfunction
RVDP	right ventricular diastolic pressure
RVE	right ventricular enlargement
RVEDP	right ventricular end-diastolic pressure
RVEDV	right ventricular end-diastolic volume
RVEF	right ventricular ejection fraction
RVET	right ventricular ejection time
RVF	Rift Valley fever right ventricular function right visual field
RVG	radionuclide ventriculography Radio VisioGraphy right ventrogluteal
RVH	renovascular hypertension right ventricular hypertrophy
RVHT	renovascular hypertension
RVI	right ventricle infarction
RVIDd	right ventricle internal dimension diastole
RVL	right vastus lateralis
RVO	relaxed vaginal outlet retinal vein occlusion right ventricular outflow right ventricular overactivity
RVOT	right ventricular outflow tract
RVOTH	right ventricular outflow tract hypertrophy
RVOTO	right ventricular outflow tract obstruction
RVP	right ventricular pressure
RVR	rapid ventricular response renal vascular resistance right ventricular rhythm
RVSP	right ventricular systolic pressure
rVSV	recombinant vesicular stomatitis virus
RVSW	right ventricular stroke work
RVSWI	right ventricular stroke work index
RVT	recurrent ventricular tachycardia renal vein thrombosis
RV/TLC	residual volume to total lung capacity ratio
RVU	relative-value units
RVV	rubella vaccine virus
RVVC	recurrent vulvovaginal candidiasis
RVVT	Russell viper venom time
RW	radiant warmer ragweed red welt respite worker rolling walker
R/W	return to work
RWIs	recreational water illnesses
RWM	regional wall motion
RWMA	regional wall motion abnormalities
RWP	ragweed pollen
RWS	ragweed sensitivity
RWT	relative wall thickness
Rx	drug medication pharmacy prescription radiotherapy take therapy treatment
RXN	reaction
RXRs	retinoid X receptors
RXT	radiation therapy right exotropia
RYGBP	Roux-en-Y gastric bypass (surgery)

S

S	sacral
	second (s)
	sensitive
	serum
	single
	sister
	son
	South (as in the location 2S would be second floor, South wing)
	sponge
	Staphylococcus
	streptomycin [part of tuberculosis regimen as in RHZ(E/S)/HR]
	subjective findings
	suicide
	suction
	sulfur
	supervision
	surgery
	susceptible
/S/	signature
$\bar{s}$	without (this is a dangerous abbreviation)
S′	shoulder
S_1	first heart sound
$S^{-1}...S^{-4}$	suicide risk classifications
S_2	second heart sound
S_3	third heart sound (ventricular filling gallop)
S_4	fourth heart sound (atrial gallop)
$S_1...S_5$	sacral vertebra or nerves 1 through 5
SI..SIV	symbols for the first to fourth heart sounds
SA	sacroanterior
	salicylic acid
	semen analysis
	Sexoholics Anonymous
	sinoatrial
	skeletal abnormalities
	sleep apnea
	slow acetylator
	Spanish American
	spinal anesthesia
	Staphylococcus aureus
	subarachnoid
	substance abuse
	suicide alert
	suicide attempt
	surface area
	surgical assistant
	sustained action
Sa	Saturday
S/A	same as
	sugar and acetone
S&A	sugar and acetone
SAA	same as above
	serum amyloid A
	Stokes-Adams attacks
	synthetic amino acids
SAAG	serum-ascites albumin gradient
SAANDs	selective apoptotic antineoplastic drugs
SAARDs	slow-acting antirheumatic drugs
SAB	serum albumin
	sinoatrial block
	Spanish-American Black
	spontaneous abortion
	Staphylococcus aureus bacteremia
	subarachnoid bleed
	subarachnoid block
SABA	short-acting beta-2 agonist
SABR	screening auditory brainstem response
SABs	side air bags
SAC	safe abortion care
	school-age children
	segmental antigen challenge
	serial abdominal closure
	serum aminoglycoside concentration
	short arm cast
	substance abuse counselor
SACC	short arm cylinder cast
SACD	subacute combined degeneration
SACH	solid ankle, cushioned heel
SACT	sinoatrial conduction time
SAD	schizoaffective disorder
	seasonal affective disorder
	Self-Assessment Depression (scale)
	social anxiety disorder
	source-axis distance
	subacromial decompression
	subacute dialysis
	sugar and acetone determination
	superior axis deviation
SADBE	squaric acid dibutyl ester
SADD	Students Against Drunk Driving
SADL	simulated activities of daily living
SADR	suspected adverse drug reaction
SADRs	serious adverse drug reactions
SADS	Schedule for Affective Disorders and Schizophrenia
	sudden arrhythmic death syndrome
SADs	severe autoimmune diseases
SADS-C	Schedule for Affective Disorders And Schizophrenia – Change Version
SAE	serious adverse event
	short above elbow (cast)
	splenic angioembolization
SAECG	signal-averaged electrocardiogram
SAEKG	signal-averaged electrocardiogram
SAESU	Substance Abuse valuating Screen Unit

SAF	Self-Analysis Form self-articulating femoral Spanish-American female subcutaneous abdominal fat
SAFA	surgical atrial fibrillation ablation
SAFE	surgery, antibiotics, facial cleanliness, and environmental change (a trachoma control program)
SAFHS	sonic accelerated fracture healing system
SAG	sodium antimony gluconate
SAGAM	Scientific Advisory Group on Antimicrobials (EMEA)
Sag D	sagittal diameter
SAGE	serial analysis of gene expression
SAH	subarachnoid hemorrhage systemic arterial hypertension
SAHA	suberoylanilide hydroxamic acid (vorinostat [Zolinza])
SAHS	sleep apnea/hypopnea (hypersomnolence) syndrome
SAI	self-administered injectable Sodium Amytal® interview
SAL	salicylate salmeterol (Serevent) *Salmonella* sensory acuity level sterility assurance level
SAL 12	sequential analysis of 12 chemistry constituents (see page 318)
SALK	surgical arthroscopy, left knee
SAM	methylprednisolone sodium succinate (Solu-Medrol), aminophylline, and metaproterenol (Metaprel) selective antimicrobial modulation self-administered medication severe acute malnutrition short arc motion sleep apnea monitor Spanish-American male systolic anterior motion
SAME	syndrome of arthralgias, myalgias, and edema
SAMe	*S*-adenosylmethionine (ademetionine)
SAMHSA	Substance Abuse and Mental Health Services Administration
SAMI	Substance Abuse, Mental Illness (program)
SAMPLE	symptoms/signs, allergies, medications, past medical history, last oral intake, and events prior to arrival (an EMT mnemonic used in initial patient questioning)
SAMU	Service d'Aide Médicale Urgente (French prehospital emergency system)
SAN	side-arm nebulizer sinoatrial node slept all night
SANC	short-arm navicular cast
SANE	Sexual Assault Nurse Examiner
sang	sanguinous
SANS	Schedule (Scale) for the Assessment of Negative Symptoms sympathetic autonomic nervous system
SAO	small airway obstruction Southeast Asian ovalocytosis
SaO_2	arterial oxygen percent saturation
SAP	Sample Accountability Program serum alkaline phosphate serum amyloid P standard automated perimetry sporadic adenomatous polyps statistical analysis plan
SAPD	self-administration of psychotropic drugs
SAPH	saphenous
SAPHO	synovitis, acne, pustulosis, hyperostosis, and osteomyelitis (syndrome)
SAPS	Scale for the Assessment of Positive Symptoms short-arm plaster splint Simplified Acute Physiology Score
SAPs	shock-absorbing pylons
SAPS II	Simplified Acute Physiology Score version II
SAPTA	stent-assisted percutaneous transluminal angioplasty
SAQ	saquinavir (Invirase) Sexual Adjustment Questionnaire short-arc quadriceps
SAQ/r	saquinavir and ritonavir
SAR	seasonal allergic rhinitis Senior Assistant Resident sexual attitudes reassessment structural activity relationships subacute rehabilitation (center)
SARA	sexually acquired reactive arthritis SQUID (superconducting quantum interference device) array for reproductive assessment system for anesthetic and respiratory administration analysis
SARAN	senior admitting resident's admission note
SARC	seasonal allergic rhinoconjunctivitis
SARK	surgical arthroscopy, right knee
SARMs	selective androgen receptor modulators

S Arrh	sinus arrhythmia
SARS	severe acute respiratory syndrome
SARS-CoV	severe acute respiratory syndrome-associated coronavirus
SART	sexual assault response team
	standard acid reflux test
SAS	saline, agent, and saline
	scalenus anticus syndrome
	Sedation-Agitation Scale
	see assessment sheet
	Self-rating Anxiety Scale
	short-arm splint
	Simpson-Angus Scale
	sleep apnea syndrome
	Social Adjustment Scale
	Specific Activity Scale
	statistical applications software
	subarachnoid space
	subaxial subluxation
	sulfasalazine (Azulfidine)
	synthetic absorbable sutures
SASA	Sex Abuse Survivors Anonymous
SASH	saline, agent, saline, and heparin
SASP	sulfasalazine (salicylazo-sulfapyridine; Azulfidine)
SASS	Social Adaptation Self-Evaluation Scale
SASSAD	six area, six sign atopic dermatitis (severity score)
SAST	slide agglutination serotyping
SAT	methylprednisolone sodium succinate (Solu-Medrol), aminophylline, and terbutaline
	saturated
	saturation
	Saturday
	self-administered therapy
	Senior Apperception Test
	speech awareness threshold
	spontaneous awakening trial
	subacute thyroiditis
	subcutaneous adipose tissue
SATC	substance abuse treatment clinic
SATL	surgical Achilles tendon lengthening
SATP	substance abuse treatment program
SATS	refers to oxygen saturation levels
SATU	substance abuse treatment unit
SAV	supra-annular valve
SaV	sapovirus
SAVD	spontaneous assisted vaginal delivery
SB	safety belt
	sandbag
	scleral buckling
	seat belt
	seen by
	Sengstaken-Blakemore (tube)
	sick boy
	side bend
	side bending
	sinus bradycardia
	slide board
	small bowel
	spina bifida
	sponge bath
	stand-by
	Stanford-Binet (test)
	sternal border
	stillbirth
	stillborn
	stone basketing
Sb	antimony
SB+	wearing seat belt
SB−	not wearing seat belt
SBA	serum bactericidal activity
	standby angioplasty
	standby assistant (assistance)
	Summary Basis of Approval
SBAC	small bowel adenocarcinoma
SBAR	Situation, Background, Assessment, and Recommendation (communication strategies)
SBB	stereotactic breast biopsy
SBBO	small-bowel bacterial overgrowth
SBC	sensory binocular cooperation
	single base cane
	standard bicarbonate
	strict bed confinement
	superficial bladder cancer
SBD	sleep-related breathing disorder
	straight bag drainage
SBE	saturated base excess
	self-breast examination
	short below-elbow (cast)
	shortness of breath on exertion
	subacute bacterial endocarditis
SBF	splanchnic blood flow
SBFT	small bowel follow through
SBG	stand-by guard
SBGM	self blood-glucose monitoring
SBH	State Board of Health
SBI	silicone (gel-containing) breast implants
	something bad inside (undiagnosed cancer etc. discovered during surgery) (Veterinary slang)
	systemic bacterial infection
SBJ	skin, bones, and joints
SBK	spinnbarkeit
SBL	sponge blood loss
sBLA	supplemental Biologic License Application
SB-LM	Stanford-Binet Intelligence Test-Form LM
SBO	small bowel obstruction
	specified bovine offals
SBOD	scleral buckle, right eye

S

SBOE	surgical blood order equation
SBOH	State Board of Health
SBOM	soybean oil meal
SBOS	scleral buckle, left eye
SBP	school breakfast program
	scleral buckling procedure
	small bowel phytobezoars
	spontaneous bacterial peritonitis
	systolic blood pressure
SBQC	small-based quad cane
SBR	sluggish blood return
	strict bed rest
SBRN	sensory branch of the radial nerve
SBRT	stereotactic body radiation therapy
SBS	serum blood sugar
	shaken baby syndrome
	short (small) bowel syndrome
	sick-building syndrome
	side-by-side
	small bowel series
SBT	serum bactericidal titers
	small bowel transplantation
	special baby Travesol
	spontaneous breathing trial
SBTB	sinus breakthrough beat
SBTs	spontaneous breathing trials
SBTT	small bowel transit time
SBV	single binocular vision
SBW	seat belts worn
SBX	symphysis, buttocks, and xiphoid
SC	schizophrenia
	Schwann cell
	self-care
	serum creatinine
	service connected
	sick call
	sickle cell
	small (blood pressure) cuff
	Snellen chart
	spinal cord
	sport cord
	sternoclavicular
	subclavian
	subclavian catheter
	subcutaneous (this is a dangerous abbreviation as it can be read as SL [sublingual]. Use subcut or spell it out.)
	succinylcholine
	sugar-coated (tablets)
	sulfur colloid
	supportive care
	surveillance cultures
$\bar{s}c$	without correction (without glasses)
S&C	sclerae and conjunctivae
SCA	sickle cell anemia
	spinocerebellar ataxia
	subclavian artery
	subcutaneous abdominal (block)
	sudden cardiac arrest
	superior cerebellar artery
SCa	serum calcium
ScA	*Scedosporium apiospermum*
SCA1	spinocerebellar ataxia type 1
SCA7	spinocerebellar ataxia type 7
SCAD	segmental colitis associated with diverticula
	short chain acyl-coenzyme A dehydrogenase
	spontaneous cervical artery dissection
SCAN	suspected child abuse and neglect
SCAP	scapula; scapulae; scapular
	stem cell apheresis
SCARMD	severe childhood autosomal recessive muscular dystrophy
SCAT	sheep cell agglutination titer
	sickle cell anemia test
SCB	stereotactic-guided core biopsy
	strictly confined to bed
SCBC	small cell bronchogenic carcinoma
SCBE	single-contrast barium enema
SCBF	spinal cord blood flow
SCC	short course chemotherapy (for tuberculosis)
	sickle cell crisis
	small cell carcinoma
	spinal cord compression
	squamous cell carcinoma
SCCA	semi-closed circle absorber
	squamous cell carcinoma antigen
SCCa	squamous cell carcinoma
SCCB	small cell cancer of the bladder
SCCE	squamous cell carcinoma of the esophagus
SCCHN	squamous cell carcinoma of the head and neck
SCCI	subcutaneous continuous infusion
SCCOT	squamous cell carcinoma of the oral tongue
SCC/T	squamous sell carcinoma of the oral tongue
SCD	sequential compression device
	service connected disability
	sickle cell disease
	spinal cord disease
	subacute combined degeneration
	sudden cardiac death
ScDA	scapulodextra anterior
SCDM	soybean-casein digest medium
ScDP	scapulodextra posterior
SCE	sister chromatid exchange
	soft cooked egg
	specialized columnar epithelium
	spinal cord ependymoma

SCEMIA self-contained enzymatic membrane immunoassay
SCEP somatosensory cortical evoked potential
SCF slow coronary flow
special care formula
stem cell factor
supra ciliochoroidal fluid
SCFA short-chain fatty acid
SCFE slipped capital femoral epiphysis
SCFGT Southern California Figure Ground Test
SCG seismocardiography
serum Chemogram
sodium cromoglycate
substitute care giver
SCH schistosomiasis (*Schistosoma* sp.) vaccine
subclinical hypothyroidism
SCh succinylcholine chloride
SCHIP State Children's Health Insurance Program
SCHISTO schistocytes
SCHIZ schizocytes
schizophrenia
SCHLP supracricord hemilaryngopharyngectomy
SCHNC squamous cell head and neck cancer
SCI silent cerebral infarct
specific COX-2 inhibitor
spinal cord injury
subcoma insulin
SCID severe combined immunodeficiency disorders (disease)
structured clinical interview for DSM-III-R
SCII Strong-Campbell Interest Inventory
SCIP Screening and Crisis Intervention Program
SCIPP sacrococcygeal to inferior pubic point
SCIT single-chain immunotoxin
subcutaneous immunotherapy
SCIU spinal cord injury unit
SCIV subclavian intravenous
SCI-WORA spinal cord injury without radiolographic abnormalities
SCJ squamocolumnar junction
sternoclavicular joint
sCJD sporadic Creutzfeldt-Jakob disease
SCL skin conductance level
symptom checklist
SCL-90 Symptoms Checklist—90 items
ScLA scapulolaeva anterior
SCLAX subcostal long axis
SCLC small cell lung cancer
SCLD sickle cell lung disease
SCLE subacute cutaneous lupus erythematosis
ScLP scapulolaeva posterior
SCLs soft contact lenses
synthetic combinatorial libraries
SCM scalene muscle
sensation, circulation, and motion
split cord malformation
spondylitic caudal myelopathy
sternocleidomastoid
supraclavicular muscle
SCMD senile choroidal macular degeneration
SCMV serogroup C meningococcal vaccine
SCN severe congenital neutropenia
special care nursery
suprachiasmatic nucleus (nuclei)
SCNB stereotactic core-needle biopsy
SCNs subepidermal calcified nodules
SCNT somatic-cell nuclear transfer
S/CO signal-to-cut-off (ratios)
SCOB Schedule-Controlled Operant Behavior
SCOH services to children in their own homes
SCOP scopolamine
SCOPE arthroscopy
SCP secondary care provider
sodium cellulose phosphate
standardized care plan
SCPF stem cell proliferation factor
S-CPK serum creatine phosphokinase
SCPP spinal cord perfusion pressure
SCQ social communication questionnaire
SCR special care room (seclusion room)
spondylitic caudal radioculopathy
standard care regimen
stem cell rescue
SCr serum creatinine
sCR soluble complement receptor
SCRIPT prescription
SC/RP scaling and root planing
SC-RNV subcutaneous radionuclide venography
SCRT sequential chemoradiation therapy
SCS spinal cord stimulation
splatter control shield
stem cell support
suspected catheter sepsis
SCSAX subcostal short axis
SCSIT Southern California Sensory Integration Tests
SCSVT Southern California Space Visualization Test
SCT Secondary Care Trust (United Kingdom)
Sertoli cell tumor
sex chromatin test

S

	sickle cell trait
	stem cell transplant
	sugar-coated tablet
SCTX	static cervical traction
SCU	self-care unit
	special care unit
	stroke care unit
SCUCP	small cell undifferentiated carcinoma of the prostate
SCUF	slow continuous ultrafiltration
SCUT	schizophrenia, chronic undifferentiated type
SCV	subclavian vein
	subcutaneous vaginal (block)
$ScvO_2$	central venous oxygen saturation
SCY	scytonemin
SD	scleroderma
	senile dementia
	sensory deficit
	severe deficit
	septal defect
	severely disabled
	shallow distance (aquatic therapy)
	shoulder disarticulation
	single dose
	skin dose
	sleep deprived
	solvent-detergent
	somatic dysfunction
	spasmodic dysphonia
	speech discrimination
	spontaneous delivery
	stable disease
	standard deviation
	standard diet
	step-down
	sterile dressing
	straight drainage
	streptozocin and doxorubicin
	sudden death
	surgical drain
S & D	seen and discussed
	stomach and duodenum
S/D	sharp/dull
	systolic-diastolic ratio
SDA	sacrodextra anterior
	same day admission
	serotonin/dopamine antagonist
	Seventh-Day Adventist
	steroid-dependent asthmatic
SDAC	single-dose activated charcoal
SDAT	senile dementia of Alzheimer type
SDB	Sabouraud dextrose broth
	self-destructive behavior
	sleep disordered breathing
SDBP	seated diastolic blood pressure
	standing diastolic blood pressure
	supine diastolic blood pressure
SDC	serum digoxin concentration
	serum drug concentration
	Sleep Disorders Center
	sodium deoxycholate
SD&C	suction, dilation, and curettage
SDD	selective digestive (tract) decontamination
	sterile dry dressing
	subantimicrobial dose doxycycline (dental; Periostat)
SDDT	selective decontamination of the digestive tract
SDE	subdural empyema
SDES	symptomatic diffuse esophageal spasm
SDF	sexual dysfunction
	stromal-cell-derived factor
SDH	spinal detrusor hyperreflexia
	subdural hematoma
SDHD	succinate dehydrogenase complex subunit D
SDI	Sandimmune (cyclosporine)
	State Disability Insurance
SDII	sudden death in infancy
SDL	serum digoxin level
	serum drug level
	speech discrimination loss
SDLE	sex-difference in life expectancy
	somatic dysfunction lower extremity
SDM	soft drusen maculopathy
	standard deviation of the mean
S/D/M	systolic, diastolic, mean
SDMC	safety and data monitoring committee
SD/N	signal-difference-to-noise ratio
SDNN	standard deviation of normal-to-normal beats
SD-NVP	single-dose nevirapine (Viramune)
SDO	surgical diagnostic oncology
SDP	sacrodextra posterior
	single donor platelets
	solvent-detergent plasma
	stomach, duodenum, and pancreas
SDPTG	second derivative of photoplethysmogram
SDR	selective dorsal rhizotomy
	short-duration response
SDS	same day surgery
	Self-Rating Depression Scale
	Sheehan Disability Scale
	Shwachman-Diamond Syndrome
	sodium dodecyl sulfate
	somatropin deficiency syndrome
	Speech Discrimination Score
	standard deviation score
	sudden death syndrome
	Symptom Distress Scale

SDSO	same day surgery overnight
SDS-PAGE	sodium dodecyl sulfate – polyacrylamide gel electrophoresis
SDT	sacrodextra transversa self-determination theory speech detection threshold
SDU	step-down unit
SDUE	somatic dysfunction upper extremity
SDV	single-dose vial
SDX/PYR	sulfadoxine; pyrimethamine (Fansidar)
SE	saline enema (0.9% sodium chloride) self-examination side effect soft exudates special education spin echo staff escort standard error Starr-Edwards (valve, pacemaker) status epilepticus surgical excision
Se	selenium
S/E	suicidal and eloper
S & E	seen and examined
SEA	sheep erythrocyte agglutination (test) side-entry (venous) access Southeast Asia Staphylococcal enterotoxin A subdural electrode array synaptic electronic activation
SEAR	Southeast Asia refugee
SEB	Staphylococcus enterotoxin B surrogate end-point biomarker
SEC	second secondary secretary size exclusion chromatography spontaneous echo contrast steric exclusion chromatography
SECG	scalp electrocardiogram
SECL	seclusion
SECPR	standard external cardiopulmonary resuscitation
SE-CPT	single-electrode current perception threshold
SED	sedimentation serious emotional disturbances skin erythema dose socially and emotionally disturbed spondyloepiphyseal dysplasia
SeDBP	seated diastolic blood pressure
SEDDS	self-emulsifying drug-delivery system
SED-NET	severely emotional disturbed - network
Sed rt	sedimentation rate
SEEG	stereoelectroencephalographic
SEER	Surveillance, Epidemiology, and End Results (program)
SEF	spectral edge frequency (anesthesia-depth monitor)
SEG	segment sonoencephalogram
SEGRA	selective glucocorticoid-receptor agonist
segs	segmented neutrophils
SEH	spinal epidural hematomas subependymal hemorrhage
SEI	subepithelial (corneal) infiltrate
SELDI	surface enhanced laser desorption/ionization
SELDI-TOF MS	surface enhanced laser desorption/ionization-time of flight mass spectrometry
SELEX	systematic evolution of ligands by exponential enrichment
SELFVD	sterile elective low forceps vaginal delivery
SEM	scanning electron microscopy semen slow eye movement standard error of mean systolic ejection murmur
SEMD	spondyloepimetaphyseal dysplasias
sEMG	surface electromyography
SEMI	subendocardial myocardial infarction
SEN	spray each nostril
SENS	sensitivity sensorium
SEOC	serous epithelial ovarian carcinoma
SEP	multiple sclerosis (French) separate serum electrophoresis somatosensory evoked potential syringe exchange program systolic ejection period
SEPS	subfascial endoscopic perforator surgery
SEQ	sequela
SER	scanning equalization radiography sertraline (Zoloft) side effects records signal enhancement ratio
SERA-TEK	technetium-99m hexametazime
SERF	Severity of Exacerbation and Risk Factors
Serial 7's	a mental status examination (starting with a 100, count backward by 7's)
SER-IV	supination external rotation, type 4 fracture
SERM	selective estrogen-receptor modulator
SERO-SANG	serosanguineous

S

SERP-ACWA Skin Exposure Reduction Paste Against Chemical Warfare Agents
SERs somatosensory evoked responses
SES sick euthyroid syndrome
sirolimus-eluting stents
socioeconomic status
standard electrolyte solution
SeSBP seated systolic blood pressure
SET signal extraction technology
skin end-point titration
social environmental therapy
systolic ejection time
SEV sevoflurane (Ultane)
SEVO Sevoflurane (Ultane)
SEWHO shoulder-elbow-wrist-hand orthosis
SF salt-free
saturated fat
scarlet fever
seizure frequency
seminal fluid
skull fracture
small finger
soft feces
sound field
spinal fluid
starch-free
stone-free
sugar-free
symptom-free
synovial fluid
S&F slip and fall
soft and flat
SF-6 sulfahexafluoride
SF 36 36-item short form health survey
SFA saturated fatty acids
superficial femoral artery
SFB single frequency bioimpedance
SFC spinal fluid count
subarachnoid fluid collection
SFD scaphoid fossa depression
small for dates
SFDA Chinese State Food and Drug Administration
SFE supercritical fluid extraction
SFEMG single-fiber electromyography
SFH schizophrenia family history
SFJ saphenofemoral junction
SFM scanning force microscopy
SF-MPQ Short-Form, McGill Pain questionnaire
SFNM subfoveal neovascular membranes
SFP simulated fluorescence process
simultaneous foveal perception
spinal fluid pressure
SFPT standard fixation preference test
SFRT stereotactic fractionated radiotherapy
SFS split function studies
SFT solitary fibrous tumor
SFTR sagittal, frontal, transverse, rotation
SFTs solitary fibrous tumors
SFUP surgical follow-up
SFV simian foamy viruses
superficial femoral vein
SFW shell fragment wound
SFWB social/family well-being
SFWD symptom-free walking distance
SG salivary gland
scrotography
serum glucose
side glide
skin graft
specific gravity
Swan-Ganz (catheter)
S/G swallow/gag
SGA small for gestational age
subjective global assessment (dietary history and physical examination)
substantial gainful activity (employment)
SGAR spectral gradient acoustic reflectometry
SGAs second-generation antihistamines
second-generation antipsychotics
SGB Swiss gym ball
SGC Swan-Ganz catheter
SGCNB stereotactic guided core-needle biopsy
SGD salivary gland dysfunction
specific granule deficiency
specific growth delay
speech generating device
straight gravity drainage
sweat gland density
SGE significant glandular enlargement
SGHL superior glenohumeral ligament
$\bar{s}$ gl without correction (without glasses)
SGM serum glucose monitoring
SGOT serum glutamic oxalo-acetic transaminase (same as AST)
SGP Schering-Plough Corporation
SGPT serum glutamate pyruvate transaminase (same as ALT)
SGRQ-A St. George's Respiratory Questionnaire translated into American English
SGS second-generation sulfonylurea
subglottic stenosis
sGS surgical Gleason score
SGTCS secondarily generalized tonic-clonic seizures
SH sclerosing hemangioma
self-help
serum hepatitis
sexual harassment
short

shoulder
shower
social history
sulfhydryl (group)
surgical history
systemic hypertension

–SH thiol

S&H speech and hearing
suicidal and homicidal

S/H suicidal/homicidal ideation

SH2 sarc homology region 2

SHA super-heated aerosol

SHAFT *s*hopping, *h*ousework, *a*ccounting (bills), *f*ood preparation, and *t*ransportation (driving); (instrumental activities of daily living)

SHAL standard hyperalimentation

SHAS supravalvular hypertrophic aortic stenosis

S Hb sickle hemoglobin screen

SHBG sex hormone-binding globulin

sHBO$_2$T systemic hyperbaric oxygen therapy

SHC subsequent hospital care

SHCP spastic hemiparetic cerebral palsy

SHEENT skin, head, eyes, ears, nose, and throat

SHG shigellosis (*Shigella* sp.) vaccine
sonohysterography

SHGT somatic-cell human gene therapy

SHI Self-Harm Inventory
standard heparin infusion

Shig *Shigella*

SHIV simian-human immunodeficiency virus

SHL sudden hearing loss
supraglottic horizontal laryngectomy

SHMB severe hypersensitivity to mosquito bites

SHO Senior House Officer

SHOX Short stature HOmeoboX (gene)

SHP secondary hypertension, pulmonary

SHPT secondary hyperparathyroidism

SHR scapulohumeral rhythm

SHRC shortened, held, resisted contraction

S-HRV short-term heart rate variability

SHS second-hand smoke
sliding hip screw
student health service

SHV short hepatic vein
sulfhydryl variant

SHx social history

SI International System of Units
sacroiliac
sagittal index
sector iridectomy
self-inflicted
sensory integration
seriously ill
sexual intercourse
signal intensity
small intestine
strict isolation
stress incontinence
stroke index
suicidal ideation

Si silicon

S & I suction and irrigation
support and interpretation

SIA small intestinal atresia

SIADH syndrome of inappropriate antidiuretic hormone secretion

SIAT supervised intermittent ambulatory treatment

SIB self-inflating bulb
self-injurious behavior

SIBC serum iron-binding capacity

SIBO small intestinal bacterial overgrowth

sibs siblings

SIC self-intermittent catherization
squamous intraepithelial cells
Standard Industrial Classification

SICD sudden infant crib death

SICOG Southern Italy Cooperative Oncology Group

SICT selective intracoronary thrombolysis

SICU surgical intensive care unit

SID strong ion difference

SID once daily (used in veterinary medicine)

SIDA French and Spanish abbreviation for AIDS
stable isotope dilution assay

SIDAM structured interview for the diagnosis of dementia of Alzheimer type

SIDAM-A structured interview for the diagnosis of dementia of the Alzheimer type, multi-infarct dementia, and dementias of other etiology according to ICD-10 and DSM-III-R

SIDD syndrome of isolated diastolic dysfunction

SIDERO siderocyte

SIDFF superimposed dorsiflexion of foot

SIDS sudden infant death syndrome

SIEA superficial inferior epigastric artery

SIEP serum immunoelectrophoresis

SIG let it be marked (appears on prescription before directions for patient)
sigmoidoscopy

Signal 99 patient in cardiac or respiratory distress

sign(s) see ABCD, ACHES, M, O, Q, STR, and VS

SI/HI suicidal/homicidal ideations

S

S

SIJ	sacroiliac joint
SIJS	sacroiliac joint syndrome
SIL	seriously ill list sister-in-law squamous intraepithelial lesion
SILFVD	sterile indicated low forceps vaginal delivery
SILV	simultaneous independent lung ventilation
SIM	selective ion monitoring Similac® surface-induced mineralization
SIMCU	surgical intermediate care unit
Sim c Fe	Similac with iron®
SIMS	secondary ion mass spectroscopy
SIMV	synchronized intermittent mandatory ventilation
SIN	salpingitis isthmica nodose
SIOD	Schimke immuno-osseous dysplasia
SIP	Sickness Impact Profile spontaneous intestinal perforation stroke in progression subcutaneously implanted ports sympathetically independent pain
SIQ	sick in quarters
SIQ-JR	Suicidal Ideation Questionnaire-Junior
SIR	standardized incidence rate (ratio)
siRNA	small interfering ribonucleic acid
SIRGE	A drug-waste collection and recycling system used in the European Union
SIRPIDs	stimulus-induced rhythmic, periodic, or ictal discharges
SIRS	systemic inflammatory response syndrome
SIRT	selective internal radiation therapy
SIS	saline infusion sonohysterography sister small intestinal submucosa Surgical Infection Stratification (system)
SISI	Short Increment Sensitivity Index
SISS	severe invasion streptococcal syndrome
SIT	serum inhibitory titers silicon-intensified target Slossen Intelligence Test specific immunotherapy (allergy) sperm immobilization test structured interrupted therapy supraspinatus, infraspinatus, teres (insertions) surgical intensive therapy
SITA	standard infertility treatment algorithm Swedish Interactive Thresholding Algorithm
SITA-SAP	Swedish Interactive Threshold Algorithm-standard automated perimetry
SIT BAL	sitting balance
SIT TOL	sitting tolerance
SIV	self-inflicted violence simian immunodeficiency virus
SIVB	self-inflicted violent behavior
SIVD	subcortical ischemic vascular dementia (disease)
SIVP	slow intravenous push
SIW	self-inflicted wound
SJ	surgical jejunostomy
SJC	swollen joint count
SJCRH	St. Jude Children's Research Hospital (preferred abbreviation "St. Jude")
SJM	St. Jude Medical (heart valve prosthesis)
S-JRA	systemic juvenile rheumatoid arthritis
SJS	Schwartz-Jampel syndrome Stevens-Johnson syndrome Swyer-James syndrome
S_{jv02}	jugular venous oxygen saturation
SK	seborrheic keratosis senile keratosis solar keratosis streptokinase
S & K	single and keeping (baby)
SKAO	supracondylar knee-ankle orthosis
SKAs	skills, knowledge, and abilities (ratings)
SKB	SmithKline Beecham
SKC	single knee to chest
SKINT	skinfold thickness
SK-SD	streptokinase streptodornase
SKU	stock keeping unit (related to product identification)
SKY	spectral karyotyping
SL	scapholunate secondary leukemia sensation level sentinel lymphadenectomy serious list shortleg side-lying staging laparoscopy slight sublingual
S/L	slit lamp (examination)
SLA	sacrolaeva anterior sex and love addictions slide latex agglutination The Satisfaction with Life Areas
SLAA	Sex and Love Addicts Anonymous
SLAC	scapholunate advanced collapse
SLat	time to onset of sleep
SLAM	Systemic Lupus Activity Measure

SLAP	serum leucine amino-peptidase
	superior labral anteroposterior (shoulder lesion)
SLB	short leg brace
SLBB	single-living baby boy
SLBG	single-living baby girl
SLC	short leg cast
SLCC	short leg cylinder cast
SLCG	sulfolithocholylglycine
SLCT	Sertoli-Leydig cell tumor
SLD	specific language disorder
	stealth liposomal doxorubicin
SLE	slit-lamp examination
	St. Louis encephalitis
	systemic lupus erythematosus
SLeA	sialyl Lewis a (antigen)
SLEDAI	Systemic Lupus Erythematosus Disease Activity Index
SLEX	slit-lamp examination (biomicroscopy)
SLex	sialyl Lewis x (antigen)
SLFVD	sterile low forceps vaginal delivery
SLGXT	symptom-limited graded exercise test
SLI	specific language impairment
SLIT	sublingual immunotherapy
SLK	superior limbic keratoconjunctivitis
SLL	second-look laparotomy
	small lymphocytic lymphoma
SLMFVD	sterile low midforceps vaginal delivery
SLMMS	slightly more marked since
SLMP	since last menstrual period
S-LMP	serous tumor(s) of low malignant potential
SLN	sentinel lymph node(s)
	superior laryngeal nerve
SLNB	sentinel lymph node biopsy
SLND	sentinel lymph node detection
SLNM	sentinel lymph node mapping
SLNTG	sublingual nitroglycerin
SLNWBC	short leg nonweight-bearing cast
SLNWC	short leg nonwalking cast
SLO	scanning laser ophthalmoscope
	second-look operation
	shark liver oil
	Smith-Lemli-Opitz (syndrome)
	streptolysin O
SLOA	short leave of absence
SLOM	serous left otitis media
SLOS	Smith-Lemli-Opitz syndrome
SLP	scanning laser polarimeter
	single-limb progression
	Speech Language Pathologist
	speech language pathology
	superficial lamina propria
SLPI	secretory leukocyte protease inhibitor
SLPMS	short-leg posterior-molded splint
SLR	straight-leg raising
SLRS	stereotactic linac radiosurgery
SLRT	straight-leg raising tenderness
	straight-leg raising test
SLS	second-look sonography
	short leg splint
	shrinking lungs syndrome
	single leg stance
	single limb support
SLT	sacrolaeva transversa
	scanning laser tomography
	single lung transplantation
	smokeless tobacco
	Speech Language Therapist
	spontaneous labor at term
	swing light test
SLT-I	Shiga-like toxin I
SLTA	severe life-threatening asthma
	standard language test for aphasia
SLTEC	Shiga-like toxin-producing *Escherichia coli*
sl. tr.	slight trace
SLUD	salivation, lacrimation, urination, and defecation
SLUDGE	salivation, **l**acrimation, **u**rination, **d**iarrhea, **g**astrointestinal upset, and **e**mesis (signs and symptoms of cholinergic excess)
SLV	since last visit
SLVD	systolic left ventricular dysfunction
SLWB	severely low birth weight
SLWC	short leg walking cast
SM	sadomasochism
	service mark (such as The Pause that Refreshes)
	setup margin (for radiotherapy)
	skim milk
	small
	sports medicine
	Stairmaster®
	streptomycin
	syringomyelia
	systolic motion
	systolic murmur
^{153}Sm	samarium 153
SMA	severe malarial anemia
	smallpox vaccine, not otherwise specified
	smooth muscle antibody
	spinal muscular atrophy
	superior mesenteric artery
SMA-II	spinal muscular atrophy type II
SMA-6	simultaneous multichannel autoanalyzer (page 318)
SMA-7	See page 318
SMA-12	See page 318
SMA-18	See page 318
SMA-23	See page 318

SMAC	sequential multiple analyzer computer
SMAO	superior mesenteric artery occlusion
SMAR	self-medication administration record
SMAS	superficial musculoaponeurotic system (graft; flat)
	superior mesenteric artery syndrome
SMAST	Short Michigan Alcoholism Screening Test
SMAvac	smallpox (vaccinia virus) vaccine
SMB	simulated moving bed (chromatography)
SMBG	self-monitoring blood glucose
SMC	skeletal myxoid chondrosarcoma
	special mouth care
SMCA	sorbitol MacConkey agar
SMCD	senile macular chorio-retinal degeneration
SMCs	smooth muscle cells
SMD	senile macular degeneration
	standardized mean difference
SMDA	Safe Medical Defice Act
SME	significant medical event
	surgical mediastinal exploration
SMF	streptozocin, mitomycin, and fluorouracil
SMFA	sodium monofluoroacetate
SMFP	sodium monofluorophosphate
SMFVD	sterile midforceps vaginal delivery
SMG	submandibular gland
SMH	state mental hospital
SMI	sensory motor integration (group)
	serious mental illness
	severely mentally impaired
	service mix index
	small volume infusion
	suggested minimum increment
	sustained maximal inspiration
SMIDS	suppertime mixed insulin and daytime sulfonylureas
SMILE	safety, monitoring, intervention, length of stay and evaluation
	sustained maximal inspiratory lung exercises
SMIs	self-management interventions
SMIT	standard mycological identification techniques
SMMVT	sustained monomorphic ventricular tachycardia
SMN	second malignant neoplasia
SMO	Senior Medical Officer
	site management organization(s)
	slip made out
SMON	subacute myelo-opticoneuropathy
SMORs	standardized mortality odds ratios
SMP	safety management plan
	self-management program
	sympathetic maintained plan
SmPC	Summary of Product Characteristics (European Union)
SMPN	sensorimotor polyneuropathy
SMQs	Standardized MedDRA (Medical Dictionary for Regulatory Activities) Queries
SMR	senior medical resident
	skeletal muscle relaxant
	sleeping metabolic rate
	standardized mortality ratio
	submucous resection
SMRR	submucous resection and rhinoplasty
SMS	scalded mouth syndrome
	senior medical student
	Smith-Magenis syndrome
	somatostatin (Zecnil)
	stiff-man syndrome
SMSA	standard metropolitan statistical area
SMT	smooth muscle tumors
	sputum methylation testing
	standard medical therapy
	study management team
SMV	stentless mitral valve
	submentovertical
	superior mesenteric vein
SMVT	sustained monomorphic ventricular tachycardia
SMX-TMP	sulfamethoxazole and trimethoprim (SMZ-TMP)
SMZL	splenic marginal-zone lymphoma
SN	sciatic notch
	sinus node
	staff nurse
	student nurse
	suprasternal notch
	superior nasal
Sn	tin
sN	sentinel lymph node
S/N	signal to noise ratio
SNA	specimen not available
	Student Nursing Assistant
SNa	serum sodium
SNAC	scaphoid nonunion advanced collapse
SNAE	*s*ustained pain-free and *n*o *a*dverse *e*vents
SNAP	scheduled nursing activities program
	Score for Neonatal Acute Physiology
	sensory nerve action potential
	Swanson, Nolan, and Pelham (rating scale)
SNAP-25	synaptosome-associated protein 25 kilodaltons
SNAP-PE	Score for Neonatal Acute Physiology-Perinatal Extension
SNARC	Spatial-Numerical Association of Response Codes

SNaRI serotonin noradrenergic reuptake inhibitor
SNASA Salford Needs Assessment Schedule for Adolescents
SNAT suspected nonaccidental trauma
SNB scalene node biopsy
sentinel (lymph) node biopsy
SNBx sentinel node biopsy
SNC skilled nursing care
SNc substantia nigra compacta
SNCV sensory nerve conduction velocity
SND selective neck dissection
single needle device
sinus node dysfunction
SNDA Supplemental New Drug Application
SNE subacute necrotizing encephalomyelopathy
SNEP student nurse extern program
SnET2 tin ethyl etiopurpurin
SNF Simon nitinol filter
skilled nursing facility
SnF_2 stannous fluoride
SNF/MR skilled nursing facility for the mentally retarded
SNGFR single nephron glomerular filtration rate
SNGP supranuclear gaze palsy
SNHL sensorineural hearing loss
SNIP silver nitrate immunoperoxidase
strict no information in paper
SNIPS single nucleotide polymorphism (SNP)
SNK Student-Newman-Keuls (test)
SNM sentinel (lymph) node mapping
serotoninergic neuroenteric modulators
student nurse midwife
SnMp tin-mesoporphyrin
SNOMED Systematized Nomenclature of Medicine
SNOMED CT Systemized Nomenclature of Medicine, Clinical Terms
SNOMED RT Systemized Nomenclature of Medicine, Reference Terminology
SNOOP Systematic Nursing Observation of Psychopathology
SNOs S-nitrosothiols
SNP simple neonatal procedure
single nucleotide polymorphism
sodium nitroprusside (Nipride)
SNP-LP single nucleotide polymorphisms – linkage disequilibrium
SNPs single nucleotide polymorphisms
SNR signal-to-noise ratio (radiology)
SNr substantia nigra reticularis
SNRB selective nerve root block
SNRI selective noradrenergic reuptake inhibitor
serotonin norepinephrine reuptake inhibitor
SNRT sinus node recovery time
SNS sacral nerve stimulation
sterile normal saline (0.9% sodium chloride, sterile)
Strategic National Stockpile
Supplemental Nursing System (for nursing mothers)
sympathetic nervous system
SNSA sympathetic nervous system activity
SNT sinuses, nose, and throat
soft, non-tender
suppan nail technique
SNU skilled nursing unit
SNUB super neurotransmitter uptake blocker
SNV Sin Nombre virus
skilled nursing visit
spleen necrosis virus
SO second opinion
sex offender
shoulder orthosis
significant other
special observation
sphincter of Oddi
standing orders
suboccipital
suggestive of
superior oblique
supraoptic
supraorbital
sutures out
sympathetic ophthalmia
S/O suggestive of
S-O salpingo-oophorectomy
S&O salpingo-oophorectomy
SO_2 sulfur dioxide
SO_3 sulfite
SO_4 sulfate
SOA serum opsonic activity
shortness of air
spinal opioid analgesia
supraorbital artery
swelling of ankles
SOAA signed out against advice
SOAM sutures out in the morning
SOAMA signed out against medical advice
SOAP subjective, objective, assessment, and plans
SOAPIE subjective, objective, assessment, plan, implementation, (intervention), and evaluation
SOAPIER **s**ubjective, **o**bjective, **a**ssessment, **p**lan, **i**ntervention, **e**valuation, and **r**evision
SOB see order book

S

S

shortness of breath (this abbreviation has caused problems)
side of bed

SOBE short of breath on exertion

SOBOE short of breath on exertion

SOC see old chart
socialization
stages of change
standard of care
start of care
state of consciousness
system organ class

S & OC signed and on chart (e.g. permit)

SOCMOB standing on corner minding own business (when inexplicable injured) (slang)

SOCs System Organ Classes

SOD sinovenous occlusive disease
sphincter of Oddi dysfunction
superoxide dismutase
surgical officer of the day

SODA Severity of Dyspepsia Assessment

SODAS spheriodal oral drug absorption system

SOE source of embolism

SOFA sepsis-related organ failure assessment
Sequential Organ Failure Assessment (score)

SOFAS Social and Occupational Functioning Assessment Scale

SOG suggestive of good

SOGS South Oaks Gambling Screen

SOH sexually oriented hallucinations

SoHx social history

SOI slipped on ice
sudden overwhelming infection
surgical orthotopic implantation (implant)
syrup of ipecac

SOL solution
space occupying lesion

SOL I special observations level one (there are also SOL II and SOL III)

SOM secretory otitis media
serous otitis media
somatization

SOMI sterno-occipital mandibular immobilizer

SONK spontaneous osteonecrosis of the knee

Sono sonogram

SONP solid organs not palpable

SOOL spontaneous onset of labor

SOP standard operating procedure

SOPM sutures out in afternoon (or evening)

SOR sign own release
strength of recommendation

SORA stable on room air

SORL1 sortilin-related receptor 1 (gene)

SOS if there is need
may be repeated once if urgently required (Latin: *si opus sit*)
self-obtained smear
Signs of Suicide (prevention program)
suicidal observation status

SOSOB sit on side of bed

SOSs standardized order sets

SOT solid organ transplant
something other than
stream of thought

SOTP Sex-Offender Treatment Provider

SOVS self-obtained vaginal swabs

SOW Scope of Work

SOZT superior oblique Z-tenotomy

SP sacrum to pubis
sequential pulse
serum protein
shoulder press
silent period (related to electromyographic responses)
spastic dysphonia
speech
Speech Pathologist
spinal
spouse
stand and pivot
stand pivot
status post
Streptococcus pneumoniae
sulfadoxine; pyrimethamine (Fansidar)
supplementary prescribing
systolic pressure

sp species

S/P status post
suprapubic

SP 1 suicide precautions number 1

SP 2 suicide precautions number 2

SPA albumin human (formerly known as salt-poor albumin)
scintillation proximity assay
serum prothrombin activity
sheep pulmonary adenomatosis
single photon absorptiometry
Speech Pathology and Audiology
stimulation produced analgesia
student physician's assistant
subperiosteal abscess
suprapubic aspiration

SpA spondyloarthropathy

SP-A surfactant-specific protein A

SPAC satisfactory postanesthesia course

SPAG small-particle aerosol generator

SPAMM spatial modulation of magnetization

SPARC	suprapubic sling operation
SPBE	saw palmetto berry extract
SPBI	serum protein bound iodine
SPBT	suprapubic bladder tap
SPC	saturated phosphatidylcholine
	second primary cancer
	sclerosing pancreatocholangitis
	single-point cane
	statistical process control
	Summary of Product Characteristics
	suprapubic catheter
SPCA	serum prothrombin conversion accelerator (factor VII)
SPCT	simultaneous prism and cover test
SPD	schizotypal personality disorder
	subcorneal pustular dermatosis
	Supply, Processing, and Distribution (department)
	suprapubic drainage
SPE	saw palmetto extract
	serum protein electrophoresis
	solid-phase extraction
	superficial punctate erosions
SPEB	streptococcal pyrogenic exotoxins B
SPEC	specimen
	streptococcal pyrogenic exotoxins C
Spec Ed	special education
SPECT	single-photon emission computed tomography
SPEEP	spontaneous positive end-expiratory pressure
SPEP	serum protein electrophoresis
SPET	single-photon emission tomography
SPF	semipermeable film
	S-phase fraction
	split products of fibrin
	sun protective factor
sp fl	spinal fluid
SPG	scrotopenogram
	sphenopalatine ganglion
SpG	specific gravity
SPH	severely and profoundly handicapped
	sighs per hour
	spherocytes
SPHERO	spherocytes
SPI	speech processor interface
	surgical peripheral iridectomy
SPIA	solid phase immunoabsor-bent assay
SPIDER	steady-state projection imaging with dynamic echo-train readout
SPIF	spontaneous peak inspiratory force
SPIFE	serum protein and immunofixation electrophoresis (system)
S-PIN	Steinmann pin
SPINK1	serine protease inhibitor Kazal type 1
SPIO	superparamagnetic iron oxide
SPK	simultaneous pancreas-kidney (transplant)
	single parent keeping (baby)
	superficial punctate keratitis
SPL	sound pressure level
	superior parietal lobule
SPL®	Staphylococcal Phage Lysate
SPLATTT	split anterior tibial tendon transfer
SPM	scanning probe microscopy
	second primary malignancy
SPM96	statistical parametric mapping 96
SPMA	spinal progressive muscle atrophy
sPMA	supplemental premarket approval application (FDA)
SPMD	scapuloperoneal muscular dystrophy
SPMDs	semipermeable membrane devices
SPME	solid-phase microextraction
SPMI	severely and persistently mentally ill
SPMS	secondary progressive multiple sclerosis
SPMSQ	Short Portable Mental Status Questionnaire
SPN	solitary pulmonary nodule
	student practical nurse
	superficial peroneal nerve
SPn	*Streptococcus pneumoniae*
SPNK	single parent not keeping (baby)
SPNP	solid pseudopapillary neoplasm of the pancreas
SPO	status postoperative
SpO_2	oxygen saturation by pulse oximeter
spont	spontaneous
SponVe	spontaneous ventilation
SPOREs	Specialized Programs of Research Excellence (National Cancer Institute)
SPP	Sexuality Preference Profile
	single presentation phenotype
	super packed platelets
	suprapubic prostatectomy
spp	species
SPQ	Schizotypal Personality Questionnaire
SPR	surface plasmon resonance
SPRAS	Sheehan Patient Rated Anxiety Scale
SP-RIA	solid-phase radioimmunoassay
SPR-MS	surface plasmon resonance mass spectrometry
SPROM	spontaneous premature rupture of membrane
SPS	shoulder pain and stiffness
	simple partial seizure
	sodium polyethanol sulfonate
	sodium polystyrene sulfonate (Kayexalate; SPS®)
	status post surgery
	stiff-person syndrome
	systemic progressive sclerosis

S

SPSU straight partial sit-up
SPT second primary tumors
skin prick test
standing pivot transfer
supportive periodontal therapy
suprapubic tenderness
surgical preparation time (start surgical preparation to incision)
SP TAP spinal tap
SPTL spontaneous preterm labor
SPTs second primary tumors
single-patient trials
SP TUBE suprapubic tube
SPTX static pelvic traction
SPU short procedure unit
SPVC Shelhigh porcine pulmonic value conduits
SPVR systemic peripheral vascular resistance
SPX smallpox vaccine, not otherwise specified
SPx spontaneous pneumothorax
SPX$_v$ smallpox vaccine (vaccinia virus)
SQ *status quo*
subcutaneous (this is a dangerous abbreviation, use subcut)
Sq CCa squamous cell carcinoma
SQE subcutaneous emphysema
SQM square meter(s)
SQUID superconducting quantum interference device
SQV saquinavir (Fortovose; Invirase)
SR screen
sedimentation rate
see report
senior resident
service record
side rails
sinus rhythm
slow release
smooth-rough
social recreation
standard risks
stretch reflex
superior rectus
sustained release
sustained response
suture removal
system review
S/R strong/regular (pulse)
S&R seclusion and restraint
smooth and rough
^{89}Sr strontium 89
SRA serotonin release assay
steroid-resistant asthma
surface replacement arthroplasty
SRAN surgical resident admission note
SRBC sheep red blood cells
sickle red blood cells
SRBD sleep-related breathing disorders
SRBOW spontaneous rupture of bag of waters
SRC sclerodermal renal crisis
SRCC sarcomatoid renal cell carcinoma
SRCS Division of Surveillance, Research, and Communication Support (FDA)
SRD service-related disability
smallest real difference
sodium-restricted diet
SRE sex and relationships education
skeletal related event
SREs skeletal related events
SRF somatotropin releasing factor
subretinal fluid
SRF-A slow-releasing factor of anaphylaxis
SRGVHD steroid-resistant graft-versus-host disease
SRH self-rated health
signs of recent hemorrhage
SRI serotonin reuptake inhibitor
SRIB severe recurrent intestinal bleeding
SRICU surgical respiratory intensive care unit
SRIF somatotropin-release inhibiting factor (somatostatin; Zecnil)
SRK smooth-rod Kaneda (implant)
SRL sirolimus (Rapamune)
SRM spontaneous rupture of membranes
SRMD stress-related mucosal damage
SRMS sustained-release morphine sulfate
SRMs specified risk materials
SR/NE sinus rhythm, no ectopy
SRNV subretinal neovascularization
SRNVM subretinal neovascular membrane
SRO sagittal ramus osteotomy
single room occupancy
smallest region of overlap
sustained-release oral
SROA sports-related osteoarthritis
SROCPI Self-Rating Obsessive-Compulsive Personality Inventory
SROM self range of motion
serous right otitis media
spontaneous rupture of membrane
SRP scaling and root planing (dental)
septorhinoplasty
stapes replacement prosthesis
SRQ-20 self-reporting questionnaire of 20 questions (mental health)
SRR surgical recovery room
SRRS social readjustment rating scale
SRS Silver-Russell syndrome
somatostatin receptor scintigraphy
$\bar{s}$RS without redness or swelling
SRS-A slow-reacting substance of anaphylaxis

SRSV small round structured viruses
SRT sedimentation rate test
sleep-related tumescence
speech reception threshold
speech recognition threshold
stereotactic radiotherapy
surfactant replacement therapy
sustained release theophylline
SRU side rails up
SRUS solitary rectal ulcer syndrome
SRVC subcutaneous reservoir and ventricular catheter
SR ↑ X2 both siderails up
SS half (this is a dangerous abbreviation as it is not understood or read as sliding scale)
sacral sulcus
sacrosciatic
saline soak (sodium chloride 0.9%)
saline solution (0.9% sodium chloride)
saliva sample
salt sensitivity (sensitive)
salt substitute
serotonin syndrome
serum sickness
sickle cell
single-session (treatment)
single-strength (as compared to double-strength)
Sjögren syndrome
sliding scale (this is a dangerous abbreviation as it is not understood or read as one half)
slip sent
Social Security
social service
somatostatin (Zecnil)
stainless steel
steady state
step stool
subaortic stenosis
susceptible
suprasciatic (notch)
Sweet syndrome
symmetrical strength
S/S Saturday and Sunday
sprain/strain
SS# Social Security number
S & S shower and shampoo
signs and symptoms
sitting and supine
sling and swathe
soft and smooth (prostate)
support and stimulation
swish and spit
swish and swallow
SSA sagittal split advancement
salicylsalicylic acid (salsalate)
Sjögren syndrome antigen A
Social Security Administration
specific surface area
Subjective Symptoms Assessment (profile)
sulfasalicylic acid (test)
SSADH succinic semialdehyde dehydrogenase
SSAs standard sedative agents
SSBP sitting systolic blood pressure
SSC sign symptom complex
silver sulfadiazine and chlorhexidine
Similac® and special care
sliding scale coverage
Special Services for Children
stainless steel crown
standard straight cane
SSc systemic sclerosis (scleroderma)
SSCA single shoulder contrast arthrography
SSCM Society of Critical Care Medicine (guidelines for the sustained use of sedatives and analgesics)
SSCP single-stranded conformational polymorphism
substernal chest pain
SSCr stainless steel crown
SSCU surgical special care unit
SSCVD sterile spontaneous controlled vaginal delivery
SSD serosanguineous drainage
sickle cell disease
silver sulfadiazine (Silvadene)
skin-to-stone distance
Social Security disability
source to skin distance
SSDI Social Security disability income
ss DNA single-stranded desoxyribonucleic acid
SSE saline solution enema (0.9% sodium chloride)
skin self-examination
soapsuds enema
sterile speculum exam
subacute spongiform encephalopathy
systemic side effects
SSEH spontaneous spinal epidural hematoma
SSEPs somatosensory evoked potentials
SSF subscapular skinfold
SSFP steady-state free precession
SSG sodium stibogluconate
sublabial salivary gland
SSHL sudden sensorineural hearing loss
SSI sliding scale insulin
Social Skills Inventory
sub-shock insulin

S

	superior sector iridectomy
	Supplemental Security Income
	surgical site infection
SSI-CCM	synthetic sentence identification with contralateral competing message
SSI-ICM	synthetic sentence identification with ipsilateral competing message
SSKI	saturated solution of potassium iodide
SSL	second stage of labor
	selective sentinel lymphadenectomy
	subtotal supraglottic laryngectomy
SSLF	sacrospinous ligament fixation
SSLR	seated straight leg raise
SSM	short stay medical
	skin-sparing mastectomy
	skin surface microscopy
	superficial spreading melanoma
SSN	severely subnormal
	Social Security number
SSNB	suprascapular nerve block
SSO	second surgical opinion
	sequence-specific oligonucleotide
	short stay observation (unit)
	Spanish speaking only
SSOP	Second Surgical Opinion Program
	sequence-specific oligonucleotide probe
SSP	sequence-specific primer
	short stay procedure (unit)
	superior spermatic plexus
	supragingival scaling and prophylaxis (dental)
SSPA	staphylococcal-slime polysaccharide antigens
SSPE	subacute sclerosing panencephalitis
SSPG	steady-state plasma glucose
SSPH	System of Social Protection in Health (Mexico)
SSPL	saturation sound pressure level
SSPU	surgical short procedure unit
SSQ	Staring Speel Questionnaire
SSR	Sleep Self-Reporting
	substernal retractions
	sympathetic skin response
SSRFC	surrounding subretinal fluid cuff
SSRI	selective serotonin reuptake inhibitor
ssRNA	single-stranded deoxyribonucleic acid
SSRO	sagittal split ramus osteotomy (dental)
SSRP	subgingival scaling and root planing (dental)
SSRs	simple sequence repeats
SSS	layer upon layer
	scalded skin syndrome
	Scandinavian Stroke Scale
	Sepsis Severity Score
	Severity Scoring System (Dart Snakebite)
	short stay service (unit)
	sick sinus syndrome
	skin and skin structures
	Spanish-speaking sometimes
	sphincter-saving surgery
	spontaneous saliva swallowing
	Stanford Sleepiness Scale
	sterile saline soak
	subclavian steal syndrome
SSSB	sagittal split setback
SSSDW	significant sharp, spike, or delta waves
SSSE	self-sustained status epilepticus
SSSIs	skin and skin structure infections
SSSS	staphylococcal scalded skin syndrome
SSSs	small short spikes (encephalography)
SST	sagittal šinus thrombosis
	Simple Shoulder Test
	somatostatin (Zecnil)
SSTI	skin and skin structure infections
SSU	short stay unit
SSX	sulfisoxazole acetyl
S/SX	signs/symptoms
ST	esotropic
	sacrum transverse
	Schiotz tonometry
	Schirmer Test (dry-eye test)
	scleral thickness
	shock therapy
	sinus tachycardia
	skin tear
	skin test
	slight trace
	slow-twitch
	smokeless tobacco
	sore throat
	spasmodic torticollis
	speech therapist
	speech therapy
	sphincter tone
	split thickness
	spondee threshold
	station (obstetrics)
	stomach
	stone (1 stone = 6.35 kg or 14 pounds)
	straight
	strength training
	stress testing
	stretcher
	subtotal
	Surgical Technologist
	survival time
	synapse time

S

S & T	sulfamethoxazole and trimethoprim (SMZ-TMP or SMX-TMP)
STA	second trimester abortion
	spike-triggered averaging
	staphylococcus vaccine, not otherwise specified
	superficial temporal artery
STA_{aur}	*Staphylococcus aureus* vaccine
stab.	polymorphonuclear leukocytes (white blood cells, in nonmature form)
STAI	State-Trait Anxiety Inventory
STAI-I	State-Trait-Anxiety Index—I
STA-MCA	superficial temporary artery-middle cerebral artery (anastomosis; bypass)
STAPES	stapedectomy
staph	*Staphylococcus aureus*
STA_{SPL}	staphylococcus vaccine, bacteriophage lysate
STAT	immediately (or as defined by the institution)
	signal transducers and activators of transcription
STATINS	HMG-CoA reductase inhibitors
STAXI	State-Trait Anger Expression Inventory
STB	stillborn
STBAL	standing balance
ST BY	stand by
STC	serum theophylline concentration
	slow-transit constipation
	soft tissue calcification
	special treatment center
	stimulate to cry
	stroke treatment center
	subtotal colectomy
	sugar tongue cast
ST CLK	station clerk
STD	sexually transmitted disease(s)
	short-term disability
	skin test dose
	skin to tumor distance
	sodium tetradecyl sulfate
STD TF	standard tube feeding
STE	ST-segment elevation
STEAM	stimulated-echo acquisition mode
STEC	shiga toxin-producing *Escherichia coli*
STEM	scanning transmission electron microscopic
STEMI	ST-segment elevation myocardial infarction
stereo	steropsis
STEPS	The System for Thalidomide Educating and Prescribing Safety
STET	single photon emission tomography
	submaximal treadmill exercise test
STETH	stethoscope
STF	slip, trip, and fall (injuries)
	special tube feeding
	standard tube feeding
STG	short-term goals
	split-thickness graft
	superior temporal gyri
STH	soft tissue hemorrhage
	somatotrophic hormone
	subtotal hysterectomy
	supplemental thyroid hormone
STHB	said to have been
STI	sexually transmitted infection
	signal transduction inhibitor((s)
	soft tissue injury
	structured treatment interruption(s)
	sum total impression
	systolic time interval
STI-571	imatinib mesylate (Gleevec)
STILLB	stillborn
STIR	short TI (tau) inversion recovery
STIs	sexually transmitted infections
	systolic time intervals
STJ	scapulothoracic joint
	subtalar joint
STK	streptokinase
STL	sent to laboratory
	serum theophylline level
STLE	St. Louis encephalitis
STLI	subtotal lymphoid irradiation
STLOM	swelling, tenderness, and limitation of motion
STLV	simian T-lymphotrophic viruses
STM	scanning tunneling microscope
	short-term memory
	soft tissue mobilization
	sternocleidomastoideus
	streptomycin
STMS	Short Test of Mental Status
STMT	Seat Movement
STN	subtalar neutral
	subthalamic nucleus
STNI	subtotal nodal irradiation
STNM	surgical evaluative staging of cancer
STNR	symmetrical tonic neck reflex
S to	sensitive to
STO_2	microvascular oxygen saturation
STOP	sensitive, timely, and organized programs (battered spouses)
STORCH	syphilis, toxoplasmosis, other agents, rubella, cytomegalovirus, and herpes (maternal infections)
STP	short-term plans
	sodium thiopental
	step training progression
STPD	standard temperature and pressure—dry
STPI	State-Trait Personality Inventory
STPS	Short-Term Performance Status

STPT second-trimester pregnancy termination
STR scotopic threshold response
short tandem repeat
signs of a stroke (ask patient to **s**mile; **t**alk [speak a simple sentence]; **r**aise both arms)
sister
small tandem repeat
stretcher
Strab strabismus
STRAWB strawberry
strep streptococcus
streptomycin
STRICU shock/trauma/respiratory intensive care unit
Str Post MI strictly posterior myocardial infarction
STS serologic test for syphilis
short-term survivors
slide thin slab
sodium tetradecyl sulfate
sodium thiosulfate
soft tissue sarcoma
soft tissue swelling
somatostatin (Zecnil)
standard threshold shift (audiology)
staurosporine
superior temporal sulcus
Surgical Technology Student
ST-SDDI short-term sequential digital dermoscopy imaging
STSG split thickness skin graft
STSS streptococcal-induced toxic shock syndrome
STS-SPT simple two-step swallowing provocation test
STT scaphoid, trapezium trapezoid
serial thrombin time
skin temperature test
soft tissue tumor
subtotal thyroidectomy
STT#1 Schirmer tear test one
STT#2 Schirmer tear test two
STTb basal Schirmer tear test
STTOL standing tolerance
STU shock trauma unit
surgical trauma unit
STV short-term variability
STV+ short-term variability-present
STV 0 short-term variability-absent
STV inter short-term variability-intermittent
STX stricture
Stx EIA Shiga toxin enzyme immunoassay
STZ streptozocin (Zanosar)
SU sensory urgency
Somogyi units
stasis ulcer
stroke unit
sulfonylurea
supine
Su Sunday
S/U shoulder/umbilicus
S&U supine and upright
SUA serum uric acid
single umbilical artery
SUB Skene urethra and Bartholin glands
Subcu subcutaneous
SUBCUT subcutaneous
Subepi M Inj subepicardial myocardial injury
SUBL sublingual
SUB-MAND submandibular
sub q subcutaneous (this is a dangerous abbreviation since the q is mistaken for every, when a number follows)
SUCC succinylcholine
SUCT suction
SUD substance use disorder(s)
sudden unexpected death
SuDBP supine diastolic blood pressure
SUDEP sudden unexpected (unexplained) death in epilepsy
SUDI sudden unexpected death in infancy
SUDS Subjective Unit of Distress (Disturbance) (Discomfort) Scale
sudden unexplained death syndrome
SUF symptomatic uterine fibroids
SUI stress urinary incontinence
suicide
SUID sudden unexplained infant death
SUIOS Simplified Urinary Incontinence Outcome Score
SULF-PRIM sulfamethoxazole and trimethoprim
SUMO small ubiquitin-like modifier
SUN serum urea nitrogen
SUNCT short-lasting unilateral neuralgiform headache attacks with conjunctival injection and tearing
SUNDS sudden unexplained nocturnal death syndrome
SUO syncope of unknown origin
SUP stress ulcer prophylaxis
superior
supination
supinator
symptomatic uterine prolapse
SUPAC Scale-Up and Post Approval Change
supp suppository
SUPRV supervision
SUR suramin (Metaret)
surgery
surgical

Surgi	Surgigator
SUSARs	suspected and unsuspected serious adverse reactions
Susp	suspension
SUUD	sudden unexpected, unexplained death
SUV	standard uptake variable
SUVs	standard uptake values
SUX	succinylcholine
	suction
SUZI	subzonal insertion
SV	scimitar vein
	seminal vesical
	severe
	sigmoid volvulus
	single ventricle
	single vessel
	snake venom
	stroke volume
	subclavian vein
Sv	sievert (radiation unit)
SV40	simian virus 40
SVA	small volume admixture
SVAB	stereotactic vacuum-assisted biopsy
SVAS	supravalvular aortic stenosis
SVB	saphenous vein bypass
SVBG	saphenous vein bypass graft
SVC	slow vital capacity
	subclavian vein compression
	superior vena cava
SVCO	superior vena cava obstruction
SVC-RPA	superior vena cava and right pulmonary artery (shunt)
SVCS	superior vena cava syndrome
SVD	singular value decomposition (analysis)
SVD	single-vessel disease
	spontaneous vaginal delivery
	structural valve deterioration (dysfunction)
SVE	sterile vaginal examination
	Streptococcus viridans endocarditis
	subcortical vascular encephalopathy
SV&E	suicidal, violent, and eloper
SVG	saphenous vein graft
SVH	subjective visual horizontal (test)
SVI	seminal vesicle invasion
	stroke volume index
S VISC	serum viscosity
SVL	severe visual loss
SVM	support vector machines
SVN	small volume nebulizer
SVO	small vessel occlusion
SVO_2	mixed venous oxygen saturation
SVOO	systemic ventricular outflow obstruction
SVP	spontaneous venous pulse
SVPB	supraventricular premature beat
SVPC	supraventricular premature contraction
SV/PP	stroke volume/pulse pressure
SVR	supraventricular rhythm
	sustained virological response
	systemic vascular resistance
SVRI	systemic vascular resistance index
SVT	splanchnic vein thrombosis
	superficial vein thrombosis
	supraventricular tachycardia
	symptom validity test(s)
SVVD	spontaneous vertex vaginal delivery
SVZ	subventricular zone
SW	sandwich
	sea water
	seriously wounded
	shallow walk (aquatic therapy)
	short wave
	Social Worker
	stab wound
	standard walker
	sterile water
	swallowing reflex
S&W	soap and water
S/W	somewhat
SWA	Social Work Associate
SWAN	statewide adoption network
SWAP	short-wavelength automated perimetry
SWAT	skin wound assessment and treatment
SWD	short wave diathermy
Sweet Milk	propofol (Diprivan) (slang)
SWFI	sterile water for injection
SWG	standard wire gauge
SWI	sterile water for injection
	surgical wound infection
S&WI	skin and wound isolation
SWL	shock wave lithotripsy
SWMA	segmental wall-motion abnormalities
SWME	Semmes-Weinstein monofilament examination
SWO	superficial white onychomycosis
SWOG	Southwest Oncology Group
SWOT	strengths, weaknesses, opportunities, threats (analysis)
SWP	small whirlpool
	southwest Pacific
SWR	surface wrinkling retinopathy
	surgical waiting room
SWS	sheltered workshop
	slow-wave sleep
	social work service
	student ward secretary
	Sturge-Weber syndrome
SWSD	shift-work sleep disorder
SWT	stab wound of the throat
	shuttle-walk test

SWU	septic work-up
SWW	static wall walk (aquatic therapy)
Sx	signs
	surgery
	symptom
SXA	single-energy x-ray absorptiometry
SXR	skull x-ray
SYN	synovial
SYN-D	synthadotin
SYN Fl	synovial fluid
SYPH	syphilis
SYR	syrup
SYS BP	systolic blood pressure
SZ	schizophrenic
	seizure
	suction
SZN	streptozocin (Zanosar)

T

T	inverted T wave
	tablespoon (15 mL) (this is a dangerous abbreviation)
	taenia
	teach (taught)
	temperature
	tender
	tension
	tesla (unit of magnetic flux density in radiology)
	testicles
	testosterone
	thoracic
	thymidine
	Toxoplasma
	trace
	transcribed
t	teaspoon (5 mL) (this is a dangerou abbreviation)
T+	increase intraocular tension
T−	decreased intraocular tension
2,4,5-T	2,4,5-trichlorophenoxyacetic acid
T°	temperature
$T_{1/2}$	half-life
T_1	tricuspid first sound
T_2	tricuspid second sound
T-2	dactinomycin, doxorubicin, vincristine, and cyclophosphamide
T_3	triiodothyronine (liothyronine)
T3	transurethral thermo-ablation therapy (Targis)
	Tylenol with codeine 30 mg (this is a dangerous abbreviation)
$T_{3/4}$ind	triiodothyronine to thyroxine index
T_4	levothyroxine
	thyroxine
T4	CD4 (helper-inducer cells)
T-7	free thyroxine factor
T-10	methotrexate, calcium leucovorin rescue, doxorubicin, cisplatin, bleomycin, cyclophosphamide, and dactinomycin
T-20	enfuvirtide (Fuzeon)
$T_1...T_{12}$	thoracic nerve 1 through 12
	thoracic vertebra 1 through 12
TA	Takayasu arteritis
	temperature axillary
	temporal arteritis
	temporal artery
	tendon Achilles
	therapeutic abortion
	tibialis anterior (muscle)
	tracheal aspirate
	traffic accident

	tricuspid atresia
	truncus arteriosus
Ta	tonometry applanation
T&A	tonsillectomy and adenoidectomy
	tonsils and adenoids
T(A)	axillary temperature
TA1	thymosin alpha-1
TA-55	stapling device
TAA	Therapeutic Activities Aide
	thoracic aortic aneurysm
	total ankle arthroplasty
	transverse aortic arch
	triamcinolone acetonide
	tumor-associated antigen (antibodies)
TAAA	thoracoabdominal aortic aneursym
TAB	tablet
	therapeutic abortion
	threatened abortion
	total androgen blockade
	triple antibiotic (bacitracin, neomycin, and polymyxin (this is a dangerous abbreviation)
TAC	docetaxel (Taxotere), doxorubicin (Adriamycin), and cyclophosphamide
	tacrolimus (Prograf, also TRL)
	tetracaine, Adrenalin® and cocaine
	total arterial compliance
	tibial artery catheter
	total abdominal colectomy
	total allergen content
	triamicinolone cream
	trigeminal autonomic cephalgias
TACC	thoracic aortic cross-clamping
TACE	transarterial chemoembolization
TACI	total anterior cerebral infarct
tac-MRA	timed arterial compression magnetic resonance angiography
TACT	tuned aperture computed tomography
TAD	thoracic asphyxiant dystrophy
	transverse abdominal diameter
TADAC	therapeutic abortion, dilation, aspiration, and curettage
TADC	tumor-associated dendritic cells
TAE	transcatheter arterial embolization
TAF	tissue angiogenesis factor
TAFI	thrombin-activatable fibrinolysis inhibitor
TAG	triacylglycerol
	tumor-associated glycoprotein
TAGA	term, appropriate for gestational age
	term, average gestational age
TA-GVHD	transfusion-associated graft-versus-host disease
TAH	total abdominal hysterectomy
	total artificial heart
TAHBSO	total abdominal hysterectomy, bilateral salpingo-oophorectomy
TAHL	thick ascending limb of Henle loop
TAI	thoracic aortic injury
T Air	air puff tonometry
TAKE	Targeting Abnormal Kinetic Effects
TAL	tendon Achilles lengthening
	total arm length
T ALCON	Alcon® tonometry
T-ALL	T-cell acute lymphoblastic leukemia
TALP	total alkaline phosphatase
TAML	therapy-related acute myelogenous leukemia
t-AML	therapy-related acute myeloid leukemia
TAM	tamoxifen (Novaldex)
	teenage mother
	total active motion
	tumor-associated macrophages
TAN	treatment-as-needed
	Treatment Authorization Number
	tropical ataxic neuropathy
TANF	Temporary Assistance for Needy Families
TANI	total axial (lymph) node irradiation
TAO	thromboangitis obliterans
	thyroid-associated ophthalmopathy
	troleandomycin
TAP	tone and positioning
	tonometry by applanation
	transabdominal preperitoneal (laparoscopic hernia repair)
	transesophageal atrial paced
	trypsinogen activation peptide
	tumor-activated prodrug
TAPP	transabdominal preperitoneal polypropylene (mesh-plasty)
T APPL	applanation tonometry
TAPVC	total anomalous pulmonary venous connection
TAPVD	total anomalous pulmonary venous drainage
TAPVR	total anomalous pulmonary venous return
TAR	thoracic aortic rupture
	thrombocytopenia with absent radius
	total ankle replacement
	total anorectal reconstruction
	treatment administration record
	treatment authorization request
TARA	total articular replacement arthroplasty
TART	tenderness, asymmetry, restricted motion, and tissue texture changes
	tumorectomy and radiotherapy
TAS	therapeutic activities specialist
	Thrombolytic Assessment System
	transabdominal sutures
	turning against self

T

	typical absence seizures
TASS	toxic anterior segment syndrome
TAT	tandem autotransplants
	tell a tale
	tetanus antitoxin
	thematic apperception test
	thrombin-antithrombin III complex
	'til all taken
	tired all the time
	total adipose tissue
	transactivator of transcription
	transfusion-associated transmission
	transplant-associated thrombocytopenia
	turnaround time
	tyrosine aminotransferase
TATT	tired all the time
TAU	tumescence activity units
TAUC	target area under the curve
	time-averaged urea concentration
TAUSA	thrombolysis and angioplasty in unstable angina
TAX	cefotaxime (Claforan)
	paclitaxel (Taxol)
TB	Tapes for the Blind
	terrible burning
	thought broadcasting
	toothbrush
	total base
	total bilirubin
	total body
	tuberculosis
TBA	to be absorbed
	to be added
	to be administered
	to be admitted
	to be announced
	to be arranged
	to be assessed
	total body (surface) area
TBAGA	term birth appropriate for gestational age
T-bar	tracheotomy bar (a device used in respiratory therapy)
TBARS	thiobarbituric acid reactive substances
TBB	transbronchial biopsy
TBBL	transblepharoplasty brow lift
TBC	to be cancelled
	total-blood cholesterol
	total-body clearance
	tuberculosis
TBD	to be determined
TBE	tick-borne encephalitis
	timed-barium esophagogram
	time to bacterial eradication
	to be evaluated
TBE_e	tick-borne encephalitis, eastern subtype (Far eastern encephalitis, Russian spring-summer e., Taiga e.) vaccine
T-berg	Trendelenburg (position)
TBEV	tick-borne encephalitis virus
TBE_w	tick-bone encephalitis, western subtype (Central European encephalitis) vaccine
TBF	total-body fat
TBG	thyroxine-binding globulin
TBI	tick-borne illness(es)
	toothbrushing instruction
	total-body irradiation
	traumatic brain injury
T bili	total bilirubin
TBK	total-body potassium
tbl	tablespoon (15 mL)
TBLB	transbronchial lung biopsy
TBLC	term birth, living child
TBLF	term birth, living female
TBLI	term birth, living infant
TBLM	term birth, living male
TBM	tracheobronchomalacia
	tuberculous meningitis
	tubule basement membrane
TBMg	total-body magnesium
TBN	total-body nitrogen
TBNA	transbronchial needle aspiration
	treated but not admitted
TBNa	total-body sodium
TBO	toluidine blue O
TBOCS	Tale-Brown Obsessive-Compulsive Scale
TBP	thyroxine-binding protein
	toe blood pressure
	total-body phosphorus
	total-body protein
	tuberculous peritonitis
TBPA	thyroxine-binding prealbumin
TBR	total-bed rest
TBRF	tick-borne relapsing fever
TBS	tablespoon (15 mL)(this is a dangerous abbreviation)
	tachycardia-bradycardia syndrome
	The Bethesda System (reporting cervical and vagina cytology)
	total-serum bilirubin
TBSA	total-body surface area
	total-burn surface area
tbsp	tablespoon (15 mL)
TBT	tolbutamide test
	tracheal bronchial toilet
	transbronchoscopic balloon tipped
TBUT	tear break-up time (dry-eye test)
TBV	thiotepa, bleomycin, and vinblastine
	total-blood volume

	transluminal balloon valvuloplasty
TBW	total-body water
TBZ	tetrabenazine (Nitoman [Canada], Xenazine [UK])
	thiabendazole (Mintezol)
TC	paclitaxel (Taxol) and cisplatin
	tactile cues
	tai chi (exercise program)
	team conference
	telephone call
	terminal cancer
	testicular cancer
	thioguanine and cytarabine
	thoracic circumference
	throat culture
	tissue culture
	tolonium chloride
	tonic-clonic
	tonsillar coblation
	total cholesterol
	total communication
	to (the) chest
	tracheal collar
	trauma center
	true conjugate
	tubocurarine
Tc	technetium
T/C	telephone call
	ticarcillin-clavulanic acid (Timentin)
	to consider
3TC	lamivudine (Epivir)
TC7	Interceed®
T&C	turn and cough
	type and crossmatch
T&C#3	Tylenol with 30 mg codeine
TCA	thioguanine and cytarabine
	tissue concentrations of antibiotic(s)
	trichloroacetic acid
	tricuspid atresia
	tricyclic antidepressant
	tumor chemosensitivity assay
	tumor clonogenic assays
TCABG	triple coronary artery bypass graft
TCAD	transplant-related coronary-artery disease
	tricyclic antidepressant
TCAR	tiazofurin
TCB	to call back
	tumor cell burden
TCBS	thiosulfate-citrate-bile salt-sucrose (agar)
TCC	total cost of care
	transitional cell carcinoma
	2,3,5-triphenyl tetrazolium chloride
TCCa	transitional cell carcinoma
TCCB	transitional cell carcinoma of bladder
TC/CL	ticarcillin-clavulanate (Timentin)
$TcCO_2$	transcutaneous carbon dioxide
TCD	T-cell depleted
	transcerebellar diameter
	transcranial Doppler (ultrasonography)
	transverse cardiac diameter
	transcystic duct
TCDB	turn, cough, and deep breath
TCDD	tetrachlorodibenzo-p-dioxin (dioxin)
^{99m}Tc DTPA	technetium Tc 99m pentetate
TCE	tetrachloroethylene
	total-colon examination
	toxicity composite endpoint
	transcatheter embolotherapy
T cell	small lymphocyte
TCES	transcranial electrical stimulation
$^{99m}TcGHA$	technetium Tc 99m gluceptate
TCFA	thin cap fibroatheroma
TCH	paclitaxel (Taxol), carboplatin, and trastuzumab (Herceptin)
	total cost of hospitalization
	turn, cough, hyperventilate
^{99m}Tc-HAS	technetium Tc 99m-labeled human serum albumin
TCHRs	traditional Chinese herbal remedies
TCI	target-control infusion
	to come in
	transcutaneous immunization
TCID	tissue culture infective dose
TCIE	transient cerebral ischemic episode
TCIT	therapeutic crisis intervention training
TCL	tibial collateral ligament
	transverse carpal ligament
TCM	tissue culture media
	traditional Chinese medicine
	transcutaneous (oxygen) monitor
^{99m}Tc-MAA	technetium Tc 99m albumin microaggregated
TCMH	tumor-direct cell-mediated hypersensitivity
TCMS	transcranial cortical magnetic stimulation
TCMZ	trichlormethiazide (Naqua)
TCN	tetracycline
	triciribine phosphate (tricyclic nucleoside)
TCNS	transcutaneous nerve stimulator
TCNU	tauromustine
TcO_2	transcutaneous oxygen pressure
TcO_4^-	pertechnetate
TCOM	transcutaneous oxygen monitor
T Con	temporary conservatorship
TCP	thrombocytopenia
	transcutaneous pacing
	tranylcypromine (Parnate)

T

	tricalcium phosphate
	tumor control probability
TCPC	total cavopulmonary connection
$TcPCO_2$	transcutaneous carbon dioxide
$TcPO_2$	transcutaneous oxygen
^{99m}TcPYP	technetium Tc 99m pyrophosphate
TCR	T-cell receptor
TCRE	transcervical resection of the endometrium
TCRFTA	temperature-controlled radiofrequency tissue ablation
TCS	tonic-clonic seizure
	topical corticosteroid
^{99m}TcSC	technetium Tc 99m sulfur colloid
TCT	thyrocalcitonin
	tincture
	transcatheter therapy
	triple combination tablet (abacavir, lamivudine, and zidovudine) (Trizivir)
TCU	transitional care unit
TCVA	thromboembolic cerebral vascular accident
TD	Takayasu disease
	tardive dyskinesia
	temporary disability
	terminal device
	test dose
	tetanus-diphtheria toxoids (pediatric use)
	tidal volume
	tolerance dose
	tone decay
	total disability
	transdermal
	transverse diameter
	travelers' diarrhea
	treatment discontinued
Td	tetanus-diphtheria toxoids (adult type)
T1D	type 1 diabetes (mellitus); (This is a dangerous abbreviation as it will be read as "three times daily" [TID]. Use DM1
TDAC	tumor-derived activated cell (cultures)
TDD	telephone device for the deaf
	thoracic duct drainage
	total daily dose
TDE	total daily energy (requirement)
TDF	tenofovir disoproxil fumarate (Virend)
	testis determining factor
	total-dietary fiber
	tumor dose fractionation
TDI	tissue Doppler imaging
	tolerable daily intake
	toluene diisocyanate
TDIs	therapist-directed interventions
TDK	tardive diskinesia
TDL	thoracic duct lymph
TDLN	tumor-draining lymph nodes
TDM	therapeutic drug monitoring
T1DM	type 1 diabetes mellitus (this is a dangerous abbreviation as it will be read as "three times daily with meals" [TIDM]. Use DM1
T2DM	type 2 diabetes mellitus
TDMAC	tridodecylmethyl ammonium chloride
TDN	totally digestible nutrients
	transdermal nitroglycerin
TDNTG	transdermal nitroglycerin
TDNWB	touchdown nonweightbearing
TdP	torsades de pointes
TDPDS	temporomandibular disorder pain dysfunction syndrome
TDPWB	touchdown partial weight-bearing
TDR	transmural dispersion of repolarization
TdR	thymidine
TDS	Teacher Drool Scale
	traveler's diarrhea syndrome
TDS	three times a day (United Kingdom)
TDT	tentative discharge tomorrow
	transmission disequilibrium test
	Trieger Dot Test
	tumor doubling time
TdT	terminal deoxynucleotidyl transferase
TDW	target dry weight
TDWB	touch down weight bearing
TDx®	fluorescence polarization immunoassay
TE	echo time
	tennis elbow
	terminal extension
	tooth extraction
	toxoplasmic encephalitis
	trace elements (chromium, copper, iodine, manganese, selenium, molybdenum and zinc)
	tracheoesophageal
	transesophageal echocardiography
	transrectal electroejaculation
*t*E	total expiratory time
T/E	testosterone to epitestosterone ratio
	testosterone/estrogen (ratio)
	trunk-to-extremity skinfold thicknes (index)
T&E	testing and evaluation
	training and evaluation
	trial and error
TEA	thoracic epidural analgesia
	thromboendarterectomy
	Time and Extent Application (FDA)

T

	total elbow arthroplasty transluminal extraction atherectomy
TEAE	treatment-emergent adverse event
TEAP	transesophageal atrial pacing
TEB	thoracic electrical bioimpedance
TEBG	testosterone-estradiol binding globulin
TeBG	testeosterone binding globulin
TeBIDA	technetium 99m trimethyl 1-bromo-imono diacetic acid
TEC	thromboembolic complication total eosinophil count toxic *Escherichia coli* transient erythroblastopenia of childhood transluminal extraction-endarterectomy catheter transpapillary endoscopic cholecystostomy triethyl citrate
T&EC	trauma and emergency center
TECA	titrated extract of *Centella asiatica*
TECAB	totally endoscopic (off-pump) coronary artery bypass grafting
TED	thromboembolic disease thyroid eye disease
TEDS	thromboembolic disease stockings transesophageal echo-Doppler system Treatment Episode Data Set
TEE	total energy expended transnasal endoscopic ethmoidectomy transesophageal echocardiography
TEEU	transesophageal endoscopic ultrasound
TEF	tracheoesophageal fistula
TEG	thromboelastogram (thromboelastography)
TEH	theophylline, ephedrine, and hydroxyzine
TEI	therapeutic equivalence interchange total episode of illness transesophageal imaging
TEL	telemetry telephone
tele	telemetry
TEM	temozolomide (Temodar) transanal endoscopic microsurgery transmission electron microscopy
TEMI	transient episodes of myocardial ischemia
TEMP	temperature temporal temporary
TEN	tension (intraocular pressure) toxic epidermal necrolysis
TEN®	Total Enteral Nutrition
TENS	transcutaneous electrical nerve stimulation
TEOAE	transient evoked otoacoustic emission (test)
TEP	total endoprosthesis total extraperitoneal (laparoscopic hernia repair) tracheoesophageal puncture tubal ectopic pregnancy
TEQ	toxic equivalents
TER	terlipressin total elbow replacement total energy requirement transnasal endoscopic resection transurethral electroresection
TERB	terbutaline
TERC	Test of Early Reading Comprehension
TERM	full-term terminal
TERT	human telomerase reverse transcriptase (also hTRT) tertiary total end-range time
TES	therapeutic electrical stimulation thoracic endometriosis syndrome thoracic endoscopic sympathectomy transcorneal electrical stimulation treatment emergent symptoms
TESA	testicular sperm aspiration
TESE	testicular sperm extraction
TESI	thoracic epidural steroid injection
TESS	Toronto Extremity Salvage Score Toxic Exposure Surveillance System treatment emergent signs and symptoms Treatment Emergent Symptom Scale
TET	transcranial electrostimulation therapy treadmill exercise test
TETE	too early to evaluate
TETig	tetanus immune globulin
TEU	token economy unit transesophageal ultrasound
TEV	talipes equinovarus (deformity)
TEVAP	transurethral electrovaporization of the prostate
TF	tactile fremitus tail flick (reflex) tetralogy of Fallot Thomsen-Friedenreich (antigen) tibiofemoral to follow trigger finger tube feeding
TFA	topical fluoride application trans fatty acids trifluoroacetic acid

T

TFB	trifascicular block
TFBC	The Family Birthing Center
TFC	thoracic fluid content
	time to following commands
TFCC	triangular fibrocartilage complex
TFESI	transforaminal epidural steroid injection
TFF	tangential flow filtration
	trefoil factor family (peptides)
TF-Fe	transferrin-bound iron
TFI	total fluid intake
	treatment-free interval
TFL	tensor fasciae latae
	transnasal fiberoptic laryngoscopy
	trimetrexate, fluorouracil, and leucovorin
	trunk-forward lean
TFM	transverse friction massage
TFN	trochanteric fixation nail
TFO	triplex-forming oligonucleotide
TFOs	triplex-forming oligonucleotides
TFPI	tissue-factor pathway inhibitor
TFR	total fertility rate
TFSI	transforaminal (epidural) steroid injection
TFT	thin-film transistor
	Thought Field Therapy
	thumb-finding test
	trifluridine (trifluorothymidine)
TFTs	thyroid function tests
TFV	tenofovir (Viread)
T25FW	timed 25-foot walk
TG	total gym
	triglycerides
Tg	thyroglobulin
6-TG	thioguanine
TGA	Therapeutic Goods Administration (Australia)
	third-generation antidepressant
	transient global amnesia
	transposition of the great arteries
TGAR	total graft area rejected
TGB	tiagabine (Gabatril)
TGCE	temperature gradient capillary electrophoresis
TGCT	testicular germ cell tumor(s)
TGD	thyroglossal duct
	tumor growth delay
TGDC	thyroglossal duct cyst
TGE	transmissible gastroenteritis
TGFA	triglyceride fatty acid
TGF	transforming growth factor
TGF-$_\beta$	transforming growth factor-beta
TGGE	temperature-gradient gel electrophoresis
TGN	trans-Golgi network
	trochanteric gamma nail
TGR	tenderness, guarding, and rigidity
TGS	tincture of green soap
TGs	triglycerides
TGT	thromboplastin generation test
TGTL	total glottic transverse laryngectomy
TGV	thoracic gas volume
	transposition of great vessels
TGXT	thallium-graded exercise test
TGZ	troglitazone (Rezulin)
TH	thrill
	thyroid hormone
	total hysterectomy
Th	thorium
	Thursday
T&H	type and hold
TH1	T helper cell, type 1
TH2	T helper cell, type 2
THA	tacrine (tetrahydroacridine; Cognex)
	total hip arthroplasty
	transient hemispheric attack
THAA	thyroid hormone autoantibodies
	tubular hypoplasia aortic arch
THAL	thalassemia
	thalidomide (Thalomid)
THAT	Toronto Hospital Alertness Test
THBI	thyroid hormone binding index
THBR	thyroid hormone-binding ratio
THAM®	tromethamine
$THBO_2$	topical hyperbaric oxygen
THC	tetrahydrocannabinol (dronabinol)
	thigh circumference
	transhepatic cholangiogram
THCT	triple-phase helical computer tomography
TH-CULT	throat culture
tHcy	total homocysteine
THDC	tunnelled hemodialysis catheter
THE	total-head excursion
	transhepatic embolization
Ther Ex	therapeutic exercise
THF	thymic humoral factor
THG	tetrahydrogestrinone
THg	total mercury
THI	transient hypogamma-globinemia of infancy
THKAFO	trunk-hip-knee-ankle-foot orthosis
THKAFO-LU	lockable joints using trunk-hip-knee-ankle-foot orthosis
THL	transvaginal hydrolaparoscopy
THLAA	tubular hypoplasia left aortic arch
THP	take home packs
	total hip prosthesis
	transhepatic portography
	trihexyphenidyl (Artane)
THR	target heart rate
	thrombin receptor
	total hip replacement
	training heart rate
THRL	total hip replacement, left

THRR	total hip replacement, right transient hyperemic response ratio
THS	Tolosa-Hunt syndrome
THTV	therapeutic home trial visit
THV	therapeutic home visit
TI	terminal ileus thallium imaging therapeutic index thought insertion time following inversion pulse (radiology) transischial transverse diameter of inlet tricuspid incompetence tricuspid insufficiency
TIA	transient ischemic attack
TIB	tibia
TIBC	total iron-binding capacity
tib-fib	tibia and fibula
TIBS	transillumination breast spectroscopy
TIC	paclitaxel (Taxol), ifosfamide, and cisplain total ion chromatograms trypsin-inhibitor capacity
TICOSMO	**t**rauma, **i**nfection, **c**hemical/drug exposure, **o**rgan systems, **s**tress, **m**usculoskeletal, and **o**ther (prompts used during history taking for possible etiologies of problems)
TICS	diverticulosis
TICU	thoracic intensive care unit transplant intensive care unit trauma intensive care unit
t.i.d.	three times a day
TIDM	three times daily with meals
TIE	transient ischemic episode
TIF	tracheal intubation fiberscope
TIG	tetanus immune globulin
TIH	tumor-inducing hypercalcemia
TKI	tyrosine kinase inhibitor
TIL	tumor-infiltrating lymphocytes
%tile	percentile
TIMI	Thrombolysis in Myocardial Infarction (studies)
TIMP	tissue inhibitor of metalloproteinase
TIMP-2	Tissue inhibitors of metallo-proteinase 2
TIN	testicular intraepithelial neoplasia three times a night (this is a dangerous abbreviation) tubulointerstitial nephritis
tinct	tincture
TIND	Treatment Investigational New Drug (application)
TINEM	there is no evidence of malignancy
TIP	toxic interstitial pneumonitis tubularized incised plate (urethroplasty)
TIPS	transvenous intrahepatic portosystemic shunt (stent-shunt)
TIPSS	transjugular intrahepatic portosystemic shunt (stent)
TIPU	tubularized-incised plate urethroplasty
TIRFM	total-internal reflection microscopy
TIS	tumor *in situ*
TISS	Therapeutic Intervention Scoring System
TIT	*Treponema* (*pallidum*) immobilization test triiodothyronine (liothyronine)
TIUP	term intrauterine pregnancy
TIV	trivalent inactivated influenza vaccine
TIVA	total intravenous anethesia
TIVC	thoracic inferior vena cava
+tive	positive
TIW	three times a week (this is a dangerous abbreviation)
TJ	tendon jerk triceps jerk
TJA	total joint arthroplasty
TJC	tender joint count
TJN	tongue jaw neck (dissection) twin-jet nebulizer
TJR	total joint replacement
TK	thymidine kinase toxicokinetics
TKA	total knee arthroplasty tyrosine kinase activity
TKD	tokodynamometer
TKE	terminal knee extension
TKIC	true knot in cord
TKNO	to keep needle open
TKP	thermokeratoplasty total knee prosthesis
TKO	to keep (vein; intravenous line) open
TKR	total knee replacement
TKRL	total knee replacement, left
TKRR	total knee replacement, right
TKVO	to keep vein open
TL	team leader thermoluminescence thoracolumbar total laryngectomy transverse line trial leave tubal ligation
T/L	terminal latency
Tl	thallium
TLA	translumbar arteriogram (aortogram) transverse ligament of atlas
TLAC	triple lumen Arrow catheter
TL BLT	tubal ligation, bilateral

T

TLC tender loving care
therapeutic lifestyle changes
thin layer chromatography
titanium linear cutter
T-lymphocyte choriocarcinoma
total lung capacity
total lymphocyte count
transitional living center
triple lumen catheter

TLD thermoluminescent dosimeter

TLE temporal lobe epilepsy

TLE-HS temporal lobe epilepsy-hippocampal sclerosis

TLESI transforaminal lumbar epidural steroid injection

TLFB timeline follow back (interview)

T-LGLL T-cell large granular lymphocyte leukemia

TLH total laparoscopic hysterectomy

TLI total lymphoid irradiation
translaryngeal intubation

TLIF transforaminal lumbar interbody fusion

TLK thermal laser keratoplasty

TLM thalidomide (Thalomid)
torn lateral meniscus

TLNB term living newborn

TLOA temporary leave of absence

TLOVR time to loss of virologic response

TLP transitional living program

TLR target lesion reintervention
target-lesion revascularization
tonic labyrinthine reflex

TLRs Toll-like receptors

TLS tumor lysis syndrome

TLSO thoracic lumbar sacral orthosis

TLSP trypsin-like serine protease

TLSSO thoracolumbosacral spinal orthosis

TLT tonsillectomy

TLTBI treatment of latent tuberculosis infection

TLUS the time elapsed from ingestion of the first dose of medication to passage of the last unformed stool

TLV threshold limit value
total lung volume

TLVAB transient left-ventricular apical ballooning

TM temperature by mouth
tetrathiomolybdate
thalassemia major
Thayer-Martin (culture)
thyromegaly
Tibetan Medicine
trabecular meshwork
trademark (unregistered)
transcendental meditation
transmetatarsal
treadmill
tropical medicine
tumor
tympanic membrane

T & M type and crossmatch

TMA thrombotic microangiopathy
tissue microarray
trained medication aid
transcription mediated amplification
transmetatarsal amputation
trimethylamine

T/MA tracheostomy mask

TMAS Taylor Manifest Anxiety Scale

TMA-uria trimethylaminuria

T_{max} temperature maximum

t_{max} time of occurrence for maximum (peak) drug concentration

TMB tetramethylberizidine
therapeutic back massage
transient monocular blindness
trimethoxybenzoates

TMC transmural colitis
Transtheoretical Model of Change
trapeziometacarpal
triamcinolone

TMCA trimethylcolchicinic acid

TMCC temporal mandibular cervical chain (of muscles)

TMCN triamcinolone

TMD temporomandibular dysfunction (disorder)
transient myeloproliferative disorder
treating physician

t-MDS therapy-related myelodysplastic syndrome

TME thermolysin-like metalloendopeptidase
total mesorectal excision

TMET treadmill exercise test

TMEV Theiler murine encephalomyelitis virus

TMG trimegestone

TMH trainable mentally handicapped

TMI threatened myocardial infarction
transmandibular implant
transmural infarct

T>MIC time above minimum inhibitory concentration

TMJ temporomandibular joint

TMJD temporomandibular joint dysfunction

TMJS temporomandibular joint syndrome

TML tongue midline
treadmill

TMLR transmyocardial laser revascularization

TMM torn medial meniscus
total muscle mass

Tmm McKay-Marg tension

TMNG	toxic multinodular goiter
TMO	transcaruncular medial orbitotomy
TMP	thallium myocardial perfusion
	transmembrane pressure
	trimethoprim
TMP/SMZ	trimethoprim and sulfamethoxazole (correct name is sulfamethoxazole and trimethoprin; SMZ-TMP)
TMR	targeted motor reinnervation
	temporary medication refill
	trainable mentally retarded
	transmyocardial revascularization
TMS	transcranial magnetic stimulation
TMSI	Task Management Strategy Index
TMST	treadmill stress test
TMT	tarsometatarsal
	teratoma with malignant transformation
	treadmill test
	tympanic membrane thermometer
TMTC	too many to count
TMTX	trimetrexate (Neutrexin)
TMUGS	Tumor Marker Utility Grading Scale
TMX	tamoxifen (Novaldex)
TMZ	temazepam (Restoril)
	temozolomide (Temodar)
TN	normal intraocular tension
	team nursing
	temperature normal
	tree nut
	trigeminal neuralgia
	triple negative
T&N	tension and nervousness
	tingling and numbness
TNA	total nutrient admixture
TNAs	transient neurological attacks
TNAB	transthoracic needle biopsy
TNB	term newborn
	transnasal butorphanol
	transrectal needle biopsy (of the prostate)
	Tru-Cut® needle biopsy
TNBP	transurethral needle biopsy of prostate
TNCC	Trauma Nursing Course Certified
TND	term, normal delivery
TNDM	transient neonatal diabetes mellitus
TNF	tumor necrosis factor
TNF-bp	tumor necrosis factor binding protein
TNG	nitroglycerin
	toxic nodular goiter
TNI	total nodal irradiation
TnI	troponin I
TNKase®	tenecteplase
TNM	primary tumor, regional lymph nodes, and distant metastasis (used with subscripts for the staging of cancer)
t-NNT	threshold number needed to treat
TNP	time to neurologic progression
TNR	tonic neck reflex
TNS	transcutaneous nerve stimulation (stimulator)
	transient neurologic symptoms
	Trauma Nurse Specialist
	Tullie-Niebörg syndrome
TNT	thiotepa, mitoxantrone (Novantrone), and paclitaxel (Taxol)
	treating to new targets
	triamcinolone and nystatin
TnT	troponin T
TNTC	too numerous to count
TNU	tobacco nonuser
TNY	trichomonas and yeast
TO	old tuberculin
	telephone order
	time off
	tincture of opium (warning: this is NOT paregoric)
	total obstruction
	transfer out
T(O)	oral temperature
T/O	time out
T&O	tandem and ovoid (insertion)
	tubes and ovaries
TOA	time of arrival
	tubo-ovarian abscess
TOAA	to affected areas
TOAST	Trial of Org 10172 (danaparoid sodium) in Acute Stroke Treatment (criteria for nonpostoperative strokes)
TOB	tobacco
	tobramycin
TOC	table of contents
	test-of-cure (post-therapy visit)
	total occlusal convergence
	total organic carbon
TOCE	transcatheter oily chemoembolization
TOCO	tocodynamometer
TOD	intraocular pressure of the right eye
	target organ damage
	target-organ disease
	time of death
	time of departure
	tubal occlusion device
TOE	transoesophageal echocardiography (United Kingdom and other countries)
TOF	tetralogy of Fallot
	time of flight (radiology)
	total of four
	train-of-four
TOFMS	time-of-flight mass spectrometry
TOGV	transposition of the great vessels
TOH	throughout hospitalization

TOI	Trial Outcome Index
TOL	tolerate
	trial of labor
TOLD	Test of Language Development
TOM	therapeutic outcomes monitoring
	tomorrow
	transcutaneous oxygen monitor
ToM	theory-of-mind
Tomo	tomography
TON	tonight
	traumatic optic neuropathy
TOP	termination of pregnancy
	Topografov (virus)
	topotecan (Hycamtin)
TOP-8	Treatment Outcome PTSD (post-traumatic stress disorder) (scale)
TOPO	topotecan (Hycamtin)
TOPO 1	topoisermerase
TOPS	Take Off Pounds Sensibly
TOPV	trivalent oral polio vaccine
TOR	toremifene (Faneston)
TORB	telephone order read back
TORC	Test of Reading Comprehension
TORCH	toxoplasmosis, others (other viruses known to attack the fetus), rubella, cytomegalovirus, and herpes simplex (maternal viral infections)
TORP	total ossicular replacement prosthesis
TOS	intraocular pressure of the left eye
	thoracic outlet syndrome
	Type of Service
TOT	tip-of-the-tongue
	transobturator tape
TOT BILI	total bilirubin
TOTM	trioctyltrimellitate
TOV	telephone order verified
	trial of void
TOW	time off work
TOWL	Test of Written Language
TOX	toxoplasmosis *(Toxoplasma gondii)* vaccine
TOXO	toxoplasmosis
TP	teaching physician
	temperature and pressure
	temporoparietal
	tender point
	therapeutic pass
	ThinPrep Pap (test)
	thought process
	thrombophlebitis
	thymidine phosphorylase
	time to progression
	Todd paralysis
	toe pressure
	toilet paper
	total protein
	"T" piece
	transverse process
	treating physician
	trigger point
T:P	trough-to-peak ratio
T & P	temperature and pulse
	turn and position
TPA	alteplase, recombinant (tissue plasminogen activator) (Activase)
	temporary portacaval anastomosis
	third-party administrator
	tissue polypeptide antigen
	total parenteral alimentation
TPAL	term infant(s), premature infant(s), abortion(s), living children
TPB	Theory of Planned Behavior
TPC	target plasma concentration
	tender-point count
	total patient care
	total plate count
	touch preparation cytology
TPD	treatable protocol depth
	tropical pancreatic diabetes
	typhoid vaccine, not otherwise specified
TPD$_{a}$	typhoid vaccine, attenuated live (oral Ty21a strain)
TPD$_{AKD}$	typhoid vaccine, acetone-killed and dried (U.S. military)
TPD$_{HP}$	typhoid vaccine, heat and phenol inactivated, dried
TPD$_{VI}$	typhoid vaccine, *Vi* capsular polysaccharide
TPE	therapeutic plasma exchange
	total placental estrogens
	total protective environment
T-penia	thrombocytopenia
TPF	docetaxel (Taxotere), cisplatin (Platinol), and fluorouracil
	trained participating father
TPG	translesional pressure gradients
TPH	thromboembolic pulmonary hypertension
	trained participating husband
TPHA	*Treponema pallidum* hemagglutination
T PHOS	triple phosphate crystals
TPI	*Treponema pallidum* immobilization
	triose phosphate isomerase
TPIT	trigger point injection therapy
t$_{pk}$	time to peak
TPL	thromboplastin
T plasty	tympanoplasty
TPLSM	two-photon laser-scanning microscope
TPM	temporary pacemaker
	topiramate (Topamax)
TPMT	thiopurine methyltransferase
TPN	total parenteral nutrition

TPO	thrombopoietin
	thyroid peroxidase
	thyroperoxidase
	trial prescription order
TPOAb	thyroid peroxidase antibodies
TPP	thiamine pyrophosphate
TpP	thrombus precursor protein
TP & P	time, place, and person
TPPN	total peripheral parenteral nutrition
TPPS	Toddler-Preschooler Postoperative Pain Scale
TPPV	trans pars plana vitrectomy
TPR	temperature
	temperature, pulse, and respiration
	termination of parental rights
	total peripheral resistance
TPRI	total peripheral resistance index
T PROT	total protein
TPS	tender point score
	typhus (*rickettsiae* sp.) vaccine
TPSA	total prostate-specific antigen
TPT	thermal perception threshold
	time to peak tension
	topotecan (Hycamtin)
	transpyloric tube
	treadmill performance test
TPTEF	time to peak tidal expiratory flow
TPU	tropical phagedenic ulcer
T-putty	Theraputty
TPV	tipranavir (Aptivus)
TPVA	tibioperoneal vessel angioplasty
TPVR	total peripheral vascular resistance
TPV/r	tipranavir (Aptivus) and ritonavir (Norvir)
TPZ	tirapazamine
TQM	total quality management
TR	therapeutic recreation
	time to repeat
	time to repetition (radiology)
	tincture
	to return
	trace
	transfusion reaction
	transplant recipients
	trapezius
	treatment
	tremor
	tricuspid regurgitation
	tumor registry
T(R)	rectal temperature
T & R	tenderness and rebound
	treated and released
	turn and reposition
TRA	therapeutic recreation associate
	to run at
	trastuzumab (Herceptin; also TRAS and H)
	tumor regression antigen
TRAb	thyrotropin-receptor antibody
TRAC	traction
TRACE	time-resolved amplified cryptate emission
TRACH	tracheal
	tracheostomy
TRAFO	tone-reducing ankle/foot orthosis
TRAIL	tumor-necrosis-factor-related apoptosis-inducing ligand
TRALI	transfusion-associated lung injury
TRAM	transverse rectus abdominis myocutaneous (flap)
	transverse rectus abdominum muscle
	Treatment Response Assessment Method
TRAMP	transversus and rectus abdominis musculo-peritoneal (flap)
TRANCE	tumor necrosis factor–related activation-induced cytokine
TRANS	transfers
Trans D	transverse diameter
TRANS Rx	transfusion reaction
TRAP	tartrate-resistant (leukocyte) acid phophatase
	Telomeric Repeat Amplification Protocol
	thrombospondin-related anonymous protein
	total radical-trapping antioxidant parameter
	trapezium
	trapezius muscle
	twin-reversed arterial perfusion
TRAS	transplant renal artery stenosis
	trastuzumab (Herceptin)
TRB	return to baseline
TRBC	total red blood cells
TRC	tanned red cells
TRD	tongue-retaining device
	total-retinal detachment
	traction retinal detachment
	treatment-related death
	treatment-resistant depression
TRD-F	treatment-related discontinuation-failure
TRDN	transient respiratory distress of the newborn
TREC	T-cell receptor-rearrangement excision circles
Tren	Trendelenburg
TRF	terminal restriction fragment
TrgEMG	triggered electromyographic (stimulation)
TRH	protirelin (thyrotropin-releasing hormone) (Relefact TRH®; Thypinone®)
TRI	transient radicular irritation
	trimester

TriA	tricuspid atresia
T_3RIA	triiodothyronine level by radioimmunoassay
TRIAC	triiodothyroacetic acid
TRIC	trachoma inclusion conjunctivitis
TRICH	*Trichomonas*
TRICKS	time-resolved imaging contrast kinetics
TRIG	triglycerides
TRISS	Trauma Related Injury Severity Score
TRL	tacrolimus (Prograf, also TAC)
TR-LSC	time-resolved liquid scintillation counting
TRM	transplant-related mortality
	treatment-related mortality
TRM-SMX	trimethoprim-sulfamethoxazole (correct name is sulfamethoxazole and trimethoprin; SMZ-TMP; SMX-TMP)
tRNA	transfer ribonucleic acid
TRNBP	transrectal needle biopsy prostate
TRND	Trendelenburg (position)
TRNG	tetracycline-resistant *Neisseria gonorrhoeae*
TRO	to return to office
TROFO	trofosfamide
TROM	torque range of motion
	total range of motion
TrOOP	true out-of-pocket costs
TRP	tubular reabsorption of phosphate
TRP-1	tyrosine-related protein-1
TRPS	trichorhinophalangeal syndrome (types I, II, and III)
TrPs	trigger points
TRPT	transplant
TRS	Therapeutic Recreation Specialist
	the real symptom
	tremor rating scale
TRT	tangential radiation therapy
	testosterone replacement therapy
	thermoradiotherapy
	thoracic radiation therapy
	tinnitus retraining therapy
	treatment-related toxicity
TR/TE	time to repetition and time to echo in spin (echo sequence of magnetic resonance imaging)
T_3RU	triiodothyronine resin uptake
TRUS	transrectal ultrasonography
TRUSP	transrectal ultrasonography of the prostate
TRUST	toluidine red unheated serum test
TRZ	triazolam (Halcion)
TS	Tay-Sachs (disease)
	telomerase
	temperature sensitive
	test solution
	thoracic spine
	throat swab
	thymidylate synthase
	timed samplings
	toe signs
	Tourette syndrome
	transsexual
	Trauma Score
	tricuspid stenosis
	triple strength
	tuberous sclerosis
	Turner syndrome
T/S	trimethoprim/sulfamethoxazole (correct name is sulfamethoxazole and trimethoprin)
T&S	type and screen
Ts	Schiotz tension
	T suppressor cell
TSAb	thyroid stimulating antibodies
TSA	toluenesulfonic acid
	total shoulder arthroplasty
	trichostatin A
	tryptone soya (blood) agar
	tumor-specific antigen
	type-specific antibody
	tyramine signal amplification
TSAR®	tape surrounded Appli-rulers
TSAS	Total Severity Assessment Score
TSAT	transferrin saturation
TSB	total serum bilirubin
	trypticase soy broth
TSBB	transtracheal selective bronchial brushing
TSC	technetium sulfur colloid
	theophylline serum concentration
	total symptom complex
	tuberous sclerosis complex
T-score	number of standard deviations from the average bone mineral density (BMD) of a 25-30 year old woman
TSD	target to skin distance
	Tay-Sachs disease
	total sleep deprivation
	T-(tumor) stage downstaging
TSDP	tapered steroid dosing package
TSE	targeted systemic exposure
	testicular self-examination
	total skin examination
	transmissible spongiform encephalopathy
TSEBT	total skin electron beam therapy
T set	tracheotomy set
TSF	tricep skin fold (thickness)
TSGA	term, small gestational age
TSGs	tumor suppressor genes
TSH	thyroid-stimulating hormone
TSH-RH	thyrotropin-releasing hormone
TSI	thyroid stimulating immunoglobulin

Abbreviation	Meaning
	tobramycin solution for inhalation (TOBI®)
TSIs	thymidylate synthase inhibitors
T-skull	trauma skull
TSM	two-spotted spider mite
tsp	teaspoon (5 mL)
TSP	thrombospondin
	total serum protein
	tropical spastic paraparesis
TSPA	thiotepa
T-spine	thoracic spine
TSR	total shoulder replacement
TSS	thumb spica splint
	total serum solids
	total symptom scores
	toxic shock syndrome
	transsphenoidal surgery
	tumor score system
TSST	toxic shock syndrome toxin
TST	titmus stereocuity test
	total sleep time
	trans-scrotal testosterone
	treadmill stress test
	tuberculin skin test(s)
TSTA	tumor-specific transplantation antigens
TSTM	too small to measure
TT	testicular torsion
	Test Tape®
	tetanus toxoid
	thiotepa (Thioplex)
	thoracostomy tube
	thrombin time
	thrombolytic therapy
	thymol turbidity
	tilt table
	tilt testing
	tonometry
	total thyroidectomy
	transit time
	transtracheal
	treponemal test
	triceps thickness
	tuberculin tested
	tuberculoid leprosy
	twitch tension
	tympanic temperature
-T	time-to-time
/T	trace of ____/trace of ____
&T	tobramycin and ticarcillin
	touch and tone
	tympantomy and tube (insertion)
T4	total thyroxine
TA	total toe arthroplasty
	transtracheal aspiration
	trauma team activation
TAT	toe touch as tolerated
	traumatic thoracic aortic transaction
TTC	transtracheal catheter
TTD	tarsal tunnel decompression
	temporary total disability
	total tumor dose
	transverse thoracic diameter
	trichothiodystrophy
TTDE	touch-tone data entry
	transthoracic color Doppler echocardiography
TTDM	thallim threadmill
TTDP	time-to-disease progression
TTE	transthoracic echocardiography
	trial terminated early
t test	Student's *t*-test
TTF	time-to-treatment failure
TTF-1	thyroid transcription factor-1
tTg	tissue transglutaminase
TTGE	timed-temperature gradient electrophoresis
TTH	tension-type headache
TTI	Teflon tube insertion
	total time to intubate
	transfer to intermediate
TTII	thyrotropin-binding inhibitory immunoglobulins
TTJV	transtracheal jet ventilation
TTM	total tumor mass
	transtelephonic monitoring
	transtheoretical model
	trichotillomania
TTMV	Torque-TenoMiniVirus
TTN	time to normalization
	transient tachypnea of the newborn
TTNA	transthoracic needle aspiration
TTNB	transient tachypnea of the newborn
TTND	time to nondetectable
TTO	tea tree oil
	time trade-off
	to take out
	transfer to open
	transtracheal oxygen
TTOD	tetanus toxoid outdated
TTOP	time to objective progression
TTOT	transtracheal oxygen therapy
TTP	tender to palpation
	tender to pressure
	thrombotic thrombocytopenic purpura
	time to pregnancy
	time to tumor progression
	time-to-progression
TTP/HUS	thrombotic thrombocytopenic purpura and hemolytic-uremic syndrome
TTR	time in therapeutic range
	transthyretin
	triceps tendon reflex
TTS	tarsal tunnel syndrome

	temporary threshold shift
	through the skin
	Toddler Temperament Scale
	transdermal therapeutic system
	transfusion therapy service
TTs	tympanostomy tubes
TTT	tilt-table test
	time to treatment termination
	tolbutamide tolerance test
	total tourniquet time
	transpupillary thermotherapy
	turn-to-turn transfusion
TTTG	tibial tuberosity to trochlear groove (distance)
TTTS	twin-twin transfusion syndrome
TTUTD	tetanus toxoid up-to-date
TTV	Torque-TenoVirus
	total tumor volume
	transfusion-transmitted virus
TTVIs	transfusion-transmitted viral infections
TTVP	temporary transvenous pacemaker
TTWB	touch-toe weight bearing
TTX	tetrodotoxin (a neurotoxin)
TTx	thrombolytic therapy
TU	Todd units
	transrectal ultrasound
	transurethral
	tuberculin units
	tumor
Tu	Tuesday
1-TU	1 tuberculin unit
5-TU	5 tuberculin units
250-TU	250 tuberculin units
TUB	tuberculosis vaccine, not BCG
tubal	tubal ligation
	tubal pregnancy
TUBS	traumatic, unidirectional instability and Bankart lesion
TUD	take as directed (this is a dangerous abbreviation as it may be read as TID [three times daily] or not understood)
TUDS	temporary ureteral drainage system
TUE	transurethral extraction
TUF	total ultrafiltration
TUG	timed Up and GO (test)
	total urinary gonadotropin
TUIBN	transurethral incision of bladder neck
TUIP	transurethral incision of the prostate
TUL	tularemia (*Francisella tularensis*) vaccine
TULIP®	transurethral ultrasound-guided laser-induced prostatectomy (system)
TULIPS	touch-up and loop incorporated primers (an alternative PCR technique)
TUMT	transurethral microwave thermotherapy
TUN	total urinary nitrogen
TUNA	transurethral needle ablation
TUNEL	terminal deoxynucleotidyl transferase-mediated dUTP-biotin nick-end labeling
TUPR	transurethral prostatic resection
TUR	transurethral resection
T_3UR	triiodothyronine uptake ratio
TURB	transurethral resection of the bladder
	turbidity
TURBN	transurethral resection bladder neck
TURBT	transurethral resection bladder tumor
TURP	transurethral resection of prostate
TURV	transurethral resection valves
TURVN	transurethral resection of vesical neck
TUTL	transuterine tubal lavage
TUU	transureteroureterostomy
TUV	transurethral valve
TUVP	transurethral vaporization of the prostate
TV	television
	temporary visit
	thyroid volume
	tidal volume
	tonic vergence
	transvenous
	trial visit
	Trichomonas vaginalis
	tricuspid valve
T/V	touch-verbal
TVC	triple voiding cystogram
	true vocal cord
TVc	tricuspid valve closure
TVD	triple vessel disease
TVDALV	triple vessel disease with an abnormal left ventricle
TVF	tactile vocal fremitus
	target vessel failure
	true vocal fold
TVH	total vaginal hysterectomy
TVI	time velocity integral
TVN	tonic vibration response
TVP	tensor veli palatini (muscle)
	transvenous pacemaker
	transvesicle prostatectomy
TVR	target vessel revascularization (rate)
	tricuspid valve replacement
TVRSS	total vasomotor rhinitis symptom score
TVS	transvaginal sonography
	transvenous system
	trigemino-vascular system
TVSC	transvaginal sector scan
TVT	tension-free vaginal tape
	transvaginal taping

	transvaginal tension-free
TVT-O	transvaginal tension-free vaginal tape-obturator
TVU	total volume of urine
	transvaginal ultrasonography
TVUS	transvaginal ultrasonography
TW	talked with
	tapwater
	test weight
	thought withdrawal
	Trophermyma whippleii
	T-wave
T1WI	T1 weighted image (magnetic resonance imaging term for short repetition time and short echo time)
T2WI	T2 weighted image (magnetic resonance imaging term for long repetition time and long echo time)
TW2	Tanner-Whitehouse mark 2 (bone-age assessment)
5TW	five times a week (this is a dangerous abbreviation)
TWA	time-weighted average
	total wrist arthroplasty
	T-wave alternans
TWAR	*Chlamydia pneumoniae*
T-wave	part of the electrocardiographic cycle, representing a portion of ventricular repolarization
TWB	total weight bearing
TWD	total white and differential count
TWE	tapwater enema
TWETC	tapwater enema 'til clear
TWG	total weight gain
TWH	transitional wall hyperplasia
TWHW ok	toe walking and heel walking all right
TWI	tooth-wear index
	T-wave inversion
TWiST	time without symptoms of progression or toxicity
TWOC	trial without catheter
TWP	twin pregnancy
TWR	total wrist replacement
TWSTRS	Toronto Western Spasmodic Torticollis Rating Scale
TWT	timed walking test
TWWD	tap water wet dressing
Tx	therapist
	therapy
	traction
	transcription
	transfuse
	transplant
	transplantation
	treatment
	tympanostomy
T & X	type and crossmatch
TXA_2	thromboxane A_2
TXB_2	thromboxane B_2
TXE	Timoptic-XE®
TXL	paclitaxel (Taxol) (this is a dangerous abbreviation as it can be read as TXT)
TXM	type and crossmatch
TXS	type and screen
TXT	docetaxel (Taxotere) (this is a dangerous abbreviation as it can be read as TXL)
TY	tympanic
T & Y	trichomonas and yeast
TYCO #3	Tylenol with 30 mg of codeine (#1=7.5 mg, #2=15 mg and #4=60 mg of codeine present)
Tyl	Tylenol (acetaminophen)
	tyloma (callus)
TYMP	tympanogram
Tyr	tyrosinase
TZ	temozolomide (Temodar)
	transition zone
TZCS	time-zone change syndrome
TZD	thiazolidinedione
TZDs	thiazolidinediones
TZM	temozolomide (Temodar)

U

U — Ultralente Insulin®
units (this is the most dangerous abbreviation—spell out "unit")
unknown
upper
uranium
urine

Ⓤ — Kosher

U/1 — 1 finger breadth below umbilicus

1/U — 1 finger over umbilicus

U/ — at umbilicus

24U — 24-hour urine (collection)

U100 — 100 units per milliliters

UA — umbilical artery
unauthorized absence
uncertain about
unstable angina
upper airway
upper arm
uric acid
urinalysis

UABD — upper airway bronchodilation

UAC — umbilical artery catheter
under active
upper airway congestion

UA/C — uric acid to creatinine (ratio)

UAD — upper airway disease
use as directed

UADE — unanticipated adverse device event

UADT — upper aerodigestive tract

UAE — urinary albumin excretion
uterine artery embolization

UACEs — unplanned acute care encounters

UAER — urinary albumin excretion rate

UAL — umbilical artery line
up *ad lib*

UA&M — urinalysis and microscopy

UA/NSTEMI — unstable angina and non-ST-segment elevation myocardial infarction

UAO — upper airway obstruction

UAP — upper abdominal pain

UAPD — Union of American Physicians and Dentists

UAPF — upon arrival patient found

UAPs — unlicensed assistive personnel

U-ARM — upper arm

UARS — upper airway resistance syndrome

UAS — upstream activating sequence

UASA — upper airway sleep apnea

UASQ — Unstable Angina Symptoms Questionnaire

UAT — up as tolerated

UAVC — univentricular atrioventricular connection

UBAs — urethral bulking agents

UBC — unicameral bone cyst
University of British Columbia (brace)

UBD — universal blood donor

UBE — upper body ergometer

UBF — unknown black female
uterine blood flow

UBI — ultraviolet blood irradiation

UBM — unknown black male

UBO — unidentified bright object

UBT — ^{13}C-urea breath test
uterine balloon therapy

UBW — usual body weight

UC — ulcerative colitis
umbilical cord
unchanged
unconscious
Unit clerk
United Church of Christ
urea clearance
urinary catheter
urine culture
usual care
uterine contraction

U&C — urethral and cervical
usual and customary

UCABG — urgent coronary artery bypass graft (surgery)

UCAD — unstable coronary artery disease

UCB — umbilical cord blood
unconjugated bilirubin (indirect)
Unicorn Campbell Boy (orthotics)

UCBT — unrelated cord-blood transplant

UCCL — ulnocarpal collateral ligament

UCD — urine collection device
usual childhood diseases

UCE — urea cycle enzymopathy

UCF — unexplained chronic fatigue

UCG — urinary chorionic gonadotropins

UCHD — usual childhood diseases

UCHI — usual childhood illnesses

UCHS — uncontrolled hemorrhagic shock

UCI — urethral catheter in
usual childhood illnesses

UCL — ulnar collateral ligament
uncomfortable loudness level

UCLP — unilateral cleft lip and palate

UCN — urocortin

UCN-01 — 7-hydroxystaurosporin

UCO — urethral catheter out

UCP — umbilical cord prolapse
uncoupling protein
urethral closure pressure

UCPs — urine collection pads

UCR	unconditioned reflex
	unconditioned response
	usual, customary, and reasonable (fees)
UCP-3	uncoupling protein −3
UCRE	urine creatinine
UCRP	universal coagulation reference plasma
UCS	unconscious
UC&S	urine culture and sensitivity
UCTD	undifferentiated connective tissue disease
UCVA	uncorrected visual acuity
UCX	urine culture
UD	as directed (this is a dangerous abbreviation as it may not be understood)
	ugly duckling (sign) (pigmented moles)
	ulnar deviation
	unit dose
	urethral dilatation
	urethral discharge
	urodynamics
	uterine distension
u.d.	as directed (this is a dangerous abbreviation as it may not be understood)
UDC	uninhibited detrusor (muscle) capacity
	usual diseases of childhood
UDCA	ursodeoxycholic acid (Ursodiol)
UDI	Urogenital Distress Inventory
UDN	updraft nebulizer
UDO	undetermined origin
UDP	unassisted diastolic pressure
UDPGT	uridinediphospho-glucuronyl transferase
UDS	uncomplicated diverticulitis of the sigmoid
	unconditioned stimulus
	urodynamic study(ies)
	urine drug screen
UDT	undescended testicle(s)
UDU	uniformity of dosage units
UE	ultrasound elastography
	under elbow
	undetermined etiology
	upper extremity
U & E	urea and electrolytes (see page 318)
UEBW	ultrasound estimated bladder weight
UEC	uterine endometrial carcinoma
UEDs	unilateral epileptiform discharges
UES	undifferentiated embryonal sarcoma
	upper esophageal sphincter
UESEP	upper extremity somatosensory evoked potential
UESP	upper esophageal sphincter pressure
UF	ultrafiltration
	until finished
UFC	urinary free cortisol
UFF	unusual facial features
UFFI	urea formaldehyde foam insulation
UFH	unfractionated heparin
UFN	until further notice
UFO	unflagged order
	unidentified foreign object
UFOV	useful field of view
UFR	ultrafiltration rate
UFT	uracil and tegafur
UFV	ultrafiltration volume
UG	until gone
	urinary glucose
	urogenital
UGA	under general anesthesia
	urogenital atrophy
UGB	upper-gastrointestinal-tract bleeding
UGCR	ultrasound-guided compression repair
UGDP	University Group Diabetes Project
UGH	uveitis, glaucoma, and hyphema (syndrome)
UGI	upper gastrointestinal series
UGIB	upper gastrointestinal bleeding
UGIE	upper gastrointestinal endoscopy
UGIH	upper gastrointestinal hemorrhage
UGIS	upper gastrointestinal series
UGIT	upper gastrointestinal tract
UGI w/SBFT	upper gastrointestinal (series) with small bowel follow through
UGK	urine, glucose, and ketones
UGP	urinary gonadotropin peptide
UGT1A1	uridine diphosphate glucuronosyltransferase
UGTI	ultrasound-guided thrombin injection
UGVA	ultrasound-guided vascular access
UH	umbilical hernia
	unfavorable history
	University Hospital
UHBI	upper hemibody irradiation
UHDDS	Uniform Hospital Discharge Data Set
UHDRS	Unified Huntington Disease Rating Scale
UHDs	ulcer-healing drugs
UHMWPE	ultra-high molecular weight polyethylene
UHP	University Health Plan
UI	urinary incontinence
UIB	Unemployment Insurance Benefits
UIBC	unbound iron binding capacity
	unsaturated iron binding capacity

UID	once daily (this is a dangerous abbreviation, spell out "once daily")
UIEP	urine (urinary) immunoelectrophoresis
UIP	usual interstitial pneumonitis (pneumonia)
UIQ	upper inner quadrant
UITN	Urinary Incontinence Treatment Network
UJ	universal joint (syndrome)
UK	United Kingdom unknown urine potassium urokinase
UK IC	urokinase intracoronary
UKE	unknown etiology
UKNDS	United Kingdom Neurological Disability Score
UKO	unknown origin
UKOSS	United Kingdom Obstetric Surveillance System
UKR	unicompartmental knee replacement
UL	Unit Leader upper left upper lid upper limb upper lobe
U/L	upper and lower
U & L	upper and lower
ULBW	ultra low birth weight (between 501 and 750 g)
ULD	Unverricht-Lundborg disease
ULDT	ultra low-dose therapy
ULL	ulnolunate ligament
ULLE	upper lid, left eye
ULN	upper limits of normal
ULPA	ultra-low particulate air
ULQ	upper left quadrant
ULRE	upper lid, right eye
ULSB	upper left sternal border
ULTT1	upper limb tension test 1 (median nerve)
ULTT2a	upper limb tension test 2a (medial nerve)
ULTT2b	upper limb tension test 2b (radial nerve)
ULTT3	upper limb tension test 3 (ulnar nerve)
ULYTES	electrolytes, urine
UM	unmarried utilization management
Umb A Line	umbilical artery line
Umb V Line	umbilical venous line
umb ven	umbilical vein
UMCD	uremic medullary cystic disease
UMLS	Unified Medical Language System
UMN	upper motor neuron (disease)
UN	undernourished urinary nitrogen
UNA	urinary nitrogen appearance
UNa	urine sodium
unacc	unaccompanied
UNC	uncrossed
UNDEL	undelivered
UNDP	United Nations Development Program
UNE	ulnar neuropathy at the elbow urinary norepinephrine
ung	ointment
UNHS	universal newborn hearing screening
UNK	unknown
UNL	upper normal levels
UNOS	United Network for Organ Sharing
UN/P	unpatched eye
UN/P OD	unpatched right eye
UN/P OS	unpatched left eye
UNS	universal neonatal screening unsatisfactory
UNSAT	unsatisfactory
uNTx	urinary N-telopeptide
UO	under observation undetermined origin ureteral orifice urinary output
UONx	unilateral optic nerve transection
UOP	urinary output
UOQ	upper outer quadrant
UORBC	uncrossmatched type-O packed red blood cells
UOS	upper oesophageal sphincter (United Kingdom and other countries)
Uosm	urinary osmolality
✓ up	check up
UP	unipolar ureteropelvic
U/P	urine to plasma (creatinine)
UPC	unknown primary carcinoma
UPD	uniparental disomy
UPDRS	Unified Parkinson Disease Rating Scale
UPEP	urine protein electrophoresis
UPG	uroporphyrinogen
UPIN	unique physician (provided) identification number
UPJ	ureteropelvic junction
UPJO	ureteropelvic junction obstruction
UPLIF	unilateral posterior lumbar interbody fusion
UPN	unique patient number
UPO	metastatic carcinoma of unknown primary origin
UPOR	usual place of residence
UPP	urethral pressure profile

	urethral pressure profilometry
	uvulopalatoplasty
UPPP	uvulopalatopharyngoplasty
U/P ratio	urine to plasma ratio
UPS	ubiquitin-dependent proteasomal system
	ubiquitin-proteasome system
UPSC	uterine papillary serous carcinoma
UPSIT	University of Pennsylvania Smell Identification Test
UPT	uptake
	urine pregnancy test
UR	unrelated
	upper respiratory
	upper right
	urinary retention
	utilization review
URA	unilateral renal agenesis
URAC	Utilization Review Accreditation Commission
UR AC	uric acid
URAS	unilateral renal artery stenosis
URD	undifferentiated respiratory disease
	unrelated donor
URE	Uniform Rules of Evidence
URG	urgent
URI	upper respiratory infection
URIC A	uric acid
url	unrelated
UR&M	urinalysis, routine and microscopic
URO	urology
UROB	urobilinogen
UROD	ultra-rapid opiate detoxification [under anesthesia]
UROL	Urologist
	urology
URQ	upper right quadrant
URR	urea reduction ratio
URS	ureterorenoscopy
URSB	upper right sternal border
URT	upper respiratory tract
	uterine resting tone
URTI	upper respiratory tract infection
US	ultrasonography
	ultrasound
	unit secretary
	United States of America
USA	unit services assistant
	United States Army
	United States of America
	unstable angina
USAF	United States Air Force
USAMRIID	United States Army Medical Research Institute of Infectious Diseases
USAN	United States Adopted Names
USAP	unstable angina pectoris
USB	upper sternal border
USC	uterine serous carcinoma
USCB	ultrasound-guided core biopsy
U-SCOPE	ureteroscopy
USCVD	unsterile controlled vaginal delivery
USDA	United States Department of Agriculture
USED-CARP	**u**reterosigmoidostomy, **s**mall bowel fistula, **e**xtra chloride, **d**iarrhea, **c**arbonic anhydrase inhibitors, **a**drenal insufficiency, **r**enal tubular acidosis, and **p**ancreatic fistula (common causes of nonanion gap metabolic acidosis)
USEIR	United States Eye Injury Registry
USG	ultrasmall gold (particles)
	ultrasonography
	urine specific gravity
USH	United Services for Handicapped
	usual state of health
USI	urinary stress incontinence
USL	uterosacral ligament
USM	ultrasonic mist
USMC	United States Marine Corps
USMLE	United States Medical Licensing Examination
USN	ultrasonic nebulizer
	United States Navy
USO	unilateral salpingo-oophorectomy
USOGH	usual state of good health
USOH	usual state of health
USP	unassisted systolic pressure
	United States Pharmacopeia
USPHS	United States Public Health Service
USS	Upshaw-Schulman syndrome
USUCVD	unsterile uncontrolled vaginal delivery
USVMD	urine specimen volume measuring device
UT	upper thoracic
UTA	urinary tract anomaly
UTC	undifferentiated thyroid carcinoma
	urinary tract calculi
UtCa	uterine cancer
UTD	unable to determine
	up to date
ut dict	as directed
UTF	usual throat flora
UTI	urinary tract infection
UTL	ulnotriquetral ligament
	unable to locate
	useful therapeutic life
UTM	urinary-tract malformations
UTMDACC	University of Texas M.D. Anderson Cancer Center
UTO	unable to obtain
	upper tibial osteotomy
UTP	uridine triphosphate

UTR	untranslated region
UTS	ulnar tunnel syndrome
	ultrasound
U/U−	uterine fundus at umbilicus (usually modified as number of finger breadths below)
U/U+	uterine fundus at umbilicus (usually modified as number of finger breadths above)
UUD	uncontrolled unsterile delivery
UUI	urge urinary incontinence
UUN	urinary urea nitrogen
UUTI	uncomplicated urinary tract infections
UV	ultraviolet
	umbilical vein
	ureterovesical
	urine volume
UVA	ultraviolet A light
	ureterovesical angle
UVB	ultraviolet B light
UVBI	ultraviolet blood irradiation
UVC	umbilical vein catheter
	ultraviolet C light
UVEB	unifocal ventricular ectopic beat
UVGI	ultraviolet germicidal irradiation
UVH	univentricular heart
UVIB	ultraviolet irradiation of blood
UVJ	ureterovesical junction
UVL	ultraviolet light
	umbilical venous line
UVR	ultraviolet radiation
UVT	unsustained ventricular tachycardia
UV-VIS	ultraviolet-visible (spectrometer)
U/WB	unit of whole blood
UW	unilateral weakness
UWF	unknown white female
UWM	unknown white male
	unwed mother
UXO	unexploded ordnance

V

V	five
	gas volume
	minute volume
	vaccinated
	vagina
	Valium (diazepam); as in vitamin V (slang)
	vein
	ventricular
	verb
	verbal
	vertebral
	very
	Viagra (sildenafil citrate) as in "vitamin V"
	viral
	vision
	vitamin
	vomiting
$\dot{V}$	ventilation (L/min)
+V	positive vertical divergence
V1	fifth cranial nerve, ophthalmic division
V2	fifth cranial nerve, maxillary division
V3	fifth cranial nerve, mandibular division
3V	3-vessel (cord)
V_1 to V_6	precordial chest leads
VA	vacuum aspiration
	valproic acid
	ventriculoatrial
	verbal autopsy
	vertebral artery
	Veterans Administration
	visual acuity
V_A	alveolar gas volume
V&A	vagotomy and antrectomy
VAAESS	Vaccine-Associated Adverse Events Surveillance System (Canada)
VAB	variable atrial blockage
	vinblastine, dactinomycin (actinomycin D), bleomycin
VABS	Vineland Adaptive Behavior Scales
VAC	etoposide (VePesid), cytarabine (ara-C), and carboplatin
	vacuum-assisted closure (dressings)
	ventriculoarterial conduction
	vincristine, dactinomycin (actinomycin D), and cyclophosphamide
	vincristine, doxorubicin (Adriamycin), and cyclophosphamide
VA cc	distance visual acuity with correction

VA ccl — near visual acuity with correction
VACE — *Vitex agnus-castus* extract (Chaste tree berry extract)
VAC EXT — vacuum extractor
VAC/IE — vincristine, doxorubicin (Adriamycin), cyclophosphamide, ifosfamide, and etoposide
VAC_{ig} — vaccinia immune globulin
VACIME — vincristine, doxorubicin (Adriamycin), cyclophosphamide, ifosfamide, mesna, and etoposide
VACO — Veterans Administration Central Office
VACTERL — **v**ertebral, **a**nal, **c**ardiac, **t**racheal, **e**sophageal, **r**enal, and **l**imb anomalies
VAD — vascular (venous) access device
ventricular assist device
vertebral artery dissection
Veterans Administration Domiciliary
vincristine, doxorubicin (Adriamycin), and dexamethasone
VaD — vascular dementia
VADCS — ventricular atrial distal coronary sinus
VADRIAC — vincristine, doxorubicin (Adriamycin), and cyclophosphamide
VAE — venous air embolism
VAERS — Vaccine Adverse Events Reporting System
VAFD — vascular access flush device
VAG — vagina
VAG HYST — vaginal hysterectomy
VAH — Veterans Administration Hospital
VAHBE — ventricular atrial His bundle electrocardiogram
VAHRA — ventricular atrial height right atrium
VAHS — virus-associated hemophagocytic syndrome
VAI — vertebral artery injury
VAIN — vaginal intraepithelial neoplasia
VALE — visual acuity, left eye
VALI — ventilator-associated lung injury
VAMC — Veterans Affairs Medical Center
VAMP® — venous-arterial management protection system
VAMS — Visual Analogue Mood Scale
VAN — vanilla
VANCO/P — vancomycin-peak
VANCO/T — vancomycin-trough
VAOD — visual acuity, right eye
VAOS — visual acuity, left eye
VA OS LP with P — visual acuity, left eye, left perception with projection
VAP — venous access port
ventilator-associated pneumonia
vincristine, asparaginase, and prednisone
VAPCS — ventricular atrial proximal coronary sinus
VAPP — vaccine-associated paralytic poliomyelitis
VAR — variant
varicella (chickenpox) (*varicella zoster* virus) vaccine (Varivax)
VARE — visual acuity, right eye
VARig — varicella-zoster immune globulin
VAS — vasectomy
vascular
Visual Analogue Scale (Score)
VASC — Visual-Auditory Screen Test for Children
VA sc — distance visual acuity without correction
VA scl — near visual acuity without correction
VASPI — Visual Analogue Self Assessment Scales For Pain Intensity
VAS RAD — vascular radiology
VAT — ventilatory anaerobic threshold
ventricular activation time
vertebral artery test
video-assist thoracoscopy
visceral adipose tissue
VATER — vertebral, anal, tracheal, esophageal, and renal anomalies
VATH — vinblastine, doxorubicin (Adriamycin), thiotepa, and fluoxymesterone (Halotestin)
VATS — video assisted thoracic surgery
VAVD — vacuum-assisted venous drainage
VAX-D — vertebral axial decompression
VB — Van Buren (catheter)
venous blood
vinblastine (Velban)
vinblastine and bleomycin
virtual bronchoscopy
VB_1 — first voided bladder specimen
VB_2 — second midstream bladder specimen
VB_3 — third voided urine specimen
VBAC — vaginal birth after cesarean
VBAI — vertebrobasilar artery insufficiency
VBAP — vincristine, carmustine (BiCNU), doxorubicin (Adriamycin), and prednisone
VBC — vinblastine, bleomycin, and cisplatin
VBG — venous blood gas
vertical banded gastroplasty
VBGP — vertical banded gastroplasty
VBI — vertebrobasilar insufficiency
VBICAD — vertebrobasilar intracranial atheromatous disease
VBL — vinblastine (Velban)
VBM — vinblastine, bleomycin, and methotrexate

	voxel-based morphometry
VBP	vinblastine, bleomycin, and cisplatin
VBR	ventricular brain ratio
VBS	vertebral-basilar system
	videofluoroscopic barium swallow (evaluation)
VC	color vision
	etoposide (VePesid) and carboplatin
	pulmonary capillary blood volume
	vena cava
	verbal cues
	vincristine (Oncovin)
	virtual colonoscopy
	vital capacity
	vocal cords
	voluntary cough
Vc	bortezomib (Velcade)
3VC	3-vessel cord
V&C	vertical and centric (a bite)
VCA	vasoconstrictor assay
VCAM	vascular cell adhesion molecule
VCAP	vincristine, cyclophosphamide, doxorubicin (Adriamycin), and prednisone
Vcc	vision with correction
VCCA	velocity common carotid artery
VCD	vocal cord dysfunction
VCDR	vertical cup-to-disc ratio
VCE	vaginal cervical endocervical (smear)
VCF	Vaginal Contraception Film™
	vertebral compression fracture(s)
VCFS	velo-cardio-facial syndrome
VCG	vectorcardiography
	voiding cystogram
VCI	vascular cognitive impairment
	vocal cord injuries
	volume contrast imaging
vCJD	variant Creutzfeldt-Jakob disease
VCO	ventilator CPAP oxyhood
V_{CO_2}	carbon dioxide output
VCP	vocal cord palsy
VCPR	veterinarian-client-patient relationship
VCR	video cassette recorder
	vincristine sulfate (Oncovin)
VCT	venous clotting time
	volumetric computed tomography
	voluntary counselling and testing
VCTS	vitreal corneal touch syndrome
VCU	voiding cystourethrogram
VCUG	vesicoureterogram
	voiding cystourethrogram
VCV	varicella virus
	volume-control ventilation
VD	vaginal delivery
	venereal disease
	vessel disease
	viral diarrhea
	voided
	voiding diary
	volume of distribution
V_D	deadspace volume
V_d	volume of distribution
V&D	vomiting and diarrhea
1-VD	one-vessel disease
VDA	venous digital angiogram
	visual discriminatory acuity
VDAC	vaginal delivery after cesarean
VDC	vincristine, doxorubicin, and cyclophosphamide
VDD	atrial synchronous ventricular inhibited pacing
VDDR I	vitamin D dependency rickets type I
VDDR II	vitamin D dependency rickets type II
VDE	vasodilatory edema
VDEPT	virus-directed enzyme prodrug therapy
VDG	venereal disease–gonorrhea
Vdg	voiding
VDH	valvular disease of the heart
VDJ	variable diversity joining
VDL	vasodepressor lipid
	visual detection level
VDO	varus derotational osteotomy
VD or M	venous distention or masses
VDP	vinblastine, dacarbazine, and cisplatin (Platinol)
VDPCA	variable-dose patient-controlled analgesia
VDR	vitamin D receptor (gene)
VDRF	ventilator dependent respiratory failure
VDRL	Venereal Disease Research Laboratory (test for syphilis)
VDRO	varus derotational osteotomy
VDRR	vitamin D-resistant rickets
VDRS	Verdun Depression Rating Scale
VDS	vasodepressor syncope
	venereal disease—syphilis
	vindesine (Eldisine)
VDT	vibration detection threshold
	video display terminal
	visual display terminal
VD/VT	dead space to tidal volume ratio
VE	vaginal examination
	vertex
	Vietnam era
	virtual endoscopy
	visual examination
	vitamin E
	vocational evaluation
V_E	minute volume (expired)
V/E	violence and eloper
VEA	ventricular ectopic activity
	viscoelastic agent
VEB	ventricular ectopic beat
VEC	vecuronium (Norcuron)

	velocity-encoded cine
VECG	vector electrocardiogram
VED	vacuum erection device
	vacuum extraction delivery
	ventricular ectopic depolarization
	vitamin E deficiency
VEE	Venezuelan equine encephalitis
VEE_a	Venezuelan equine encephalitis vaccine, attenuated live
VEE_I	Venezuelan equine encephalitis vaccine, inactivated
VEEV	Venezuelan equine encephalitis virus
VEF	visually evoked field
VEG	vegetation (bacterial)
VEGF	vascular endothelial growth factor
VeIP	vinblastine (Velban), ifosfamide, and cisplatin (Platinol)
VEMP	vestibular evoked myogenic potentials
VENC	velocity encoding value (radiology)
VENT	ventilation
	ventilator
	ventral
	ventricular
VEP	visual evoked potential
VER	ventricular escape rhythm
	visual evoked responses
VERDICT	Veterans Evidence-based Research Dissemination Implementation Center
VERP	ventricular effective refractory period
VERT	velocity-enhanced resistance training
VES	ventricular extrasystoles
	video-endoscopic surgery
	vitamin E succinate
	Vulnerable Elders Survey (UK)
VESS	video endoscopic swallowing study
VET	veteran
	Veterinarian
	veterinary
VF	left leg (electrode)
	ventricular fibrillation
	vertical float (aquatic therapy)
	videofluoroscopic
	virologic failure
	visual field
	vocal fremitus
VFC	Vaccines for Children (program)
VFCB	vertical flow clean bench
VFD	ventilator-free days
	visual fields
VFFC	visual fields full to confrontation
VFI	visual fields intact
	Visual Functioning index
V. Fib	ventricular fibrillation
VFL	vinflunine
VFMI	vocal fold motion impairment
VFP	vertical float progression (aquatic therapy)
	vitreous fluorophotometry
	vocal fold paralysis
VFPN	Volu-feed premie nipple
VFQ-25	National Eye Institute 25-item Visual Function Questionnaire
VFR	visiting friends and relatives (possible contacts for communicable diseases)
VFRN	Volu-feed regular nipple
VFSS	videofluoroscopic swallowing study
VFT	venous filling time
	ventricular fibrillation threshold
VG	vein graft
	ventricular gallop
	ventrogluteal
	very good
V&G	vagotomy and gastroenterotomy
VGAD	vein of Galen aneurysmal dilatation
VGAM	vein of Galen aneurysmal malformation
VGB	vigabatrin (Sabril)
VGE	viral gastroenteritis
VGH	very good health
VGKC	voltage-gated potassium channel
VGM	vein graft myringoplasty
VGPO	volume-guaranteed pressure option
VH	vaginal hysterectomy
	Veterans Hospital
	viral hepatitis
	visual hallucinations
	vitreous hemorrhage
	von Herrick (grading system)
VH I	very narrow anterior chamber angles
VH II	moderately narrow anterior chamber angles
VH III	moderately wide open anterior chamber angles
VH IV	wide open anterior chamber angles
VHA	Veterans Health Administration
	Voluntary Hospitals of America
VHC	valved-holding chamber
VHD	valvular heart disease
	vascular hemostatis device
VHF	viral hemorrhagic fever
VHI	Voice Handicap Index
VHL	von Hippel-Lindau disease (complex)
VHP	vaporized hydrogen peroxide
VI	six
	velocity index
	volume index
VIA	visual inspection (of the cervix) with 4% acetic acid
via	by way of
vib	vibration
VIBS	Victim's Information Bureau Service

V

VICA velocity internal carotid artery
VICH International Cooperation on Harmonization of Technical Requirements for Registration of Veterinary Products
VICP Vaccine Injury Compensation Program
Vi CPs typhoid Vi (capsular) polysaccharide vaccine (Typhim Vi)
VID videodensitometry
VIG vaccinia immune globulin
vinblastine, ifosfamide, and gallium nitrate
VIH human immunodeficiency virus (Spanish and French abbreviation)
VILI visual inspection (of the cervix) with Lugol's iodine
VIN vibration-induced nystagmus
vulvar intraepithelial neoplasm
VIP etopside (VePesid), ifosfamide, and cisplatin (Platinol)
vasoactive intestinal peptide
vasoactive intracorporeal pharmacotherapy
Vattikuti Institute prostatectomy
very important patient
vinblastine, ifosfamide, and cisplatin (Platinol)
voluntary interruption of pregnancy
VIPomas vasoactive intestinal peptide-secreting tumors
VIQ Verbal Intelligence Quotient (part of Wechsler tests)
VIS Vaccine Information Statement
Visual Impairment Service
VISA vancomycin-intermediate-resistant *Staphylococcus aureus*
VISC vitreous infusion suction cutter
VISI Vaccine Identification Standards Initiative
volar intercalated segmental instability
VISN Veterans Integrated Service Networks
VISs Vaccine Information Statements
VIT venom immunotherapy
vital
vitamin
vitreous
Vitamin see individual letters such as B, D, G, H, K, P, R, V, etc.
VIT CAP vital capacity
VIU visual internal urethrotomy
VIZ namely
V-J ventriculo-jugular (shunt)
VKA vitamin K antagonists
VKC vernal keratoconjunctivitis
VKDB vitamin K deficiency bleeding
VKH Vogt-Koyanagi-Harada disease
VKORC1 vitamin K epoxide reductase complex, subunit 1 (gene)
VL left arm (electrode)
vial
viral load
visceral leishmaniasis (kala-azar)
VLA very-late antigen
VLAD variable life-adjusted display
VLAP vaporization laser ablation of the prostate
VLBW very low birth weight (less than 1500 g)
VLBWPN very low birth weight preterm neonate
VLCAD very-long-chain acyl coenzyme A dehydrogenase
VLCD very low calorie diet
VLCFA very-long-chain fatty acids
VLDL very-low-density lipoprotein
VLE vision left eye
VLED very-low-energy diet
VLH ventrolateral nucleus of the hypothalamus
VLK vascularized limbal keratitis
VLL vastus lateralis longus
VLM visceral larva migrans
VLP virus-like particle
VLPFC ventrolateral prefrontal cortex
VLPP Valsalva lead-point pressure
VLR vastus lateralis release
VM venous malformation
ventilated mask
ventimask
Venturi mask
vestibular membrane
VM 26 teniposide (Vumon)
VMA vanillylmandelic acid
VMATs Veterinary Medical Assistance Teams
VMCP vincristine, melphalan, cyclophosphamide, and prednisone
VMD Doctor of Veterinary Medicine (DVM)
vertical maxillary deficiency
VME vertical maxillary excess
VMH ventromedial hypothalamus
VMI vendor-managed inventory
visual motor integration
VMO vaccinia melanoma oncolysate
vastus medialis oblique
VMR vasomotor rhinitis
VMS vanilla milkshake
VMU vertebral motion unit
VN vestibular neuritis
visiting nurse
VNA Visiting Nurses' Association
VNB vinorelbine (Navelbine)
VNC vesicle neck contracture
VNS vagal nerve stimulation (stimulator)

VNTR	variable number of tandem repeats
VO	verbal order
	visual observation
VO_2	oxygen consumption
VOC	vaso-occlusive crisis
VOCA	voice-output communication aid
VOCAB	vocabulary
VOCOR	vaso-occlusive crisis
	void on-call to operating room
VOCs	volatile organic compounds
VOCTOR	void on-call to operating room
VOD	veno-occlusive disease
	vision right eye
VOE	vascular occlusive episode
VO_2I	oxygen consumption index
VOL	Valuation of Life
	volume
	voluntary
VOM	vomited
VOO	continuous ventricular asynchronous pacing
VOOD	vesico-outlet obstructive disease
VOR	vestibular ocular reflex
VORB	verbal order read back
VOS	vision left eye
VOSS	visual observation shivering score
VOT	Visual Organization Test
VOU	vision both eyes
VOV	verbal order verified
VP	etoposide (VePesid) and cisplatin (Platinol)
	vagal paraganglioma
	variegate porphyria
	venipuncture
	venous pressure
	ventriculoperitoneal
	visual perception
	voiding pressure
V & P	vagotomy and pyloroplasty
	ventilation and perfusion
VP-16	etoposide (VePesid)
VPA	valproic acid
	ventricular premature activation
	vigorous physical activity
V-Pad	sanitary napkin
VPB	ventricular premature beat
VPC	ventricular premature contractions
VPD	ventricular premature depolarization
VPDC	ventricular premature depolarization contraction
VPDF	vegetable protein diet plus fiber
VPDs	ventricular premature depolarizations
VPI	velopharyngeal incompetence
	velopharyngeal insufficiency
VPL	ventro-posterolateral
VPLN	vaccine-primed lymph node (cells)
VPLS	ventilation-perfusion lung scan
VPM	venous pressure module

VPR	virtual patient record
	volume pressure response
VPS	valvular pulmonic stenosis
	ventriculoperitoneal shunt
VPT	vascularized patellar tendon
	vibration perception threshold
VQ	ventilation perfusion
VQM	voice quality measurements
VR	right arm (electrode) valve replacement
	venous resistance
	ventricular rhythm
	verbal reprimand
	vocational rehabilitation
$V_3R \cdot\cdot V_6R$	right sided precordial leads
VRA	visual reinforcement audiometry
	visual response audiometry
VRB	vinorelbine (Navelbine)
VRC	vocational rehabilitation counselor
VRE	vancomycin-resistant enterococci
	vision right eye
VREF	vancomycin-resistant *Enterococcus faecium*
VRI	viral respiratory infection
VRL	ventral root, lumbar
	vinorelbine (Navelbine)
VRP	vocational rehabilitation program
VRS	viral rhinosinusitis
VRSA	vancomycin-resistant *Staphylococcus aureus*
VRT	variance of resident time
	ventral root, thoracic
	vertical radiation topography
	visual restoration therapy
	Visual Retention Test
	vocational rehabilitation therapy
VRTA	Vocational Rehabilitation Therapy Assistant
VRU	ventilator rehabilitation unit
VS	vagal stimulation
	vegetative state
	versus *(vs)*
	very sensitive
	vestibular schwannomas
	visit
	visited
	vital signs (temperature, pulse, and respiration)
VSA	variant surface antigens
VSADP	vocational skills assessment and development program
VSBE	very short below elbow (cast)
VSCC	vertical semicircular canal
VSD	Vaccine Safety Datalink
	ventricular septal defect
	vesicosphincter dyssynergia
VSGP	vertical supranuclear gaze palsy
VSI	visual motor integration

VSLI	vincristine sulfate liposomal injection
VSMC	vascular smooth muscle cell
VSN	visuospatial neglect
	vital signs normal
VSO	vertical subcondylar oblique
VSOK	vital signs normal
VSP	vertical stabilization program
VSQOL	Vital Signs Quality of Life
VSR	venous stasis retinopathy
	ventricular septal rupture
VSS	variable spot scanning
	visual sexual stimulation
	vital signs stable
V_{SS}	apparent volume of distribution
VSSAF	vital signs stable, afebrile
VST	visual search task
VSTM	visual short-term memory
VSULA	vaccination scar, upper left arm
VSV	vesicular stomatitis virus
VT	validation therapy
	ventricular tachycardia
V_t	tidal volume
VTA	vascular targeting agents
	ventral tegmentum area
VTBI	volume to be infused
v. tach.	ventricular tachycardia
VTD	bortezomib (Velcade), thalidomide and dexamethasone
VTE	venous thromboembolic events
	venous thromboembolism
VTEC	verotoxin-producing *Escherichia coli*
VTED	venous thromboembolic disease
VT-NS	ventricular tachycardia nonsu stained
VTOP	voluntary termination of pregnancy
VTP	voluntary termination of pregnancy
VTS	Volunteer Transport Service
VT-S	ventricular tachycardia sustained
VTSRS	Verdun Target Symptom Rating Scale
VT/VF	ventricular tachycardia/fibrillation
VTX	vertex
VU	venous ulcer
	vesicoureteral (reflux)
V/U	verbalize understanding
VUC	voided-urine cytology
VUD-BMT	volunteer unrelated-donor bone marrow transplantation
VUJ	vesico ureteral junction
VUR	vesicoureteric reflux
VV	vaccina virus
	varicose veins
	vulvar vestibulitis
V-V	ventriculovenous (shunt)
V&V	vulva and vagina
V/V	volume to volume ratio
VVB	venovenous bypass
VVC	vulvovaginal candidiasis
VVD	vaginal vertex delivery
VVETP	Vietnam Veterans Evaluation and Treatment Program
VVFR	vesicovaginal fistula repair
VVI	vector velocity imaging
	venous valvular insufficiency
	ventricular demand pacing
V/VI	grade 5 on a 6 grade basis
VVI-40	ventricular backup pacing at 40/minute
VVIR	ventricular demand inhibited pacemaker (V = chamber paced-ventricle, V = chamber sensed-ventricle, I = response to sensing-inhibited, R = programmability–rate modulation)
VVL	varicose veins ligation
	verruca vulgaris of the larynx
VVOR	visual-vestibulo-ocular-reflex
VVR	ventricular response rate
VVS	vasovagal syncope
	vulvar vestibulitis syndrome
VVs	varicose veins
VVT	ventricular synchronous pacing
VW	vessel wall
VWD	ventral wall defect
vWD	von Willebrand disease
VWF	vibration-induced white finger (syndrome)
vWF	von Willebrand factor
VWM	ventricular wall motion
V_x	vaccination
	vitrectomy
V-XT	V-pattern exotropia
VY	surgical replacement flap
VZ	varicella zoster
VZIG	varicella zoster immune globulin
VZV	varicella zoster virus (Varivax)

W

W	wash
	watts
	wearing glasses
	Wednesday
	week
	weight
	well
	West (as in the location e.g. 2W, is second floor, West wing)
	white
	widowed
	wife
	with
	work
w/	with
W-1	insignificant (allergies)
W-3	minimal (allergies)
W-5	moderate (allergies)
W-7	moderate-severe (allergies)
W-9	severe (allergies)
W-10	Interagency Transfer Form
W 22	Central Institute for the Deaf 22 Word List
WA	when awake
	while awake
	White American
	wide awake
	with assistance
W-A	Wyeth-Ayerst Laboratories
W & A	weakness and atrophy
W or A	weakness or atrophy
WAC	wholesale acquisition cost
WACH	wedge adjustable cushioned heel
WADA	World Anti-Doping Agency
WAF	weakness, atrophy, and fasciculation
	white adult female
WAGR	Wilm tumor, aniridia, genitourinary malformations, and mental retardation (syndrome)
WAIS	Wechsler Adult Intelligence Scale
WAIS-R	Wechsler Adult Intelligence Scale-Revised
WAL	Wyeth-Ayerst Laboratories
WALK	weight-activated locking knee (prosthesis)
WAM	white adult male
WAP	wandering atrial pacemaker
WAPRT	whole-abdominopelvic radiation therapy
WARI	wheezing associated respiratory infection
WAS	whiplash-associated disorders
	Wiskott-Aldrich syndrome
WASI	Wechsler Abbreviated Scale of Intelligence
WASO	wakefulness after sleep onset
WASP	Wiskott-Aldrich syndrome protein
WASS	Wasserman test
WAT	word association test
WAZ	weight-for-age Z scores
WB	waist belt
	weight bearing
	well baby
	Western blot
	whole blood
WBACT	whole-blood activated clotting time
WBAT	weight bearing as tolerated
WBC	weight bearing with crutches
	well baby clinic
	white blood cell (count)
WBCT	whole-blood clotting time
WBD	weeks by dates (for gestational age)
WBDOs	waterborne disease and outbreaks
WBE	weeks by examination (for gestational age)
	whole-body extract
WBGD	whole-body glucose disposal
WBH	weight-based heparin (dosing)
	whole-body hyperthermia
WBI	whole-bowel irrigation
W Bld	whole blood
WBN	wellborn nursery
WBNAA	whole-brain *N*-acetylaspartate
WBOS	wide base of support
WBPTT	whole-blood partial thromboplastin time
WBQC	wide-base quad cane
WBR	whole-body radiation
WBRT	whole-brain radiotherapy
WBS	weeks by size (for gestational age)
	whole body scan
	Williams-Beuren syndrome
WBTF	Waring Blender tube feeding
WBTT	weight bearing to tolerance
WBUS	weeks by ultrasound
WBV	whole blood volume
WC	waist circumference
	ward clerk
	ward confinement
	warm compress
	wet compresses
	wheelchair
	when called
	white count
	whooping cough
	will call
	workers' compensation
WCA	work capacity assessment
WCB	Workers' Compensation Board
WCC	well-child care
	white cell count

W

WCE	white coat effect
	wireless capsule endoscopy
	work capacity evaluation
WCH	white coat hypertension
WCHE	well-child health examination
WC/LC	warm compresses and lid scrubs
WCM	whole cow's milk
WCS	work capacity specialist
WCST	Wisconsin Card Sorting Test
WCT	wide-complex tachycardia
WCV	within-subject coefficient of variation
WCVs	well-child visits
WD	ward
	well developed
	well differentiated
	wet dressing
	Wilson disease
	word
	working distance
	wound
W/D	warm and dry
	withdrawal
W → D	wet to dry
W4D	Worth four-dot (test for fusion)
WDCC	well-developed collateral circulation
WDEIA	wheat-dependent, exercise-induced anaphylaxis
WDF	white divorced female
WDHA	watery diarrhea, hypokalemia, and achlorhydria
WDHH	watery diarrhea, hypokalemia, and hypochlorhydria
WDL	within defined limits
WDLL	well-differentiated lymphocytic lymphoma
WDM	white divorced male
WDP	within defined parameters
WDR	weighed dietary records
WDS	word discrimination score
WDTC	well-differentiated thyroid cancer
WDWG	well dressed, well groomed
WDWN-AAF	well-developed, well-nourished African-American female
WDWN-BM	well-developed, well-nourished black male
WDWN-WF	well-developed, well-nourished white female
WDXRF	wavelength-dispersive x-ray fluorescence
WE	weekend
	wide excision
W/E	weekend
WEBINO	wall-eyed bilateral internuclear ophthalmoplegia
WE-D	withdrawal-emergent dyskinesia
WEE	Western equine encephalitis
WEMINO	wall-eyed monocular internuclear ophthalmoplegia
WEP	weekend pass
WESR	Westergren erythrocyte sedimentation rate
	Wintrobe erythrocyte sedimentation rate
WEUP	willful exposure to unwanted pregnancy
WF	well flexed
	wet film
	white female
W/F	weakness and fatigue
WFB	wooden foreign body
WFE	Williams flexion exercises
W FEEDS	with feedings
WFH	white-faced hornet
WFI	water for injection
WFL	within full limits
	within functional limits
WFLC	white female living child
WFNS	World Federation of Neurosurgical Societies (grade or scale)
WF-O	will follow in office
WFR	wheel-and-flare reaction
WG	Wegener granulomatosis
WGA	wheat germ agglutinin
	whole genome amplification
WGL	wire-guide localization
WH	walking heel (cast)
	well healed
	well hydrated
	work hardening (physical therapy)
WHA	warmed humidified air
WHAS	Women's Health Assessment Scale
WHI	Women's Health Initiative
WHIM	Worts, Hypogammaglobulinamia, Infections, and Myelokathexis (syndrome)
WHIS	War Head-Injury Score
whites	white blood cells
WHNP	Women's Healthcare Nurse Practitioner
WHNR	well-healed, no residuals
WHNS	well-healed, no sequelae
	well-healed, nonsymptomatic
WHO	World Health Organization
	wrist-hand orthosis
WHOART	World Health Organization Adverse Reaction Terms (Terminology)
WHOQOL-100	World Health Organization Quality of Life 100-Item (instrument)
WHP	whirlpool
WHPB	whirlpool bath
WHpR	waist-to-hip ratio
WHR	ratio of waist to hip circumference
WHV	woodchuck hepatitis virus

Abbreviation	Meaning
WHVP	wedged hepatic venous pressure
WH/WD	withholding/withdrawal (of life support)
WHZ	wheezes
WI	ventricular demand pacing
	walk-in
W/I	within
W+I	work and interest
WIA	wounded in action
WIC	Women, Infants, and Children (program)
WID	widow
	widower
WIED	walk-in emergency department
WIP	work in progess
WIQ	Walking Impairment Questionnaire
WIS	Ward Incapacity Scale
	Wister Institute
WISC	Wechsler Intelligence Scale for Children
WISC-R	Wechsler Intelligence Scale for Children-Revised
WIT	warm ischemia time
	water-induced thermotherapy
WK	week
	work
WKHL	Weck hem-o-lock (suture clip)
WKI	Wakefield Inventory
WKS	Wernicke-Korsakoff Syndrome
WL	waiting list
	wave length
	weight loss
WLE	wide local excision
WLI	weight-length index
WLM	working level months
WLQ	Work Limitation Questionnaire
WLS	weight-loss surgery
	wet lung syndrome
WLST	withdrawal of life-sustaining therapy
WLT	waterload test
WM	Waldenstrom macroglobulinemia
	wall motion
	warm, moist
	weight maintenance
	wet mount
	white male
	white matter
	whole milk
	working memory
WMA	wall motion abnormality
WMD	warm moist dressings (sterile)
	weapons of mass destruction
	weighted mean differences
WMF	white married female
WMFT	Wolf Motor Function Test
WMH	white matter hyperintensities
WMH-CIDI	World Mental Health Composite International Diagnostic Interview
WMI	wall motion index
	weighted mean index
WML	white matter lesions (cerebral)
WMLC	white male living child
WMM	white married male
WMP	warm moist packs (unsterile)
	weight management program
WMS	Wechsler Memory Scale
	Wilson-Mikity syndrome
WMSI	wall-motion score index
WMT	Word Memory Test
WMTS	wireless medical telemetry service
WMX	whirlpool, massage, and exercise
WN	well nourished
WND	wound
WNE	West Nile encephalitis
WNF	well-nourished female
	West Nile fever
WNL	within normal limits
WNL x 4	upper and lower extremities within normal limits
WNLS	weighted nonlinear least squares
WNM	well-nourished male
WNND	West Nile neuroinvasive disease
WNR	within normal range
WNt^{50}	Wagner-Nelson time 50 hours
WNV	West Nile virus
WO	weeks old
	wide open
	written order
W/O	water-in-oil (emulsion)
	without
WOB	work of breathing
WOCF	worst observation carried forward
WOCN	Wound, Ostomy and Continence Nurses (Society)-formerly known as the International Association for Enterostomal Therapy (IEAT)
WOMAC	Western Ontario and McMaster Universities Osteoarthritis Index
WOP	without pain
W or A	weakness or atrophy
WORD	Wechsler objective reading dimensions
WORLD/ DLROW	a test used in mental status examinations (patient is asked to spell WORLD backwards)
WP	whirlpool
WPAI	Work Productivity and Activity Impairment (Questionnaire)
WPBT	whirlpool, body temperature
WPCs	washed packed cells
WPFM	Wright peak flow meter
WPOA	wearing patch on arrival
WPP	Wechsler Preschool and Primary Scale of Intelligence

WPPSI	Wechsler Preschool and Primary Scale of Intelligence
WPPSI-R	WPPSI revised
WPR	written progress report
WPS	Worker Protection Standard
WPV	wild poliovirus
	within-person variability
	workplace violence
WPW	Wolff-Parkinson-White (syndrome)
WR	Wassermann reaction
	word recognition
	wrist
WRA	with-the-rule astigmatism
WRAIR	Walter Reed Army Institute of Research
WRAMC	Walter Reed Army Medical Center
WRARU	Walter Reed AFRIMS (Armed Forces Research Institute of Medical Sciences) Research Unit
WRAT	Wide Range Achievement Test
WRAT-R	The Wide Range Achievement Test, Revised
WRBC	washed red blood cells
WRC	washed red (blood) cells
WRF	worsening renal function
WRIOT	Wide Range Interest-Opinion Test (for career planning)
WRL	World Reference Laboratory for Foot-and-Mouth Disease (Institute for Animal Health, Survey, United Kingdom)
WRN	Werner syndrome protein
WRT	weekly radiation therapy
	with respect (regards) to
WRUED	work-related upper-extremity disorder
WS	Waardenburg syndrome (classified into four subtypes, WS1-WS4)
	walking speed
	ward secretary
	watt seconds
	Werner syndrome
	West syndrome
	Williams syndrome
	work simplification
	work simulation
	work status
W&S	wound and skin
WSCP	Williams Syndrome Cognitive Profile
WSEP	Williams syndrome, early puberty
WSepF	white separated female
WSepM	white separated male
WSF	white single female
WSLP	Williams syndrome, late puberty
WSM	white single male
WSO	white superficial onychomycosis
WSOC	water-soluble organic compounds
WSP	wearable speech processor
WSW	women who have sex with women
WST	Wheelchair Skills Test
	Wheelchair Skills Training
WSTP	Wheelchair Skills Training Program
WT	wait times
	walking tank
	walking training
	weight (wt)
	wild type
	Wilms tumor
	wisdom teeth
0WT	zero work tolerance
WTC	World Trade Center
W-T-D	wet to dry
WTP	willingness to pay
WTS	whole tomography slice
WU	Wunsch units
W/U	work-up
WV	whispered voice
W/V	weight-to-volume ratio
WW	watchful waiting
	Weight Watchers
	wheeled walker
WWI	World War One
WWII	World War Two
W/W	weight-to-weight ratio
W ∅ W	wet-to-wet
WWAC	walk with aid of cane
WW Brd	whole wheat bread
WWidF	white widowed female
WWidM	white widowed male
WWTP	wastewater treatment plant
WWW	World Wide Web
WYOU	women years of usage

X

X — break
capecitabine (Xeloda) (This is a dangerous abbreviation)
cross
crossmatch
exophoria for distance
Ecstasy (methylenedioxy-methamphetamine; MDMA)
extra
female sex chromosome
start of anesthesia
ten
times
xylocaine

$\bar{x}$ — except
mean

X′ — exophoria at 33 cm

X^2 — chi-square

X+# — xyphoid plus number of fingerbreadths

X3 — orientation as to time, place and person

X-ALD — X-linked adrenoleukodystrophy

XBT — xylose breath test

XC — excretory cystogram

XCCL — crossed-coupled-cavity-laser
exaggerated craniocaudal lateral

XCF — aortic cross clamp off

XCO — aortic cross clamp on

XD — times daily
xanthoma dissemination

X&D — examination and diagnosis

X2d — times two days

XDP — xeroderma pigmentosum

XDR — extensively drug-resistant (tuberculosis)

XDR-TB — extensively drug-resistant tuberculosis

XE — capecitabine (Xeloda)

Xe — xenon

^{133}Xe — xenon, isotope of mass 133

XeCl — xenon chloride

XeCT — xenon-enhanced computed tomography

X-ed — crossed

XELIRI — capecitabine (Xeloda) and irinotecan

XEM — xonics electron mammography

XES — x-ray energy spectrometer

XFER — transfer

XFS — exfoliation syndrome

XGP — xanthogranulomatous pyelonephritis

XI — eleven

XII — twelve

XIAP — X-linked inhibitor of apoptosis

XIP — x-ray in plaster

XKO — not knocked out

XL — extended release (once a day oral solid dosage form)
extra large
forty

XLA — X-linked infantile agammaglobulinemia

X-leg — cross leg

XLFDP — cross-linked fibrin degradation products

XLH — X-linked hypophos-phatemia

XLIF — extreme lateral interbody fusion

XLJR — X-linked juvenile retinoschisis

XLMR — X-linked mental retardation

XLOA — X-linked optic atrophy

XLP — X-linked proliferative (syndrome)

XLRS — X-linked retinoschisis

XM — crossmatch

X-mat. — crossmatch

XMG — mammogram

XML — extensible markup language

XMM — xeromammography

XMR — magnetic resonance and X-rays

XMT — cross matched

XNA — xenoreactive natural antibodies

XOM — extraocular movements

XOP — x-ray out of plaster

XP — xeroderma pigmentosum

XR — x-ray

XRF — x-ray fluorescence

XRT — radiation therapy

XS — excessive

X-SCID — X-linked severe combined immunodeficiency

XS-LIM — exceeds limits of procedure

X-STOP — an interspinous process decompression system

XT — exotropia
extract
extracted

X(T′) — intermittent exotropia at 33 cm

X(T) — intermittent exotropia

XTLE — extratemporal-lobe epilepsy

XU — excretory urogram

XULN — times upper limit of normal

XV — fifteen

3X/WK — three times a week

XX — normal female sex chromosome type
twenty

XX/XY — sex karyotypes

XXX — thirty

XY — normal male sex chromosome type

XYL — xylose

XYLO — lidocaine (Xylocaine)

Y

Y	male sex chromosome year yellow
YAC	yeast artificial chromosome
YACs	yeast artificial chromosomes
YACP	young adult chronic patient
YAG	yttrium aluminum garnet (laser)
YAS	youth action section (police)
Yb	ytterbium
YBOCS	Yale-Brown Obsessive-Compulsive Scale
Yel	yellow
YEPQ	Yale Eating Patterns Questionnaire
YF	yellow fever
YFH	yellow-faced hornet
YFI	yellow fever immunization
YFV	yellow-fever virus
YHL	years of healthy life
YJV	yellow jacket venom
Y2K	year 2,000
YLC	youngest living child
YLD	years of life with disability
YLL	years of life lost
YMC	young male Caucasian
YMRS	Young Mania Rating Scale
Y/N	yes/no
YO	years old
YOB	year of birth
YOD	year of death
YORA	younger-onset rheumatoid arthritis
YPC	YAG (yttrium aluminum garnet) posterior capsulotomy
YPLL	years of potential life lost before age 65
yr	year
YRI	Yoruba from Ibadan, Nigeria (populations included in HapMap - see HapMap)
YSC	yolk sac carcinoma
YTD	year to date
YTDY	yesterday

Z

Z	impedance pyrazinamide [part of tuberculosis regimen, see RHZ(E/S)/HR]
ZAL	zaleplon (Sonata)
ZAP	zoster-associated pain
ZD	Zenker diverticulum zinc-deficient
ZDV	zidovudine (Retrovir)
Z-E	Zollinger-Ellison (syndrome)
ZEEP	zero end-expiratory pressure
ZES	Zollinger-Ellison syndrome
Z-ESR	zeta erythrocyte sedimentation rate
ZIFT	zygote intrafallopian (tube) transfer
ZIG	zoster serum immune globulin
ZIP	zoster immune plasma
ZMC	zygomatic zygomatic maxillary compound (complex)
Zn	zinc
ZnO	zinc oxide
ZnOE	zinc oxide and eugenol
ZnPc	zinc phthalocyanine
ZnPP	zinc protoporphyrin
ZNS	zolmitriptan nasal spray (Zomig) zonisamide (Zonegran)
$ZnSO_4$	zinc sulfate
ZOI	zone of inhibition
ZOOM	Guarana
ZOT	zonula occludens toxin
ZPC	zero point of charge zopiclone
z-Plasty	surgical relaxation of contracture
ZPO	zinc peroxide
ZPP	zinc protoporphyrin
ZPS	Zubrod performance status
ZPT	zinc pyrithione
ZSB	zero stools since birth
ZSR	zeta sedimentation rate
ZSRDS	Zung Self-Rating Depression Scale

Chapter 7
Symbols and Numbers

Symbols

Symbol	Meaning
↑	above
	alive
	elevated
	greater than
	high
	improved
	increase
	rising
	up
	upper
↑g	increasing
↓	dead
	decrease
	depressed
	diminished
	down
	falling
	lower
	lowered
	normal plantar reflex
	restricted
↓g	decreasing
→	causes to
	greater than
	progressing
	results in
	showed
	to
	to the right
	transfer to
←	less than
	resulted from
	to the left
↔	same as
	stable
	to and from
	unchanging
↓↓	flexor
	plantar response (Babinski)
	testes descended
↑↑	extensor
	extensor response (positive Babinsky)
	testes undescended
‖	parallel
	parallel bars
√	check
	flexion
√'d	checked
√'ing	checking
#	fracture
	number
	pound
	weight
∴	therefore
∵	because
Δ scan	delta scan (computed tomography scan)
+	plus
	positive
	present
−	absent
	minus
	negative
/	extend
	extended
	slash mark signifying per, and, over, as a blood pressure of 160 over 100, or with (this is a dangerous symbol as it is mistaken for a one)
±	either positive or negative
	no definite cause
	plus or minus
	very slight trace

└	right lower quadrant
┌	right upper quadrant
┐	left upper quadrant
┘	left lower quadrant
>	greater than (can be confused with <, use "greater than")
	left ear-bone conduction threshold
≥	greater than or equal to
<	caused by
	less than (can be confused with >, use "less than")
	right ear-bone conduction threshold
≤	less than or equal to
≮	not less than
≯	not more than
V	above
	diastolic blood pressure
	increased
	below
	systolic blood pressure
≠	not equal to
≅	approximately equal to
=	equal
	equal to
′	feet
	minutes (as in 30′)
″	inches
	seconds
~	about
	approximately
	difference
≈	approximately equal to
≡	identical
×	left ear-air conduction threshold
	ten
]	left ear-masked bone conduction threshold
[	right ear-masked bone conduction
△	right ear-masked air conduction threshold
	change
○	threshold
	reversible
?	questionable
—	not tested
Ø	no
	none
	without
⊙	start of an operation
⊗	end of anesthesia
@	at
ṫ	one
ṫṫ	two
♂	male
♀	female
⚣	gay
⚢	lesbian
■	deceased male
●	deceased female
□	living male
	left ear-masked air conduction threshold
○	living female
	respiration
	right ear-air conduction threshold
◇	sex unknown
(□)	adopted living male
*	birth
†	dead
	death
⚲	standing
o—<	recumbent position
	sitting position
♥	heart

Numbers (Arabic and Roman)

1/2 and 1/2	half Dakin solution and half glycerin
1°	first degree
	primary
1:1	one-to-one (individual session with staff)
2°	second degree
	secondary
2×2	gauze dressing folded 2″×2″
222	aspirin, caffeine, and codeine (8 mg) tablets (Canada)
282	aspirin, caffeine, codeine, and meprobamate (Canada)
3°	tertiary
	third degree

3×	three times
4×4	gauze dressing folded 4″×4″
5+2	5 days of cytarabine and 2 days of daunorubicin leukemia therapy
642	propoxyphene tablets (Canada)
7+3	7 days of cytarabine and 3 days of daunorubicin leukemia therapy
Serial 7's	a mental status examination (starting with 100, count backward by 7's)
24°	twenty-four hours (24 hr is safer as the ° is seen as a zero)
777	Ortho Novum 777® (a triphasic oral contraceptive)
1500	Health Insurance Claim Form HCFA 1500
1,000	one thousand (1×10^3)
10,000	ten thousand (1×10^4)
100,000	one hundred thousand (1×10^5)
1,000,000	one million (1×10^6)
10,000,000	ten million (1×10^7)
100,000,000	one hundred million (1×10^8)
1,000,000,000	one billion (1×10^9)
i	one (Roman numerals are dangerous expressions and should not be used because they are not universally understood)
ii	two
iii	three
iiii	four
iv	four (this is a dangerous abbreviation as it is read as intravenous, use 4)
v	five
vi	six
vii	seven
viii	eight
ix	nine
x	ten
xi	eleven
xii	twelve
XL	forty
	extended release dosage form
L	fifty
C	hundred
M	thousand

Greek Letters

Α α	alpha
β Β	beta
Γ γ	gamma
Δ δ	anion gap
	change
	delta
	delta gap
	prism diopter
	temperature
	trimester
Ε ϵ	epsilon
Ζ ζ	zeta
Η η	eta
Θ θ	negative
	theta
Ι ι	iota
Κ κ	kappa
Λ λ	lambda
Μ μ	micro
	mu
Ν ν	nu
Ξ ξ	xi
Ο ο	omicron
Π π	pi
Ρ ρ	rho
Σ σ	sigma
	sum of
	summary
Τ τ	tau
Υ υ	upsilon
Φ ϕ	phenyl
	phi
	thyroid
Χ χ	chi
Ψ ψ	psi
	psychiatric
Ω ω	omega
	ohm

Miscellaneous

L M / K Ō / S T (crossed-lines diagram)	liver, kidneys, and spleen negative, no masses, or tenderness

#

Additions, Corrections, and Suggestions are Welcomed

Please send them via any means shown below:

Neil M Davis
2049 Stout Drive, B-3
Warminster PA 18974-3861

FAX 1 888 333 4915 or 1 215 442 7432
Email med@neilmdavis.com
Web site www.medabbrev.com

Thank you for your help in the past.

Have You Used the Internet Version of This Book?

- It is instantaneously searchable for the meanings of abbreviations
- It is reverse searchable (search for all the abbreviations containing a particular word)
- Each month, about 80 new entries are added

See the preface (page vii) for access instructions. A one-year, single-user access is included in the purchase price of the book. Also one-year subscriptions are available for purchase (see page 377).

PDA and BlackBerry Versions are Available

See pricing and ordering information in the pricing section on page 379.

Multi-User Site Licenses are Available

Medical facilities can substitute their own "Do Not Use" list of dangerous abbreviations for the one present. The ability also exists to list abbreviations that are unique to your region and/or organization which would normally not appear in any national list. These lists would be controlled by the facility or company. A no-cost, 3-week trial and pricing information are available by calling 1 888 333 1862 or 1 215 442 7430 or via an e-mail request to ev@neilmdavis.com

Chapter 8

Tables, Lists, and Conversions

Numbers and letters for teeth

Two adult numbering systems and a deciduous system are shown. The adult systems are shown as numbers, whereas deciduous teeth are lettered. The system commonly used in the U.S. is 1 to 32 (shown in bold face type).

1 (18) upper right 3rd molar
2 (17) (A) upper right 2nd molar
3 (16) (B) upper right 1st molar
4 (15) upper right 2nd bicuspid
5 (14) upper right 1st bicuspid
6 (13) (C) upper right canine (eyetooth)
7 (12) (D) upper right lateral incisor
8 (11) (E) upper right central incisor
9 (21) (F) upper left central incisor
10 (22) (G) upper left lateral incisor
11 (23) (H) upper left canine
12 (24) upper left 1st bicuspid
13 (25) upper left 2nd bicuspid
14 (26) (I) upper left 1st molar
15 (27) (J) upper left 2nd molar
16 (28) upper left 3rd molar
17 (38) lower left 3rd molar
18 (37) (K) lower left 2nd molar
19 (36) (L) lower left 1st molar
20 (35) lower left 2nd bicuspid
21 (34) lower left 1st bicuspid
22 (33) (M) lower left canine
23 (32) (N) lower left lateral incisor
24 (31) (O) lower left central incisor
25 (41) (P) lower right central incisor
26 (42) (Q) lower right lateral incisor
27 (43) (R) lower right canine
28 (44) lower right 1st bicuspid
29 (45) lower right 2nd bicuspid
30 (46) (S) lower right 1st molar
31 (47) (T) lower right 2nd molar
32 (48) lower right 3rd molar

UPPER																	UPPER
	1	**2**	**3**	**4**	**5**	**6**	**7**	**8**	**9**	**10**	**11**	**12**	**13**	**14**	**15**	**16**	
	18	17	16	15	14	13	12	11	21	22	23	24	25	26	27	28	
		A	B			C	D	E	F	G	H			I	J		
Right																	**Left**
		T	S			R	Q	P	O	N	M			L	K		
	48	47	46	45	44	43	42	41	31	32	33	34	35	36	37	38	
	32	**31**	**30**	**29**	**28**	**27**	**26**	**25**	**24**	**23**	**22**	**21**	**20**	**19**	**18**	**17**	
LOWER																	LOWER

#

#

Laboratory Test Panels*

	Cl CO_2 K Na	BUN Ca Creat Gluc	Alb Alk P AST(SGOT) ALT(SGPT) T Bili TP	ANA ESR RF Ur Ac	Calc LDL HDL T Chol Trig VLDL	Alb Phos	HAAb, IgM Ab HbcAb, IgM Ab HbsAG HCAb
Lytes (electrolyte panel)	X						
BMP (basic metabolic panel) or MBP, MPB	X	X					
CMP (comprehensive metabolic panel)	X	X	X				
HFP (hepatic function panel)			X plus D Bili				
AP (arthritis panel)				X			
LP (lipid Panel)					X		
RFP (renal function panel)	X	X				X	
AHP (acute hepatitis panel)							X

*These can vary from institution to institution and from year to year

Abbreviation Key

Ab-antibody
Alb-albumin
Alk P-alkaline phosphate
ALT (SGPT)-alanine aminotransferase (serum glutamate pyruvate)
ANA-antinuclear antibody
AST (SGOT)-aspartate-aminotransferase (serum glutamate oxaloacetic transaminase)
BUN-blood urea nitrogen
Ca-calcium
Calc LDL-calculated low-density lipoprotein
LDL-low density lipoprotein
Cl-chloride
CO_2-carbon dioxide
Creat-creatinine
D Bili-direct bilirubin
ESR-erythrocyte sedimentation rate
Gluc-glucose
HAAb-hepatitis A antibody
HBcAb-hepatitis B core antibody
HBsAg-hepatitis B surface antigen
HCAb-hepatitis C antibody
HDL-high-density lipoprotein
IgM-immunoglobulin M
K-potassium
Na-sodium
Phos-phosphate
RF-rheumatoid factor
T Bili-total bilirubin
T Chol-total cholesterol
TP-total protein
Trig-triglycerides
Ur Ac-uric acid
VLDl-very low-density lipoprotein

See text for meaning of the abbreviations shown

Complete Blood Count

```
                11.7   / 50S, 25B, 35L, 5M 2N, 3E
10,000 >-------------<   83/29/30
                36.5   \ 290,00

          HgB        / Segs/Bands/Lymphs/Monos/Basos/Eos
WBC  >-------------<   MCV-MCH-MCHC
          HCT        \ platelet count
```

Electrolyte Panel

142	99	sodium	chloride
4.7	25	potassium	carbon dioxide

Blood Gases

7.4/80/48/98/25 pH/PO_2/PCO_2/% O_2 saturation/bicarbonate

Obstetrical shorthand

2 cm | 80%
−2 Vtx

2 cm = dilation of cervix

80% = degree of cervix effacement

Vtx = vertex; presentation of fetus, (breech = Br)

−2 = station; distance above (+) or below (−) the spine of the ischium measured in cm

Reflexes

Reflexes are usually graded on a 0 to 4+ scale. The designations +, ++, +++, and ++++ should not be used.

4+ may indicate disease often associated with clonus
very brisk, hyperactive
3+ brisker than average
possibly but not necessarily indicative of disease
2+ average
normal
1+ low normal
somewhat diminished
0 may indicate neuropathy
no response

Muscle strength[1]

0—No muscular contraction detected
1—A barely detectable flicker or trace of contraction
2—Active movement of the body part with gravity eliminated
3—Active movement against gravity
4—Active movement against gravity and some resistance
5—Active movement against full resistance without evident fatigue. This is normal muscle strength

#

Pulse[1]

0 completely absent
+1 markedly impaired (or 1+)
+2 modererately impaired (or 2+)
+3 slightly impaired (or 3+)
+4 normal (or 4+)

Gradation of intensity of heart murmurs[1]

1/6 or I/VI	may not be heard in all positions very faint, heard only after the listener has "tuned in"
2/6 or II/VI	quiet, but heard immediately upon placing the stethoscope on the chest
3/6 or III/VI	moderately loud
4/6 or IV/VI	loud
5/6 orV/VI	very loud, may be heard with a stethoscope partly off the chest (thrills are associated)
6/6 or VI/VI	may be heard with the stethoscope entirely off the chest (thrills are associated)

Tonsil Size

0 no tonsils
1 less than normal
2 normal
3 greater than normal
4 touching

Metric Prefixes and Symbols

Prefix	Symbol	
tera-	T	1,000,000,000,000 or (10^{12}) one trillion
giga-	G	1,000,000,000 or (10^{9}) one billion
mega-	M	1,000,000 or (10^{6}) one million
kilo-	k	1,000 or (10^{3}) one thousand
hecto-	h	100 or (10^{2}) one hundred
deka-	da	10 or (10^{1}) ten
deci-	d	0.1 or (10^{-1}) one-tenth
centi-	c	0.01 or (10^{-2}) one-hundredth
milli-	m	0.001 or (10^{-3}) one-thousandth
micro-	μ	0.000,001 or (10^{-6}) one-millionth
nano-	n	0.000,000,001 or (10^{-9}) one-billionth
pico-	p	0.000,000,000,000,001 or (10^{-12}) one-trillionth
femto-	f	0.000,000,000,000,001 or (10^{-15}) one-quadrillionth
atto-	a	0.000,000,000,000,000,001 or (10^{-18}) one-quintillionth

#

Kilograms/Pounds Conversions

To convert pounds to kilograms, divide by 2.2
To convert kilograms to pounds, multiply by 2.2

After carrying out a calculation, always make sure your answer is reasonable by checking with the table below.

kilograms	pounds
0.5	1.1
1	2.2
5	11
10	22
25	55
50	110
75	165
100	220

Fahrenheit/Centigrade Conversions

To convert Centigrade to Fahrenheit

°F = 32 plus (9/5 times °C)   or   °F = 32 plus (1.8 times °C)

To convert Fahrenheit to Centigrade

°C = 5/9 times (°F minus 32)   or   °C ≈ 0.556 times (°F minus 32)

After carrying out a calculation, always make sure your answer is reasonable by checking with the table below.

°Centigrade	°Fahrenheit
0	32
2	36
8	46
15	59
20	68
25	77
30	86
36	96.8
37	98.6
38	100.4
39	102.2
40	104
41	105.8
50	122
100	212

Apothecary symbols (Should never be used)

The symbols presented below are for informational use. The apothecary system should **not** be used. Only the metric system should be used. The methods of expressing the symbols, the meanings, and the equivalence are not the classic ones, nor are they precise, but reflect the usual intended meanings when used by some older physicians in writing prescription directions.

Symbol	Meaning	Symbol	Meaning
ʒ or ʒi̇	dram, teaspoonful, (5 mL)	℥ or ℥i̇	ounce, (30 mL)
		gr	grain (approximately 65 mg)
ʒi̇i̇	two drams, 2 teaspoonfuls, (10 mL)		
		♏	minim (approximately 0.06 mL)
℥ss	half ounce, tablespoonful, (15 mL)	**gtt**	drop

Reference

1. Adopted from Bates, B., *Bates' Guide to Physical Examinations and History Taking,* 9th ed. Philadelphia: Lippincott Williams and Wilkins; 2007.

Additions, Corrections, and Suggestions are Welcomed

Please send them via any means shown below:

Neil M Davis
2049 Stout Drive, B-3
Warminster PA 18974-3861

FAX 1 888 333 4915 or 1 215 442 7432
Email med@neilmdavis.com
Web site www.medabbrev.com

Thank you for your help in the past.

Have You Used the Internet Version of This Book?

- It is instantaneously searchable for the meanings of abbreviations
- It is reverse searchable (search for all the abbreviations containing a particular word)
- Each month, about 80 new entries are added

See the preface (page vii) for access instructions. A one-year, single-user access is included in the purchase price of the book. Also one-year subscriptions are available for purchase (see page 377).

PDA and BlackBerry Versions are Available

See pricing and ordering information in the pricing section on page 379.

Multi-User Site Licenses are Available

Medical facilities can substitute their own "Do Not Use" list of dangerous abbreviations for the one present. The ability also exists to list abbreviations that are unique to your region and/or organization which would normally not appear in any national list. These lists would be controlled by the facility or company. A no-cost, 3-week trial and pricing information are available by calling 1 888 333 1862 or 1 215 442 7430 or via an e-mail request to ev@neilmdavis.com

Chapter 9

Cross-Referenced List of Generic and Brand Drug Names

Listed below is a cross-referenced index of generic and brand drug names. Generic names begin with a lower case letter while brand names begin with a capital letter. This partial list consists of frequently prescribed drugs, new drugs, and recently discontinued drugs.

The meanings of abbreviated and coded drug names can be found in Chapter 6 (Lettered Abbreviations and Acronyms).

This listing is intended to allow readers to reference generic and trade drug names. Since products are added and taken off the market daily, this listing can not be relied on for accuracy of availability. The best reference for checking on availability is the web version of Drug Facts and Comparisons[1] as it has a complete and current listing for drugs available as well as those no longer available.

Complete indices of United States drug names can be found in current editions of Drug Facts and Comparisons[1] and the American Drug Index[2]. A complete list of world-wide names may be found in Martindales.[3] These and other references should be used to determine the equivalence of products, strengths, and dosage forms. Although several products may be listed under one generic name they may differ in strength, dosage form, or concentration available, as is the case with estradiol transdermal (Climara, Estraderm, and Vivelle).

Some products are marketed without a brand name, as in the case of thioguanine. In such cases only the generic name is listed. When a product is often prescribed and/or labeled generically, the generic name is shown in italics.

The following abbreviations are used in this listing:

EC	enteric coated	SR	sustained release tablets or capsules, and other designations for extended release dosage forms such as CR, LX, SA, LA, CC, XR, SR, CD, XT, etc.
HCl	hydrochloride		
IM	intramuscular	susp	suspension
IV	intravenous	(W)	withdrawn or discontinued from US market
inj	injection	(WA)	withdrawn or discontinued from U.S. Market but available under it's generic name and/or another brand name from another manufacturer
oint	ointment		
ophth	ophthalmic		
soln	solution		

A

abacavir sulfate	Ziagen
abarelix	Plenaxis
abatacept	Orencia
Abbokinase (W)	urokinase (W)
abciximab	ReoPro
Abelcet	amphotericin B lipid complex
Abilify	aripiprazole
Abraxane	paclitaxel, albumin-bound inj
ACAM 2000	smallpox (vaccinia)
acamprosate calcium	Campral
acarbose	Precose

Accolate	zafirlukast
AccuNeb	albuterol inhalation soln
Accupril	quinapril HCl
Accuretic	quinapril; hydrochlorothiazide
Accutane	isotretinoin
Accuzyme	papain; urea oint
acebutolol HCl	Sectral
Aceon	perindopril erbumine
acetaminophen	paracetamol
	Tylenol
acetaminophen 300 mg with Codeine Phosphate (15, 30, and 60 mg)	Phenaphen with Codeine (#2, 3, and 4) (WA)
	Tylenol with Codeine (#2, 3, and 4)
acetazolamide	Diamox
acetohexamide (W)	Dymelor (W)
acetohydroxamic acid	Lithostat
acetylcholine ophth	Miochol E
acetylcysteine	Mucomyst
Achromycin (WA)	tetracycline HCl
Aciphex	rabeprazole sodium
acitretin	Soriatane
Acora	argatroban
Acthar (W)	corticotropin (W)
ActHIB/Tripedia	*Haemophilus b* conjugate vaccine reconstituted with diphtheria and tetanus toxoids and acellular pertussis vaccine adsorbed
Acthrel	corticorellin ovine triflutate
Actifed	triprolidine HCl; pseudoephedrine HCl
Actigall	ursodiol
Actimmune	interferon gamma 1-b
Actiq	fentanyl oral transmucosal
Activase	alteplase, recombinant
Activella (WA)	norethindrone acetate; estradiol
Actonel	risedronate sodium
Actos	pioglitazone HCl
Acular	ketorolac tromethamine ophth
acyclovir	Zovirax
Adacel	diphtheria, tetanus, and acellular pertussis (TdaP) vaccine (adult type)
Adalat CC	nifedipine SR
adalimumab	Humira
adapalene	Differin
Adapin	doxepin HCl
Adderall	amphetamine; dextroamphetamine mixed salts
adefovir dipivoxil	Hepsera
	Preveon
Adenocard	adenosine
adenosine	Adenocard
Adrenalin	epinephrine
Adriamycin	doxorubicin HCl
Advair Diskus	fluticasone propionate; salmeterol inhalation powder
Advicor	lovastatin; niacin
Advil	ibuprofen
AeroBid	flunisolide
Afluria	influenza vaccine
Afrin nasal spray	oxymetazoline HCl
agalsidase beta	Fabrazyme
Agenerase (W)	amprenavir (W)
Aggrastat	tirofiban HCl
Aggrenox	aspirin; extended-release dipyridamole
Agrylin	anagrelide HCl
Akineton	biperiden
Alamast	pemirolast potassium ophth soln
alatrofloxacin mesylate IV (W)	Trovan inj (W)
albendazole	Albenza
Albenza	albendazole
albumin human	Albuminar
	Albutein
	Buminate
	Plasbumin
albumin (human), sonicated	Albunex
Albuminar	albumin human
Albunex	albumin (human), sonicated
Albutein	albumin human
albuterol	AccuNeb
	Proventil
	salbutamol
	Ventolin
albuterol SR	Proventil Repetabs
	Volmax
albuterol sulfate inhalation aerosol	Proventil HFA
Aldactazide	spironolactone; hydrochlorothiazide
Aldactone	spironolactone
Aldara	imiquimod cream
aldesleukin	Proleukin
Aldomet	methyldopa

Aldoril	methyldopa; hydrochlorothiazide
Aldurazyme	laronidase
alefacept	Amevive
alemtuzumab	Campath
alendronate sodium	Fosamax
Alesse	levonorgestrel; ethinyl estradiol
Alfenta	alfentanil HCl
alfentanil HCl	Alfenta
alfuzosin	UroXatral
alglucerase	Ceredase
alglucosidase alfa	Myozyme
Alimta	pemetrexed disodium
aliskiren hemifumarate	Tekturna
alitretinoin	Panretin
Allegra	fexofenadine HCl
Alinia	nitazoxanide
Alkeran	melphalan
allopurinol	Zyloprim
almotriptan malate	Axert
Alocril	nedocromil ophth soln
Alomide	lodoxamide tromethamine ophth soln
Alora	estradiol transdermal
alosetron	Lotronex
Aloxi	palonosetron HCl
Alphagan (W)	brimonidine tartrate ophth (W)
alpha$_1$-proteinase inhibitor (human)	Prolastin
alprazolam	Xanax
alprostadil	Caverject Edex Prostin VR
alprostadil urethral suppository	Muse
Alrex	loteprednol etabonate ophth susp
Altabax	retapamulin oint
Altace	ramipril
alteplase, recombinant	Activase
alteplase (for catheter occlusions)	Cathflo Activase
altretamine	Hexalen
aluminum acetate	Domeboro
aluminum carbonate (W)	Basaljel (W)
aluminum hydroxide	Amphojel
aluminum hydroxide; magnesium hydroxide	Maalox
Alupent	metaproterenol sulfate
Alustra (W)	hydroquinone topical susp (W)
Alvesco	ciclesonide inhalation
alvimopam	Entereg
amantadine HCl	Symmetrel
Amaryl	glimepiride
Ambien	zolpidem tartrate
AmBisome	liposomal amphotericin B
ambrisentan	Letairis
amcinonide (W)	Cyclocort (W)
Amerge	naratriptan HCl
Amevive	alefacept
Amicar	aminocaproic acid
Amidate	etomidate
amifostine	Ethyol
amikacin sulfate	Amikin
Amikin	amikacin sulfate
amiloride HCl	Midamor
amiloride; hydrochlorothiazide	Moduretic
amino acid inj	Aminosyn Travasol TrophAmine
amino acid with electrolytes in dextrose with calcium inj (various concentrations) (W)	Clinimix E (W)
aminocaproic acid	Amicar
aminocaproic acid gel	Caprogel
aminoglutethimide	*aminoglutethimide*
aminolevulinic acid HCl topical soln	Levulan Kerastick
aminophylline	aminophylline
aminosalicylic acid	Paser
Aminosyn	amino acid inj
amiodarone HCl	Cordarone
Amitiza	lubiprostone
amitriptyline HCl	*amitriptyline HCl*
AmLactin	ammonium lactate lotion
amlexanox oral paste	Aphthasol
amlodipine besylate	Norvasc

amlodipine besylate; atorvastatin calcium	Caduet
amlodipine besylate; benazepril HCl	Lotrel
amlodipine; valsartan	Exforge
ammonium lactate lotion	AmLactin
amobarbital sodium	Amytal
amoxapine	*amoxapine*
amoxicillin	Amoxil
	Trimox
	Wymox
amoxicillin; clavulanic acid	Augmentin
amoxicillin; clavulanate potassium SR	Augmentin XR
Amoxil	amoxicillin
amphetamine resins (W)	Biphetamine (W)
amphetamine; dextroamphetamine mixed salts	Adderall
Amphojel	aluminum hydroxide
Amphotec	amphotericin B cholesteryl sulfate
amphotericin B (W)	Fungizone (W)
amphotericin B cholesteryl sulfate	Amphotec
amphotericin B lipid complex	Abelcet
ampicillin	Principen
ampicillin sodium; sulbactam sodium	Unasyn
amprenavir (W)	Agenerase (W)
amrinone (former name)	inamrinone (new name)
Amrix	cyclobenzaprine SR
amsacrine	Amsidyl
Amsidyl	amsacrine
Amvisc	sodium hyaluronate
Amytal	amobarbital sodium
Anadrol-50	oxymetholone
Anafranil	clomipramine HCl
anagrelide HCl	Agrylin

anakinra	Kineret
Anaprox	naproxen sodium
anastrozole	Arimidex
Anbesol	benzocaine
Ancef (WA)	*cefazolin sodium*
Ancobon	flucytosine
Androderm	testosterone transdermal system
AndroGel	testosterone gel
Androgel-DHT	dihydrotestosterone transdermal
Anectine	succinylcholine chloride
Anexsia	hydrocodone bitartrate; acetaminophen
Angiomax	bivalirudin
anidulafungin IV	Eraxis
Ansaid	flurbiprofen
Antabuse	disulfiram
Antagon	ganirelix acetate
antihemophilic factor (recombinant)	Kogenate
	ReFacto
Antilirium	physostigmine salicylate
antipyrine otic (W)	Auralgan (W)
antithrombin III (human)	Thrombate III
antithymocyte globulin, (rabbit)	Thymoglobulin
Antivert	meclizine
Antizol	fomepizole
Anturane	sulfinpyrazone
Anzemet	dolasetron mesylate
Aphthasol	amlexanox oral paste
Apidra	insulin glulisine [rDNA origin]
A.P.L. (WA)	*chorionic gonadotropin*
apligraf (W)	Graftskin (W)
Aplisol	tuberculin skin test
Apokyn	apomorphine HCl inj
apomorphine HCl inj	Apokyn
Aposyn (W)	exisulind (W)
aprepitant	Emend capsules
Apresazide	hydralazine HCl; hydrochloro-thiazide
Apresoline	hydralazine HCl
aprotinin	Trasylol
Aptivus	tipranavir
AquaMEPHY-TON (W)	phytonadione inj (W)
Aralen	chloroquine phosphate
Aramine	metaraminol bitartrate
Aranesp	darbepoetin alfa
Arava	leflunomide
arbutamine HCl (W)	GenEsa (W)

Arcalyst	rilonacept
arcitumomab	CEA-Scan
ardeparin sodium (W)	Normiflo (W)
Arduan (W)	pipecuronium bromide (W)
Aredia	pamidronate disodium
Arestin	minocycline HCl dental microspheres
Arfonad (W)	trimethaphan camsylate (W)
argatroban	argatroban
arginine HCl	R-Gene
Aricept	donepezil HCl
Arimidex	anastrozole
aripiprazole	Abilify
Aristocort	triamcinolone
Arixtra	fondaparinux sodium
armodafinil	Nuvigil
Aromasin	exemestane
Arranon	nelarabine
arsenic trioxide	Trisenox
Artane (WA)	*trihexyphenidyl HCl*
Arthrotec	diclofenac; misoprostol
articaine; epinephrine	Septocaine
Asacol	mesalamine
Asendin (WA)	*amoxapine*
Aslera (W)	prasterone (W)
asparaginase	Elspar
aspirin 325 mg with codeine phosphate (30 and 60 mg)	Empirin with codeine #3 and #4
aspirin buffered	Bufferin
aspirin EC	Ecotrin
aspirin; extended-release dipyridamole	Aggrenox
Astelin	azelastine HCl nasal spray
astemizole (W)	Hismanal (W)
Atacand	candesartan cilexetil
Atarax (WA)	hydroxyzine HCl
atazanavir (W) sulfate	Reyataz (W)
atenolol	Tenormin
atenolol; chlorthalidone	Tenoretic
Atgam	lymphocyte imimmune globulin
Atacand HCT	candesartan cilexetil; hydrochlorothiazide
atazanavir (W)	Revetaz (W)
Ativan	lorazepam
Atomoxetine HCl	Strattera
atorvastatin calcium	Lipitor
atovaquone	Mepron
atovaquone; proguanil HCl	Malarone
atracurium besylate	Tracrium
Atridox	doxycycline hyclate gel
Atripla	efavirenz, emtricitabine, and tenofovir
Atromid-S (W)	clofibrate (W)
atropine sulfate tablets	Sal-Tropine
Atrovent	ipratropium bromide
Augmentin	amoxicillin; clavulanic acid
Augmentin XR	amoxicillin; clavulanate potassium SR
Auralgan (W)	antipyrine otic (W)
auranofin	Ridaura
Aurolate	gold sodium thiomalate
aurothioglucose	Solganal
Avalide	irbesartan; hydro-chlorothiazide
Avandamet	rosiglitazone maleate; metformin HCl
Avandia	Rosiglitazone maleate
Avanir (W)	docosanol cream (W)
Avapro	irbesartan
Avastin	bevacizumab
Avelox	moxifloxacin HCl
Aventyl	nortriptyline HCl
Avinza	morphine sulfate tab SR
Avita	tretinoin cream 0.025%
Avitene	collagen hemostat
Avodart	dutasteride
Avonex	interferon beta-la
Axert	almotriptan malate
Axid	nizatidine
azacitidine	Vidaza
Azactam	aztreonam
AzaSite	azithromycin ophth soln
azatadine maleate	Optimine
azathioprine	Imuran
azelaic acid cream	Azelex Finevin
azelastine HCl nasal spray	Astelin
azelastine HCl ophth soln	Optivar
Azelex	azelaic acid cream
Azilect	rasagiline mesylate
azithromycin	Zithromax
azithromycin ophth soln	AzaSite
Azmacort	triamcinolone acetonide aerosol
Azopt	brinzolamide ophth susp
aztreonam	Azactam
Azulfidine	sulfasalazine

B

Baciguent	bacitracin ointment
bacitracin ointment	*bacitracin ointment*
baclofen	Lioresal
Bactrim	sulfamethoxazole; trimeth-oprim
Bactroban	mupirocin nasal ointment
BAL in Oil	dimercaprol
Baraclude	entecavir
Basaljel (W)	aluminum carbonate (W)
balsalazide disodium	Colazal
basiliximab	Simulect
Baycol (W)	cerivastatin sodium (W)
BCG intravesical	Pacis TheraCys TICE BCG
becaplermin gel	Regranex
beclomethasone dipropionate	Beclovent (W) Beconase AQ Nasal Qvar Vancenase (W) Vancenase AQ Nasal (W) Vanceril (W)
Beclovent (WA)	beclomethasone dipropionate
Beconase AQ Nasal	beclomethasone dipropionate
belladonna alkaloids; phenobarbital	Donnatal (W)
Bellergal-S	phenobarbital; ergotamine; belladonna
Benadryl	diphenhydramine HCl
benazepril HCl	Lotensin
bendamustine HCl inj	Treanda
BeneFix	factor IX, (recombinant)
Benemid (WA)	*probenecid*
Benicar	olmesartan medoxomil
Benicar HCT	olmesartan medoxomil; hydrochlorothiazide
bentoquatam	IvyBlock
Bentyl	dicyclomine HCl
Benzamycin	erythromycin; benzoyl peroxide topical gel
benzocaine	Anbesol Hurricaine Orabase Orajel
benzocaine; tetracaine HCl	Cetacaine
benztropine mesylate	Cogentin
bepridil (W)	Vascor (W)
beractant	Survanta
Berroca	vitamin B complex; folic acid; vitamin C
Betadine	povidone iodine
17β-estradiol; norgestimate	Ortho-Prefest
Betagan	levobunolol HCl
betaine anhydrous	Cystadane
betamethasone	Celestone
betamethasone dipropionate	Diprosone
betamethasone; clotrimazole cream	Lotrisone
betamethasone valerate (foam)	Luxiq
Betapace	sotalol
Betaseron	interferon beta-1b
betaxolol	Kerlone
betaxolol HCl ophth soln	Betoptic
betaxolol HCl ophth susp	Betoptic S
betaxolol HCl; pilocarpine HCl ophth soln (W)	Betoptic Pilo (W)
bethanechol chloride	Urecholine
Betoptic	betaxolol HCl ophth soln
Betoptic Pilo (W)	betaxolol HCl; pilocarpine HCl, ophth soln (W)
Betoptic S	betaxolol HCl ophth suspension
bevacizumab	Avastin
bexarotene gel	Targretin
Bextra (W)	valdecoxib (W)
Bexxar	tositumomab and I-131 tositumomab
Biaxin	clarithromycin
Biaxin XL	clarithromycin SR
bicalutamide	Casodex
Bicillin C-R	penicillin G benzathine; penicillin G procaine (for IM use only)
Bicillin L-A	penicillin G benzathine (for IM use only)
Bicitra	sodium citrate; citric acid
BiCNU	carmustine
BiDil	isosorbide dinitrate; hydralazine
Bilopaque (W)	tyropanoate sodium (W)
bimatoprost ophth soln (W)	Lumigan (W)
biperiden	Akineton
Biphetamine (W)	amphetamine resins (W)
bisacodyl	Dulcolax

bismuth subsalicylate; metronidazole; tetracycline HCl	Helidac
bisoprolol fumarate; hydrochlorothiazide	Ziac
bitolterol mesylate	Tornalate
bivalirudin	Angiomax
Blenoxane	bleomycin sulfate
bleomycin sulfate	Blenoxane
Blocadren	timolol maleate
Boniva	ibandronate
bortezomib	Velcade
bosentan	Tracleer
B & O Supprettes	opium; belladonna suppositories
Botox	botulinum toxin type A
botulinum toxin type A	Botox
botulinum toxin type B	Myobloc
Bravelle	urofollitropin
Brethaire	terbutaline sulfate aerosol
Brethine	terbutaline sulfate tablets and inj
bretylium tosylate	Bretylol
Bretylol	bretylium tosylate
Brevibloc	esmolol HCl
Brevital Sodium	methohexital sodium
Bricanyl (WA)	*terbutaline sulfate tablets and inj*
brimonidine tartrate ophth	Alphagan
brinzolamide ophth suspension	Azopt
bromfenac ophth soln	Xibrom
bromocriptine mesylate	Parlodel
brompheniramine maleate	*brompheniramine maleate*
brompheniramine maleate; phenylpropanolamime	Dimetapp Extentabs (WA)
Bronkometer (WA)	*isoetharine HCl aerosol*
Bronkosol (WA)	*isoetharine HCl soln*
Bucladin-S	buclizine HCl
buclizine HCl	Bucladin-S
budesonide capsule SR	Entocort EC
budesonide inhalation powder	Pulmicort Turbuhaler
budesonide nasal inhaler	Rhinocort
Bufferin	aspirin buffered
bumetanide	Bumex
Bumex	bumetanide
Buminate	albumin human
Buphenyl	phenylbutyrate sodium
bupivacaine HCl	Marcaine HCl
buprenorphine HCl	Subutex
buprenorphine HCl; naloxone HCl	Suboxone
bupropion HCl	Wellbutrin
bupropion HCl SR	Wellbutrin SR Zyban
BuSpar	buspirone HCl
buspirone HCl	BuSpar
busulfan	Myleran
busulfan inj	Busulfex
Busulfex	busulfan inj
butabarbital sodium	Butisol
butalbital; acetaminophen; caffeine	Fioricet
butalbital; aspirin; caffeine	Fiorinal
butenafine HCl	Mentax
Butisol	butabarbital sodium
butoconazole nitrate vaginal cream	Gynazole
butorphanol tartrate inj	Stadol
butorphanol tartrate nasal spray	Stadol NS
Byetta	exenatide inj

C

cabergoline (W)	Dostinex (W)
Ca-DTPA	calcium trisodium (trisodium calcium diethylenetriamine-pentaacetate)
Caduet	amlodipine besylate; atorvastatin calcium
Cafcit	caffeine citrate inj
Cafergot	ergotaminetartrate; caffeine
caffeine citrate inj	Cafcit

Calan SR	verapamil HCl SR
Calciferol	ergocalciferol
Calcimar	calcitonin
calcipotriene cream	Dovonex
calcitonin	Calcimar
calcitonin-salmon	Miacalcin
calcitriol	Rocaltrol
calcium carbonate	Os-Cal 500
	Tums
calcium carbonate; vitamin D and K chewable	Viactiv
calcium trisodium (trisodium calcium diethylenetriaminepentaacetate)	Ca-DTPA
calfactant intratracheal susp	Infasurf
Campath	alemtuzumab
camphorated tincture of opium	paregoric
Campral	acamprosate calcium
Camptosar	irinotecan HCl
candesartan cilexetil	Atacand
candesartan cilexetil; hydrochlorothiazide	Atacand HCT
Cancidas	caspofungin acetate
Capastat Sulfate	capreomycin sulfate
capecitabine	Xeloda
Capital w/ Codeine Suspension	codeine phosphate; acetaminophen suspension
Capitrol	chloroxine
Capoten	captopril
capreomycin sulfate	Capastat Sulfate
Caprogel	aminocaproic acid gel
capromab pendetide	ProstaScint
captopril	Capoten
Carac	fluorouracil cream
Carafate	sucralfate
carbachol (W)	Isopto Carbachol (W)
carbamazepine	Tegretol
carbamazepine SR	Carbatrol
	Tegretol-XR

carbamide peroxide otic	Debrox
Carbatrol	carbamazepine SR
carbenicillin (W)	Geocillin (W)
Carbex	selegiline
Carbocaine	mepivacaine HCl
carboplatin	*carboplatin*
Cardene	nicardipine HCl
Cardiolite	technetium Tc99m sestamibi
Cardiotec	technetium Tc-99m teboroxime kit
Cardizem	diltiazem HCl
Cardizem CD	diltiazem HCl SR
Cardura	doxazosin mesylate
carisoprodol	Soma
carmustine	BiCNU
carmustine implantable wafer	Gliadel
Carnitor	levocarnitine
Cartia XR (WA)	*diltiazem HCl SR*
carvedilol	Coreg
Casodex	bicalutamide
caspofungin acetate	Cancidas
Cataflam	diclofenac potassium
Catapres	clonidine HCl
Cathflo Activase	alteplase (for catheter occlusions)
Caverject	alprostadil
CEA-SCAN	arcitumomab
Ceclor	cefaclor
Cedax	ceftibuten
CeeNu	lomustine
cefaclor	Ceclor
cefadroxil	Duricef
Cefadyl (W)	cephapirin sodium
cefamandole nafate (W)	Mandol (W)
cefazolin sodium	*cefazolin sodium*
cefdinir	Omnicef
cefditoren pivoxil	Spectracef
cefepime HCl	Maxipime
cefixime	Suprax
Cefizox	ceftizoxime sodium
Cefobid (W)	cefoperazone sodium (W)
cefonicid sodium (W)	Monocid (W)
cefoperazone sodium (W)	Cefobid (W)
Cefotan	cefotetan
cefotaxime sodium	Claforan
cefotetan	Cefotan
cefoxitin sodium	Mefoxin

cefpodoxime proxetil	Vantin
cefprozil	Cefzil
ceftazidime	Ceptaz
	Fortaz
	Tazicef
	Tazidime
ceftibuten	Cedax
Ceftin	cefuroxime axetil
ceftizoxime sodium	Cefizox
ceftriaxone sodium	Rocephin
cefuroxime axetil	Ceftin
cefuroxime sodium	Kefurox (W)
	Zinacef
Cefzil	cefprozil
Celebrex	celecoxib
celecoxib	Celebrex
Celestone	betamethasone
Celexa	citalopram hydrobromide
CellCept	mycophenolate mofetil
Cenestin	synthetic conjugated estrogens, A
Centrum	vitamins; minerals
cephalexin	*cephalexin HCl*
	Keflex
cephalothin sodium (W)	Keflin (W)
cephapirin sodium (W)	Cefadyl (W)
cephradine (W)	Velosef (W)
Cephulac	lactulose
Ceprotin	protein C concentrate (human)
Ceptaz	ceftazidime
Cerebyx	fosphenytoin sodium
Ceredase	alglucerase
Cerezyme	imiglucerase
cerivastatin sodium (W)	Baycol (W)
Cernevit-12	multivitamins for infusion
certolizumab pegol	Cimzia
Cerubidine	daunorubicin HCl
Cervidil	dinoprostone vaginal insert
Cesamet	nabilone
Cetacaine	benzocaine; tetracaine HCl
cetirizine HCl	Zyrtec
cetirizine HCL; pseudoephedrine HCl SR	Zyrtec-D
cetrorelix	Cetrotide
Cetrotide	cetrorelix
cetuximab	Erbitux
cevimeline HCl	Evoxac
Chantix	varenicline

Chirocaine (W)	levobupivacaine (W)
chloral hydrate	chloral hydrate
chlorambucil	Leukeran
chloramphenicol	Chloromycetin
chloramphenicol ophth (W)	Chloroptic ophth (W)
chlordiazepoxide HCl	Librium
chlordiazepoxide HCl; amitriptyline HCl	Limbitrol
chlorhexidine gluconate	Hibiclens
	PerioChip
chlorhexidine gluconate mouth rinse	Peridex
Chloromycetin	chloramphenicol
chloroprocaine HCl	Nesacaine
Chloroptic ophth (W)	chloramphenicol ophth (W)
chloroquine phosphate	Aralen
chlorothiazide	Diuril
chloroxine	Capitrol
chlorpheniramine maleate	Chlor-Trimeton
chlorpheniramine maleate SR	*chlorpheniramine maleate SR*
chlorpromazine	*chlorpromazine*
chlorpropamide	Diabinese
chlorthalidone	Hygroton
chlorthalidone; reserpine (W)	Regroton (W)
Chlor-Trimeton	*chlorpheniramine maleate*
chlorzoxazone 250 mg	Paraflex
chlorzoxazone 500 mg	Parafon Forte DSC
Cholebrine	iocetamic acid
Choledyl (W)	oxtriphylline (W)
cholestyramine (W)	Questran (W)
choline chloride inj	Intrachol
choline (W) magnesium trisalicylate	Trilisate (W)
Choloxin (W)	dextrothyroxine sodium (W)
chorionic gonadotropin	*chorionic gonadotropin*
choriogona-dotropin alfa	Ovidrel
Chronulac	lactulose
Chymodiactin	chymopapain
chymopapain	Chymodiactin
Cialis	tadalafil
Cibalith-S	lithium citrate

ciclesonide inhalation	Alvesco
ciclopirox cream and lotion	Loprox
ciclopirox soln	Penlac Nail Lacquer
cidofovir	Vistide
cilostazol	Pletal
Ciloxan	ciprofloxacin ophth soln
cimetidine HCl	Tagamet
Cimzia	certolizumab pegol
cinacalcet HCl	Sensipar
Cipro	ciprofloxacin HCl
ciprofloxacin HCl	Cipro
ciprofloxacin; hydrocortisone otic	Cipro HC Otic
ciprofloxacin ophth soln	Ciloxan
Cipro HC Otic	ciprofloxacin; hydrocortisone otic
cisapride (W)	Propulsid (W)
cisatracurium besylate	Nimbex
cisplatin	*cisplatin*
citalopram hydrobromide	Celexa
cladribine	Leustatin
Claforan	cefotaxime sodium
Clarinex	desloratadine
clarithromycin	Biaxin
clarithromycin SR	Biaxin XL
Claritin	loratadine
Claritin D	loratadine; pseudoephedrine sulfate
clemastine fumarate	Tavist
Cleocin	clindamycin HCl
clidinium (W) bromide	Quarzan (W)
clidinium; chlordiazepoxide	Librax
Climara	estradiol transdermal
clindamycin; benzoyl peroxide gel	BenzaClin
clindamycin HCl	Cleocin
clindamycin phosphate pledgets	Clindets
Clindets	clindamycin phosphate pledgets
Clinimix E (W)	amino acid with electrolytes in dextrose with calcium inj (various concentrations) (W)
Clinoril	sulindac

clioquinol (W)	Vioform (W)
clobetasol foam	Olux
clobetasol propionate gel (W)	Clobevate (W)
Clobevate (W)	clobetasol propionate gel (W)
clofarabine	Clolar
clofibrate (W)	Atromid-S (W)
Clolar	clofarabine
Clomid	clomiphene citrate
clomiphene citrate	Clomid
clomipramine HCl	Anafranil
clonazepam	Klonopin
clonidine HCl	Catapres
clonidine HCl inj	Duraclon
clopidogrel bisulfate	Plavix
clorazepate dipotassium	Tranxene
Clorpactin WCS-90	oxychlorosene sodium
clotrimazole	Gyne-Lotrimin Lotrimin Mycelex
clozapine	Clozaril
Clozaril	clozapine
coagulation factor IX (recombinant)	BeneFix
coagulation factor VII a (recombinant)	NovoSeven
coal tar product	Zetar
codeine phosphate; acetaminophen suspension	Capital w/ Codeine Suspension
coenzyme Q10	UbiQGel
Cogentin	benztropine mesylate
Cognex	tacrine HCl
Colace	docusate sodium
Colazal	balsalazide disodium
ColBENEMID (W)	probenecid; colchicine (W)
colchicine tablets	*colchicine tablets*
colchinine inj (W)	*colchicine inj* (W)
colesevelam HCl	Welchol
Colestid	colestipol HCl
colestipol HCl	Colestid
colistimethate sodium	Coly-Mycin M
colistin sulfate; hydrocortisone, and neomycin otic soln	Coly-Mycin S

collagen hemostat	Avitene
collagenase	Santyl
Collyrium	tetrahydrozoline HCl ophth
Colomed	short chain fatty acids enema
Coly-Mycin M	colistimethate sodium
Coly-Mycin S	colistin sulfate; hydrocortisone, and neomycin otic soln
CoLyte	polyethylene glycol-electrolyte soln
CombiPatch	norethindrone acetate; estradiol transdermal
Combivent	ipratropium bromide; albuterol sulfate
Combivir	lamivudine; zidovudine
Combunox	oxycodone HCl, ibuprofen
Compazine	prochlorperazine
Comtan	entacapone
Comvax	*Haemophilus b* conjugate; Hepatitis B vaccine
Concerta	methylphenidate HCl SR
Condylox	podofilox gel
conivaptan HCl	Vaprisol
Copaxone	glatiramer acetate
Cordarone	amiodarone HCl
Coreg	carvedilol
Corgard (WA)	*nadolol*
Corlopam	fenoldopam mesylate
Cortef	hydrocortisone
corticorellin ovine triflutate	Acthrel
corticotropin (W)	Acthar (W)
cortisone acetate	Cortone Acetate
Cortone Acetate	cortisone acetate
Cortrosyn	cosyntropin
Corvert	ibutilide fumarate
Cosmegen	dactinomycin
Cosopt	dorzolamide HCl; timolol maleate ophth soln
cosyntropin	Cortrosyn
Cotazym (W)	*pancrelipase*
Cotazym-S (W)	*pancrelipase EC*
Cotrim	sulfamethoxazole; trimethoprim
co-trimoxazole	Bactrim Cotrim Septra sulfamethoxazole; trimethoprim
Coumadin	warfarin sodium
Covera HS	verapamil HCl SR bedtime formulation
Cozaar	losartan potassium
Crestor	rosuvastatin calcium

Crinone	progesterone gel
Crixivan	indinavir
CroFab	crotalidae polyvalent immune fab (ovine)
cromolyn sodium	Gastrocrom Nasalcrom Opticrom
crotalidae polyvalent immune fab (ovine)	CroFab
crotamiton	Eurax
Cubicin	daptomycin
Cuprimine	penicillamine
Curosurf	poractant alpha intratracheal susp
Cutivate	fluticasone propionate cream & ointment
cyanocobalamin nasal gel	Nascobal
cyclobenzaprine HCl	Flexeril
cyclobenzaprine SR	Amrix
Cyclocort (W)	amcinonide (W)
Cyclogyl	cyclopentolate HCl
cyclopentolate HCl	Cyclogyl
cyclophosphamide	Cytoxan Neosar
cycloserine	Seromycin
cyclosporine	Sandimmune
cyclosporine capsules (modified) and oral soln	Neoral
cyclosporine capsules, (modified)	Gengraf
cyclosporine ophth emulsion	Restasis
Cycrin (WA)	*medroxyprogesterone acetate*
Cylert (WA)	pemoline
Cymbalta	duloxetine HCl
Cypher stent	sirolimus-eluting stent
cyproheptadine HCl	*cyproheptadine HCl*
Cystadane	betaine anhydrous
Cytadren (W)	*aminoglutethimide*
cytarabine	*cytarabine*
cytarabine, liposomal inj	DepoCyt
Cytomel	liothyronine sodium
Cytosar-U (W)	*cytarabine*
Cytotec	misoprostol
Cytovene	ganciclovir
Cytoxan	cyclophosphamide

D

dacarbazine	DTIC-Dome
daclizumab	Zenapax
Dacogen	decitabine inj
dactinomycin	Cosmegen
Dalmane (WA)	*flurazepam HCl*
dalteparin sodium	Fragmin
danaparoid sodium	Orgaran
danazol (W)	Danocrine (W)
Danocrine (W)	danazol (W)
Dantrium	dantrolene sodium
dantrolene sodium	Dantrium
dapsone	dapsone
daptomycin	Cubicin
Daranide (W)	dichlorphenamide (W)
Daraprim	pyrimethamine
darbepoetin alfa	Aranesp
darifenacin	Enablex
darunavir	Prezista
Darvocet-N 100	propoxyphene napsylate; acetaminophen
Darvon	propoxyphene HCl
Darvon Compound 65	propoxyphene HCl; aspirin; caffeine
dasatinib	Sprycel
daunorubicin citrate liposomal	DaunoXome
daunorubicin HCl	Cerubidine
DaunoXome	daunorubicin citrate liposomal
Daypro	oxaprozin
DDAVP	desmopressin acetate
Debrox	carbamide peroxide otic
Decadron	dexamethasone
Deca-Durabolin (W)	nandrolone decanoate (W)
decitabine inj	Dacogen
Declomycin	*demeclocycline HCl*
deferasirox	Exjade
deferoxamine mesylate	Desferal
delavirdine mesylate	Rescriptor
Delestrogen	estradiol valerate
Deltasone (WA)	*prednisone*
Demadex	torsemide
demecarium bromide (W)	Humorsol (W)
demeclocycline HCl	Declomycin
Demerol	meperidine HCl
Demser	metyrosine
Demulen (WA)	ethynodiol diacetate; ethinyl estradiol
Denavir	penciclovir cream
denileukin diftitox	Ontak
Depacon	valproate sodium inj
Depakene	valproic acid
Depakote	divalproex sodium
Depakote ER	divalproex sodium SR
DepoCyt	cytarabine, liposomal inj
DepoDur	morphine sulfate extended-release liposome inj
Depo-Medrol	methylprednisolone acetate SR
Depo-Provera	medroxyprogesterone acetate SR
Depo-Testosterone	testosterone cypionate SR
Desferal	deferoxamine mesylate
desflurane	Suprane
desipramine HCl	Norpramin
Desirudin	iprivask
desloratadine	Clarinex
desmopressin acetate	DDAVP
Desogen	desogestrel; ethinyl estradiol
desogestrel; ethinyl estradiol	Desogen Ortho-Cept
desogestrel and ethinyl estradiol; ethinyl estradiol	Mircette
desonide	Tridesilon
desoximetasone	Topicort
Desoxyn	methamphetamine HCl
desvenlafaxine succinate	Pristiq
Desyrel (WA)	*trazodone HCl*
Detrol	tolterodine tartrate
Detrol LA	tolterodine tartrate (SR)
dexamethasone	Decadron Hexadrol
dexamethasone-eluting stent	Dexamet stent
Dexamet stent	dexamethasone-eluting stent
dexchlorphenir-amine maleate SR	*dexchlorpheniramine maleate* SR
Dexedrine (WA)	*dextroamphetamine sulfate*
dexfenfluramine HCl (W)	Redux (W)
Dexferrum	iron dextran inj
dexmedetomidine HCl inj	Precedex

dexmethylphenidate HCl	Focalin
dexrazoxane	Zinecard
dextroamphetamine sulfate	*dextroamphetamine sulfate*
dextrothyroxine sodium (W)	Choloxin (W)
D.H.E. 45	dihydroergotamine mesylate inj
DiaBeta	glyburide
Diabinese	chlorpropamide
Diamox	acetazolamide
Diapid (W)	lypressin (W)
Diastat	diazepam rectal gel
diazepam	Valium
diazepam emulsified inj	Dizac
diazepam rectal gel	Diastat
diazoxide	Hyperstat
Dibenzyline	phenoxybenzamine HCl
dibucaine	Nupercainal
dichlorphenamide (W)	Daranide (W)
diclofenac gel	Solaraze
diclofenac potassium	Cataflam
diclofenac sodium	Voltaren
diclofenac sodium; misoprostol	Arthrotec
diclofenac sodium SR	Voltaren-XR
dicloxacillin sodium	*dicloxacillin sodium*
dicyclomine HCl	Bentyl
didanosine	Videx
didanosine SR	Videx EC
Didronel	etidronate disodium
diethylcarbamazine citrate	Hetrazan
diethylpropion HCl	*diethylpropion HCl*
Differin	adapalene
diflorasone diacetate	Florone
Diflucan	fluconazole
diflunisal	*diflunisal*
difluprednate ophth emulsion	Durezol
Digibind	digoxin immune fab
digoxin	Lanoxin
digoxin capsules (W)	Lanoxicaps (W)

digoxin immune fab	Digibind
dihydroergotamine mesylate inj	D.H.E. 45
dihydroergotamine mesylate nasal spray	Migranol
dihydrotestosterone transdermal	Androgel2DHT
Dilacor XR	diltiazem HCl SR
Dilantin	phenytoin
Dilaudid	hydromorphone HCl
diltiazem HCl	Cardizem
diltiazem HCl SR	Cardizem CD Cartia XR (WA) Dilacor XR Tiazac
diltiazem maleate SR	Tiamate
dimenhydrinate	Dramamine
dimercaprol	BAL in Oil
Dimetane (WA)	*brompheniramine maleate*
dinoprostone gel	Prepidil
dinoprostone vaginal insert	Cervidil
dinoprostone vaginal suppositories	Prostin E2
Diovan	valsartan
Diovan HCT	valsartan; hydrochlorothiazide
Dipentum	olsalazine sodium
diphenhydramine HCl	Benadryl
diphenoxylate HCl; atropine sulfate	Lomotil
diphtheria, tetanus, and acellular pertussis (TdaP) vaccine (adult type)	Adacel
dipivefrin	Propine
Diprivan	propofol
Diprosone	betamethasone dipropionate
dipyridamole	Persantine
dirithromycin	Dynabac
Disalcid	salsalate
disopyramide phosphate	Norpace
disulfiram	Antabuse
Ditropan	oxybutynin chloride
Diulo (WA)	metolazone
Diuril	chlorothiazide
divalproex sodium	Depakote

divalproex sodium SR	Depakote ER
Dizac	diazepam emulsified inj
dobutamine HCl	Dobutrex
Dobutrex	dobutamine HCl
docetaxel	Taxotere
docosanol cream (W)	Avanir (W)
docusate sodium	Colace
docusate sodium; casanthranol	Peri-Colace
dofetilide	Tikosyn
dolasetron mesylate	Anzemet
Dolobid (WA)	*diflunisal*
Dolophine	methadone HCl
Domeboro	aluminum acetate
donepezil HCl	Aricept
Donnatal (W)	belladonna alkaloids; phenobarbital
dopamine HCl	Intropin (WA)
Dopar	levodopa
Dopram	doxapram HCl
Doribax	doripenem
doripenem	Doribax
dornase alpha	Pulmozyme
Doryx	doxycycline hyclate SR
dorzolamide HCI	Trusopt
dorzolamide HCl; timolol maleate ophth soln	Cosopt
Dostinex (W)	cabergoline (W)
Dovonex	calcipotriene cream
doxacurium chloride (W)	Nuromax (W)
doxapram HCl	Dopram
doxazosin mesylate	Cardura
doxepin HCl	*doxepin HCl* Sinequan
doxepin HCl cream	Prudoxin
doxercalciferol	Hectorol
Doxil	doxorubicin, liposomal
doxorubicin HCl	Adriamycin Rubex
doxorubicin, liposomal	Doxil
doxycycline hyclate	Vibramycin
doxycycline hyclate 20 mg tab & cap	Periostat
doxycycline hyclate gel	Atridox
doxycycline hyclate SR	Doryx
Dramamine	dimenhydrinate
Drisdol	ergocalciferol
Dristan Long Lasting	oxymetazoline HCl
Drixoral Syrup	pseudoephedrine HCl; bromphiramine maleate
dronabinol	Marinol
droperidol	Inapsine
drospirenone; ethinyl estradiol	Yasmin
drotrecogin alfa	Xigris
Droxia	hydroxyurea
DTIC-Dome	dacarbazine
Dulcolax	bisacodyl
duloxetine HCl	Cymbalta
Durabolin (W)	nandrolone phenpropionate (W)
Duraclon	clonidine HCl inj
Duragesic	fentanyl transdermal
Durezol	difluprednate ophth emulsion
Duramorph	morphine sulfate inj
Duranest (W)	etidocaine HCl (W)
Duricef	cefadroxil
dutasteride	Avodart
Dyazide	triamterene 37.5 mg; hydrochlorothiazide 25 mg
Dymelor (W)	acetohexamide (W)
Dynabac	dirithromycin
DynaCirc	isradipine
Dynapen (WA)	*dicloxacillin sodium*
dyphylline	Lufyllin
Dyrenium	triamterene

E

EchoGen	perflenapent emulsion
echothiophate iodide (W)	Phospholine Iodide (W)
Ecotrin	aspirin EC
eculizumab	Soliris
Edecrin	ethacrynic acid
edetate disodium	Endrate
Edex	alprostadil inj
edrophonium chloride	Tensilon
E.E.S. 400	erythromycin ethylsuccinate
efalizumab	Raptiva
efaproxiral	Efaproxyn
Efaproxyn	efaproxiral
efavirenz	Sustiva

efavirenz, emtricitabine, and tenofovir	Atripla
Effexor	venlafaxine HCl
Effexor XR	venlafaxine HCl SR
eflornithine HCl cream	Vaniqa
Efudex	fluorouracil cream; soln
Elaprase	idursulfase
Elavil (WA)	*amitriptyline HCl*
Eldepryl	selegiline HCl
Eldisine	vindesine sulfate
Elestat	epinastine
eletriptan hydrobromide	Relpax
Elidel	pimecrolimus cream
Eligard	leuprolide acetate
Elitek	rasburicase
Elixophyllin	theophylline
Ellence	epirubicin HCl
Elmiron	pentosan polysulfate sodium
Elocon	mometasone furoate topical
Eloxatin	oxaliplatin
Elspar	asparaginase
Emadine	emedastine difumarate opthth soln
Emcyt	estramustine phosphate sodium
emedastine difumarate opthth soln	Emadine
Emend capsule	aprepitant
Emend inj	fosaprepitant
EMLA Cream	lidocaine; prilocaine cream
Empirin with codeine #3 and #4	aspirin 325 mg with codeine phosphate (30 and 60 mg)
emtricitabine	Emtriva
emtricitabine, efavirenz, and tenofovir	Atripla
emtricitabine; tenofovir disoproxil	Truvada
Emtriva	emtricitabine
E-Mycin (WA)	*erythromycin*
Enablex	darifenacin
enalapril maleate	Vasotec
enalapril maleate; diltiazem malate (W)	Teczem (W)
enalapril maleate; felodipine SR (W)	Lexxel (W)

enalapril maleate; hydrochlorothiazide	Vaseretic
Enbrel	etanercept
encainide HCl (W)	Enkaid (W)
Endep	amitriptyline HCl
Endocet	oxycodone HCl; acetaminophen
Endrate	edetate disodium
Enduron	methyclothiazide
enflurane	Ethrane
enfuvirtide	Fuzeon
Engerix-B	hepatitis B vaccine
Enkaid (W)	encainide HCl (W)
enoxaparin sodium	Lovenox
entacapone	Comtan
entecavir	Baraclude
Entereg	alvimopam
Entex LA	phenylpropanolamine HCl; guaifenesin SR
Entocort EC	budesonide capsule SR
Eovist	gadoxetate disodium inj
epinastine	Elestat
epinephrine	Adrenalin
epinephrine racemic (W)	Vaponefrin (W)
epirubicin HCl	Ellence
Epivir	lamivudine
Epivir HBV	lamivudine
eplerenone	Inspra
epoetin alfa	Epogen Procrit
Epogen	epoetin alfa
epoprostenol sodium	Flolan
eprosartan mesylate	Teveten
eprosartan mesylate; hydrochlorothiazide	Teveten HCT
eptifibatide	Integrilin
Epzicom	lamivudine; abacavir sulfate
Equanil (WA)	meprobamate
Eraxis	anidulafungin IV
Erbitux	cetuximab
Ergamisol (W)	levamisole HCl (W)
ergocalciferol	Calciferol Drisdol
ergoloid mesylates	Hydergine
ergotamine tartrate; caffeine	Cafergot
ergotamine tartrate	Ergostat

Ergotrate	ergonovine maleate
erlotinib	Tarceva
Ertaczo	sertaconazole
ertapenem sodium	Invanz
Ery-Tab	erythromycin EC
Erythrocin Stearate	erythromycin stearate
erythromycin	*erythromycin*
erythromycin base coated particles	PCE Dispertab
erythromycin; benzoyl peroxide topical gel	Benzamycin
erythromycin EC	Ery-Tab
erythromycin estolate (W)	Ilosone (W)
erythromycin ethylsuccinate	E.E.S. 400
erythromycin ethylsuccinate; sulfisoxazole	Pediazole
erythromycin stearate	Erythrocin Stearate
escitalopram oxalate	Lexapro
Esclim	estradiol transdermal
Eserine Sulfate	physostigmine ophth ointment
Esidrix (WA)	hydrochlorothiazide
Esimil (W)	guanethidine monosulfate; hydrochlorothiazide (W)
Eskalith (WA)	*lithium carbonate*
esmolol HCl	Brevibloc
esomeprazole magnesium	Nexium
estazolam	*estazolam*
Estinyl (WA)	*ethinyl estradiol*
Estrace	estradiol
Estraderm	estradiol transdermal
estradiol	Estrace
estradiol hemihydrate vaginal tab	Vagifem
estradiol transdermal	Alora
	Climara
	Esclim
	Estraderm
	FemPatch (W)
	Menostar
	Vivelle
estradiol vaginal ring	Estring
estradiol valerate	Delestrogen
estramustine phosphate sodium	Emcyt
Estratest	estrogens, esterified; methyltestosterone
Estratest H.S.	estrogens, esterified; methyltestosterone, half strength
Estring	estradiol vaginal ring
estrogens, conjugated	Premarin
estrogens conjugate, A synthetic	Cenestin
estrogens, conjugated; medroxyprogesterone acetate	Premphase
	Prempro
estrogens, esterified; methyltestosterone	Estratest
estrogens, esterified methyltestosterone, half strength	Estratest H.S.
estropipate	Ogen
Estrostep	norethindrone acetate; ethinyl estradiol
eszopiclone	Lunesta
etanercept	Enbrel
ethacrynic acid	Edecrin
ethambutol HCl	Myambutol
ethchlorvynol (W)	Placidyl (W)
Ethezyme	papain; urea oint
ethinyl estradiol	Estinyl (WA)
ethinyl estradiol; levonorgestrel (91 day cycle)	Seasonale
ethionamide	Trecator-SC
Ethmozine	moricizine
ethopropazine HCl	Parsidol
ethosuximide	Zarontin
Ethrane	enflurane
ethyl chloride	ethyl chloride
ethynodiol diacetate; ethinyl estradiol	Demulen
Ethyol	amifostine
etidocaine HCl (W)	Duranest (W)
etidronate disodium	Didronel
etodolac	*etodolac*
etodolac SR	*etodolac SR*
etomidate	Amidate

etonogestrel; ethinyl estradiol vagina ring	NuvaRing
etonogestrel implant	Implanon
Etopophos	etoposide phosphate diethanolate
etoposide	VePesid
etoposide phosphate diethanolate	Etopophos
Etrafon	perphenazine; amitriptyline HCl
etravirine	Intelence
Eulexin (W)	flutamide (W)
Eurax	crotamiton
Euthroid (WA)	liotrix
Eutonyl	pargyline HCl
Evista	raloxifene HCl
Evithrom	thrombin, topical (human)
Evoxac	cevimeline HCl
Exelon	rivastigmine tartrate
exemestane	Aromasin
exenatide inj	Byetta
Exforge	amlodipine; valsartan
exisulind (W)	Aposyn (W)
Exjade	deferasirox
Ex-Lax	sennosides
Extraneal	icodextrin 7.5% with electrolyte peritoneal dialysis soln
ezetimibe	Zetia
ezetimibe; simvastatin	Vytorin

F

Fabrazyme	agalsidase beta
Factive	gemifloxacin mesylate
factor IX, concentrate	BeneFix
Factrel	gonadorelin HCl
famciclovir	Famvir
famotidine	Pepcid
famotidine, oral disintegrating tablet	Pepcid RPD
Famvir	famciclovir
Fansidar	sulfadoxine; pyrimethamine
Fareston	toremifene citrate
Faslodex	fulvestrant
Fastin	phentermine HCl
fat emulsion	Intralipid Liposyn II and III
felbamate	Felbatol
Felbatol	felbamate
Feldene	piroxicam
felodipine	Plendil
Femara	letrozole
Femhrt	norethindrone acetate; ethinyl estradiol
FemPatch (WA)	estradiol transdermal
fenfluramine HCl (W)	Pondimin (W)
fenofibrate	Tricor
fenoldopam mesylate	Corlopam
fenoprofen calcium	Nalfon
fentanyl citrate	Sublimaze
fentanyl citrate; droperidol (W)	Innovar (W)
fentanyl iontophoretic transdermal system	Ionsys
Fentanyl Oralet (W)	fentanyl transmucosal (W)
fentanyl transdermal	Duragesic
fentanyl transmucosal (W)	Actiq Fentanyl Oralet (W)
Feosol	ferrous sulfate
Fer-In-Sol	ferrous sulfate
Fergon	ferrous gluconate
Feridex	ferumoxide HCl
Ferrlecit	sodium ferric gluconate complex in sucrose inj
ferrous gluconate	Fergon
ferrous sulfate	Feosol Fer-In-Sol
ferrous sulfate SR	SlowFe
Fertinex	urofollitropin for inj
ferumoxetil oral suspension (W)	Gastromark (W)
ferumoxide HCl	Feridex
fexofenadine HCl	Allegra
filgrastim	Neupogen
finasteride	Propecia 1 mg tablet Proscar 5 mg tablet
Finevin	azelaic cream
Fioricet	butalbital; acetaminophen; caffeine
Fiorinal	butalbital; aspirin; caffeine
Flagyl	metronidazole
Flagyl ER	metronidazole SR
flavocoxid	Limbrel
flavoxate HCl	Urispas
Flaxedil	gallamine triethiodide
flecainide acetate	Tambocor

Flexeril	cyclobenzaprine HCl
Flolan	epoprostenol sodium
Flomax	tamsulosin HCl
Flonase	fluticasone propionate spray
Florinef	fludrocortisone acetate
Florone	diflorasone diacetate
Floropryl (W)	isoflurophate (W)
Florotag (W)	synopinine (W)
Flovent (WA)	fluticasone propionate spray
Floxin	ofloxacin
Floxin Otic	ofloxacin otic soln
floxuridine	FUDR
fluconazole	Diflucan
flucytosine	Ancobon
Fludara	fludarabine phosphate
fludarabine phosphate	Fludara
fludrocortisone acetate	Florinef
Flumadine	rimantadine
flumazenil	Romazicon
flunisolide	Aero Bid
fluocinolone acetonide	Synalar
fluocinonide	Lidex
Fluor-I-Strip	fluorescein sodium strips
fluorescein sodium soln	Fluorescite
fluorescein sodium strips	Fluor-I-Strip
Fluorescite	fluorescein sodium soln
fluorometholone	FML
Fluoroplex	fluorouracil cream; soln
fluorouracil cream	Carac
fluorouracil inj	*fluorouracil inj*
fluorouracil cream; soln	Efudex Fluoroplex
Fluothane	halothane
fluoxetine HCl	Prozac Sarafem
fluoxymesterone (W)	Halotestin (W)
fluphenazine HCl	*fluphenazine HCl*
flurazepam HCl	*flurazepam HCl*
flurbiprofen	Ansaid
flutamide (W)	Eulexin (W)
fluticasone propionate spray	Flonase Flovent (WA)
fluticasone propionate cream & ointment	Cutivate
fluticasone propionate; salmeterol inhalation powder	Advair Diskus

fluvastatin sodium	Lescol
fluvoxamine maleate SR	Luvox CR
FML	fluorometholone
Focalin	dexmethylphenidate HCl
Folex PFS	methotrexate inj
folic acid	Folvite
Follistim	follitropin beta
follitropin alfa	Gonal-F
follitropin beta	Follistim
Folvite	folic acid
fomepizole	Antizol
fomivirsen sodium inj (W)	Vitravene (W)
fondaparinux sodium	Arixtra
Foradil	formoterol fumarate
Forane	isoflurane
formoterol fumarate	Foradil
Fortaz	ceftazidime
Forteo	teriparatide
Fortovase (W)	saquinavir soft gel capsule (W)
Fosamax	alendronate sodium
fosamprenavir calcium	Lexiva
fosaprepitant	Emend inj
foscarnet	Foscavir
Foscavir	foscarnet
fosfomycin tromethamine	Monurol
fosinopril sodium	Monopril
fosphenytoin sodium	Cerebyx
Fosrenol	lanthanum carbonate
Fragmin	dalteparin sodium
Frova	frovatriptan succinate
frovatriptan succinate	Frova
FUDR	floxuridine
fulvestrant	Faslodex
Fulvicin P/G	griseofulvin
Fungizone (W)	amphotericin B (W)
Furacin	nitrofurazone
furosemide	Lasix
Fuzeon	enfuvirtide

G

gabapentin	Neurontin
Gabitril	tiagabine HCl
gadoteridol	ProHance

gadoversetamide	OptiMark
gadoxetate disodium inj	Eovist
galantamine HBr	Razadyne (formerly called Reminyl)
gallamine triethiodide (W)	Flaxedil (W)
gallium nitrate	Ganite
galsulfase	Naglazyme
Galzin	zinc acetate
Gamimune N	immune globulin intravenous
Gammagard S/D	immune globulin intravenous
ganciclovir	Cytovene
ganciclovir ophthalmic implant (W)	Vitrasert (W)
ganirelix acetate	Antagon
Ganite	gallium nitrate
Gantanol (W)	sulfamethoxazole (W)
Garamycin	*gentamicin sulfate*
Gardasil	quadrivalent human papillomavirus (types 6, 11, 16, 18) recombinant vaccine
Gastrocrom	cromolyn sodium
Gastromark (W)	ferumoxetil oral suspension (W)
gatifloxacin (W)	Tequin (W)
gatifloxacin ophth soln	Zymar
gefitinib	Iressa
gemcitabine HCl	Gemzar
gemfibrozil	*gemfibrozil*
gemifloxacin mesylate	Factive
gemtuzumab ozogamicin	Mylotarg
Gemzar	gemcitabine HCl
GenEsa (W)	arbutamine HCl (W)
Gengraf	cyclosporine capsules, (modified)
Genotropin	somatropin for inj
gentamicin sulfate	Garamycin
Geocillin (W)	carbenicillin (W)
Geodon	ziprasidone HCl
Geref	sermorelin acetate
glatiramer acetate	Copaxone
Gleevec	imatinib mesylate
Gliadel	carmustine implantable wafer
glimepiride	Amaryl
glipizide	Glucotrol
glipizide SR	Glucotrol XL

glipizide; metformin	Metaglip
GlucaGen	glucagon (rDNA origin)
glucagon	glucagon
glucagon (rDNA origin)	GlucaGen
Glucophage	metformin HCl
Glucophage XR	metformin HCl SR
Glucotrol	glipizide
Glucotrol XL	glipizide SR
Glucovance	glyburide; metformin HCl
glyburide	DiaBeta Micronase
glyburide; metformin HCl	Glucovance
glyburide micronized	Glynase
glycerin ophth soln	Ophthalgan
glycopyrrolate	Robinul
Glynase	glyburide micronized
Glyset	miglitol
gold sodium thiomalate	Aurolate Myochrysine
GoLYTELY	polyethylene glycol-electrolyte soln
gonadorelin HCl	Factrel
Gonal-F	follitropin alfa
goserelin acetate implant	Zoladex
graftskin (W)	Apligraf (W)
granisetron HCl	Kytril
grepafloxacin HCl (W)	Raxar (W)
Grifulvin V	griseofulvin microsize
griseofulvin microsize	Grifulvin V
guaifenesin	Organidin NR Robitussin
guaifenesin; codeine phosphate	Robitussin A-C Tussi-Organidin NR
guaifenesin; dextromethorphan	Robitussin-DM
guanabenz acetate	Wytensin
guanadrel sulfate	Hylorel
guanethidine monosulfate (W)	Ismelin (W)
guanethidine monosulfate; hydrochlorothiazide	Esimil
guanfacine HCl	Tenex

Gynazole	butoconazole nitrate vaginal cream
Gyne-Lotrimin	clotrimazole

H

Habitrol	nicotine transdermal system
Haemophilus b conjugate vaccine reconstituted with diphtheria and tetanus toxoids and acellular pertussis vaccine adsorbed	ActHIB/Tripedia
Haemophilus b conjugate; Hepatitis B vaccine	Comvax
halcinonide	Halog
Halcion	triazolam
Haldol	haloperidol
Halfan	halofantrine HCl
halofantrine HCl	Halfan
Halog	halcinonide
haloperidol	Haldol
haloprogin (W)	Halotex (W)
Halotestin (W)	fluoxymesterone (W)
Halotex (W)	haloprogin (W)
halothane	Fluothane
Havrix	hepatitis A vaccine, inactivated
Healon	sodium hyaluronate
Hectorol	doxercalciferol
Helidac	bismuth subsalicylate; metronidazole; tetracycline HCl
heparin sodium	*heparin sodium*
hepatitis A inactivated; hepatitis B (recombinant) vaccine	Twinrix
hepatitis A vaccine, inactivated	Havrix Vaqta
hepatitis B immune globulin (human)	NABI-HB
hepatitis B vaccine	Engerix-B Recombivax HB
Hepsera	adefovir dipivoxil
Herceptin	trastuzumab
Herplex (W)	idoxuridine (W)
Hespan	hetastarch
hetastarch	Hespan
hetastarch in lactated electrolyte inj (W)	Hextend (W)
Hetrazan	diethylcarbamazine citrate
Hexadrol	dexamethasone
Hexalen	altretamine
Hextend (W)	hetastarch in lactated electrolyte inj (W)
Hibiclens	chlorhexidine gluconate
Hiprex	methenamine hippurate
Hismanal (W)	astemizole (W)
Hivid (W)	zalcitabine (W)
homatropine hydrobromide ophth	Isopto Homatropine
Humalog	insulin, lispro (human)
Humalog Mix75/25	insulin lispro protamine susp 75%; insulin lispro inj 25% [rDNA origin]
Humatin	paromomycin sulfate
Humatrope	somatropin
Humira	adalimumab
Humorsol (W)	demecarium bromide (W)
Humulin 70/30	isophane insulin suspension 70%, insulin inj 30% (human)
Humulin L (W)	insulin zinc suspension (Lente) (human) (W)
Humulin N	isophane insulin suspension (NPH) (human)
Humulin R	insulin inj (human)
Humulin U Ultralente (W)	insulin zinc suspension, extended, (human) (W)
Hurricane	benzocaine
Hyalgan	sodium hyaluronate
hyaluronidase	Wydase
Hycamtin	topotecan HCl
Hydergine	ergoloid mesylates
hydralazine HCl	Apresoline
hydralazine HCl; hydrochlorothiazide	Apresazide
hydralazine; hydrochlorothiazide; reserpine (W)	Ser-Ap-Es (W)
Hydrea	hydroxyurea
hydrochlorothiazide	Esidrix (WA) HydroDIURIL Microzide Oretic (WA)

hydrocodone bitartrate; acetaminophen	Anexsia 5/500 Anexsia 7.5/650 Lorcet 10/650 Lorcet-HD (5/500) Lorcet plus (7.5/650) Lortab 2.5/500; 5/500; 7.5/500; 10/500 Norco Vicodin Vicodin ES Zydone 5/400, 7.5/400, 10/400
hydrocodone bitartrate 7.5 mg; ibuprofen 200 mg	Vicoprofen
hydrocodone polistirex; chlorphenira-mine	Tussionex
hydrocortisone	Cortef Hydrocortone
hydrocortisone buteprate cream	Pandel
hydrocortisone sodium succinate	Solu-Cortef
Hydrocortone	hydrocortisone
HydroDIURIL	hydrochlorothiazide
hydroflumethia-zide (W)	Saluron (W)
hydromorphone HCl	Dilaudid
hydromorphone HCl SR	*hydromorphone HCl SR*
Hydromox (W)	quinethazone (W)
hydroquinone topical susp (W)	Alustra (W)
hydroquinone; tretinoin; fluocinolone cream	Tri-Luma
hydroxychloro-quine sulfate	Plaquenil
hydroxyurea	Droxia Hydrea
hydroxyzine HCl	Atarax (WA)
hydroxyzine pamoate	Vistaril
Hygroton	chlorthalidone
hylan G-F 20	Synvisc
Hylorel	guanadrel sulfate
hyoscyamine sulfate orally disintegrating tab	NuLev
hyoscyamine sulfate SR	Cystospaz-M (WA) Levbid
Hyperab (W)	rabies immune globulin, human
Hyperstat	diazoxide
Hyper-Tet (W)	tetanus immune globulin (human) (W)
Hytrin	terazosin HCl
Hyzaar	losartan potassium; hydrochlorothiazide

I

ibandronate	Boniva
ibritumomab tiuxetan	Zevalin
ibuprofen	Advil Motrin
ibutilide fumarate	Corvert
icodextrin 7.5% with electro-lyte peritoneal dialysis soln	Extraneal
Idamycin	idarubicin
idarubicin	Idamycin
idoxuridine (W)	Herplex (W)
idursulfase	Elaprase
IFEX	ifosfamide
ifosfamide	IFEX
iloprost	Ventavis
Ilosone	erythromycin estolate
Imagent GI	perflubron
imatinib mesylate	Gleevec
imciromab pentetate	Myoscint
Imdur	isosorbide mononitrate SR
imiglucerase	Cerezyme
imipenem-cilastatin sodium	Primaxin
imipramine HCl	Tofranil
imiquimod cream	Aldara
Imitrex	sumatriptan
immune globulin intravenous	Gamimune N Gammagard S/D
Imodium	loperamide HCl
Imogam	rabies immune globulin, human
Implanon	etonogestrel implant
Imuran	azathioprine
inamrinone lactate	*inamrinone lactate*

Inapsine	droperidol
indapamide	Lozol
Inderal	propranolol HCl
Inderide (W)	propranolol HCl; hydrochlorothiazide (W)
indinavir	Crixivan
indium In-111 pentetreotide	OctreoScan
Indocin	indomethacin
indomethacin	Indocin
Infasurf	calfactant intratracheal susp
INFeD	iron dextran inj
Infergen	interferon alfacon-1
infliximab	Remicade
influenza vaccine	Afluria
Innohep	tinzaparin sodium
Innovar (W)	fentanyl citrate; droperidol (W)
Inocor (WA)	*inamrinone lactate*
INOmax	nitric oxide for inhalation
Inspra	eplerenone
insulin aspart (rDNA origin)	NovoLog
insulin detemir [rDNA origin]	Levemir
insulin glargine (rDNA origin)	Lantus
insulin glulisine [rDNA origin]	Apidra
insulin inj (human)	Humulin R Novolin R Velosulin Human
insulin lispro (human)	Humalog
insulin lispro protamine susp 75%; insulin lispro inj 25% [rDNA origin]	Humalog Mix75/25
insulin zinc suspension (Lente) (human) (W)	Humulin L (W) Novolin L (W)
insulin zinc suspension, extended (beef)	Ultralente U
insulin zinc suspension, extended, (human)	Humulin U Ultralente
Integrilin	eptifibatide
Intelence	etravirine
interferon alfa-2a (W)	Roferon-A (W)

interferon alfa-2b	Intron A
interferon alfa-n[1] lymphoblastoid	Wellferon
interferon alfa-n3 (human leukocyte derived)	Alferon
interferon alfacon-1	Infergen
interferon beta-la	Avonex Rebif
interferon beta-1b	Betaseron
interferon gamma 1-b	Actimmune
Intrachol	choline chloride inj
Intralipid	fat emulsion
Intron A	interferon alfa-2b
Intropin (WA)	dopamine HCl
Invanz	ertapenem sodium
Invega	paliperidone
Inversine	mecamylamine HCl
Invirase	saquinavir mesylate
iocetamic acid	Cholebrine
iodamide meglumine	Renovue 65
iodixanol	Visipaque
iohexol	Omnipaque
Ionamin	phentermine resin
Ionsys	fentanyl iontophoretic transdermal system
iopamidol	Isovue
iopanoic acid (W)	Telepaque (W)
iopromide	Ultravist
iotrolan	Osmovist
ioversol	Optiray
ioxilan (W)	Oxilan (W)
Iplex	mecasermin rinfabate
Ipol	poliovirus vaccine inactivated
ipratropium bromide	Atrovent
ipratropium bromide; albuterol sulfate	Combivent
iprivask	Desirudin
irbesartan	Avapro
irbesartan; hydrochlorothiazide	Avalide
Iressa	gefitinib
irinotecan HCl	Camptosar
iron dextran inj	INFeD Dexferrum
iron sucrose inj	Venofer
Isentress	raltegravir

Ismelin	guanethidine monosulfate
ISMO	isosorbide mononitrate
isocarboxazid	Marplan
isoetharine HCl aerosol	*isoetharine HCl aerosol*
isoetharine HCl soln	*isoetharine HCl soln*
isoflurane	Forane
isoflurophate (W)	Floropryl (W)
isoniazid	Nydrazid
isoniazid; rifampin	Rifamate
isophane insulin suspension (NPH) (human)	Humulin N Novolin N
isophane insulin suspension (NPH) 70%, insulin inj 30% (human)	Humulin 70/30 Novolin 70/30
isoproterenol HCl	Isuprel
Isoptin	verapamil HCl
Isopto Carbachol	carbachol ophth
Isopto Carpine	pilocarpine HCl ophth
Isopto Homatropine	homatropine hydrobromide ophth
Isopto Hyoscine	scopolamine hydrobromide ophth
Isordil	isosorbide dinitrate
isosorbide dinitrate	Isordil
isosorbide dinitrate; hydralazine	BiDil
isosorbide mononitrate	ISMO
isosorbide mononitrate SR	Imdur
isotretinoin	Accutane
Isovue	iopamidol
isoxsuprine HCl	Vasodilan
isradipine	DynaCirc
Isuprel	isoproterenol HCl
itraconazole	Sporanox
ivermectin	Stromectol
IvyBlock	bentoquatam
ixabepilone	Ixempra
Ixempra	ixabepilone

J

Januvia	sitagliptin

K

Kadian	morphine sulfate SR
Kaletra	lopinavir; ritonavir
kanamycin sulfate	Kantrex
Kantrex	kanamycin sulfate
Kaon	potassium gluconate
Kaon-Cl	potassium chloride SR
Kayexalate	polystyrene sulfonate sodium
K-Dur	potassium chloride SR
Keflex	cephalexin
Keflin (W)	cephalothin sodium (W)
Keftab (W)	cephalexin HCl (W)
Kefurox (W)	cefuroxime sodium
Kefzol (WA)	*cefazolin sodium*
Kemadrin	procyclidine HCl
Kenalog	triamcinolone acetonide
Kepivance	palifermin
Keppra	levetiracetam
Kerlone	betaxolol
Ketalar	ketamine HCl
ketamine HCL	Ketalar
Ketek	telithromycin
ketoconazole	Nizoral
ketoprofen	Orudis (WA)
ketoprofen SR	Oruvail (WA)
ketorolac tromethamine	Toradol
ketorolac tromethamine ophth	Acular
ketotifen fumarate ophth soln	Zaditor
Kineret	anakinra
Klaron	sodium sulfacetamide lotion
Klonopin	clonazepam
Klor-Con 10	potassium chloride SR
K-Lyte	potassium bicarbonate; potassium citrate effervescent
K-Lyte/Cl	potassium chloride potassium bicarbonate effervescent
Kogenate	antihemophilic factor (recombinant)
Kolyum	potassium chloride; potassium gluconate
Konsyl-D	psyllium
Kuvan	sapropterin dihydrochloride
Kwell (WA)	*lindane*
Kytril	granisetron HCl

L

labetalol HCl	Normodyne Trandate
Lac-Hydrin	lactic acid; ammonium lactate lotion
lactic acid; ammonium lactate lotion	Lac-Hydrin
lactulose	Cephulac Chronulac
Lamictal	lamotrigine
Lamisil	terbinafine HCl
lamivudine	Epivir Epivir HBV
lamivudine; abacavir sulfate	Epzicom
lamivudine; zidovudine	Combivir
lamivudine; zidovudine; abacavir sulfate	Trizivir
lamotrigine	Lamictal
Lanoxicaps (W)	digoxin capsules (W)
Lanoxin	digoxin
lanreotide	Somatuline
lansoprazole	Prevacid
lansoprazole; amoxicillin; clarithromycin	Prevpac
lanthanum carbonate	Fosrenol
Lantus	insulin glargine (rDNA origin)
lapatinib	Tykerb
Lariam	mefloquine HCl
Larodopa	levodopa
laronidase	Aldurazyme
Lasix	furosemide
latanoprost	Xalatan
leflunomide	Arava
lenalidomide	Revlimid
lepirudin	Refludan
Lescol	fluvastatin sodium
Letairis	ambrisentan
letrozole	Femara
leucovorin calcium	Wellcovorin (WA)
Leukeran	chlorambucil
Leukine	sargramostim
leuprolide acetate	Eligard Lupron
leuprolide acetate implant	Viadur (WA)
Leustatin	cladribine
levalbuterol HCl inhalation soln	Xopenex
levamisole HCl (W)	Ergamisol (W)
Levaquin	levofloxacin
Levbid	hyoscyamine sulfate SR
Levemir	insulin detemir [rDNA origin]
levetiracetam	Keppra
Levitra	vardenafil HCl
Levlite	levonorgestrel; ethinyl estradiol
levobupivacaine	Chirocaine
levocabastine HCl ophth susp (W)	Livostin (W)
levocetirizine	Xylzal
Levo-Dromoran	levorphanol tartrate
levobunolol HCl	Betagan
levocarnitine	Carnitor
levodopa	Dopar Larodopa
levodopa; carbidopa	Parcopa Sinemet
levodopa; carbidopa SR	Sinemet CR
levodopa, carbidopa, and entacapone	Stalevo
levofloxacin	Levaquin
levofloxacin ophth soln	Quixin
levomethadyl acetate HCl (W)	Orlaam (W)
levonorgestrel	Plan B
levonorgestrel; ethinyl estradiol	Alesse Levlite Nordette Preven Emergency Contraceptive Kit Tri-Levlen Triphasil
levonorgestrel implant (W)	Norplant (W)
levonorgestrel-releasing intrauterine system	Mirena
Levophed	norepinephrine bitartrate
levorphanol tartrate	Levo-Dromoran
levothyroxine sodium	Levoxyl Synthroid
Levoxyl	levothyroxine sodium
Levulan Kerastick	aminolevulinic acid HCl topical soln

Lexapro	escitalopram oxalate
Lexiscan	regadenoson inj
Lexiva	fosamprenavir calcium
Lexxel	enalapril maleate; felodipine SR
Lialda	mesalamine multimatrix tablets
Librax	*clidinium; chlordiazepoxide*
Librium	chlordiazepoxide HCl
Lidex	fluocinonide
lidocaine HCl	Xylocaine HCl
lidocaine patch	Lidoderm
lidocaine; prilocaine cream	EMLA Cream
Lidoderm	lidocaine patch
Limbitrol	chlordiazepoxide HCl; amitriptyline HCl
Limbrel	flavocoxid
Lincocin	lincomycin HCl
lincomycin HCl	Lincocin
lindane	*lindane*
linezolid	Zyvox
Lioresal	baclofen
liothyronine sodium	Cytomel
liothyronine sodium inj	Triostat
liotrix	Thyrolar
Lipitor	atorvastatin calcium
liposomal amphotericin B	AmBisome
Liposyn II and III	fat emulsion
isdexamfetamine dimesylate	Vyvanse
isinopril	Prinivil Zestril
isinopril; hydrochlorothiazide	Zestoretic
ithium carbonate	*lithium carbonate*
ithium citrate	*lithium citrate*
ithobid	*lithium carbonate*
ithostat	*acetohydroxamic acid*
ivostin (W)	levocabastine HCl ophth susp (W)
odine (WA)	*etodolac*
odine XL (WA)	*etodolac SR*
odoxamide tromethamine ophth soln	Alomide
oestrin	norethindrone acetate; ethinyl estradiol
omefloxacin	Maxaquin

Lomotil	diphenoxylate HCl; atropine sulfate
lomustine	CeeNu
Loniten (W)	minoxidil tablets (W)
Lo/Ovral	norgestrel; ethinyl estradiol
loperamide HCl	Imodium
Lopid	gemfibrozil
lopinavir; ritonavir	Kaletra
Lopressor	metoprolol tartrate
Loprox	ciclopirox cream and lotion
loratadine	Claritin
loratadine; pseudoephedrine sulfate	Claritin D
lorazepam	Ativan
Lorcet (various combinations)	hydrocodone bitartrate; acetaminophen
Lortab (various combinations)	hydrocodone bitartrate; acetaminophen
losartan potassium	Cozaar
losartan potassium; hydrochlorothiazide	Hyzaar
Lotemax	loteprednol etabonate ophth susp
Lotensin	benazepril HCl
loteprednol etabonate ophth susp	Alrex Lotemax
Lotrel	amlodipine besylate; benazepril HCl
Lotrimin	clotrimazole
Lotrisone	betamethasone; clotrimazole cream
Lotronex (W)	alosetron (W)
lovastatin	Mevacor
lovastatin; niacin	Advicor
Lovaza	omega-3-acid ethyl esters
Lovenox	enoxaparin sodium
loxapine succinate	Loxitane
Loxitane	loxapine succinate
Lozol	indapamide
lubiprostone	Amitiza
Lucentis	ranibizumab inj
Ludiomil (WA)	*maprotiline HCl*
Lufyllin	dyphylline
LumenHance	manganese chloride
Lunelle (W)	medroxyprogesterone acetate; estradiol cypionate inj (W)
Lunesta	eszopiclone
Lupron	leuprolide acetate

Luride	sodium fluoride
lutropin alfa	Luveris
Luveris	lutropin alfa
Luvox CR	fluvoxamine maleate SR
Luxiq	betamethasone valerate (foam)
Lyrica	pregabalin
Lyme disease vaccine (W)	LYMErix (W)
LYMErix (W)	Lyme disease vaccine (W)
lymphocyte immune globulin	Atgam
lypressin (W)	Diapid (W)
Lysodren	mitotane

M

Maalox	aluminum hydroxide; magnesium hydroxide
Macrobid	nitrofurantoin macrocrystals and monohydrate
Macrodantin	nitrofurantoin macrocrystals
Macugen	pegaptanib
magaldrate	Riopan
manganese chloride	LumenHance
Magnacet	oxycodone; acetaminophen
magnesium chloride SR	Slow-Mag
magnesium oxide	MAG-OX 400
magnesium sulfate	magnesium sulfate
MAG-OX 400	magnesium oxide
Malarone	atovaquone; proguanil HCl
Mandol (W)	cefamandole nafate (W)
mangafodipir trisodium	Teslascan
maprotiline HCl	*maprotiline HCl*
maraviroc	Selzentry
Marcaine HCl	bupivacaine HCl
Marinol	dronabinol
Marplan	isocarboxazid
Matulane	procarbazine HCl
Mavik	trandolapril
Maxalt	rizatriptan benzoate
Maxalt-MLT	rizatriptan oral disintegrating tablet
Maxaquin	lomefloxacin
Maxipime	cefepime HCl
Maxzide	triamterene 75 mg; hydrochlorothiazide 50 mg
Maxzide-25MG	triamterene 37.5 mg; hydrochlorothiazide 25 mg

mazindol	Sanorex
measles, mumps, rubella vaccines, combined	M-M-R II
Mebaral	mephobarbital
mebendazole	Vermox
mecamylamine HCl	Inversine
mecasermin rinfabate	Iplex
mechlorethamine HCl	Mustargen
Meclan (W)	meclocycline sulfosalicylate (W)
meclizine	Antivert
meclocycline sulfosalicylate (W)	Meclan (W)
meclofenamate sodium	*meclofenamate sodium*
Meclomen (W)	*meclofenamate sodium*
Medrol	methylprednisolone
medroxyprogesterone acetate	Cycrin (W) Provera
medroxyprogesterone acetate; estradiol cypionate inj (W)	Lunelle (W)
medroxyprogesterone acetate SR	Depo-Provera
mefenamic acid	Ponstel
mefloquine HCl	Lariam
Mefoxin	cefoxitin sodium
Megace	megestrol acetate
megestrol acetate	Megace
Mellaril (WA)	thioridazine HCl
meloxicam	Mobic
melphalan	Alkeran
memantine HCl	Namenda
Menactra	meningococcal vaccine
menadiol sodium diphosphate	Synkayvite
meningococcal vaccine	Menactra Menomune
Menomune	meningococcal vaccine
Menostar	estradiol transdermal system
menotropins	Pergonal (WA) Repronex
Mentax	butenafine HCl
meperidine HCl	Demerol
mephentermine sulfate (W)	Wyamine (W)
mephenytoin (W)	Mesantoin (W)
mephobarbital	Mebaral
Mephyton	phytonadione

mepivacaine HCl	Carbocaine
meprobamate	Equanil (WA) Miltown
Mepron	atovaquone
mequinol; tretinoin	Solage
mercaptopurine	Purinethol
Meridia	sibutramine HCl monohydrate
meropenem	Merrem
Merrem	meropenem
Meruvax II	rubella virus vaccine live attenuated
mesalamine	Asacol Rowasa
mesalamine multimatrix tablets	Lialda
Mesantoin (W)	mephenytoin (W)
mesna	Mesnex
Mesnex	mesna
mesoridazine (W)	Serentil (W)
Mestinon	pyridostigmine bromide
Metadate ER	methylphenidate HCl SR
Metaglip	glipizide; metformin
Metamucil	psyllium
Metaprel	metaproterenol sulfate
metaproterenol sulfate	Alupent Metaprel
metaraminol bitartrate	Aramine
Metaret	suramin
Metastron	strontium-89 chloride inj
metformin HCl	Glucophage
metformin HCl SR	Glucophage XR
methadone HCl	Dolophine
methamphetamine HCl	Desoxyn
methazolamide	Neptazane
methenamine combination	Urised
methenamine hippurate	Hiprex
Methergine	methylergon-ovine maleate
methicillin sodium (W)	Staphcillin (W)
methimazole	Tapazole
methocarbamol	Robaxin
methohexital sodium	Brevital Sodium
methotrexate	Rheumatrex Trexall
methotrexate, sodium preservative-free inj	Folex PFS (WA)
methoxamine HCl (W)	Vasoxyl (W)
methoxsalen	Oxsoralen
methoxsalen extracorporeal administration	Uvadex
methoxy polyethylene glycol-epoetin beta	Mircera
methscopolamine bromide	Pamine
methyclothiazide	Enduron
methyldopa	Aldomet
methyldopa; hydrochlorothiazide	Aldoril
methylergonovine maleate (W)	Methergine (W)
Methylin	methylphenidate HCl
Methylin ER	methylphenidate HCl SR
methylnaltrexone bromide inj	Relistor
methylphenidate HCl	Methylin Ritalin
methylphenidate SR	Concerta Metadate ER Methylin ER Ritalin SR
methylprednisolone	Medrol
methylprednisolone acetate SR inj	Depo-Medrol
methylprednisolone sodium succinate inj	Solu-Medrol
methyltestosterone	*methyltestosterone*
methysergide maleate (W)	Sansert (W)
Meticorten	prednisone
metoclopramide HCl	Reglan
metolazone	Zaroxolyn
Metopirone	metyrapone
metoprolol succinate SR	Toprol XL
metoprolol tartrate	Lopressor
MetroGel-Vaginal	metronidazole vaginal gel
metronidazole	Flagyl
metronidazole SR	Flagyl ER
metronidazole vaginal gel	MetroGel-Vaginal
metyrapone	Metopirone
metyrosine	Demser

Mevacor	lovastatin
Mexate (WA)	*methotrexate*
mexiletine HCl	Mexitil
Mexitil	mexiletine HCl
Mezlin (W)	mezlocillin (W)
mezlocillin (W)	Mezlin (W)
Miacalcin	calcitonin-salmon
mibefradil dihydrochloride (W)	Posicor (W)
micafungin sodium	Mycamine
Micardis	telmisartan
Micro K	potassium chloride SR
miconazole nitrate	Monistat
Micronase	glyburide
Micronor	norethindrone
Microzide	hydrochlorothiazide
Midamor	amiloride HCl
midazolam HCl	*midazolam HCl*
midodrine HCl	ProAmatine
Mifeprex	mifepristone
mifepristone	Mifeprex
miglitol	Glyset
miglustat	Zavesca
Migranol	dihydroergotamine mesylate nasal spray
milrinone lactate	Primacor
Miltown	meprobamate
Minipress	prazosin HCl
Minocin	minocycline HCl
minocycline HCl	Minocin
minocycline HCl dental microspheres	Arestin
minoxidil tablets (W)	Loniten (W)
minoxidil topical	Rogaine
Mintezol	thiabendazole
Miochol E	acetylcholine ophth
MiraLax	polyethylene glycol 3350 powder
Mirapex	pramipexole dihydrochloride
Mircera	methoxy polyethylene glycol-epoetin beta
Mircette	desogestrel; ethinyl estradiol and ethinyl estradiol
Mirena	levonorgestrel-releasing intrauterine system
mirtazapine	Remeron
misoprostol	Cytotec
Mithracin (W)	plicamycin (W)
mitomycin	Mutamycin
mitotane	Lysodren

mitoxantrone HCl	Novantrone
Mivacron (W)	mivacurium chloride (W)
mivacurium chloride (W)	Mivacron (W)
M-M-R II	measles, mumps, rubella vaccines, combined
Moban	molindone HCl
Mobic	meloxicam
modafinil	Provigil
Moduretic	amiloride HCl; hydrochlorothiazide
moexipril HCl	Univasc
moexipril HCl; hydrochloro-thiazide	Uniretic
molindone HCl	Moban
mometasone furoate topical	Elocon
Mometasone furoate monohydrate nasal spray	Nasonex
Monistat	miconazole nitrate
Monocid (W)	cefonicid sodium (W)
Monopril	fosinopril sodium
montelukast sodium	Singulair
Monurol	fosfomycin tromethamine
moricizine	Ethmozine
morphine sulfate	Roxanol
morphine sulfate extended-release liposome inj	DepoDur
morphine sulfate, immediate release concentrated oral soln	Roxanol-T
morphine sulfate inj	Duramorph
morphine sulfate SR	Avinza Kadian MS Contin Oramorph SR Roxanol SR
Motrin	ibuprofen
moxifloxacin HCl	Avelox
MS Contin	morphine sulfate SR
Mucomyst	acetylcysteine
multivitamins for infusion	Cernevit-12 Multi-12 (vial 1 and vial 2)
mupirocin nasal ointment	Bactroban
muromonab-CD3	Orthoclone OKT3
Muse	alprostadil urethral suppository

Mustargen	mechlorethamine HCl
Mutamycin	mitomycin
M.V.I.-12	vitamin, multiple inj
Myambutol	ethambutol HCl
Mycamine	micafungin sodium
Mycelex	clotrimazole
Mycifradin Sulfate	neomycin sulfate oral soln
Myciguent (W)	neomycin sulfate ointment and cream (W)
Mycolog Cream	nystatin; triamcinolone cream
mycophenolate mofetil	CellCept
mycophenolic acid	Myfortic
Mycostatin	nystatin
Mydriacyl	tropicamide
Myfortic	mycophenolic acid
Mykrox	metolazone
Myleran	busulfan
Mylicon	simethicone
Mylotarg	gemtuzumab ozogamicin
Myobloc	botulinum toxin type B
Myochrysine	gold sodium thiomalate
Myoscint	imciromab pentetate
Myozyme	alglucosidase alfa
Mysoline	primidone

N

NABI-HB	hepatitis B immune globulin (human)
nabilone	Cesamet
nabumetone	Relafen
nadolol	*nadolol*
Nafcil (W)	*nafcillin sodium*
nafcillin sodium	Nafcil (W)
	Unipen (W)
Naglazyme	galsulfase
nalbuphine HCl	Nubain
Nalfon	fenoprofen calcium
nalidixic acid	NegGram
nalmefene HCl	Revex
naloxone HCl	Narcan (WA)
naltrexone	ReVia
Namenda	memantine HCl
nandrolone phenpropionate (W)	Durabolin (W)
nandrolone decanoate	Deca-Durabolin
naphazoline ophth soln	Vasocon
Naprelan	naproxen sodium SR
Naprosyn	naproxen
naproxen	Naprosyn
naproxen sodium	Anaprox
naproxen sodium SR	Naprelan
naratriptan HCl	Amerge
Narcan (WA)	naloxone HCl
Nardil	phenelzine sulfate
Naropin	ropivacaine HCl
Nasacort	triamcinolone acetonide nasal inhaler
Nasalcrom	cromolyn sodium
Nascobal	cyanocobalamin nasal gel
Nasonex	Mometasone furoate monohydrate nasal spray
natalizumab (W)	Tysabri (W)
nateglinide	Starlix
Natrecor	nesiritide
Navane	thiothixene
Navelbine	vinorelbine tartrate
Nebcin (WA)	*tobramycin sulfate*
nebivolol	Bystolic
NebuPent	pentamidine isethionate aerosol
nedocromil inhalation	Tilade
nedocromil ophth soln	Alocril
nefazodone HCl (W)	Serzone (W)
NegGram	nalidixic acid
nelarabine	Arranon
nelfinavir mesylate	Viracept
Nembutal	pentobarbital sodium
Neo-Synephrine	phenylephrine HCl
neomycin sulfate ointment and cream (W)	Myciguent (W)
neomycin sulfate oral soln	Mycifradin Sulfate
Neoral	cyclosporine capsules (modified) and oral soln
Neosar	cyclophosphamide
Neosporin Cream	polymyxin; neomycin
Neosporin Ointment	polymyxin; neomycin; bacitracin
Neosporin ophth Ointment	polymyxin; neomycin; bacitracin
Neosporin ophth soln	polymyxin; neomycin
neostigmine methylsulfate	Prostigmin
nepafenac	Nevanac
Neptazane	methazolamide
Nesacaine	chloroprocaine HCl

nesiritide	Natrecor
netilmicin sulfate (W)	Netromycin (W)
Netromycin (W)	netilmicin sulfate (W)
Neulasta	pegfilgrastim
Neumega	oprelvekin
Neupogen	filgrastim
Neupro	rotigotine transdermal system
Neurolite	technetium Tc-99m bicisate kit
Neurontin	gabapentin
Neutrexin	trimetrexate glucuronate
Nevance	nepafenac
nevirapine	Viramune
Nexavar	sorafenib tosylate
Nexium	esomeprazole magnesium
niacin SR	Niaspan
Niaspan	niacin SR
nicardipine HCl	Cardene
Niclocide (W)	niclosamide (W)
niclosamide (W)	Niclocide (W)
Nicobid	niacin SR
Nicorette	nicotine polacrilex
nicotine nasal spray	Nicotrol NS
nicotine polacrilex	Nicorette
nicotine transdermal	Habitrol Nicotrol Prostep
Nicotrol	nicotine transdermal
Nicotrol NS	nicotine nasal spray
nifedipine	Procardia
nifedipine SR	Adalat CC Procardia XL
Nilandron	nilutamide
nilotinib	Tasigna
nilutamide	Nilandron
Nimbex	cisatracurium besylate
nimodipine	Nimotop
Nimotop	nimodipine
Nipent	pentostatin inj
Nipride (WA)	*nitroprusside sodium*
nisoldipine SR	Sular
nitazoxanide	Alinia
nitisinone	Orfadin
Nitrek	nitroglycerin transdermal
nitric oxide for inhalation	INOmax
Nitro-Bid	nitroglycerin oint
Nitro-Dur	nitroglycerin transdermal
nitrofurantoin macrocrystals	Macrodantin
nitrofurantoin macrocrystals and monohydrate	Macrobid

nitrofurazone	Furacin
nitroglycerin transdermal	Transderm-Nitro
nitroglycerin inj	*nitroglycerin inj*
nitroglycerin ointment	Nitrol Nitro-Bid
nitroglycerin sublingual tablets	Nitrostat
nitroglycerin transdermal	Nitrek Nitro-Dur
Nitro-BID	nitroglycerin ointment
nitroprusside sodium	*nitroprusside sodium inj*
Nitrostat	nitroglycerin sublingual tablets
Nix	permethrin
nizatidine	Axid
Nizoral	ketoconazole
nofetumomab (W)	Verluna (W)
nolatrexed dihydrochloride	Thymitaq
Nolvadex (WA)	*tamoxifen citrate*
Norco	hydrocodone bitartrate; acetaminophen
Norcuron	vecuronium bromide
Nordette	levonorgestrel; ethinyl estradiol
Norditropin	somatropin inj
norelgestromin; ethinyl estradiol transdermal system	Ortho Evra
norepinephrine bitartrate	Levophed
norethindrone	Micronor
norethindrone acetate; ethinyl estradiol	Estrostep Loestrin
norethindrone; ethinyl estradiol (or mestranol)	Femhrt Ortho-Novum (products)
norethindrone acetate; estradiol transdermal	CombiPatch
Norflex	orphenadrine citrate
norfloxacin	Noroxin
Norgesic	orphenadrine citrate; aspirin; caffeine
norgestimate; ethinyl estradiol	Ortho Tri-Cyclen

norgestrel; ethinyl estradiol	Lo/Ovral Ovral
Normiflo (W)	ardeparin sodium (W)
Normodyne	labetalol HCl
Noroxin	norfloxacin
Norpace	disopyramide phosphate
Norplant (W)	levonorgestrel implant (W)
Norpramin	desipramine HCl
nortriptyline HCl	Aventyl Pamelor
Norvasc	amlodipine besylate
Norvir	ritonavir
Novantrone	mitoxantrone HCl
Novocain HCl	procaine HCl
Novolin 70/30	isophane insulin suspension (NPH) 70%, insulin inj 30% (human)
Novolin N	isophane insulin suspension (NPH) (human)
Novolin R	insulin inj (human)
NovoLog	insulin aspart (rDNA origin)
NovoSeven	coagulation factor VII a (recombinant)
Noxafil	posaconazole
Nubain	nalbuphine HCl
NuLev	hyoscyamine sulfate orally disintegrating tab
Numorphan	oxymorphone HCl
Nupercainal	dibucaine
Nuromax	doxacurium chloride
Nuprin (WA)	*ibuprofen*
Nutropin	somatropin for inj
Nutropin AQ	somatropin inj
NuvaRing	etonogestrel; ethinyl estradiol vagina ring
Nuvigil	armodafinil
Nydrazid	isoniazid
nystatin	Mycostatin
nystatin topical powder	Nystop
nystatin; triamcinolone cream	Mycolog Cream
Nystop	nystatin topical powder

O

OctreoScan	indium In-111 pentetreotide
octreotide acetate	Sandostatin
octreotide acetate susp for inj	Sandostatin LAR Depot
ofloxacin	Floxin
ofloxacin otic soln	Floxin Otic
Ogen	estropipate
olanzapine	Zyprexa
olanzapine; fluoxetine	Symbyaz
olmesartan medoxomil	Benicar
olmesartan medoxomil; hydrochloro-thiazide	Benicar HCT
olopatadine HCl ophth soln	Patanol
olsalazine sodium	Dipentum
Olux	clobetasol foam
Omacor (name changed to Lovaza)	omega-3-acid ethyl esters
omalizumab	Xolair
omega-3-acid ethyl ester	Lovaza (formerly called Omacor)
omeprazole	Prilosec
Omnicef	cefdinir
Omnipaque	iohexol
Oncaspar	pegaspargase
OncoScint	satumomab pendetide
Oncovin	vincristine sulfate
ondansetron	Zofran
ondansetron orally disintegrating tab	Zofran ODT
Ontak	denileukin diftitox
Onxol	paclitaxel inj
Opana	oxymorphone HCl
Opana ER	oxymorphone HCl extended release tablets
Ophthaine (WA)	proparacaine
Ophthalgan	glycerin ophth soln
Ophthetic	proparacaine HCl
opium; belladonna suppositories	B & O Supprettes
oprelvekin	Neumega
Opticrom	cromolyn sodium
OptiMark	gadoversetamide
Optimine	azatadine maleate
Optiray	ioversol
Optivar	azelastine HCl ophth soln
Orabase	benzocaine
Orajel	benzocaine
Oramorph SR	morphine sulfate SR
Orap	pimozide
OraVerse	phentolamine mesylate inj
Orencia	abatacept
Oretic	hydrochlorothiazide
Orfadin	nitisinone
Organidin NR	guaifenesin

Orgaran	danaparoid sodium
Orinase	tolbutamide
Orlaam (W)	levomethadyl acetate HCl (W)
orlistat	Xenical
Ornade Spansules (W)	phenylpropanolamine HCl; chlorpheniramine maleate SR (W)
orphenadrine citrate	Norflex
orphenadrine citrate; aspirin; caffeine	Norgesic
Ortho-Cept	desogestrel; ethinyl estradiol
Orthoclone OKT3	muromonab-CD3
Ortho Evra	norelgestromin; ethinyl estradiol transdermal system
Ortho-Novum (products)	norethindrone; ethinyl estradiol (or mestranol)
Ortho-Prefest	17β-estradiol; norgestimate
Ortho Tri-Cyclen	norgestimate; ethinyl estradiol (combinations)
Orudis (WA)	*ketoprofen*
Oruvail (WA)	*ketoprofen SR*
Os-Cal 500	calcium carbonate
oseltamivir phosphate	Tamiflu
Osmovist	iotrolan
Otrivin	xylometazoline
Ovidrel	choriogonadotropin alfa
ovine hyaluronidase (W)	Vitrase (W)
Ovral	norgestrel; ethinyl estradiol
oxaliplatin	Eloxatin
Oxandrin	oxandrolone
oxandrolone	Oxandrin
oxaprozin	Daypro
oxazepam	Serax
oxcarbazepine	Trileptal
oxiconazole nitrate cream	Oxistat
Oxilan (W)	ioxilan (W)
Oxistat	oxiconazole nitrate cream
Oxsoralen	methoxsalen
oxtriphylline	*oxtriphylline*
oxybate sodium	Xyrem
oxybutynin chloride	Ditropan
oxychlorosene sodium	Clorpactin WCS-90
oxycodone HCl	Percolone (WA) Roxicodone
oxycodone HCl SR	OxyContin
oxycodone HCl; acetaminophen	Percocet 5/325; 7.5/500; 10/650 Endocet Magnacet Roxicet
oxycodone HCl; aspirin	Percodan
oxycodone HCl; ibuprofen	Combunox
OxyContin	oxycodone HCl SR
oxymetazoline HCl	Afrin nasal spray Dristan Long Lasting
oxymetholone	Anadrol-50
oxymorphone HCl	Numorphan Opana tablets
oxymorphone HCl extended release tablets	Opana ER
oxytocin	Pitocin

P

Pacis	BCG intravesical
paclitaxel	Onxol Taxol
paclitaxel, albumin-bound inj	Abraxane
paclitaxel-eluting stent	Taxus Express2 stent V-Flex plus PTX stent
palifermin	Kepivance
paliperidone	Invega
palivizumab	Synagis
Palladone XL	hydromorphone HCl SR
palonosetron HCl	Aloxi
Pamelor	nortriptyline HCl
pamidronate disodium	Aredia
Pamine	methscopolamine bromide
Pancrease	pancrelipase EC
pancrelipase	*pancrelipase*
pancrelipase EC	*pancrelipase EC* Pancrease
pancuronium bromide	Pavulon
Pandel	hydrocortisone buteprate cream
Panretin	alitretinoin
panitumumab	Vectibix
pantoprazole	Protonix
papain; urea oint	Accuzyme Ethezyme
papaverine HCl SR (W)	Pavabid (W)

papillomavirus quadrivalent human (types 6, 11, 16, 18) recombinant vaccine	Gardasil
paracetamol	acetaminophen
Paradione (W)	paramethadione (W)
Paraflex	chlorzoxazone 250 mg
Parafon Forte DSC	chlorzoxazone 500 mg
paramethadione (W)	Paradione (W)
Paraplatin (WA)	*carboplatin*
Parathar	teriparatide acetate
Parcopa	levodopa; carbidopa
paregoric	camphorated tincture of opium
pargyline HCl	Eutonyl
paricalcitol	Zemplar
Parlodel	bromocriptine mesylate
Parnate	tranylcypromine sulfate
paromomycin sulfate	Humatin
paroxetine HCl	Paxil
Parsidol	ethopropazine HCl
Paser	aminosalicylic acid
Patanol	olopatadine HCl ophth soln
Pavabid (W)	papaverine HCl SR (W)
Pavulon	pancuronium bromide
Paxil	paroxetine HCl
PBZ (W)	tripelennamine HCl (W)
PCE Dispertab	erythromycin base coated particles
Pediazole	erythromycin ethylsuccinate; sulfisoxazole
pegaptanib	Macugen
pegaspargase	Oncaspar
Pegasys	peginterferon alfa-2a
pegfilgrastim	Neulasta
peginterferon alfa-2a	Pegasys
peginterferon alfa-2b (recombinant)	PEG-Intron
PEG-Intron	peginterferon alfa-2b (recombinant)
pegvisomant	Somavert
pemetrexed disodium	Alimta
pemirolast potassium ophth soln	Alamast
pemoline	Cylert (WA)
penicillamine	Cuprimine

penciclovir cream	Denavir
penicillin G benzathine	Bicillin L-A (for IM use only) Permapen (for IM use only)
penicillin G benzathine; penicillin G procaine	Bicillin C-R (for IM use only)
penicillin G procaine	Wycillin (for IM use only)
penicillin V potassium	*penicillin V potassium*
Penlac Nail Lacquer	ciclopirox soln
pentaerythritol tetranitrate (W)	Peritrate (W)
pentagastrin (W)	Peptavlon (W)
Pentam 300	pentamidine isethionate inj
pentamidine isethionate aerosol	NebuPent
pentamidine isethionate inj	Pentam 300
Pentaspan	pentastarch
pentastarch	Pentaspan
pentazocine HCl	Talwin
pentazocine HCl; naloxone HCl	Talwin Nx
pentetate zinc trisodium (trisodium zinc diethylenetriaminepentaacetate)	Zn-DTPA
pentobarbital sodium	Nembutal
pentosan polysulfate sodium	Elmiron
pentostatin inj	Nipent
Pentothal	thiopental sodium
pentoxifylline	Trental
Pen Vee K (WA)	*penicillin V potassium*
Pepcid	famotidine
Pepcid RPD	famotidine, oral disintegrating tablet
Peptavlon (W)	pentagastrin (W)
Percocet 5/325; 7.5/500; 10/650	oxycodone HCl; acetaminophen
Percodan	oxycodone HCl; aspirin
Percolone (WA)	oxycodone HCl
perflenapent emulsion	EchoGen
perflubron	Imagent GI
Pergonal (WA)	menotropins
Periactin (WA)	*cyproheptadine HCl*
Peri-Colace	docusate sodium; senna concentrate

Peridex	chlorhexidine gluconate mouth rinse
perindopril erbumine	Aceon
PerioChip	chlorhexidine gluconate
Periostat	doxycycline hyclate 20 mg tab & cap
Peritrate (W)	pentaerythritol tetranitrate (W)
Permapen	penicillin G benzathine (for IM use only)
permethrin	Nix
Permitil	fluphenazine HCl
perphenazine	*perphenazine*
perphenazine; amitriptyline HCl	Etrafon Triavil (WA)
Persantine	dipyridamole
petrolatum, white	Vaseline
Phenaphen with Codeine (#2, 3, and 4) (WA)	acetaminophen 300 mg with Codeine Phosphate (15, 30, and 60 mg)
phenazopyridine HCl	Pyridium
phendimetrazine tartrate	Plegine
phenelzine sulfate	Nardil
Phenergan	promethazine HCl
phenobarbital	phenobarbital
phenobarbital, ergotamine; belladonna	Bellergal-S
phenoxybenzamine HCl	Dibenzyline
phentermine HCl	Fastin
phentermine resin	Ionamin
phentolamine mesylate	OraVerse Regitine (WA)
phenylbutyrate sodium	Buphenyl
phenylephrine HCl	Neo-Synephrine
phenylpropanolamine HCl; guaifenesin SR	Entex LA
Phenytek	phenytoin sodium extended
phenytoin	Dilantin
phenytoin sodium extended	Phenytek
Phospholine Iodide (W)	echothiophate iodide (W)
Photofrin	porfimer sodium
physostigmine ophth ointment	Eserine Sulfate
physostigmine salicylate	Antilirium
phytonadione	Mephyton
pilocarpine HCl ophth	Isopto Carpine
pilocarpine HCl tablet	Salagen
pimecrolimus cream	Elidel
pimozide	Orap
pindolol	Visken
pioglitazone HCl	Actos
pipecuronium bromide (W)	Arduan (W)
piperacillin sodium (W)	Pipracil (W)
piperacillin sodium; tazobactam sodium	Zosyn
Pipracil (W)	piperacillin sodium (W)
piroxicam	Feldene
Pitocin	oxytocin
Pitressin	vasopressin
Placidyl (W)	ethchlorvynol (W)
Plan B	levonorgestrel
Plaquenil	hydroxychloroquine sulfate
Plasbumin	albumin human
plasma protein fraction	Plasma-Plex Plasmanate Plasmatein Protenate
Plasma-Plex	plasma protein fraction
Plasmanate	plasma protein fraction
Plasmatein	plasma protein fraction
Platinol AQ (WA)	cisplatin
Plavix	clopidogrel bisulfate
Plegine	phendimetrazine tartrate
Plenaxis	abarelix
Plendil	felodipine
Pletal	cilostazol
Plexion	sulfacetamide sodium and sulfur lotion
plicamycin (W)	Mithracin (W)
pneumococcal vaccine	Pneumovax
pneumococcal 7-valent conjugate vaccine	Prevnar
Pneumovax	pneumococcal vaccine
podofilox gel	Condylox
Polaramine Repetabs (WA)	*dexchlorpheniramine-maleate SR*

P ℞

poliovirus vaccine inactivated	Ipol
polyethylene glycolelectro-lyte soln	CoLyte GoLYTELY
polyethylene glycol 3350 powder	MiraLax
poly-l-lactic acid	Sculptra
polymyxin B sulfate; trimethoprim ophth soln	Polytrim
polymyxin; neomycin	Neosporin Cream Neosporin ophth soln
polymyxin; neomycin; bacitracin	Neosporin Ointment Neosporin ophth Ointment
polystyrene sulfonate sodium	Kayexalate
polythiazide (W)	Renese (W)
Polytrim	polymyxin B sulfate; trimethoprim ophth soln
Pondimin (W)	fenfluramine HCl (W)
Ponstel	mefenamic acid
Pontocaine	tetracaine HCl
poractant alpha intratracheal susp	Curosurf
porfimer sodium	Photofrin
posaconazole	Noxafil
Posicor (W)	mibefradil dihydrochloride (W)
potassium bicarbonate; potassium citrate effervescent	K-Lyte
potassium chloride; potassium bicarbonate effervescent	K-Lyte/Cl
potassium chloride SR	Kaon-Cl K-Dur Klor-Con 10 Slow-K (WA) Micro K
potassium chloride; potassium gluconate	Kolyum
potassium citrate tab	Urocit-K
potassium gluconate	Kaon
povidone iodine	Betadine
pralidoxime chloride	Protopam
pramipexole dihydrochloride	Mirapex
pramlintide acetate	Symlin
pramoxine HCl	Tronothane HCl
Prandin	repaglinide
prasterone (W)	Aslera (W)
Pravachol	pravastatin sodium
pravastatin sodium	Pravachol
prazosin HCl	Minipress
Precedex	dexmedetomidine HCl inj
Precose	acarbose
prednisolone syrup	Prelone
prednisone	*prednisone*
pregabalin	Lyrica
Prelone	prednisolone syrup
Premarin	estrogens, conjugated
Premphase Prempro	estrogens, conjugated; medroxyprogesterone acetate
Prepidil	dinoprostone gel
Preven Emergency Contraceptive Kit	levonorgestrel; ethinyl estradiol
Prevacid	lansoprazole
Prevnar	pneumococcal 7-valent conjugate vaccine
Preveon	adefovir dipivoxil
Prevpac	lansoprazole; amoxicillin; clarithromycin
Prezista	darunavir
Prialt	ziconotide
Priftin	rifapentine
Prilosec	omeprazole
Primacor	milrinone lactate
Primaxin	imipenemcilastatin sodium
primidone	Mysoline
Primsol (W)	trimethoprim (W)
Principen	ampicillin
Prinivil	lisinopril
Priscoline (W)	tolazoline (W)
Pristiq	desvenlafaxine succinate
ProAmatine	midodrine HCl
Pro-Banthine	propantheline bromide
probenecid	*probenecid*
probenecid; colchicine	ColBENEMID (W)

procainamide	Pronestyl
procainamide HCl SR	Procanbid
procaine HCl	Novocain HCl
Procan SR (WA)	*procainamide HCl SR*
Procanbid	procainamide HCl SR
procarbazine HCl	Matulane
Procardia	nifedipine
Procardia XL	nifedipine SR
Prochieve	progesterone gel
prochlorperazine	Compazine
Procrit	epoetin alfa
procyclidine HCl	Kemadrin
progesterone gel	Crinone Prochieve
progesterone micronized	Prometrium
Prograf	tacrolimus
ProHance	gadoteridol
ProHIBiT	haemophilus b vaccine
Prokine (WA)	sargramostim
Prolastin	alpha$_1$-proteinase inhibitor (human)
Proleukin	aldesleukin
Prolixin (WA)	*fluphenazine HCl*
Proloid (W)	thyroglobulin (W)
promethazine HCl	Phenergan
Prometrium	progesterone micronized
Pronestyl	procainamide
Propacet-100	propoxyphene napsylate; acetaminophen
propafenone HCl	Rythmol
propantheline bromide	Pro-Banthine
proparacaine HCl	Ophthaine (WA) Ophthetic
Propecia	finasteride tablets 1 mg
Propine	dipivefrin
propofol	Diprivan
propoxyphene HCl	Darvon
propoxyphene HCl; acetaminophen	*propoxyphene HCl; acetaminophen*
propoxyphene HCl; aspirin; caffeine	Darvon Compound 65
propoxyphene napsylate; acetaminophen	Darvocet-N 100 Propacet-100
propranolol HCl	Inderal
propranolol HCl; hydrochlorothiazide	Inderide
Propulsid (W)	cisapride (W)
Proscar	finasteride tablets 5 mg

ProSom (W)	*estazolam*
ProstaScint	capromab pendetide
Prostep	nicotine transdermal system
Prostigmin	neostigmine methylsulfate
Prostin E_2	dinoprostone vaginal suppositories
Prostin VR	alprostadil
protamine sulfate	protamine sulfate
protein C concentrate (human)	Ceprotin
Protenate	plasma protein fraction
Protonix	pantoprazole
Protopam	pralidoxime chloride
Protopic	tacrolimus oint
protriptyline HCl	*protriptyline HCl*
Protropin	somatrem
Protropin II	somatropin for inj
Proventil	albuterol
Proventil HFA	albuterol sulfate inhalation aerosol
Proventil Repetabs	albuterol SR
Provera	medroxyprogesterone acetate
Provigil	modafinil
Prozac	fluoxetine HCl
Prudoxin	doxepin HCl cream
Prussian blue	Radiogardase
pseudoephedrine HCl	Sudafed
pseudoephedrine HCl; bromphiramine maleate	Drixoral Syrup
psyllium	Konsyl-D Metamucil
Pulmicort Turbuhaler	budesonide inhalation powder
Pulmozyme	dornase alfa
Purinethol	mercaptopurine
Pyridium	phenazopyridine HCl
pyridostigmine bromide	Mestinon
pyrimethamine	Daraprim
pyrimethamine; sulfadoxine	Fansidar

Q

Quadramet	samarium SM 153 lexidronam
Qualaquin	quinine sulfate
Quarzan (W)	clidinium bromide (W)
Questran (W)	cholestyramine (W)

quetiapine fumerate	Seroquel
Quinaglute (WA)	*quinidine gluconate SR*
quinapril HCl	Accupril
quinapril; hydrochlorothiazide	Accuretic
quinethazone (W)	Hydromox (W)
Quinidex Extentabs	quinidine sulfate SR
quinidine gluconate SR	*quinidine gluconate SR*
quinidine sulfate	quinidine sulfate
quinidine sulfate SR	Quinidex Extentabs
quinine sulfate	Qualaquin
quinupristin; dalfopristin	Synercid
Quixin	levofloxacin ophth soln
Qvar	beclomethasone diproprionate inhalation aerosol

R

RabAvert	rabies vaccine for human use
rabeprazole sodium	Aciphex
rabies immune globulin, human	Hyperab (W) Imogam
rabies vaccine for human use	RabAvert
Radiogardase	Prussian blue
raloxifene HCl	Evista
raltegravir	Isentress
ramelteon	Rozerem
ramipril	Altace
Ranexa	ranolazine
ranibizumab inj	Lucentis
ranitidine bismuth citrate (W)	Tritec (W)
ranitidine HCl	Zantac
ranolazine	Ranexa
rapacuronium bromide (W)	Raplon (W)
Rapamune	sirolimus
Raplon (W)	rapacuronium bromide (W)
Raptiva	efalizumab
rasagiline mesylate	Azilect
rasburicase	Elitek
rattlesnake anti-venom	CroFab
Raxar (W)	grepafloxacin HCl (W)
Razadyne	galanthamine HBr
Rebetol	ribavirin
Rebetron	ribavirin; interferon alfa-2b
Rebif	interferon beta-1a
reboxetine mesylate	Vestra
Reclast intravenous infusion	zoledronic acid inj
Recombivax HB	hepatitis B vaccine
Recothrom	thrombin, topical (recombinant)
Redux (W)	dexfenfluramine HCl (W)
Refacto	antihemophilic factor (recombinant)
Refludan	lepirudin
regadenoson inj	Lexiscan
Regitine (WA)	phentolamine mesylate
Reglan	metoclopramide HCl
Regranex	becaplermin gel
Regroton (W)	chlorthalidone; reserpine (W)
Relafen	nabumetone
Relenza	zanamivir for inhalation
Relistor	methylnaltrexone bromide inj
Relpax	eletriptan hydrobromide
Remeron	mirtazapine
Remicade	infliximab
remifentanil HCl	Ultiva
Reminyl	name changed to Razadyne
Remodulin	treprostinil sodium
Renagel (W)	sevelamer HCl (W)
Renese (W)	polythiazide (W)
Renova	tretinion topical
Renovue 65	iodamide meglumine
ReoPro	abciximab
repaglinide	Prandin
Repronex	menotropins
Requip	ropinirole HCl
Rescriptor	delavirdine mesylate
Rescula (W)	unoprostone isopropyl ophth soln (W)
reserpine	Serpasil (WA)
RespiGam	respiratory syncytial virus immune globulin intravenous (human)
respiratory syncytial virus immune globulin intravenous (human)	RespiGam
Restasis	cyclosporine ophth emulsion

Restoril	temazepam
retapamulin oint	Altabax
Retavase	reteplase
reteplase	Retavase
Retin-A	tretinoin topical
Retin-A Micro	tretinoin gel
Retrovir	zidovudine
Revex	nalmefene HCl
ReVia	naltrexone
Revlimid	lenalidomide
Reyataz (W)	atazanavir sulfate (W)
Rezulin (W)	troglitazone (W)
R-Gene	arginine HCl
Rheumatrex	methotrexate tablets
Rhinocort	budesonide nasal inhaler
RH_O (D) immune globulin	RhoGAM
RH_O (D) immune globulin IV (human)	WinRho SD
RhoGAM	RH_O (D) immune globulin
ribavirin	Rebetol Virazole
ribavirin; interferon alfa-2b	Rebetron
Ridaura	auranofin
Rifadin	rifampin
Rifamate	isoniazid; rifampin
rifampin	Rifadin Rimactane
rifapentine	Priftin
rifaximin	Xifaxan
rilonacept	Arcalyst
Rilutek	riluzole
riluzole	Rilutek
Rimactane	rifampin
rimantadine	Flumadine
rimexolone	Vexol
Riopan	magaldrate
risedronate sodium	Actonel
Risperdal	risperidone
risperidone	Risperdal
Ritalin	methylphenidate HCl
Ritalin SR	methylphenidate SR
ritodrine HCl (W)	Yutopar (W)
ritonavir	Norvir
Rituxan	rituximab
rituximab	Rituxan
rivastigmine tartrate	Exelon
rizatriptan benzoate	Maxalt
rizatriptan oral disintegrating tablet	Maxalt-MLT
Robaxin	methocarbamol

R ℞

Robinul	glycopyrrolate
Robitussin	guaifenesin
Robitussin A-C	guaifenesin; codeine phosphate
Robitussin-DM	guaifenesin; dextromethorphan
Rocaltrol	calcitriol
Rocephin	ceftriaxone sodium
rofecoxib (W)	Vioxx (W)
Roferon-A (W)	interferon alfa-2a (W)
Rogaine	minoxidil topical
Romazicon	flumazenil
ropinirole HCl	Requip
ropivacaine HCl	Naropin
Rosiglitazone maleate	Avandia
rosiglitazone maleate; metformin HCl	Avandamet
rosuvastatin calcium	Crestor
Rotashield (W)	rotavirus (W) vaccine, live, oral, tetravalent
rotavirus vaccine, live, oral, (W) tetravalent	Rotashield (W)
rotigotine transdermal system	Neupro
Rowasa	mesalamine
Roxanol	morphine sulfate
Roxanol SR	morphine sulfate SR
Roxanol-T	morphine sulfate, immediate release concentrated oral soln
Roxicet	oxycodone HCl; acetaminophen
Roxicodone	oxycodone HCl
Rozerem	ramelteon
rubella virus vaccine live attenuated	Meruvax II
Rubex	doxorubicin HCl
Rythmol	propafenone HCl

S

sacrosidase	Sucraid
Saizen	somatropin
Salagen	pilocarpine HCl tablet
salbutamol sulfate	albuterol sulfate
salmeterol xinafoate	Serevent

salmeterol xinafoate inhalation powder	Serevent Diskus
salsalate	Disalcid
Sal-Tropine	atropine sulfate tablets
Saluron (W)	hydroflumethiazide (W)
samarium SM 153 lexidronam	Quadramet
Sanctura	trospium chloride
Sandimmune	cyclosporine
Sandoglobulin (WA)	immune globulin intravenous
Sandostatin	octreotide acetate
Sandostatin LAR Depot	octreotide acetate susp for inj
Sanorex	mazindol
Sansert (W)	methysergide maleate (W)
Santyl	collagenase
sapropterin dihydrochloride	Kuvan
saquinavir mesylate	Invirase
saquinavir soft gel capsule (W)	Fortovase (W)
Sarafem	fluoxetine
sargramostim	Leukine
	Prokine (WA)
satumomab pendetide	OncoScint
Sclerosol	talc, sterile aerosol
Scopace	scopolamine hydrobromide, soluble tab
scopolamine hydrobromide ophth	Isopto Hyoscine
scopolamine hydrobromide, soluble tab	Scopace
scopolamine transdermal	Transderm Scop
Sculptra	poly-l-lactic acid
Seasonale	ethinyl estradiol; levonorgestrel (91 day cycle)
Sectral	acebutolol HCl
Seldane (W)	terfenadine (W)
Seldane D (W)	terfenadine; pseudoephedrine HCl (W)
selegiline HCl	Carbex
	Eldepryl
selenium sulfide	Selsun Blue
Selsun Blue	selenium sulfide
Selzentry	maraviroc
Sensipar	cinacalcet
sennosides	Ex Lax
sennosides	Senokot
sennosides; docusate sodium	Senokot-S
Senokot	senna concentrates
Senokot-S	sennosides; docusate sodium
Sensipar	cinacalcet HCl
Septocaine	articaine; epinephrine
Septra	sulfamethoxazoletrimethoprim
Ser-Ap-Es (W)	hydralazine; hydrochlorothiazide; reserpine (W)
Serax	oxazepam
Serentil (W)	mesoridazine (W)
Serevent	salmeterol xinafoate
Serevent Diskus	salmeterol xinafoate inhalation powder
Serlect	sertindole
sermorelin acetate	Geref
Seromycin	cycloserine
Seroquel	quetiapine fumerate
Serostim	somatropin (rDNA origin) for inj
Serpasil (WA)	*reserpine*
sertaconazole	Ertaczo
sertindole	Serlect
sertraline HCl	Zoloft
Serzone (W)	nefazodone HCl (W)
sevelamer HCl (W) (W)	Renagel (W)
sevoflurane	Ultane
short chain fatty acids enema	Colomed
sibutramine HCl monohydrate	Meridia
sildenafil citrate	Viagra
Silvadene	silver sulfadiazine
silver sulfadiazine	Silvadene
simethicone	Mylicon
Simulect	basiliximab
simvastatin	Zocor
Sinemet	levodopa; carbidopa
Sinemet CR	levodopa; carbidopa SR
Sinequan	doxepin HCl
Singulair	montelukast sodium
sirolimus	Rapamune
sirolimus-eluting stent	Cypher stent
sitagliptin	Januvia
Skelid	tiludronate disodium
Slo-bid	theophylline SR
Slo-Phyllin	theophylline
Slow Fe	ferrous sulfate SR
Slow-K (WA)	*potassium chloride SR*
Slow-Mag	magnesium chloride SR

smallpox (vaccinia)	ACAM 2000
sodium citrate; citric acid	Bicitra
sodium ferric gluconate complex in sucrose inj	Ferrlecit
sodium fluoride	Luride
sodium hyaluronate	Amvisc Healon Hyalgan
sodium oxybate	Xyrem
sodium phenylbutyrate	Buphenyl
sodium phosphate tab	Visicol
sodium sulfacetamide lotion	Klaron
sodium tetradecyl sulfate	Sotradecol
Solage	mequinol; tretinoin
Solaraze	diclofenac gel
Solganal	aurothioglucose
solifenacin succinate	Vesicare
Soliris	eculizumab
Solu-Cortef	hydrocortisone sodium succinate
Solu-Medrol	methylprednisolone sodium succinate
Soma	carisoprodol
somatostatin	Zecnil
Somatuline	lanreotide
somatrem	Protropin
somatropin for inj	Genotropin Humatrope Norditropin Nutropin Protropin II Saizen
somatropin inj	Nutropin AQ
somatropin (rDNA origin) for inj	Serostim
Somavert	pegvisomant
Sonata	zaleplon
sorafenib tosylate	Nexavar
Soriatane	acitretin
sotalol	Betapace
Sotradecol	sodium tetradecyl sulfate
sparfloxacin (W)	Zagam (W)
stavudine	Zerit
spectinomycin HCl	Trobicin
Spectracef	cefditoren pivoxil

Spiriva HandiHaler	tiotropium bromide inhalation powder
spironolactone	Aldactone
spironolactone; hydrochlorothiazide	Aldactazide
Sporanox	itraconazole
Sprycel	dasatinib
Stadol	butorphanol tartrate inj
Stadol NS (W)	butorphanol tartrate nasal spray (W)
Stalevo	levodopa; carbidopa; entacapone
stanozolol (W)	Winstrol (W)
Staphcillin	methicillin sodium
Starlix	nateglinide
stavudine SR	Zerit XR
Stelazine (WA)	*trifluoperazine HCl*
Strattera	Atomoxetine HCl
Streptase (W)	streptokinase (W)
streptokinase (W)	Streptase (W)
streptomycin sulfate	streptomycin sulfate
streptozocin	Zanosar
Striant	testosterone buccal
Stromectol	ivermectin
strontium-89 chloride inj	Metastron
Sublimaze	fentanyl citrate
Suboxone	buprenorphine HCl; naloxone HCl
Subutex	buprenorphine HCl
succinylcholine chloride	Anectine
Sucraid	sacrosidase
sucralfate	Carafate
Sudafed	pseudoephedrine HCl
Sufenta	sufentanil citrate
sufentanil citrate	Sufenta
Sulamyd sodium (WA)	*sulfacetamide sodium ophth*
Sular	Nisoldipine SR
sulfacetamide sodium and sulfur lotion	Plexion
sulfacetamide sodium ophth	*sulfacetamide sodium ophth*
sulfadoxine; pyrimethamine	Fansidar
sulfamethoxazole (W)	Gantanol (W)
sulfamethoxazole-trimethoprim	Bactrim Cotrim co-trimoxazole Septra
sulfasalazine	Azulfidine
sulfinpyrazone	Anturane

sulindac	Clinoril
Sultrin	triple sulfa vaginal cream
sumatriptan	Imitrex
sumatriptan; naproxen sodium	Treximet
Sumycin	tetracycline HCl
sunitinib malate	Sutent
Suprane	desflurane
Suprax	cefixime
suramin	Metaret
Surmontil	trimipramine maleate
Survanta	beractant
Sustiva	Efavirenz
Sutent	sunitinib malate
Symbyax	olanzapine; fluoxetine
Symlin	pramlintide acetate
Symmetrel	amantadine HCl
Synagis	palivizumab
Synalar	fluocinolone acetonide
Synercid	quinupristin; dalfopristin
Synkayvite	menadiol sodium diphosphate
synopinine (W)	Florotag (W)
synthetic conjugated estrogens, A	Cenestin
Synthroid	levothyroxine sodium
Synvisc	hylan G-F 20

T

tacrine HCl	Cognex
tacrolimus	Prograf
tacrolimus oint	Protopic
tadalafil	Cialis
Tagamet	cimetidine HCl
talc, sterile aerosol	Sclerosol
Talwin	pentazocine HCl
Talwin Nx	pentazocine HCl; naloxone HCl
Tambocor	flecainide acetate
Tamiflu	oseltamivir phosphate
tamoxifen citrate	*tamoxifen citrate*
tamsulosin HCl	Flomax
Tapazole	methimazole
Tarceva	erlotinib
Targretin	bexarotene gel
Tarka	trandolapril; verapamil SR
tarzarotene gel	Tazorac
Tasigna	nilotinib
Tasmar	tolcapone
tasosartan (W)	Verdia (W)
Tavist	clemastine fumarate
Taxol	paclitaxel
Taxotere	docetaxel
Taxus Express2 stent	paclitaxel-eluting stent
Tazicef	ceftazidime
Tazidime	ceftazidime
Tazorac	tarzarotene gel
technetium Tc-99m bicisate kit	Neurolite
technetium Tc-99m red blood cell kit	Ultratag
technetium Tc-99m	Cardiotec
technetium Tc99m sestamibi teboroxime kit	Cardiolite
Teczem	enalapril maleate; diltiazem malate
tegaserod maleate (W)	Zelnorm (W)
Tegretol	carbamazepine
Tekturna	aliskiren hemifumarate
telbivudine	Tyzeka
Teldrin	chlorpheniramine maleate SR
Telepaque (W)	iopanoic acid (W)
telithromycin	Ketek
telmisartan	Micardis
temazepam	Restoril
Temodar	temozolomide
temozolomide	Temodar
temsirolimus	Torisel
tenecteplase	TNKase
Tenex	guanfacine HCl
teniposide	Vumon
tenofovir disoproxil fumarate	Viread
tenofovir, efavirenz, and emtricitabine	Atripla
Tenoretic	atenolol; chlorthalidone
Tenormin	atenolol
Tensilon	edrophonium chloride
Tenuate	diethylpropion HCl
Tequin (W)	gatifloxacin (W)
Terazol	terconazole
terazosin HCl	Hytrin
terbinafine HCl	Lamisil
terbutaline sulfate aerosol	Brethaire
terbutaline sulfate tablets and inj	Brethine Bricanyl

terconazole	Terazol
terfenadine (W)	Seldane (W)
terfenadine; pseudoephedrine HCl (W)	Seldane D (W)
teriparatide	Forteo
teriparatide acetate	Parathar
Teslac (W)	testolactone (W)
Teslascan	mangafodipir trisodium
Testim	testosterone gel
Testoderm (WA)	testosterone transdermal
Testoderm TTS (WA)	testosterone transdermal
testolactone (W)	Teslac (W)
testosterone buccal	Striant
testosterone cypionate SR	DEPO-Testosterone
testosterone gel	AndroGel Testim
testosterone transdermal	Androderm Testoderm (WA) Testoderm TTS (WA)
tetrabenazine	Xenazine
tetracaine HCl	Pontocaine
tetracycline HCl	Achromycin (WA) Sumycin
tetrahydrozoline HCl ophth	Collyrium Visine Extra
Teveten	eprosartan mesylate
Teveten HCT	eprosartan mesylate; hydrochlorothiazide
thalidomide	Thalomid
Thalomid	thalidomide
Tham	tromethamine
Theo-Dur (WA)	theophylline SR
theophylline	Elixophyllin Slo-Phyllin
theophylline SR	Slo-bid Theo-Dur (WA) Uniphyl
TheraCys	BCG intravesical
Theragran	vitamins
thiabendazole	Mintezol
thiethylperazine maleate	Torecan
thioguanine	thioguanine
thiopental sodium	Pentothal
Thioplex	thiotepa
thioridazine HCl	Mellaril (WA)
thiotepa	Thioplex
thiothixene	Navane
Thorazine (WA)	*chlorpromazine*
Thrombate III	antithrombin III (human)
thrombin, topical (human)	Evithrom

thrombin, topical (recombinant)	Recothrom
thymalfasin	Zadaxin
Thymitaq (W)	nolatrexed dihydrochloride (W)
Thymoglobulin	anti-thymocyte globulin, (rabbit)
thyroglobulin (W)	Proloid (W)
thyroid	thyroid
Thyrogen	thyrotropin alpha
Thyrolar	liotrix
thyrotropin (W)	Thytropar (W)
thyrotropin alpha	Thyrogen
Thytropar (W)	thyrotropin (W)
tiagabine HCl	Gabitril
Tiamate	diltiazem maleate SR
Tiazac	diltiazem HCl SR
Ticar	ticarcillin disodium
ticarcillin disodium	Ticar
ticarcillin; clavulanic acid	Timentin
TICE BCG	BCG intravesical
Ticlid	ticlopidine
ticlopidine	Ticlid
Tigan	trimethobenzamide HCl
tigecycline inj	Tygacil
Tikosyn	dofetilide
Tilade	nedocromil inhalation
tiludronate disodium	Skelid
Timentin	ticarcillin; clavulanic acid
timolol maleate ophth soln	Timoptic
timolol maleate ophth soln, gel forming	Timoptic-XE
timolol maleate	Blocadren
timolol maleate; dorzolamide HCl	Cosopt
Timoptic-XE	timolol maleate ophth soln, gel forming
Timoptic	timolol maleate ophth soln
Tinactin	tolnaftate
Tindamax	tinidazole
tinidazole	Tindamax
tinzaparin sodium	Innohep
TNKase	tenecteplase
tioconazole	Vagistat-1
tiotropium bromide inhalation powder	Spiriva HandiHaler
tipranavir	Aptivus

tirofiban HCl	Aggrastat
tizanidine HCl	Zanaflex
TOBI	tobramycin soln for inhalation
TobraDex	tobramycin; dexamethasone oint and susp
tobramycin sulfate inj	*tobramycin sulfate inj*
tobramycin sulfate ophth	Tobrex
tobramycin; dexamethasone oint and susp	TobraDex
tobramycin soln for inhalation	TOBI
Tobrex	tobramycin sulfate ophth
tocainide HCl	Tonocard
Tofranil	imipramine HCl
tolazamide	Tolinase
tolazoline (W)	Priscoline (W)
tolbutamide	Orinase
tolcapone	Tasmar
Tolectin	tolmetin sodium
Tolinase (W)	tolazamide (W)
tolmetin sodium	Tolectin
tolnaftate	Tinactin
tolterodine tartrate	Detrol
tolterodine tartrate (SR)	Detrol LA
Tonocard	tocainide HCl
Topamax	topiramate
Topicort	desoximetasone
topiramate	Topamax
topotecan HCl	Hycamtin
Toprol XL	metoprolol succinate SR
Toradol	ketorolac tromethamine
Torecan	thiethylperazine maleate
toremifene citrate	Fareston
Torisel	temsirolimus
Tornalate	bitolterol mesylate
torsemide	Demadex
tositumomab and I-131 tositumomab	Bexxar
Totacillin-N	ampicillin sodium
Tracleer	bosentan
Tracrium	atracurium besylate
tramadol; acetaminophen	Ultracet
tramadol HCl	Ultram
Trandate	labetalol HCl
trandolapril	Mavik
trandolapril; verapamil SR	Tarka
Transderm Scop	scopolamine transdermal
Transderm-Nitro	nitroglycerin transdermal
Tranxene	clorazepate dipotassium
tranylcypromine sulfate	Parnate
trastuzumab	Herceptin
Trasylol	aprotinin
Travasol	amino acid inj
Travatan	travoprost ophth soln
travoprost ophth soln	Travatan
trazodone HCl	*trazodone HCl*
Treanda	bendamustine HCl inj
Trecator-SC	ethionamide
Trelstar Depot	triptorelin pamoate
Trelstar LA	triptorelin pamoate (3 month inj)
Trental	pentoxifylline
treprostinil sodium	Remodulin
tretinoin cream 0.025%	Avita
tretinoin gel	Retin-A Micro
tretinion topical	Renova Retin-A
tretinoin capsules	Vesanoid
Trexall	methotrexate tablets
Treximet	sumatriptan; naproxen sodium
triamcinolone	Aristocort Kenalog
triamcinolone acetonide aerosol	Azmacort
triamcinolone acetonide nasal inhaler	Nasacort
triamcinolone acetonide nasal spray	Tri-Nasal
triamcinolone acetonide ophth inj	Trivaris
triamterene	Dyrenium
triamterene 37.5 mg; hydro-chlorothiazide 25 mg	Maxzide -25MG Dyazide
triamterene 75 mg; hydro-chlorothiazide 50 mg	Maxzide
Triavil (WA)	perphenazine; amitriptyline HCl
triazolam	Halcion
Tricor	fenofibrate
Tri-Cyclen	norgestimate; ethinyl estradiol
Tridesilon	desonide
Tridil	nitroglycerin inj

Tridione	trimethadione
trifluoperazine HCl	*trifluoperazine HCl*
trifluridine	Viroptic
trihexyphenidyl HCl	*trihexyphenidyl HCl*
Trileptal	oxcarbazepine
Trilafon (WA)	*perphenazine*
Tri-Levlen	levonorgestrel; ethinyl estradiol
Trilisate (W)	choline magnesium trisalicylate (W)
Tri-Luma	hydroquinone; tretinoin; fluocinolone cream
trimethadione	Tridione
trimethaphan camsylate (W)	Arfonad (W)
trimethobenzamide HCl	Tigan
trimethoprim (W)	Primsol (W)
trimetrexate glucuronate	Neutrexin
trimipramine maleate	Surmontil
Trimox	amoxicillin
Tri-Nasal	triamcinolone acetonide nasal spray
Triostat	liothyronine sodium inj
tripelennamine HCl (W)	PBZ (W)
Triphasil	levonorgestrel; ethinyl estradiol
triple sulfa vaginal cream	Sultrin
triprolidine HCl; pseudoephedrine HCl	Actifed
triptorelin pamoate	Trelstar Depot
triptorelin pamoate (3 month inj)	Trelstar LA
Trisenox	arsenic trioxide
Tritec (W)	ranitidine bismuth citrate (W)
Trivaris	triamcinolone acetonide ophth inj
Tri-Vi-Flor	vitamins A, D, & C; fluoride
Trizivir	lamivudine; zidovudine; abacavir sulfate
Trobicin	spectinomycin HCl
troglitazone (W)	Rezulin (W)
tromethamine	Tham
Tronothane HCl	pramoxine HCl
TrophAmine	amino acid inj
Tropicacyl	tropicamide
tropicamide	Mydriacyl
	Tropicacyl
trospium chloride	Sanctura
trovafloxacin (W)	Trovan tablets (W)
Trovan tablet (W)	trovafloxacin mesylate (W)
Trovan inj (W)	alatrofloxacin mesylate IV (W)
Trusopt	dorzolamide HCl
Truvada	emtricitabine; tenofovir disoproxil
trypan blue ophth soln	VisionBlue
tuberculin skin test	Aplisol
tubocurarine	tubocurarine
Tucks	witch hazel pads
Tums	calcium carbonate
Tussi-Organidin NR	guaifenesin; codeine phosphate
Tussionex	hydrocodone polistirex; chlorpheniramine
Twinrix	hepatitis A inactivated; hepatitis B (recombinant) vaccine
Tygacil	tigecycline inj
Tykerb	lapatinib
Tylenol	acetaminophen
Tylenol with Codeine (#2, 3, and 4)	acetaminophen 300 mg with Codeine Phosphate (15, 30, and 60 mg)
Typhim Vi	typhoid Vi polysaccharide vaccine
typhoid Vi polysaccharide vaccine	Typhim Vi
tyropanoate sodium	Bilopaque
Tysabri	natalizumab
Tyzeka	telbivudine

U

UbiQGel	coenzyme Q10
Ultane	sevoflurane
Ultiva	remifentanil HCl
Ultracet	tramadol HCl; acetaminophen
Ultralente U	insulin zinc suspension, extended (beef)
Ultram	tramadol HCl
Ultratag	technetium Tc-99m red blood cell kit
Ultravist	iopromide

Unasyn	ampicillin sodium; sulbactam sodium
Unipen (W)	nafcillin sodium (W)
Uniphyl	theophylline SR
Uniretic	moexipril HCl; hydrochlorothiazide
Univasc	moexipril HCl
Urecholine	bethanechol chloride
Urised	methenamine combination
Urispas	flavoxate HCl
urofollitropin	Bravelle
urofollitropin for inj	Fertinex
urokinase (W)	Abbokinase (W)
unoprostone isopropyl ophth soln (W)	Rescula (W)
UroXatral	alfuzosin
Uprima	apomorphine HCl
Urocit-K	potassium citrate tab
URSO	ursodiol
ursodiol	Actigall URSO
Uvadex	methoxsalen extracorporeal administration

V

Vagifem	estradiol hemihydrate vaginal tab
Vagistat-1	tioconazole
valacyclovir	Valtrex
Valcyte	valganciclovir
valdecoxib (W)	Bextra (W)
valganciclovir	Valcyte
Valium	diazepam
valproate sodium inj	Depacon
valproic acid	Depakene
valrubicin, (for intravesical use)	Valstar
valsartan	Diovan
valsartan; hydro-chlorothiazide	Diovan HCT
Valstar	valrubicin, (for intravesical use)
Valtrex	valacyclovir
Vancenase	beclomethasone dipropionate
Vancenase AQ Nasal (WA)	beclomethasone dipropionate
Vanceril (WA)	beclomethasone dipropionate
Vancocin	vancomycin HCl
vancomycin HCl	Vancocin
Vaniqa	eflornithine HCl cream
Vantin	cefpodoxime proxetil
Vaponefrin (W)	epinephrine racemic (W)
Vaprisol	conivaptan HCl
Vaqta	hepatitis A vaccine, inactivated
vardenafil HCl	Levitra
varicella virus vaccine	Varivax
varenicline	Chantix
Varivax	varicella virus vaccine
Vascor (W)	bepridil (W)
Vaseline	petrolatum, white
Vaseretic	enalapril maleate; hydrochlorothiazide
Vasocon	naphazoline ophth soln
Vasodilan	isoxsuprine HCl
vasopressin	Pitressin
Vasotec	enalapril maleate
Vasoxyl (W)	methoxamine HCl (W)
Vectibix	panitumumab
vecuronium bromide	Norcuron
Velban	vinblastine sulfate
Velcade	bortezomib
Velosef (W)	cephradine (W)
Velosulin Human	insulin inj (human)
venlafaxine HCl	Effexor
venlafaxine HCl SR	Effexor XR
Venofer	iron sucrose inj
Ventavis	iloprost
Ventolin	albuterol
VePesid	etoposide
verapamil HCl	Isoptin
verapamil HCl SR	Calan SR Verelan
verapamil HCl SR bedtime formulation	Covera HS Verelan PM
Verdia (W)	tasosartan (W)
Verelan	verapamil HCl SR
Verelan PM	verapamil HCl SR bedtime formulation
Verluna (W)	nofetumomab (W)
Vermox	mebendazole
Versed	midazolam HCl
verteporfin inj	Visudyne
Vesanoid	tretinoin capsules
Vesicare	solifenacin succinate
Vestra	reboxetine mesylate
Vexol	rimexolone
Vfend	voriconazole
V-Flex plus PTX stent	paclitaxel-eluting stent
Viactiv	calcium carbonate; vitamin D and K chewable
Viadur (WA)	leuprolide acetate implant

Viagra	sildenafil citrate
Vibramycin	doxycycline hyclate
Vicodin	hydrocodone bitartrate; acetaminophen
Vicoprofen	hydrocodone bitartrate 7.5 mg; ibuprofen 200 mg
vidarabine monohydrate (W)	Vira-A (W)
Vidaza	azacitidine
Videx	didanosine
Videx EC	didanosine SR
vinblastine sulfate	Velban
vincristine sulfate	Oncovin
vindesine sulfate	Eldisine
vinorelbine tartrate	Navelbine
Vioform	clioquinol
Vioxx (W)	rofecoxib (W)
Vira-A (W)	vidarabine monohydrate (W)
Viracept	nelfinavir mesylate
Viramune	nevirapine
Virazole	ribavirin
Viread	tenofovir disoproxil fumarate
Viroptic	trifluridine
Visicol	sodium phosphate tab
Visine Extra	tetrahydrozoline HCl ophth
VisionBlue	trypan blue ophth soln
Visipaque	iodixanol
Visken	pindolol
Vistaril	hydroxyzine pamoate
Vistide	cidofovir
Visudyne	verteporfin inj
Vitrase	ovine hyaluronidase
Vitravene (W)	fomivirsen sodium inj (W)
Vivactil (WA)	*protriptyline HCl*
Vivelle	estradiol transdermal system
Volmax	albuterol SR
Voltaren	diclofenac sodium
Voltaren-XR	diclofenac sodium SR
voriconazole	Vfend
vorinostat	Zolinza
Vumon	teniposide
Vytorin	ezetimibe; simvastatin
Vyvanse	lisdexamfetamine dimesylate

warfarin sodium	Coumadin
Welchol	colesevelam HCl
Wellbutrin	bupropion HCl
Wellbutrin SR	bupropion HCl SR
Wellcovorin (WA)	*leucovorin calcium*
Wellferon	interferon ALFA-n^{1} lymphoblastoid
WinRho SD	RH_{O} (D) immune globulin IV (human)
Winstrol (W)	stanozolol (W)
witch hazel pads	Tucks
Wyamine (W)	mephentermine sulfate (W)
Wycillin (for IM use only)	penicillin G procaine (for IM use only)
Wydase (W)	hyaluronidase (W)
Wygesic (WA)	*propoxyphene HCl; acetaminophen*
Wymox	amoxicillin
Wytensin	guanabenz acetate

XYZ

Xalatan	latanoprost
Xanax	alprazolam
Xeloda	capecitabine
Xenazine	tetrabenazine
Xenical	orlistat
Xibrom	bromfenac ophth soln
Xifaxan	rifaximin
Xigris	drotrecogin alfa
Xolair	omalizumab
Xopenex	levalbuterol HCl inhalation soln
Xylocaine HCl	lidocaine HCl
xylometazoline	Otrivin
Xylzal	levocetirizine
Xyrem	oxybate sodium
Yasmin	drospirenone; ethinyl estradiol
Yutopar (W)	ritodrine HCl (W)
Zadaxin	thymalfasin
Zaditor	ketotifen fumarate ophth soln
zafirlukast	Accolate
Zagam (W)	sparfloxacin (W)
zalcitabine (W)	Hivid (W)
zaleplon	Sonata
Zanaflex	tizanidine HCl
zanamivir for inhalation	Relenza
Zanosar	streptozocin
Zantac	ranitidine HCl
Zarontin	ethosuximide
Zaroxolyn	metolazone
Zavesca	miglustat

Zecnil	somatostatin
Zelnorm (W)	tegaserod maleate (W)
Zemplar	paricalcitol
Zenapax	daclizumab
Zerit XR	stavudine SR
Zestoretic	lisinopril; hydrochlorothiazide
Zestril	lisinopril
Zetar	coal tar product
Zetia	ezetimibe
Zevalin	ibritumomab tiuxetan
Ziac	bisoprolol fumarate; hydrochlorothiazide
Ziagen	abacavir sulfate
ziconotide	Prialt
zidovudine	Retrovir
zidovudine; lamivudine	Combivir
zileuton	Zyflo
Zinacef	cefuroxime sodium
zinc acetate	Galzin
Zinecard	dexrazoxane
ziprasidone HCl	Geodon
Zithromax	azithromycin
Zn-DTPA	pentetate zinc trisodium (trisodium zinc diethylenetriamine-pentaacetate)
Zocor	simvastatin
Zofran	ondansetron
Zofran ODT	ondansetron orally disintegrating tab
Zoladex	goserelin acetate implant
zoledronic acid for inj	Zometa
zoledronic acid inj	Reclast intravenous infusion
Zolinza	vorinostat
zolmitriptan	Zomig
zolmitriptan orally disintegrating tablet	Zomig-ZMT
Zoloft	sertraline HCl
zolpidem tartrate	Ambien
Zometa	zoledronic acid for inj
Zomig	zolmitriptan
Zomig-ZMT	zolmitriptan orally disintegrating tablet
Zonegran	zonisamide
zonisamide	Zonegran
Zosyn	piperacillin sodium; tazobactam sodium
Zovirax	acyclovir
Zyban	bupropion HCl SR
Zydone 5/400, 7.5/400, 10/400	hydrocodone bitartrate; acetaminophen
Zyflo	zileuton
Zyloprim	allopurinol
Zymar	gatifloxacin opth soln
Zyprexa	olanzapine
Zyrtec	cetirizine HCl
Zyrtec-D	cetirizine HCl; pseudo-ephedrine HCl SR
Zyvox	linezolid

References

1. Facts and Comparisons. St. Louis: Wolters Kluwer Health; Facts and Comparisons, Inc. (published monthly and online)

2. Billup NF, Billup SM. American drug index. St. Louis: Wolters Kluwer Health; Facts and Comparisons. Inc.yw (published yearly)

3. Sweetman SC. Ed. Martindale: 35th edition. The Pharmaceutical Press. London, 2006.

Additions, Corrections, and Suggestions are Welcomed

Please send them via any means shown below:

Neil M Davis
2049 Stout Drive, B-3
Warminster PA 18974-3861

FAX 1 888 333 4915 or 1 215 442 7432
Email med@neilmdavis.com
Web site www.medabbrev.com

Thank you for your help in the past.

Have You Used the Internet Version of This Book?

- It is instantaneously searchable for the meanings of abbreviations
- It is reverse searchable (search for all the abbreviations containing a particular word)
- Each month, about 80 new entries are added

See the preface (page vii) for access instructions. A one-year, single-user access is included in the purchase price of the book. Also one-year subscriptions are available for purchase (see page 377).

PDA and BlackBerry Versions are Available

See pricing and ordering information in the pricing section on page 379.

Multi-User Site Licenses are Available

Medical facilities can substitute their own "Do Not Use" list of dangerous abbreviations for the one present. The ability also exists to list abbreviations that are unique to your region and/or organization which would normally not appear in any national list. These lists would be controlled by the facility or company. A no-cost, 3-week trial and pricing information are available by calling 1 888 333 1862 or 1 215 442 7430 or via an e-mail request to ev@neilmdavis.com

Chapter 10

L A B

Normal Adult Laboratory Values*

In the following tables, normal reference values for commonly requested laboratory tests are listed in traditional units and in SI units. The tables are a guideline only. Values are method dependent and "normal values" may vary between laboratories.

Blood, Plasma or Serum		
	Reference Value	
Determination	**Conventional Units**	**SI Units**
Ammonia (NH_3) – diffusion	20–120 mcg/dl	12–70 mcmol/L
Ammonia Nitrogen	15–45 mcg/dl	11–32 μmol/L
Amylase	35–118 IU/L	0.58–1.97 mckat/L
Anion Gap (Na^+ – [Cl^- + HCO_3^-]) (P)	7–16 mEq/L	7–16 mmol/L
Antinuclear antibodies	negative at 1:10 dilution of serum	negative at 1:10 dilution of serum
Antithrombin III (AT III)	80–120 units/dl	800–1200 units/L
Bicarbonate: Arterial Venous	21–28 mEq/L 22–29 mEq/L	21–28 mmol/L 22–29 mmol/L
Bilirubin: Conjugated (direct) Total	≤0.2 mg/dl 0.1–1 mg/dl	≤4 mcmol/L 2–18 mcmol/L
Calcitonin <100 pg/mL	<100 pg/mL	<100 pg/mL
Calcium: Total Ionized	8.6–10.3 mg/dl 4.4–5.1 mg/dl	2.2–2.74 mmol/L 1–1.3 mmol/L
Carbon dioxide content (plasma)	21–32 mmol/L	21–32 mmol/L
Carcinoembryonic antigen	<3 ng/mL	<3 mcg/L
Chloride	95–110 mEq/L	95–110 mmol/L
Coagulation screen: Bleeding time Prothrombin time Partial thromboplastin time (activated) Protein C Protein S	 3–9.5 min 10–13 sec 22–37 sec 0.7–1.4 μ/mL 0.7–1.4 μ/mL	 180–570 sec 10–13 sec 22–37 sec 700–1400 units/mL 700–1400 units/mL
Copper, total	70–160 mcg/dl	11–25 mcmol/L
Corticotropin (ACTH adrenocorticotropic hormone) – 0800 hr	<60 pg/mL	<13.2 pmol/L
Cortisol: 0800 hr 1800 hr 2000 hr	5–30 mcg/dl 2–15 mcg/dl ≤50% of 0800 hr	138–810 nmol/L 50–410 nmol/L ≤50% of 0800 hr
Creatine kinase: Female Male	20–170 IU/L 30–220 IU/L	0.33–2.83 mckat/L 0.5–3.67 mckat/L
Creatine kinase isoenzymes, MB fraction	0–12 IU/L	0–0.2 mckat/L
Creatinine	0.5–1.7 mg/dl	44–150 mcmol/L
Fibrinogen (coagulation factor I)	150–360 mg/dl	1.5–3.6 g/L

Normal Adult Laboratory Values (Cont.) Blood*

Blood, Plasma or Serum (Cont.)		
	Reference Value	
Determination	Conventional Units	SI Units
Follicle-stimulating hormone (FSH): Female Midcycle Male	 2–13 mIU/mL 5–22 mIU/mL 1–8 mIU/mL	 2–13 IU/L 5–22 IU/L 1–8 IU/L
Glucose, fasting	65–115 mg/dl	3.6–6.3 mmol/L
Glucose Tolerance Test (Oral) Fasting 60 min 90 min 120 min Fasting 60 min 90 min 120 min	mg/dL Normal 70–105 120–170 100–140 70–120 Diabetic >140 ≥200 ≥200 ≥140	mmol/L Normal 3.9–5.8 6.7–9.4 5.6–7.8 3.9–6.7 Diabetic >7.8 ≥11.1 ≥11.1 ≥7.8
(γ) – Glutamyltransferase (GGT): Male Female	 9–50 units/L 8–40 units/L	 9–50 units/L 8–40 units/L
Haptoglobin	44–303 mg/dl	0.44–3.03 g/L
Hematologic tests: Fibrinogen Hematocrit (Hct), female male Hemoglobin A_{1C} Hemoglobin (Hb), female male Leukocyte count (WBC) Erythrocyte count (RBC), female male Mean corpuscular volume (MCV) Mean corpuscular hemoglobin (MCH) Mean corpuscular hemoglobin concentrate (MCHC) Erythrocyte sedimentation rate (sedrate, ESR)	 200–400 mg/dl 36%–44.6% 40.7%–50.3% 5.3%–7.5% of total Hgb 12.1–15.3 g/dl 13.8–17.5 g/dl 3800–9800/mcl 3.5–5 × 10^6/mcl 4.3–5.9 × 10^6/mcl 80–97.6 mcm^3 27–33 pg/cell 33–36 g/dl ≤30 mm/hr	 2–4 g/L 0.36–0.446 fraction of 1 0.4–0.503 fraction of 1 0.053–0.075 121–153 g/L 138–175 g/L 3.8–9.8 × 10^9/L 3.5–5 × 10^{12}/L 4.3–5.9 × 10^{12}/L 80–97.6 fl 1.66–2.09 fmol/cell 20.3–22 mmol/L ≤30 mm/hr
Erythrocyte enzymes: Glucose-6-phosphate dehydrogenase (G-6-PD) Ferritin Folic acid: normal Platelet count Reticulocytes Vitamin B_{12}	250–5000 units/10^6 cells 10–383 ng/mL >3.1–12.4 ng/mL 150–450 × 10^3/mcl 0.5%–1.5% of erythrocytes 223–1132 pg/mL	250–5000 mcunits/cell 23–862 pmol/L 7–28.1 nmol/L 150–450 × 10^9/L 0.005–0.015 165–835 pmol/L
Iron: Female Male	30–160 mcg/dl 45–160 mcg/dl	5.4–31.3 mcmol/L 8.1–31.3 mcmol/L
Iron binding capacity	220-420 mcg/dl	39.4–75.2 mcmol/L
Isocitrate Dehydrogenase	1.2–7 units/L	1.2–7 units/L
Isoenzymes Fraction 1 Fraction 2 Fraction 3 Fraction 4 Fraction 5	 14%–26% of total 29%–39% of total 20%–26% of total 8%–16% of total 6%–16% of total	 0.14–0.26 fraction of total 0.29–0.39 fraction of total 0.20–0.26 fraction of total 0.08–0.16 fraction of total 0.06–0.16 fraction of total
Lactate dehydrogenase	100–250 IU/L	1.67–4.17 mckat/L

Normal Adult Laboratory Values (Cont.) Blood*

Blood, Plasma or Serum (Cont.)		
	Reference Value	
Determination	**Conventional Units**	**SI Units**
Lactic acid (lactate)	6–19 mg/dl	0.7–2.1 mmol/L
Lead	≤50 mcg/dl	≤2.41 mcmol/L
Lipase	10–150 units/L	10–150 units/L
Lipids:		
Total Cholesterol		
Desirable	<200 mg/dl	<5.2 mmol/L
Borderline-high	200–239 mg/dl	<5.2–6.2 mmol/L
High	>239 mg/dl	>6.2 mmol/L
LDL		
Desirable	<130 mg/dl	<3.36 mmol/L
Borderline-high	130–159 mg/dl	3.36–4.11 mmol/L
High	>159 mg/dl	>4.11 mmol/L
HDL (low)	<35 mg/dl	<0.91 mmol/L
Triglycerides		
Desirable	<200 mg/dl	<2.26 mmol/L
Borderline-high	200–400 mg/dl	2.26–4.52 mmol/L
High	400–1000 mg/dl	4.52–11.3 mmol/L
Very high	>1000 mg/dl	>11.3 mmol/L
Magnesium	1.3–2.2 mEq/L	0.65–1.1 mmol/L
Osmolality	280–300 mOsm/kg	280–300 mmol/kg
Oxygen saturation (arterial)	94%–100%	0.94–1 fraction of 1
PCO_2, arterial	35–45 mm Hg	4.7–6 kPa
pH, arterial	7.35–7.45	7.35–7.45
PO_2, arterial: Breathing room air[1]	80–105 mm Hg	10.6–14 kPa
On 100% O_2	>500 mm Hg	
Phosphatase (acid), total at 37°C	0.13–0.63 IU/L	2.2–10.5 IU/L or 2.2–10.5 mckat/L
Phosphatase alkaline[2]	20–130 IU/L	20–130 IU/L or 0.33–2.17 mckat/L
Phosphorus, inorganic,[3] (phosphate)	2.5–5 mg/dl	0.8–1.6 mmol/L
Potassium	3.5–5 mEq/L	3.5–5 mmol/L
Progesterone		
Female	0.1–1.5 ng/mL	0.32–4.8 nmol/L
Follicular phase	0.1–1.5 ng/mL	0.32–4.8 nmol/L
Luteal phase	2.5–28 ng/mL	8–89 nmol/L
Male	<0.5 ng/mL	<1.6 nmol/L
Prolactin	1.4–24.2 ng/mL	1.4–24.2 mcg/L
Prostate specific antigen	0–4 ng/mL	0–4 ng/mL
Protein: Total	6–8 g/dl	60–80 g/L
Albumin	3.6–5 g/dl	36–50 g/L
Globulin	2.3–3.5 g/dl	23–35 g/L
Rheumatoid factor	<60 IU/mL	<60 kIU/L
Sodium	135–147 mEq/L	135–147 mmol/L
Testosterone: Female	6–86 ng/dl	0.21–3 mmol/L
Male	270–1070 ng/dl	9.3–37 nmol/L

[1]Age dependent
[2]Infants and adolescents up to 104 IU/L
[3]Infants in the first year up to 6 mg/dl

L A B

Normal Adult Laboratory Values (Cont.) Blood*

Blood, Plasma or Serum (Cont.)		
	Reference Value	
Determination	**Conventional Units**	**SI Units**
Thyroid Hormone Function Tests: Thyroid-stimulating hormone (TSH) Thyroxine-binding globulin capacity Total triiodothyronine (T_3) Total thyroxine by RIA (T_4) T_3 resin uptake	 0.35–6.2 mcU/mL 10–26 mcg/dl 75–220 ng/dl 4–11 mcg/dl 25%–38%	 0.35–6.2 mU/L 100–260 mcg/L 1.2–3.4 nmol/L 51–142 nmol/L 0.25–0.38 fraction of 1
Transaminase, AST (aspartate aminotransferase, SGOT)	11–47 IU/L	0.18–0.78 mckat/L
Transaminase, ALT (alanine aminotransferase, SGPT)	7–53 IU/L	0.12–0.88 mckat/L
Transferrin	220–400 mg/dL	2.20–4.00 g/L
Urea nitrogen (BUN)	8–25 mg/dl	2.9–8.9 mmol/L
Uric acid	3–8 mg/dl	179–476 mcmol/L
Vitamin A (retinol)	15–60 mcg/dl	0.52–2.09 mcmol/L
Zinc	50–150 mcg/dl	7.7–23 mcmol/L

Normal Laboratory Values—Urine

Urine		
	Reference Value	
Determination	**Conventional Units**	**SI Units**
Calcium[1]	50–250 mcg/day	1.25–6.25 mmol/day
Catecholamines: Epinephrine Norepinephrine	<20 mcg/day <100 mcg/day	<109 nmol/day <590 nmol/day
Catecholamines, 24-hr	<110 mcg	<650 nmol
Copper[1]	15–60 mcg/day	0.24–0.95 mcmol/day
Creatinine: Child Adolescent Female Male	8–22 mg/kg 8–30 mg/kg 0.6–1.5 g/day 0.8–1.8 g/day	71–195 μmol/kg 71–265 μmol/kg 5.3–13.3 mmol/day 7.1–15.9 mmol/day
pH	4.5–8	4.5–8
Phosphate[1]	0.9–1.3 g/day	29–42 mmol/day
Potassium[1]	25–100 mEq/day	25–100 mmol/day
Protein Total At rest	 1–14 mg/dL 50–80 mg/day	 10–140 mg/L 50–80 mg/day
Protein, quantitative	<150 mg/day	<0.15 g/day
Sodium[1]	100–250 mEq/day	100–250 mmol/day
Specific Gravity, random	1.002–1.030	1.002–1.030
Uric Acid, 24-hr	250–750 mg	1.48–4.43 mmol

[1]Diet dependent

Normal Adult Laboratory Values—Drug Levels*

LAB

Drug Levels†			
		Reference Value	
	Drug Determination	Conventional Units	SI Units
Aminoglycosides	Amikacin		
	(trough)	1–8 mcg/mL	1.7–13.7 mcmol/L
	(peak)	20–30 mcg/mL	34–51 mcmol/L
	Gentamicin		
	(trough)	0.5–2 mcg/mL	1–4.2 mcmol/L
	(peak)	6–10 mcg/mL	12.5–20.9 mcmol/L
	Kanamycin		
	(trough)	5–10 mcg/mL	nd
	(peak)	20–25 mcg/mL	nd
	Netilmicin		
	(trough)	0.5–2 mcg/mL	nd
	(peak)	6–10 mcg/mL	nd
	Streptomycin		
	(trough)	<5 mcg/mL	nd
	(peak)	5–20 mcg/mL	nd
	Tobramycin		
	(trough)	0.5–2 mcg/mL	1.1–4.3 mcmol/L
	(peak)	5–20 mcg/mL	12.8–21.8 mcmol/L
Antiarrhythmics	Amiodarone	0.5–2.5 mcg/mL	1.5–4 mcmol/L
	Bretylium	0.5–1.5 mcg/mL	nd
	Digitoxin	9–25 mcg/L	11.8–32.8 nmol/L
	Digoxin	0.8–2 ng/mL	0.9–2.5 nmol/L
	Disopyramide	2–8 mcg/mL	6–18 mcmol/L
	Flecainide	0.2–1 mcg/mL	nd
	Lidocaine	1.5–6 mcg/mL	4.5–21.5 mcmol/L
	Mexiletine	0.5–2 mcg/mL	nd
	Procainamide	4–8 mcg/mL	17–34 mcmol/mL
	Propranolol	50–200 ng/mL	190–770 nmol/L
	Quinidine	2–6 mcg/mL	4.6–9.2 mcmol/L
	Tocainide	4–10 mcg/mL	nd
	Verapamil	0.08–0.3 mcg/mL	nd
Anti-convulsants	Carbamazepine	4–12 mcg/mL	17–51 mcmol/L
	Phenobarbital	10–40 mcg/mL	43–172 mcmol/L
	Phenytoin	10–20 mcg/mL	40–80 mcmol/L
	Primidone	4–12 mcg/mL	18–55 mcmol/L
	Valproic acid	40–100 mcg/mL	280–700 mcmol/L
Antidepressants	Amitriptyline	110–250 ng/mL[3]	500–900 nmol/L
	Amoxapine	200–500 ng/mL	nd
	Bupropion	25–100 ng/mL	nd
	Clomipramine	80–100 ng/mL	nd
	Desipramine	115–300 ng/mL	nd
	Doxepin	110–250 ng/mL[3]	nd
	Imipramine	225–350 ng/mL[3]	nd
	Maprotiline	200–300 ng/mL	nd
	Nortriptyline	50–150 ng/mL	nd
	Protriptyline	70–250 ng/mL	nd
	Trazodone	800–1600 ng/mL	nd
Antipsychotics	Chlorpromazine	50–300 ng/mL	150–950 nmol/L
	Fluphenazine	0.13–2.8 ng/mL	nd
	Haloperidol	5–20 ng/mL	nd
	Perphenazine	0.8–1.2 ng/mL	nd
	Thiothixene	2–57 ng/mL	nd

The values given are generally accepted as desirable for treatment without toxicity for most patients. However, exceptions are not uncommon.
24 hour trough values
Toxic: 50–100 mg/dl (10.9–21.7 mmol/L)
Parent drug plus N-desmethy7l metabolite
d – No data available

L
A
B

Normal Adult Laboratory Values (Cont.) Drug Levels*

Drug Levels†			
		Reference Value	
	Drug Determination	Conventional Units	SI Units
Miscellaneous	Amantadine	300 ng/mL	nd
	Amrinone	3.7 mcg/mL	nd
	Chloramphenicol	10–20 mcg/mL	31–62 mcmol/L
	Cyclosporine[1]	250–800 ng/mL (whole blood, RIA)	nd
		50–300 ng/mL (plasma, RIA)	nd
	Ethanol[2]	0 mg/dl	0 mmol/L
	Hydralazine	100 ng/mL	nd
	Lithium	0.6–1.2 mEq/L	0.6–1.2 mmol/L
	Salicylate	100–300 mg/L	724–2172 mcmol/L
	Sulfonamide	5–15 mg/dl	nd
	Terbutaline	0.5–4.1 ng/mL	nd
	Theophylline	10–20 mcg/mL	55–110 mcmol/L
	Vancomycin		
	(trough)	5–15 ng/mL	nd
	(peak)	20–40 mcg/mL	nd

†The values given are generally accepted as desirable for treatment without toxicity for most patients. However, exceptions are not uncommon.
[1]24 hour trough values
[2]Toxic: 50–100 mg/dl (10.9–21.7 mmol/L)
nd – No data available

#1 in the Field

Order Form and Prices for the 14th Edition of

Medical Abbreviations: 30,000 Conveniences at the Expense of Communication and Safety
Authored by Neil M Davis
ISBN 978-0-931431-14-2

THE BOOK (prices shown include a 1-year single-user access license to the Internet version of the book which is updated with 80 new entries per month)

1–19 copies	**$28.95 each plus S & H**
20 or more copies	**$20.25 each plus S & H**

Plus shipping and handling charges to the 48 contiguous US states as shown below

Number of books ordered	For the 48 contiguous US states
1	$7.00 + the price shown above
2	$9.00 + the price shown above
3–6	$12.00 + the price shown above
7–11	$15.00 + the price shown above
12–20	$19.00 + the price shown above
21–40	$36.00 + the price shown above
41 or more	$48.00 + the price shown above

For S & H costs to Hawaii, Alaska, Puerto Rico, or countries other than the USA, contact one of the sites shown below.

- Orders shipped to Pennsylvania, add 6% sales tax.
- No sales tax for other US states (subject to change)
- Purchase orders are accepted

1-YEAR SINGLE-USER ACCESS LICENSE TO THE INTERNET VERSION OF THE BOOK WHICH IS UPDATED WITH 80 NEW ENTRIES PER MONTH (no book, just the Internet version)

1-year Single-User Access License (Internet version only—no book)	$20.00

- Orders from Pennsylvania, add 6% sales tax.
- No sales tax for other US states (subject to change)
- No S & H charges
- Credit Cards or other forms of prepayment only (secure web site)

PAYABLE BY–

Visa	MasterCard	Discover
American Exp.	Check	Money Order

ORDER FROM AND MAKE CHECK PAYABLE TO–

Neil M Davis Associates
2049 Stout Drive, B-3
Warminster PA 18974-3861

(continued)

Order and Price Information—continued

ORDERS MAY BE MAILED TO THE ADDRESS ON PREVIOUS PAGE OR

Phone 1 215 442 7430 or 1 888 333 1862
Fax 1 215 442 7432 or 1 888 333 4915
Secure Web site www.medabbrev.com
E-mail ev@neilmdavis.com

Where applicable, please have ready your credit card number and expiration date, phone number and mailing address.

COUNTRIES OTHER THAN THE UNITED STATES

- Pay by credit card or in US dollars through corresponding US bank or an International Money Order in US currency.
- Prices shown on previous page
- To obtain shipping costs or provide shipping instructions call 1 215 442 7430, FAX 1 215 442 7432 or E-mail to ev@neilmdavis.com

Information Needed on Order Form

PLEASE PRINT OR TYPE

Name ____________________

Address ____________________

____

City ____________ State ______ Zip Code ______

Phone ( ) ____________________

Attention (If Applicable) ____________________

Number of **books** ordered (**includes** a 1-year single-user Internet access license) ________

Number of 1-year single-user Internet access licenses (No book wanted) ________

PO # (If applicable) ________

Method of payment:

______ Check or money order enclosed

______ Visa ______ MasterCard

______ Discover ______ American Express

Card Number ____________________

Exp. Date ____________

Cardholder's Name ____________________

Signature ____________________

MULTI-USER ACCESS LICENSES TO THE INTERNET VERSION are available. The ability exists for you to add and control a list on abbreviations which are unique to your locale and/or organization, that would not normally appear in a national list. Hospitals and other healthcare facilities have the ability to add and control their own list of dangerous abbreviations which should not be used. To obtain a price list, a copy of the license agreement, and a 3-week free trial call 1 215 442 7430, FAX 1 215 442 7432 or E-mail ev@neilmdavis.com

To Order the PDA and BlackBerry Versions

Palm OS or Pocket PC PDA, and BlackBerry versions of "Medical Abbreviations: 30,000 Conveniences at the Expense of Communication and Safety," the 14th edition, 2009, by Neil M Davis, are available from Lexi-Comp Inc., at either:

Phone 1 800 837 5394 or 1 330 650 6506
Fax 1 330 656 4307
Lexi-Comp, Inc.
1100 Terex Road
Hudson, Ohio, USA 44236

These versions are updated with 80 new entries per month.

Pricing: If you mention the Promotion Code **"KT8BK"** you will be given a 10% discount, lowering the price to $31.50 for one year. The normal price is $35.00.

Additions

Please forward additional meanings for these abbreviations, additional abbreviations and their meanings, or corrections to the author so that the Internet version, PDA versions, and book can be updated. Thank you. Dr. Neil M Davis, 2049 Stout Drive, B-3, Warminster, PA 18974. FAX 215 442 7432 or 888 333 4915. E-mail med@neilmdavis.com

Additions

(See the preface (page vii) for instructions on how to access to the Internet version of this book which is updated each month with about 80 new entries. Your suggestions are appreciated.)

Additions

(See the preface (page vii) for instructions on how to access to the Internet version of this book which is updated each month with about 80 new entries. Your suggestions are appreciated.)

Additions

(See the preface (page vii) for instructions on how to access to the Internet version of this book which is updated each month with about 80 new entries. Your suggestions are appreciated.)

Additions

(See the preface (page vii) for instructions on how to access to the Internet version of this book which is updated each month with about 80 new entries. Your suggestions are appreciated.)

Additions, Corrections, and Suggestions are Welcomed

Please send them via any means shown below:

Neil M Davis
2049 Stout Drive, B-3
Warminster PA 18974-3861

FAX 1 888 333 4915 or 1 215 442 7432
Email med@neilmdavis.com
Web site www.medabbrev.com

Thank you for your help in the past.

Have You Used the Internet Version of This Book?

- It is instantaneously searchable for the meanings of abbreviations
- It is reverse searchable (search for all the abbreviations containing a particular word)
- Each month, about 80 new entries are added

See the preface (page vii) for access instructions. A one-year, single-user access is included in the purchase price of the book. Also one-year subscriptions are available for purchase (see page 377).

PDA and BlackBerry Versions are Available

See pricing and ordering information in the pricing section on page 379.

Multi-User Site Licenses are Available

Medical facilities can substitute their own "Do Not Use" list of dangerous abbreviations for the one present. The ability also exists to list abbreviations that are unique to your region and/or organization which would normally not appear in any national list. These lists would be controlled by the facility or company. A no-cost, 3-week trial and pricing information are available by calling 1 888 333 1862 or 1 215 442 7430 or via an e-mail request to ev@neilmdavis.com